Clinical Atlas of 3D Printing Bone Reconstruction

Hyun-Guy Kang

Clinical Atlas of 3D Printing Bone Reconstruction

Springer

Hyun-Guy Kang
Orthopaedic Oncology Clinic
National Cancer Center
Goyang
Republic of Korea

ISBN 978-981-16-2042-3 ISBN 978-981-16-2043-0 (eBook)
https://doi.org/10.1007/978-981-16-2043-0

This Springer imprint is published by the registered company Springer Nature Singapore Pte Ltd.
The registered company address is: 152 Beach Road, #21-01/04 Gateway East, Singapore 189721, Singapore

Preface

The medical use of advanced 3D printing technology is being tried in various fields. Printing the desired model using the desired material in a short period of time is very attractive. The 3D printing technology that enables patient-specific bone reconstruction is now becoming the key in musculoskeletal tumor surgery. Current bone reconstruction surgery involves a ready-made artificial joint forcibly inserted into the body. On the contrary, the use of 3D printing technology enables customized artificial joint to be perfectly fitted in the patient's body.

Using the 3D printing technology requires a lot of time and effort before the surgery, and collaboration with multiple engineering teams is required. One must design optimal reconstruction that allows strength and function, beyond designing structural similarity. While it is complex, I have found out that 3D printing design has infinite possibilities, like the art of painting.

This book is composed of photos with minimum descriptions so that the readers can develop their imaginative view. Express your freedom in the limitless 3D printing design. I hope this book will give you courage in your new challenges.

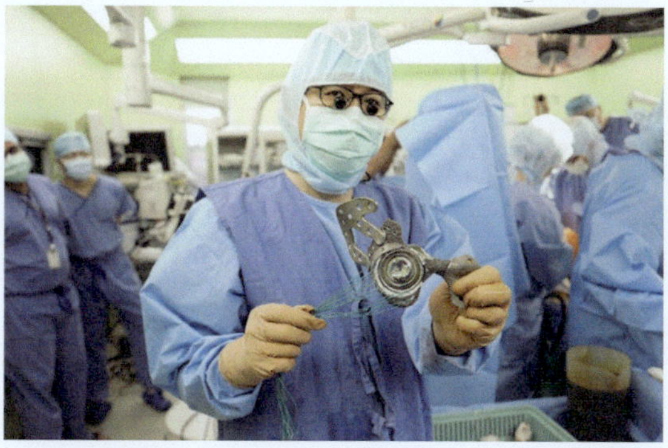

Hyun-Guy Kang, MD, PhD, National Cancer Center

Goyang-si, Republic of Korea

Hyun-Guy Kang, MD, PhD

Acknowledgment

My teacher and mentor who guided me to walk on this path

Han-Soo Kim, MD, PhD

Professor, Seoul National University College of Medicine & Hospital

My beloved Orthopaedic colleagues

Jong-Woong Park, MD and June-Hyuk Kim, MD

Staff Surgeon, Orthopedic Oncology Clinic, National Cancer Center

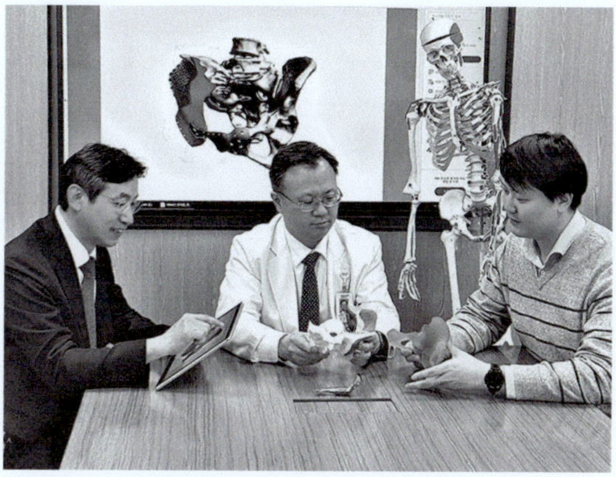

Dr. HG Kang, HS Kim, JW Park

Orthopaedic Department, National Cancer Center

Sung-Keun Kim, Ju-Yeon Han: Registered Nurse

Sung-Eun Oh, Tae-Il Um and Se-Bin Kim: Researcher

MEDYSSEY Company

Hyo-Bok Jeong and Hyun-Woo Jung: 3D printing engineer

Springer Nature Korea Limited

Jenny Chun: Editor of medicine and life sciences books

Government, Republic of Korea

The Ministry of Health and Welfare

The Ministry of Trade, Industry and Energy

Lastly, I would like to express my deepest love and gratitude to dentist Eun-Ha Kim for giving me a lot of ideas and courage in every moment.

Contents

Part I

Pelvis

Patient Case 1: Unique Iliac Plate, Combined with Total Hip Arthroplasty

1

1.1 Patient Case 1

Age/sex	54/female
Location/site	Pelvis, femur/left
Diagnosis	Undifferentiated spindle cell sarcoma of bone
Preoperative symptom	Wheelchair ambulation
Preoperative pain score	Resting 5/activity 7
BMI (height/weight)	20.8 (155.5/50.3)
Past history	32 years old: Lt breast cancer, mastectomy and chemotherapy
	47 years old: Lt femur neck pathologic fracture, malignant fibrous histiocytoma of bone, radiation therapy
	49 years old: Rt breast cancer, mastectomy and chemotherapy
	54 years old: incisional biopsy pelvis, sarcoma
Present illness	Visit after refusing amputation at several other hospitals

1.2 Preoperative Images

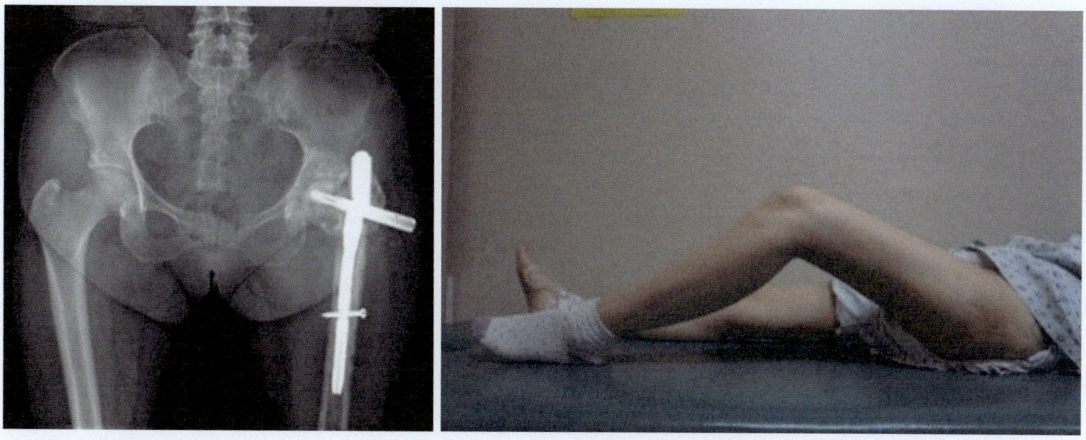

Fig. 1.1 Preoperative X-ray image and photograph: The range of motion restricted hip, knee, and ankle

H.-G. Kang, *Clinical Atlas of 3D Printing Bone Reconstruction*,
https://doi.org/10.1007/978-981-16-2043-0_1

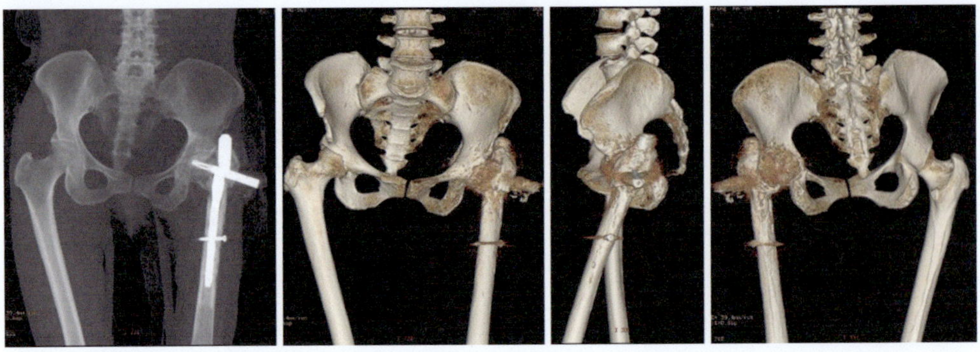

Fig. 1.2 Preoperative CT images

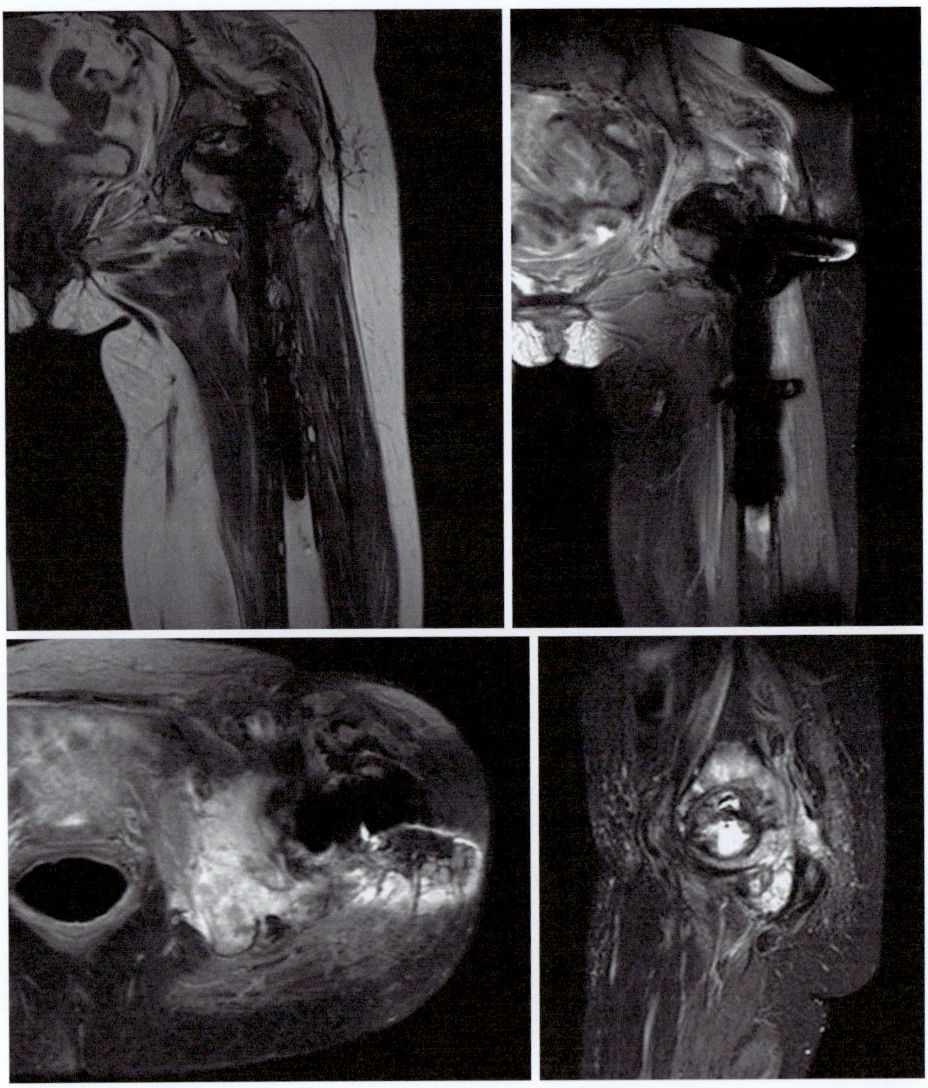

Fig. 1.3 Preoperative MRI images

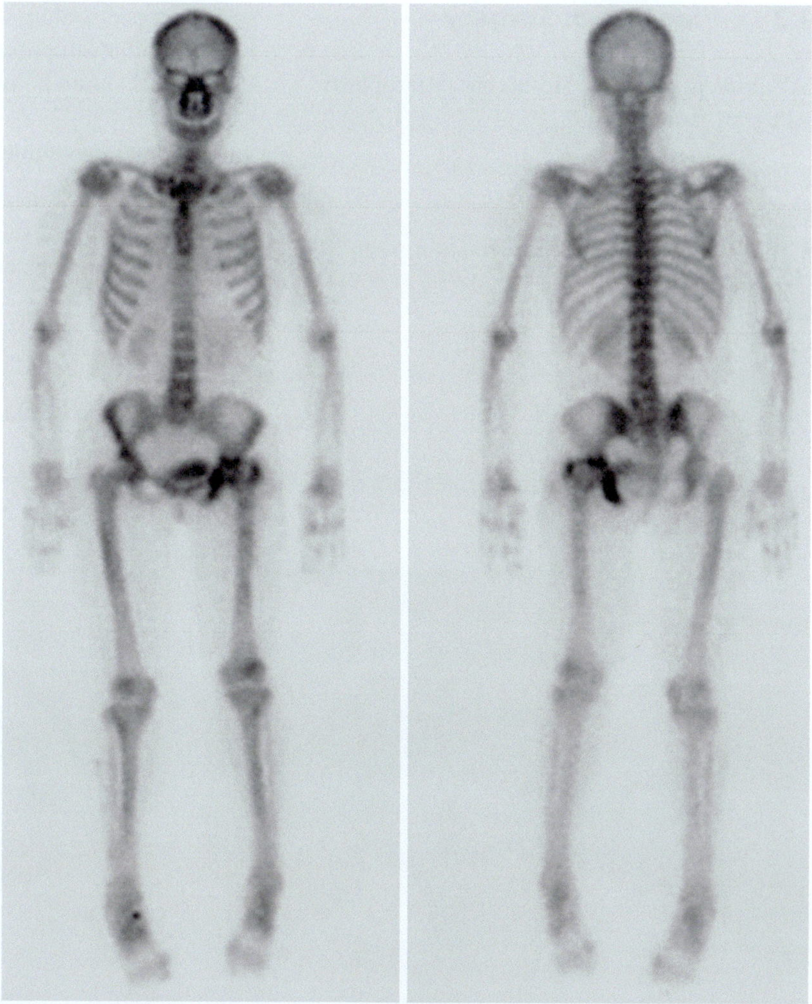

Fig. 1.4 Preoperative bone scan images

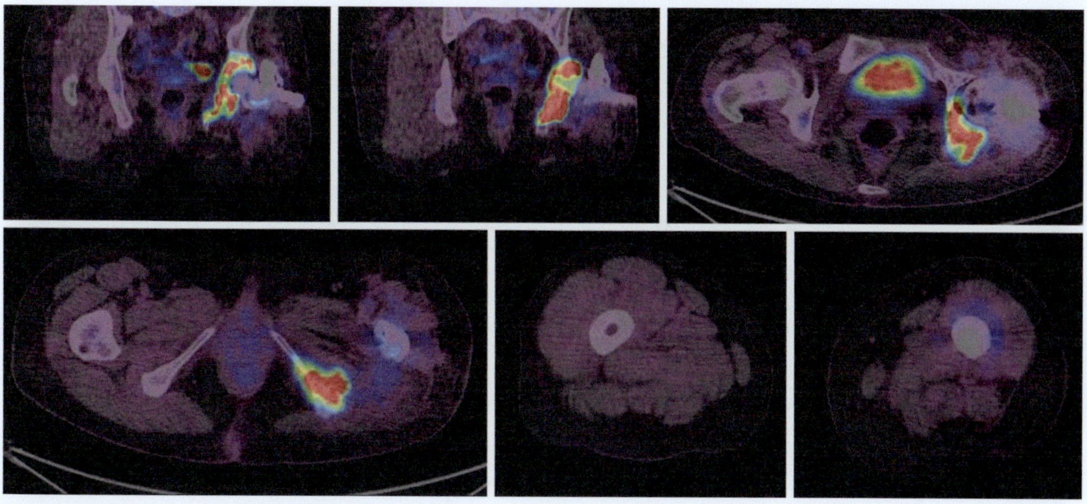

Fig. 1.5 Preoperative PET-CT images

1.3 Planning of Surgery

3D printed pelvis + Total hip arthroplasty + Allograft femur

3D printed pelvis Implant:

- Reverse V-shaped iliac bone cut
- Inter-bridging plate for fixation with iliac bone
- Lateral side screw fixation
- Bigger acetabulum
- Acetabular rim prominent
- Multiple suture holes

Total hip cup conjugation:

- MDM Stryker Acetabular cup (Fig. 1.6)
- Acetabular metal shell: 50 mm diameter
- 3D printed pelvic acetabular diameter: 54 mm

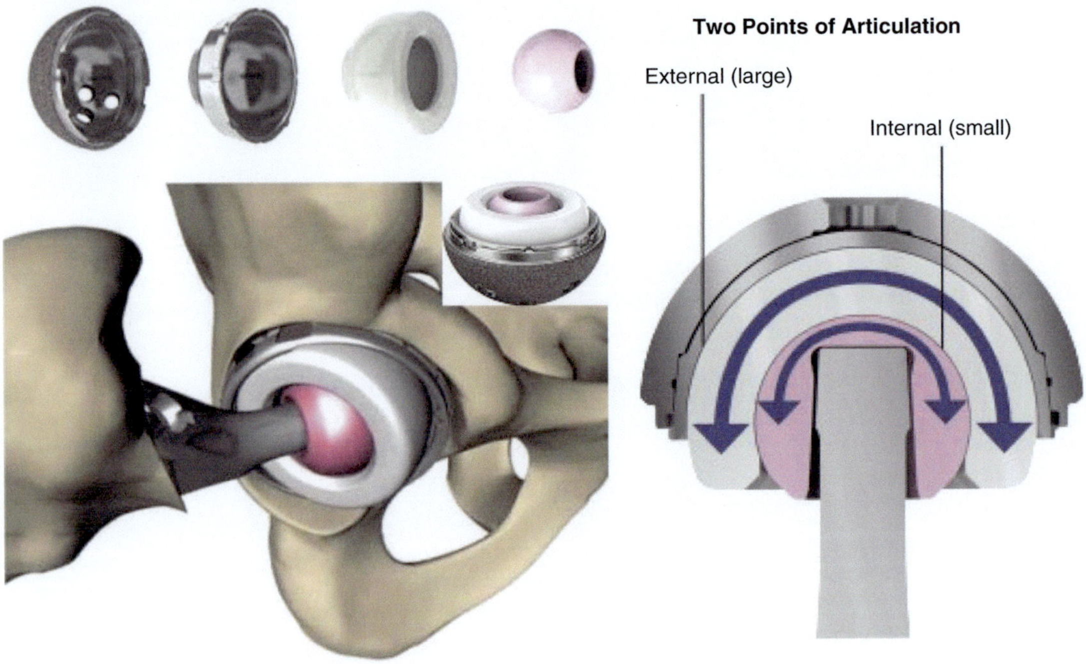

Fig. 1.6 Select Modular Dual Mobility (MDM®) Stryker MedEd

1.4 Design and Fabrication

Use mirror image of normal right pelvis

Iliac bone cutting—Both medial and lateral cutting guides makes more accurate cortical cut

Iliac crest and greater sciatic notch are reference points of guide

Pubic ramus cutting—flat bone contoured itself can be touching reference points (Fig. 1.7)

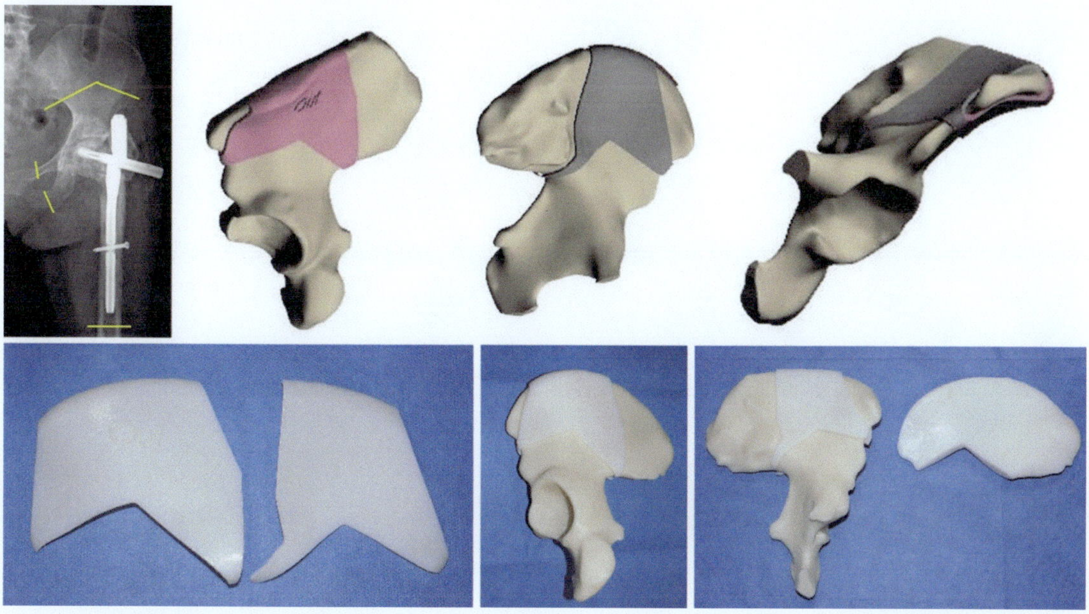

Fig. 1.7 Cutting guide design

1.5 Fixation with Iliac Bone

- Implant measurement
- Implant weight (g): 573
- Size (mm): 126

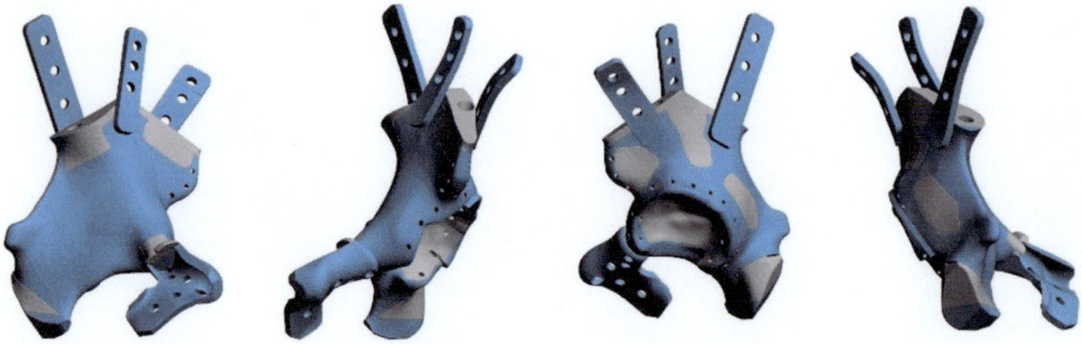

Fig. 1.8 Initial implant design: difficult insert bone between the medial and lateral plate wing and difficult screwing on the medial wing

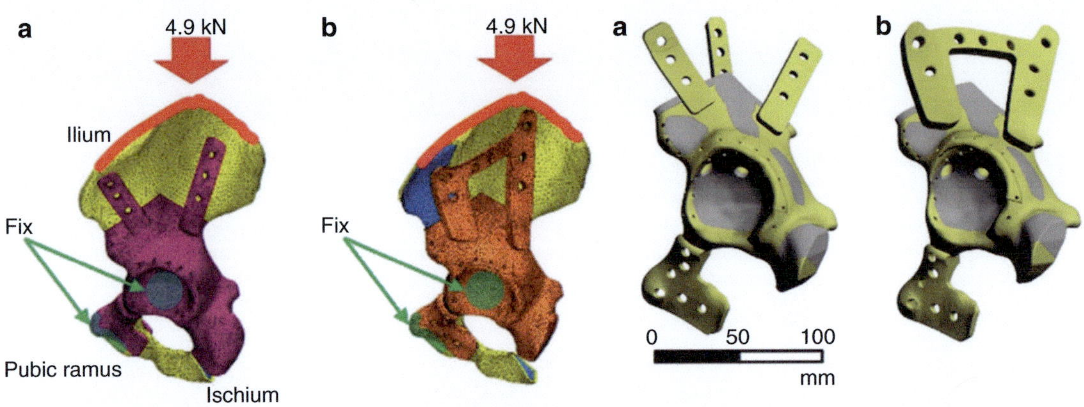

Fig. 1.9 Simulation study: (**a**) three independent plate wings, (**b**) inter-bridging horseshoe-shaped plate wing

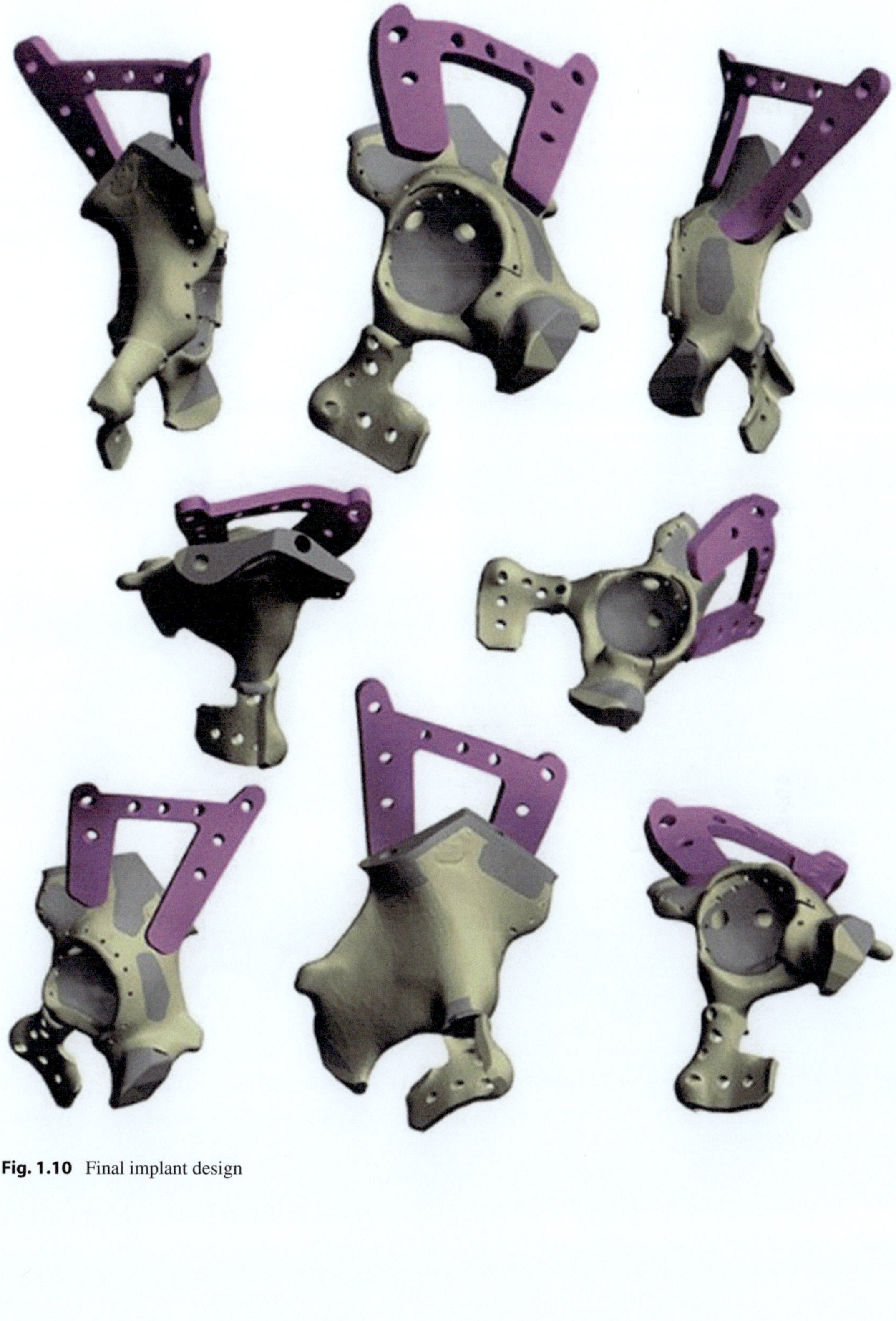

Fig. 1.10 Final implant design

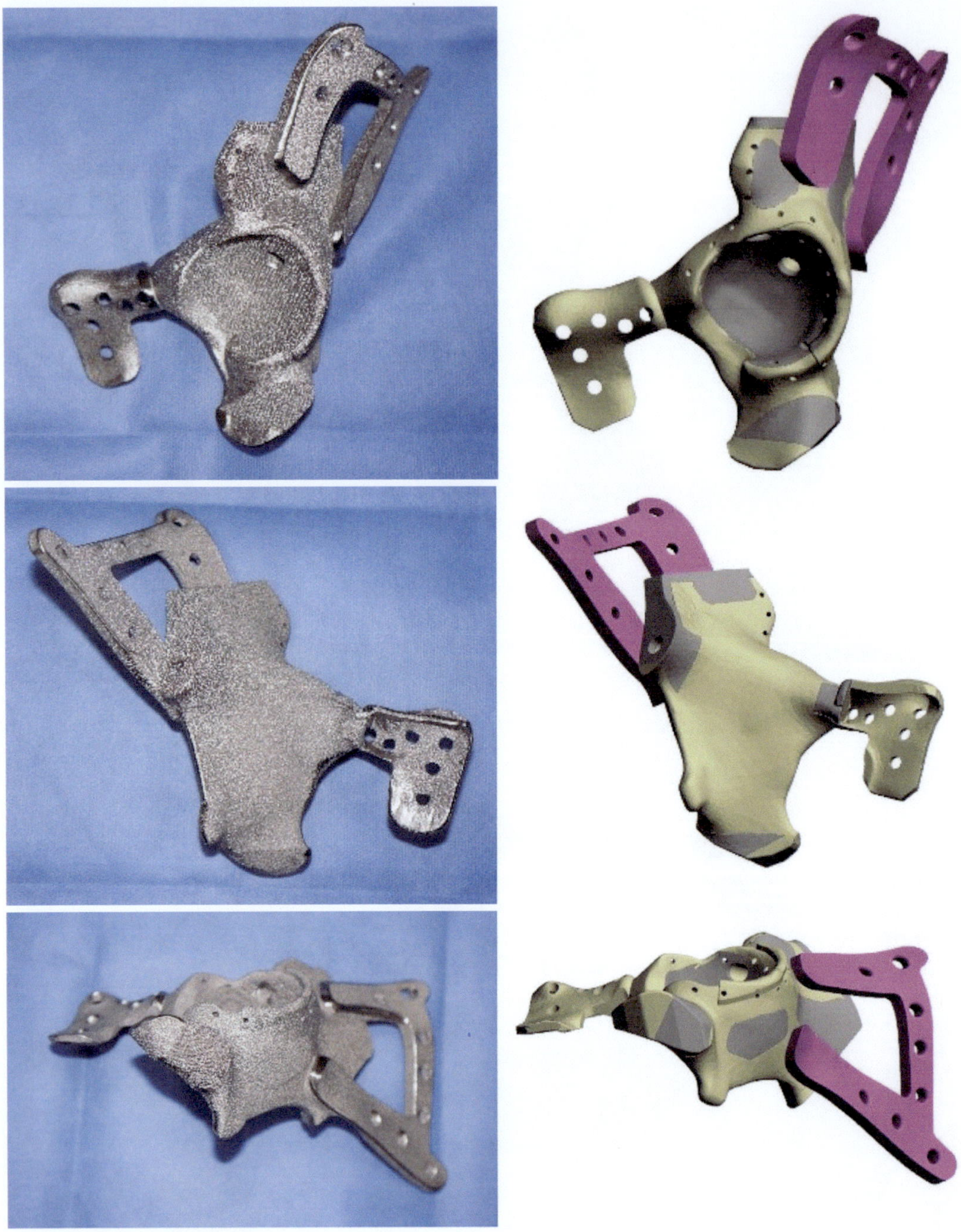

Fig. 1.11 Printed implant

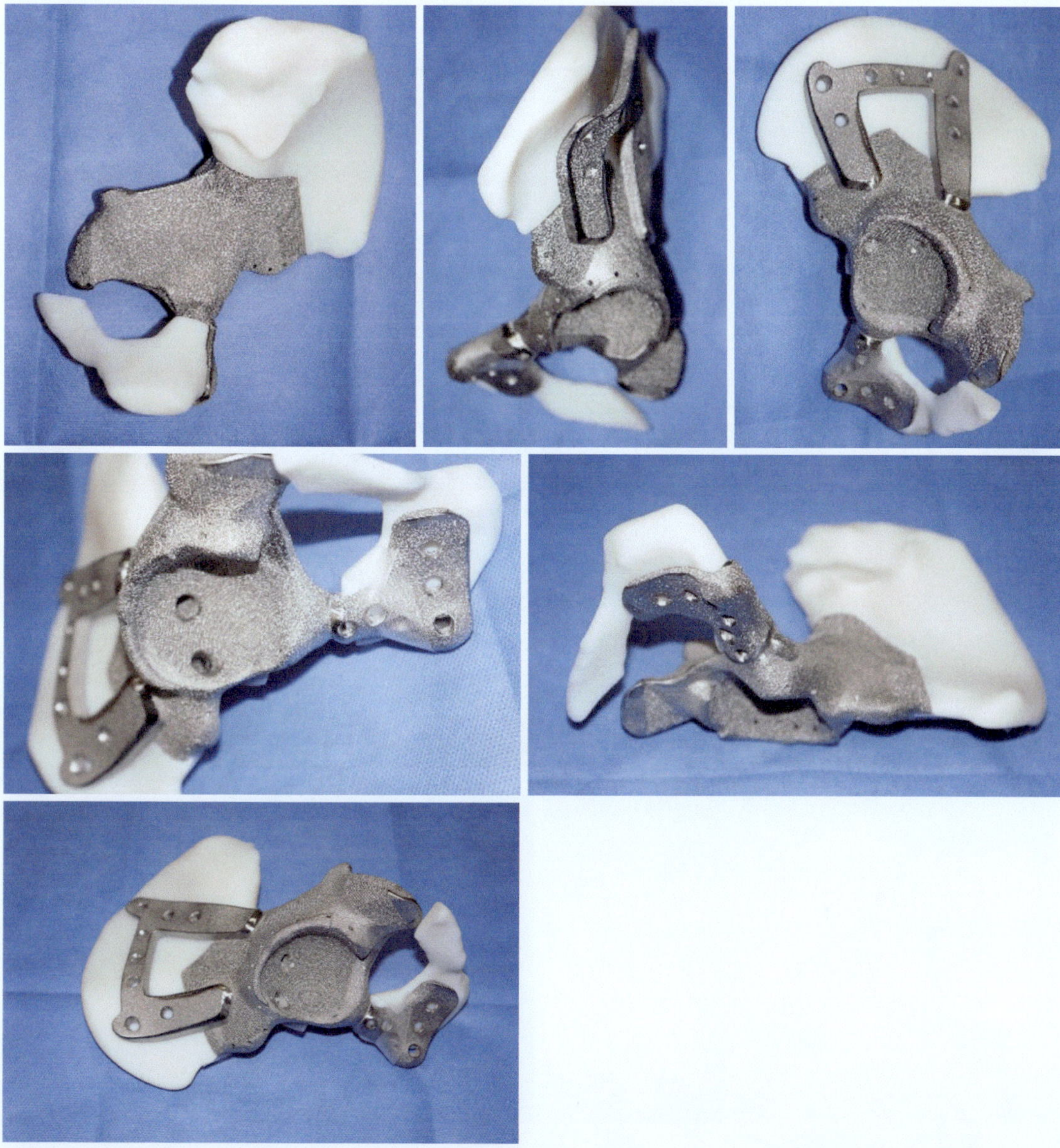

Fig. 1.11 (continued)

1.6 Operation

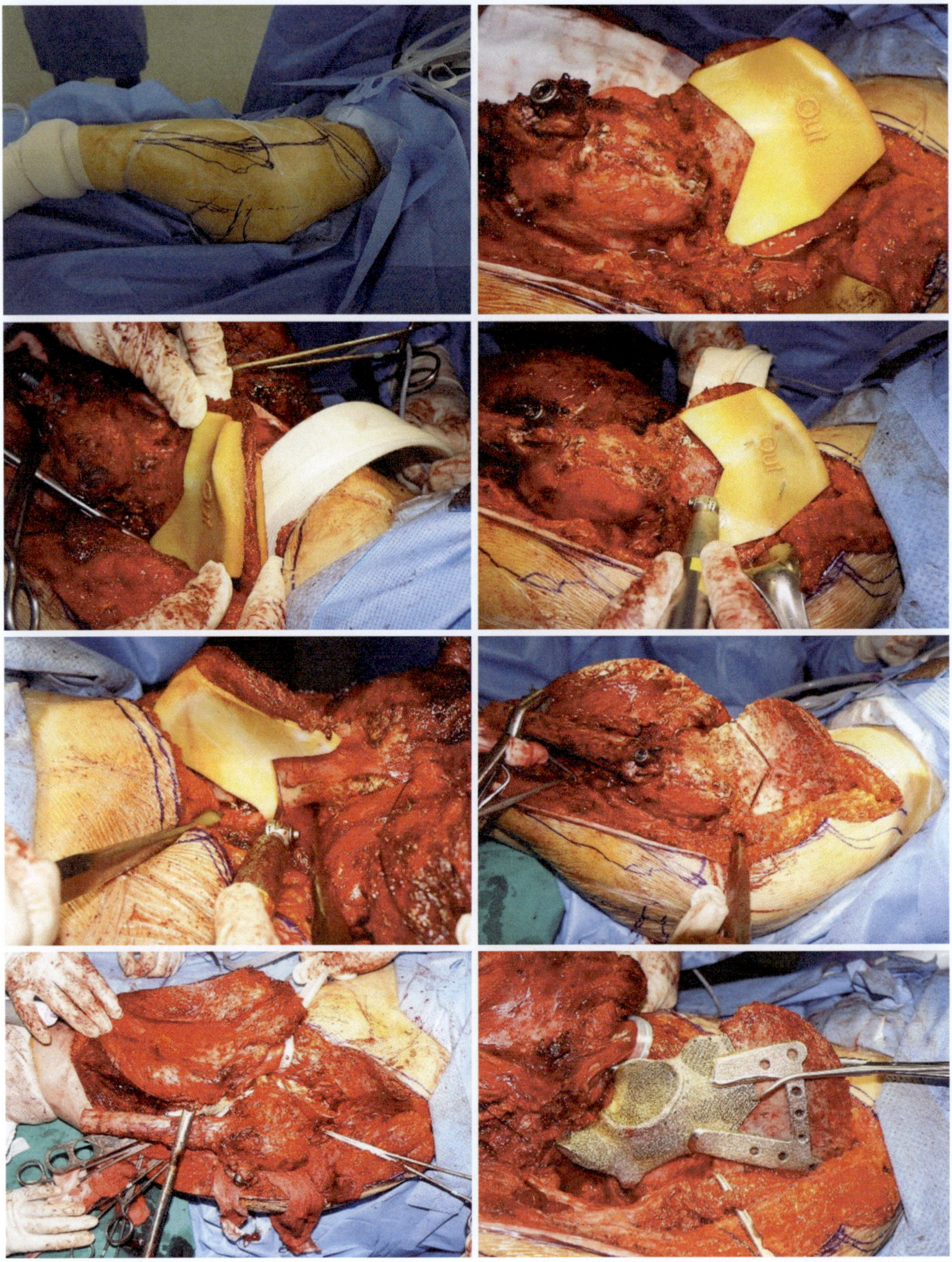

Fig. 1.12 Intraoperative photographs

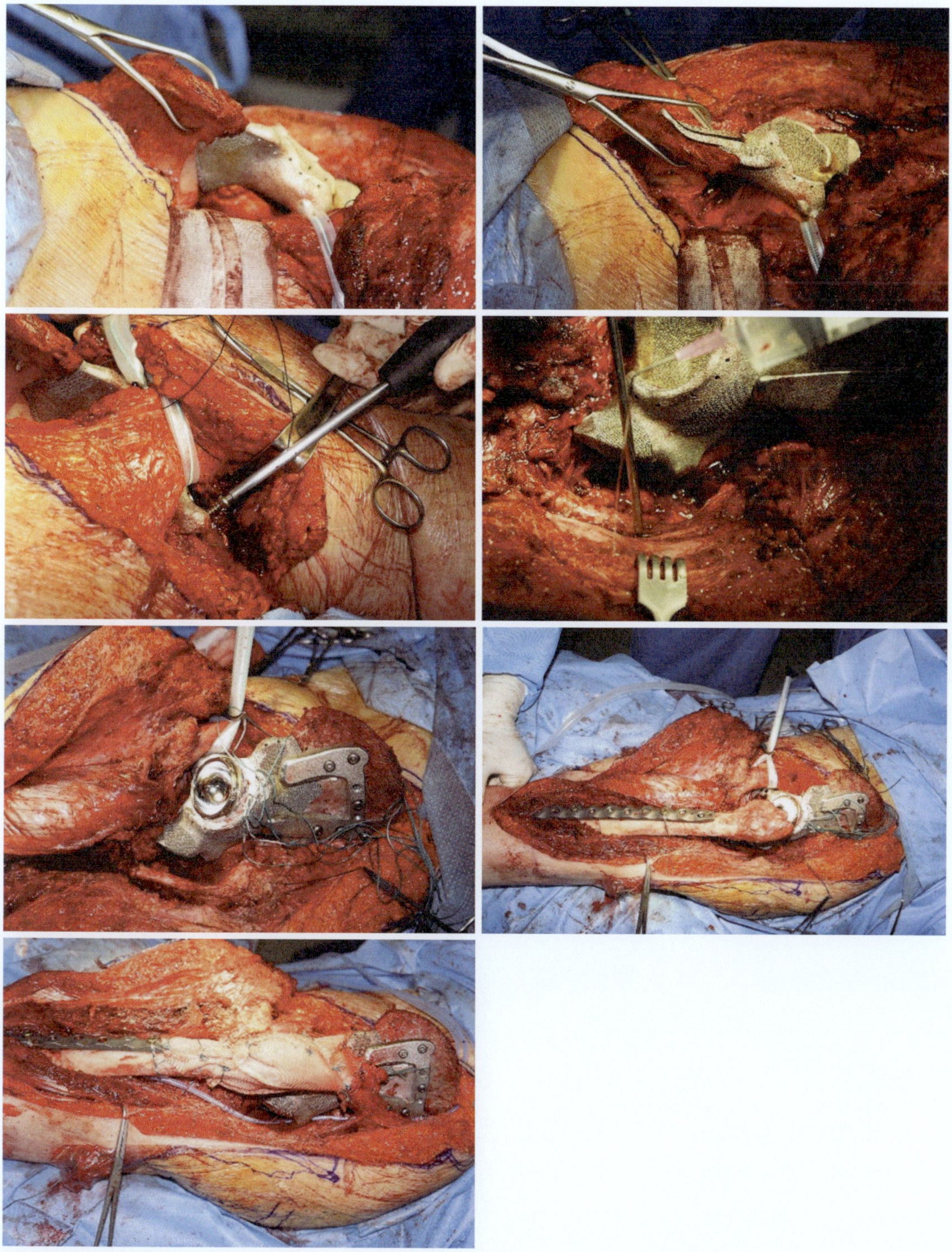

Fig. 1.12 (continued)

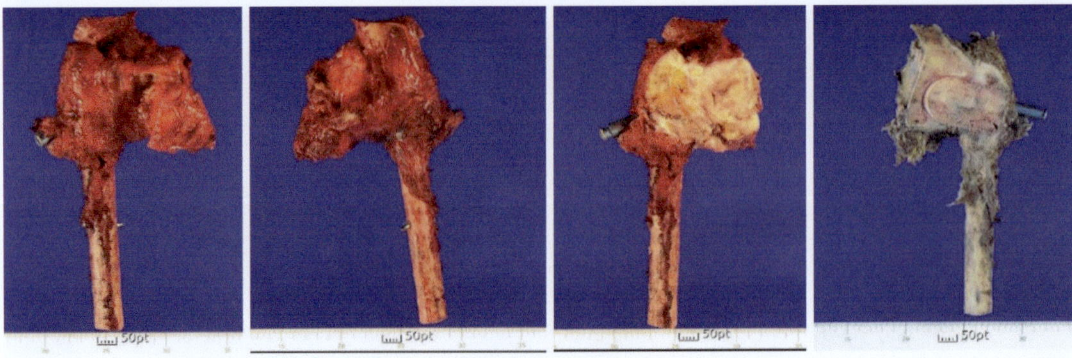

Fig. 1.13 Resected tumor

1.7 Postoperative Images

Since metal artifacts are present in the MRI, it is better to take a bone scan, PET-CT before surgery

The recurrence of tumor in the metal artifacts can be diagnosed with comparing several images

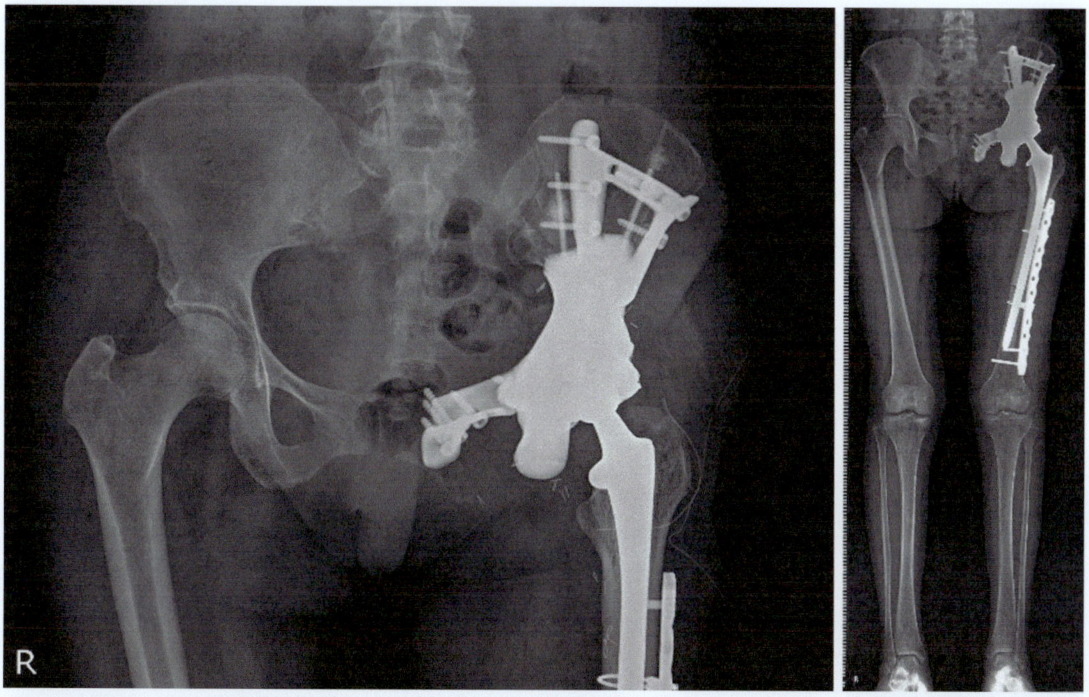

Fig. 1.14 Postoperative X-ray images

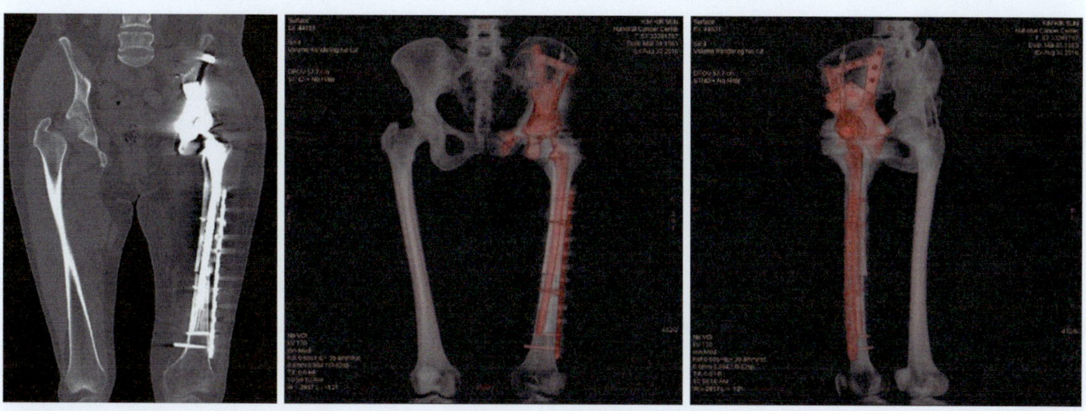

Fig. 1.15 Postoperative CT images

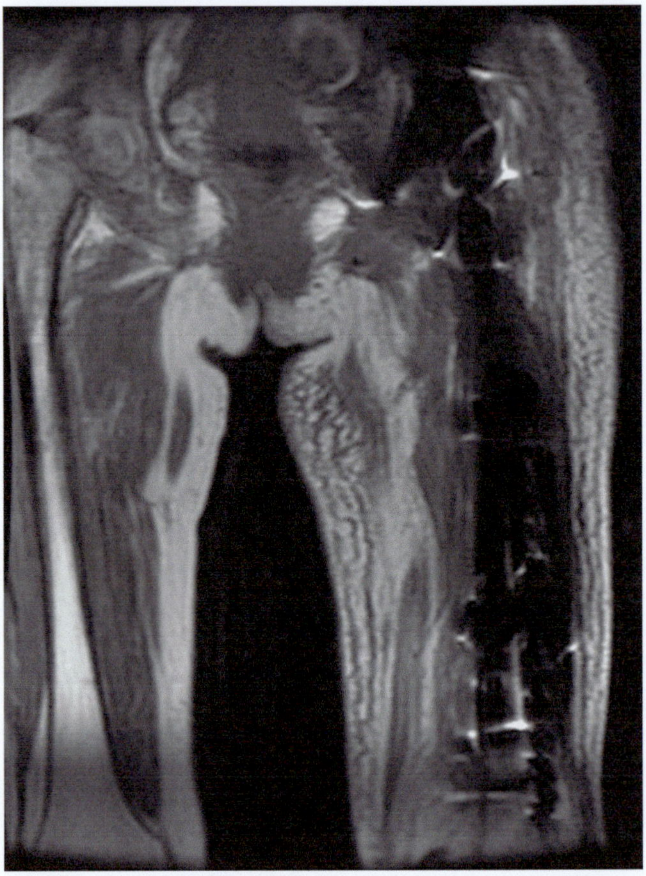

Fig. 1.16 Postoperative MRI image

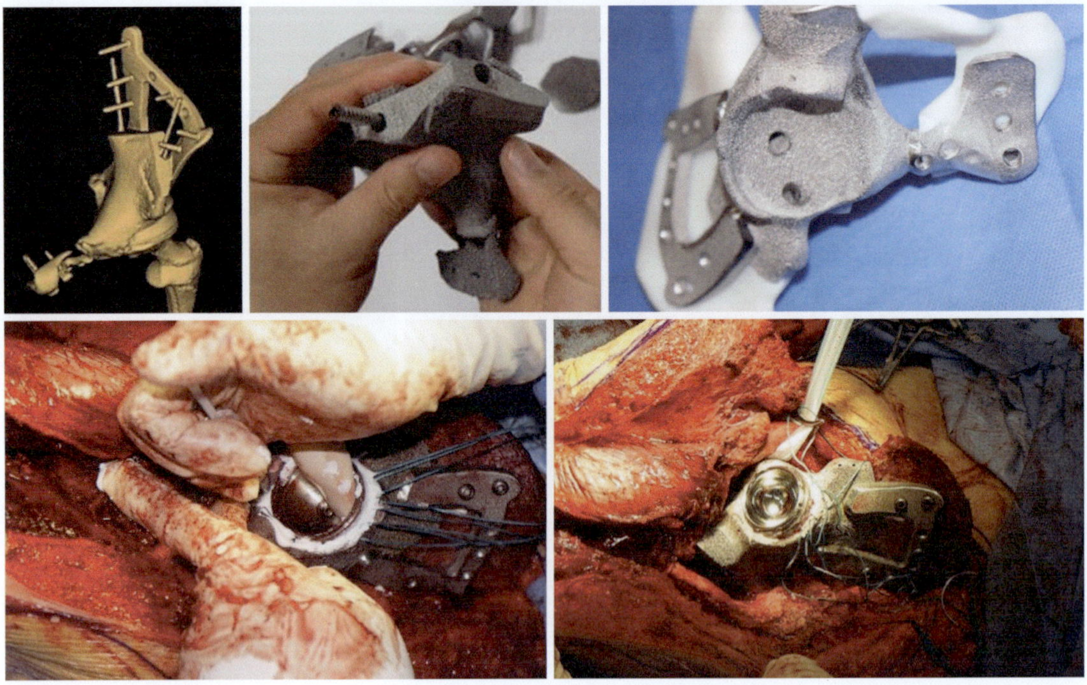

Fig. 1.17 Difficult acetabular metal shell combination at a small intraoperative field, difficult long screw fixation from acetabular cup to iliac bone through hollow holes of 3D printed implant body

Patient Case 2: Unique Acetabulum for Easy Assembly of Total Hip Cup

2

2.1 Patient Case 2

Age/sex	45/male
Location/site	Pelvis/left
Diagnosis	Chondrosarcoma, grade 2
Preoperative symptom	Sciatica and radiating pain with limping gait
Preoperative pain score	Resting 2/activity 6
BMI (height/weight)	21.98 (172.1/65.1)
Past history	Pain clinic treatment for 1 year Several lumbar spinal root block
Present illness	Visit after refusing allograft reconstruction at another hospital

2.2 Preoperative Images

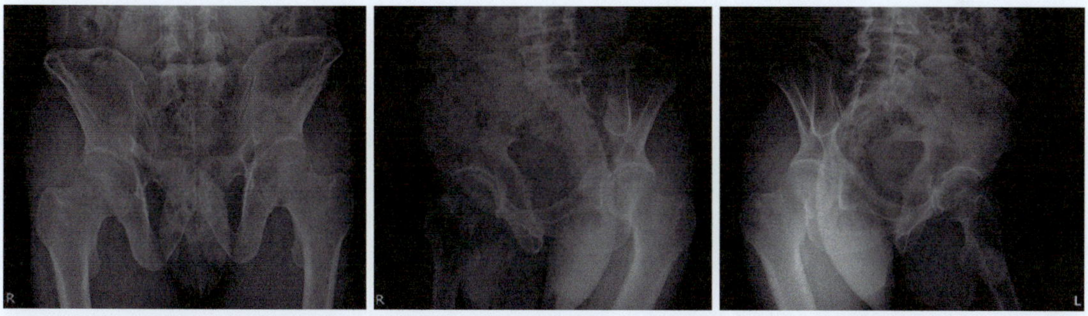

Fig. 2.1 Preoperative X-ray images

H.-G. Kang, *Clinical Atlas of 3D Printing Bone Reconstruction*,
https://doi.org/10.1007/978-981-16-2043-0_2

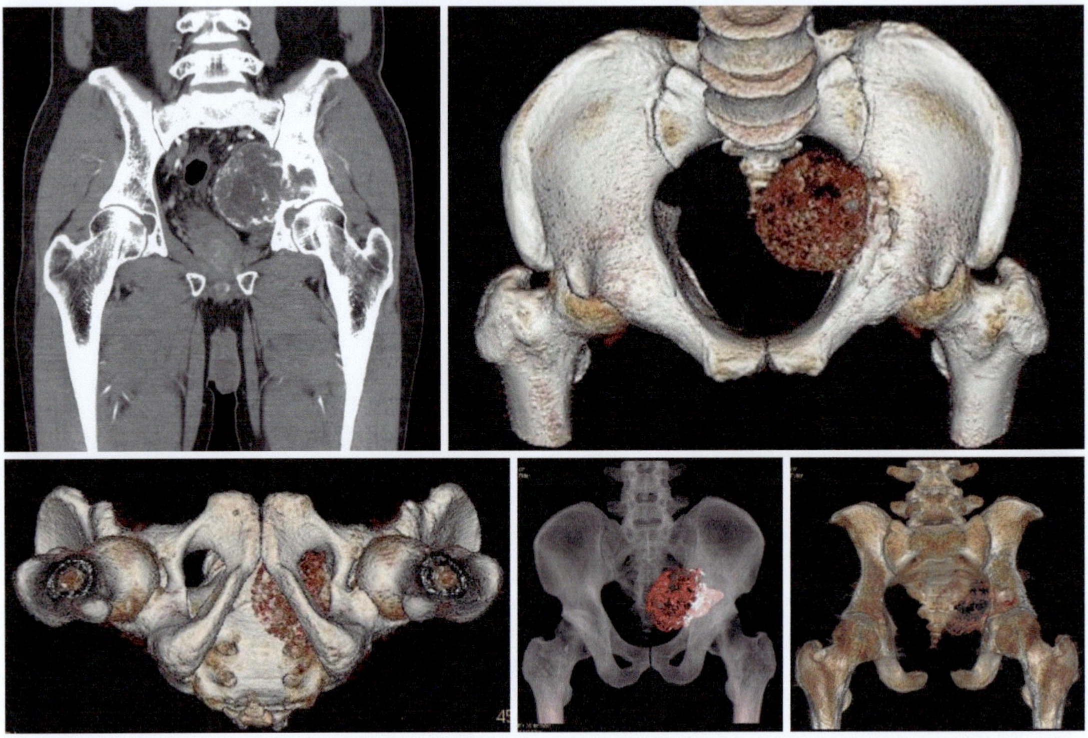

Fig. 2.2 Preoperative CT images

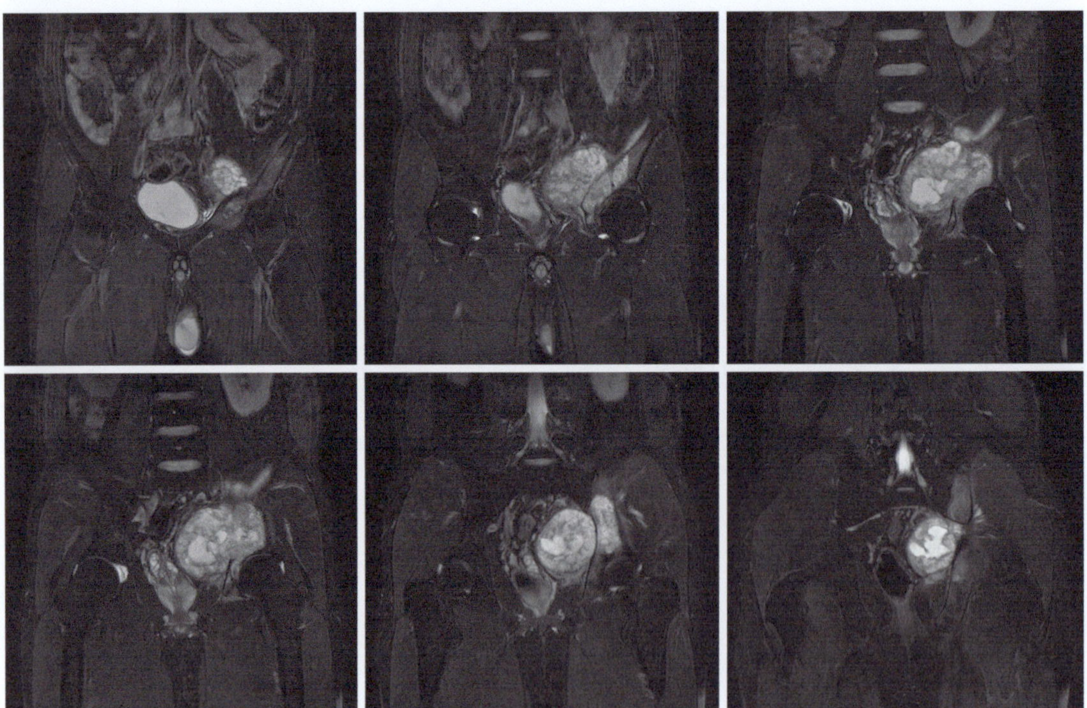

Fig. 2.3 Preoperative MRI images

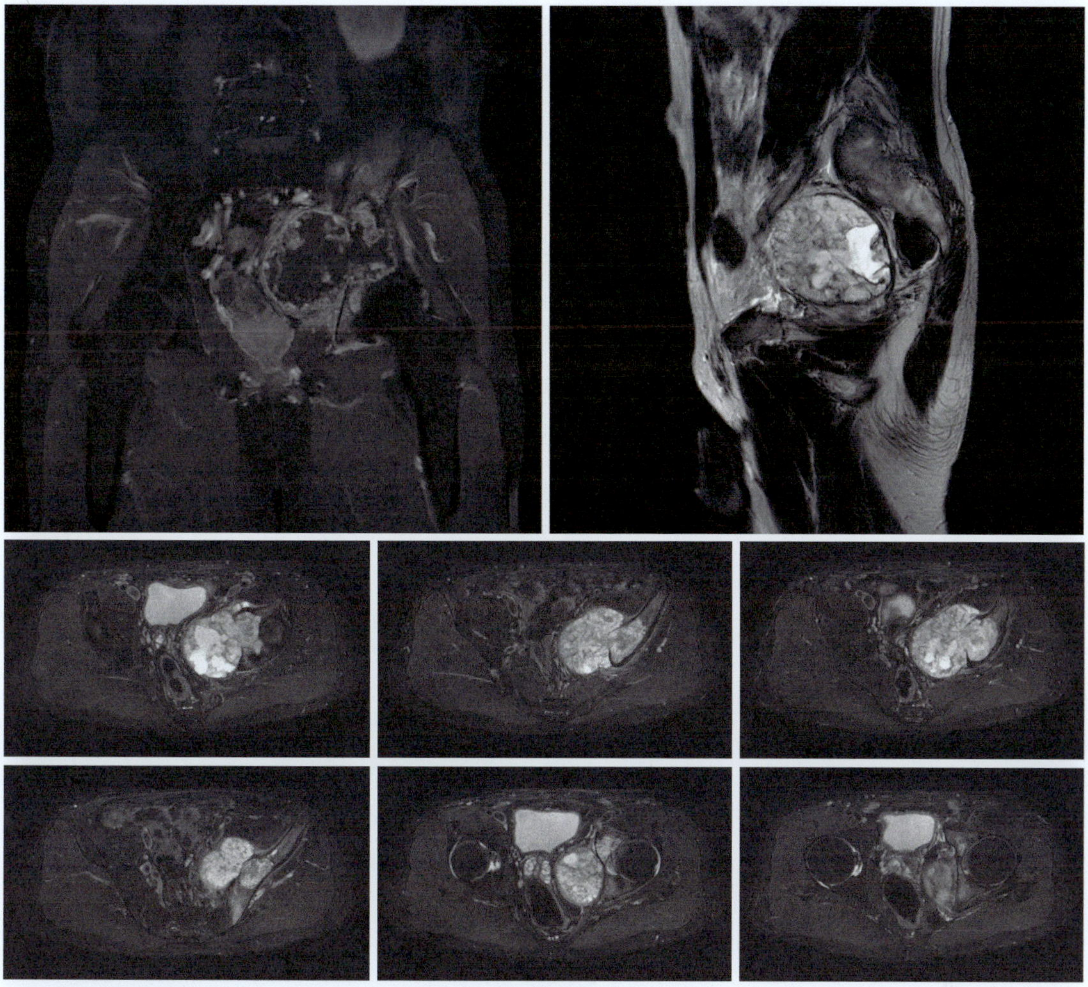

Fig. 2.3 (continued)

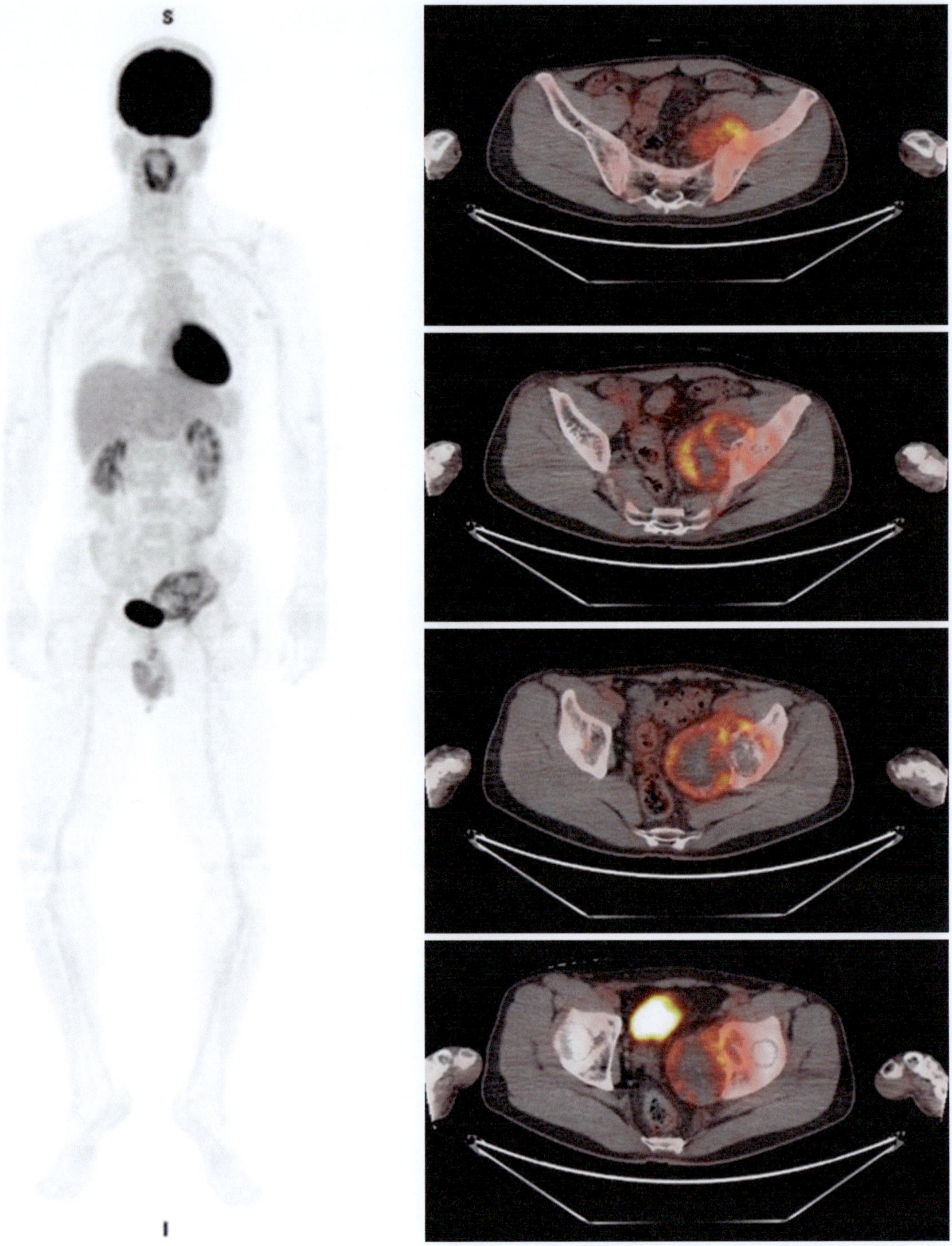

Fig. 2.4 Preoperative PET-CT images

2.3 Planning of Surgery

3D printed pelvis + Total hip arthroplasty

2.4 Design and Fabrication

The saw capture wing for iliac bone cutting
Guide designed to orient the saw blade

- Implant measurement
- Implant weight (g): 649
- Size (mm): 178

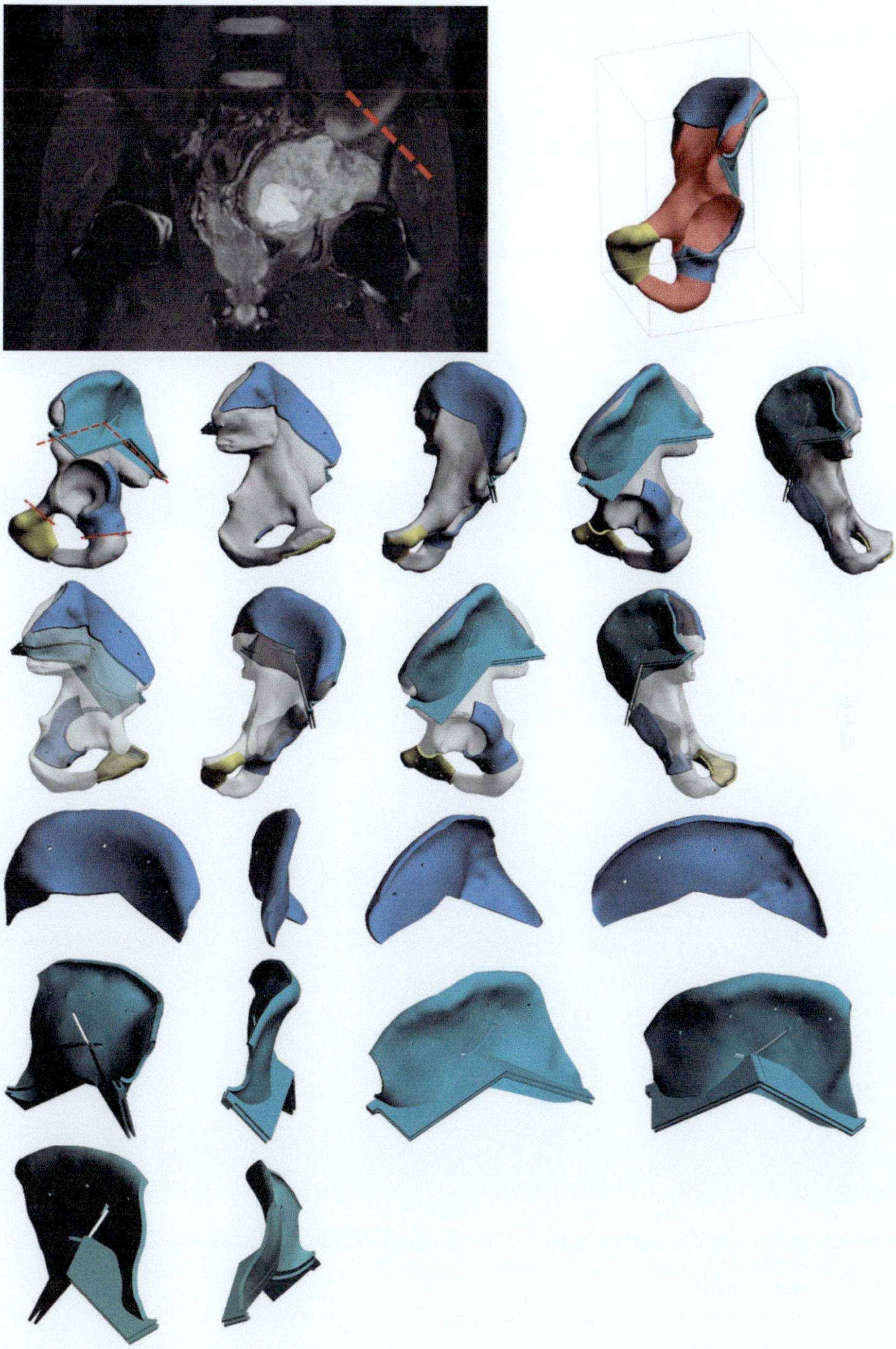

Fig. 2.5 Cutting guide design of ilium

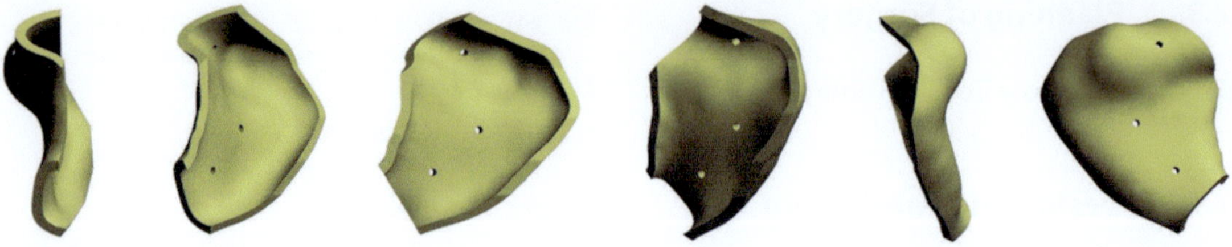

Fig. 2.6 Cutting guide design of pubis

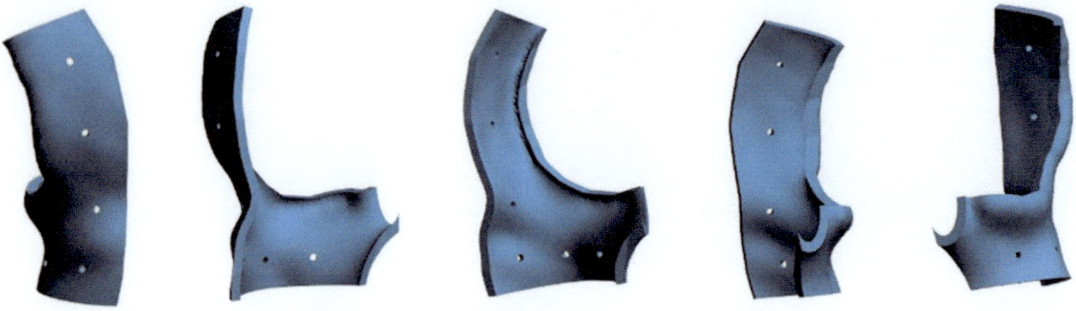

Fig. 2.7 Cutting guide design of ischium

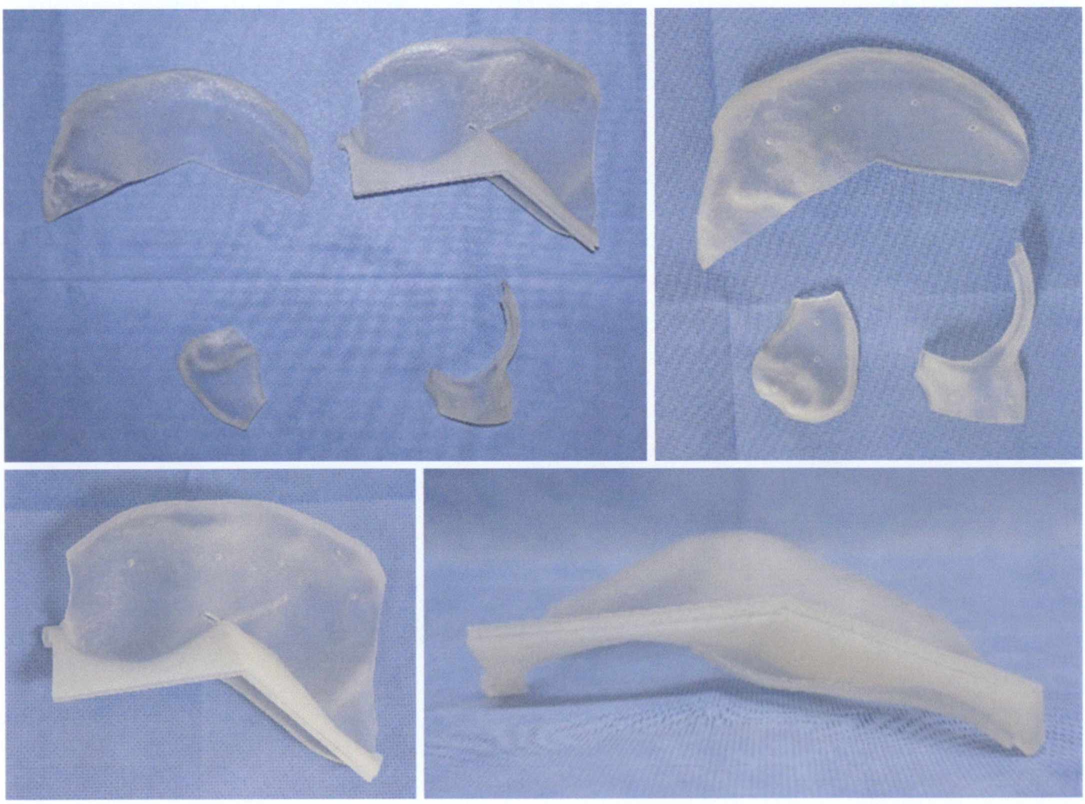

Fig. 2.8 Printed cutting guide

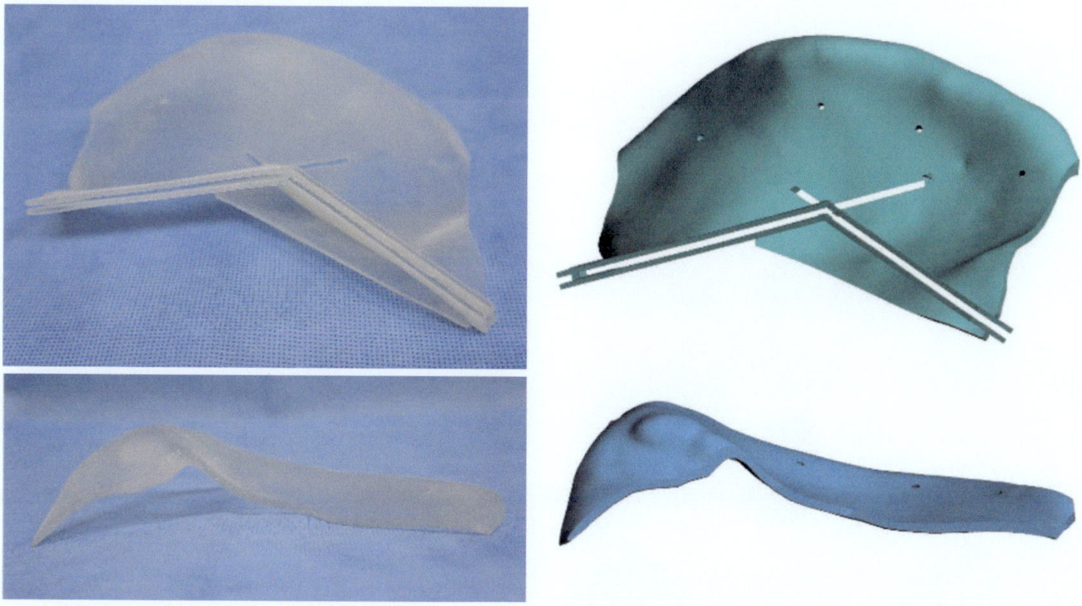

Fig. 2.8 (continued)

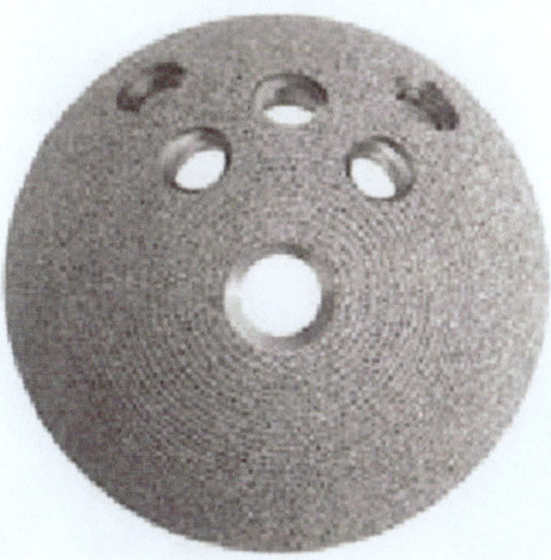

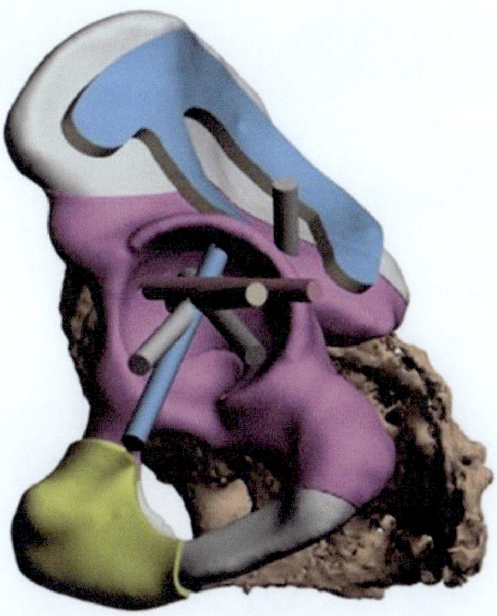

Fig. 2.9 New acetabular design (right) has 5 matching cup screw holes comparing previous (left)

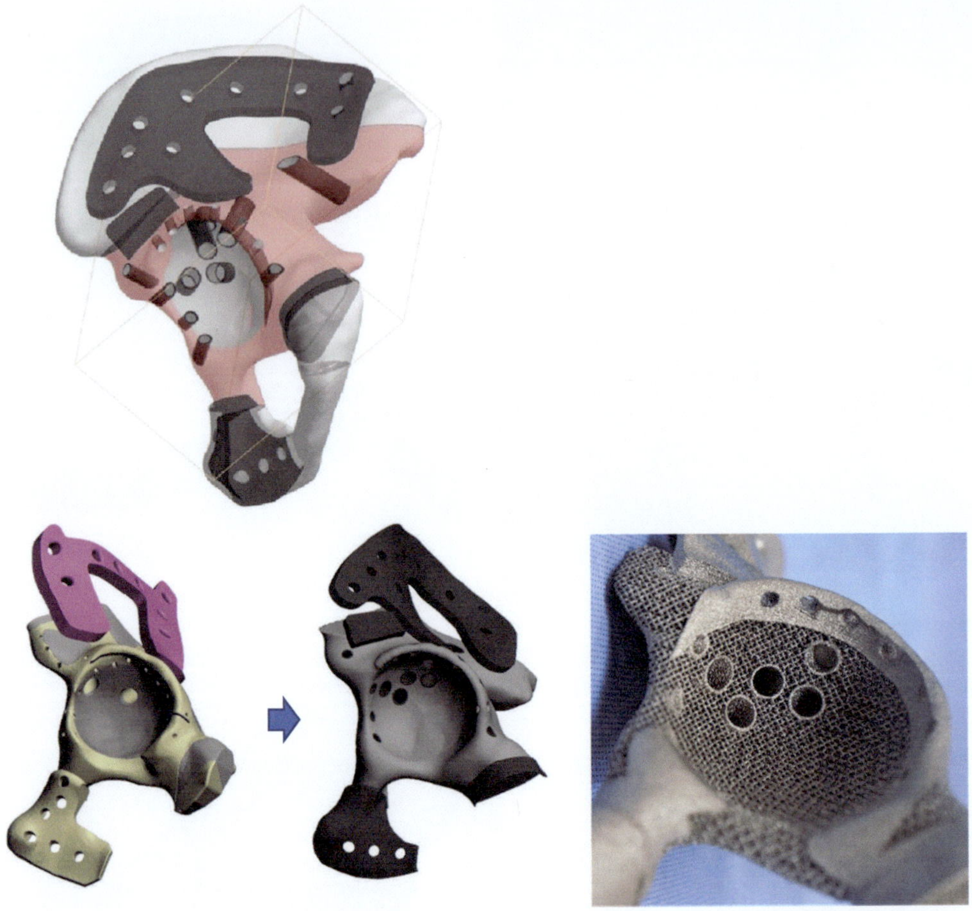

Fig. 2.9 (continued)

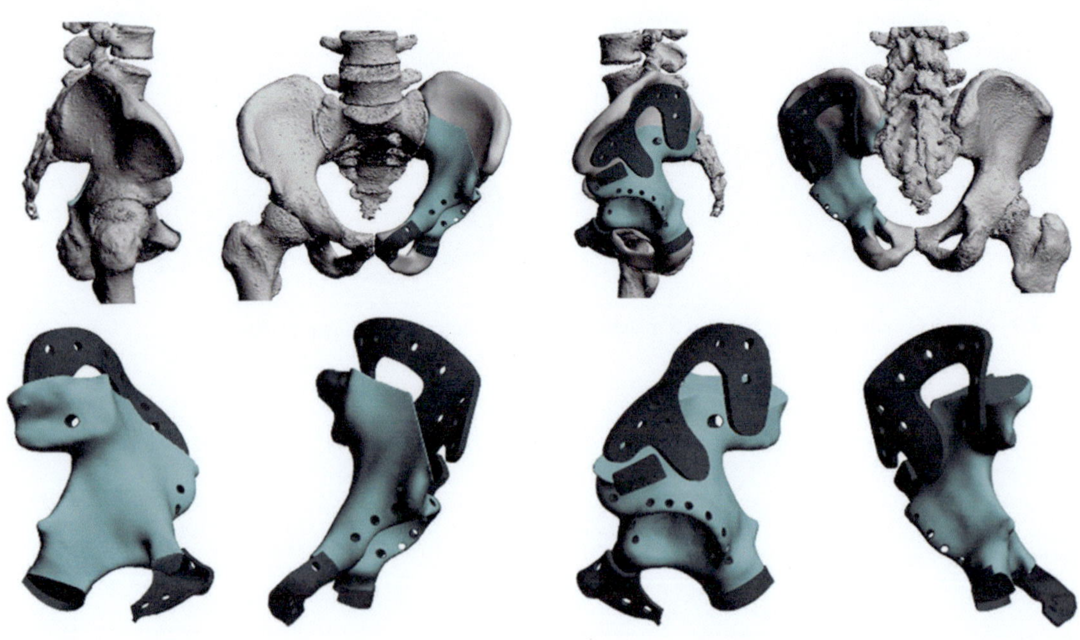

Fig. 2.10 Implant design

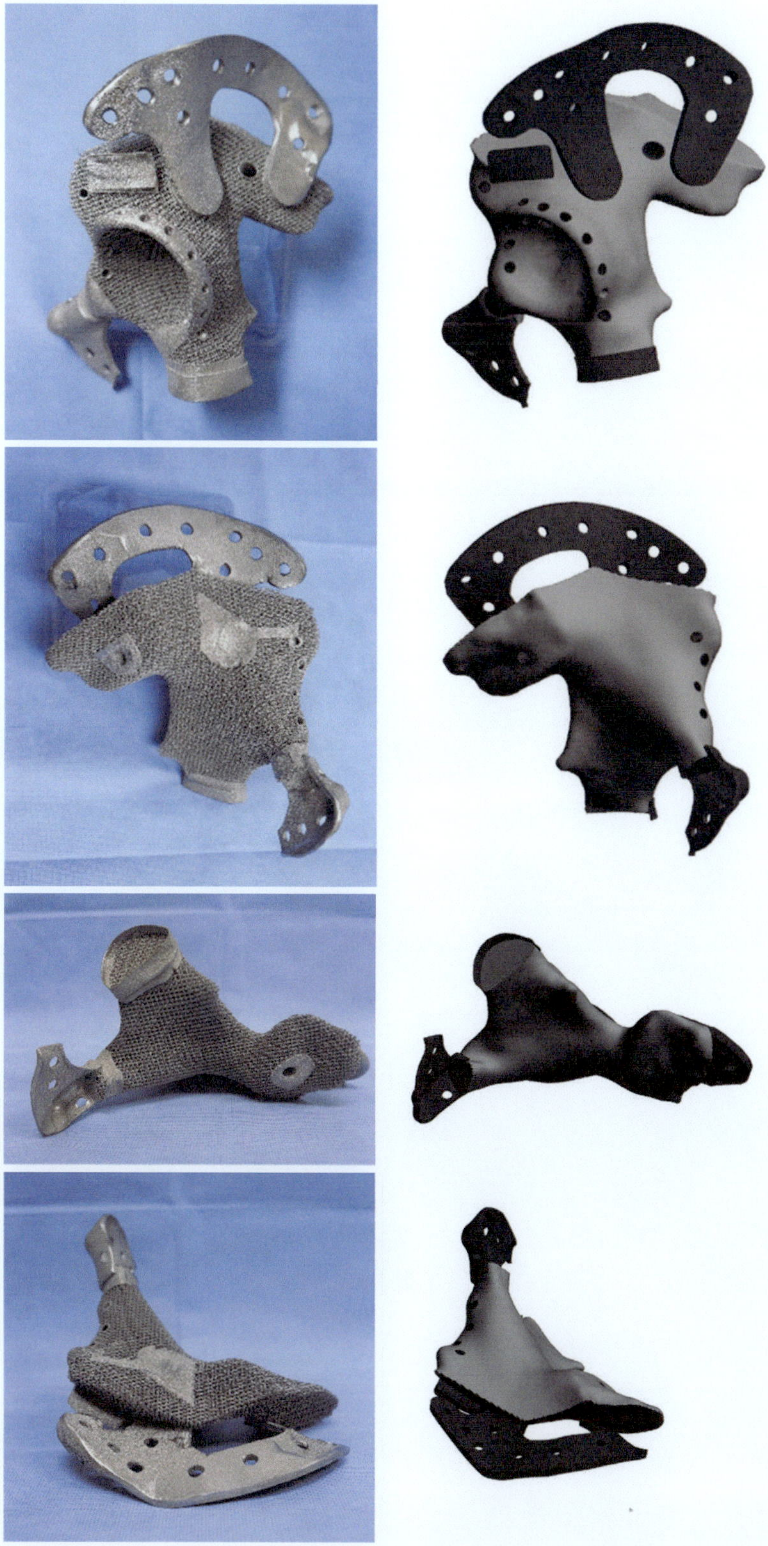

Fig. 2.11 Printed implant, light is transmitted through mesh style body

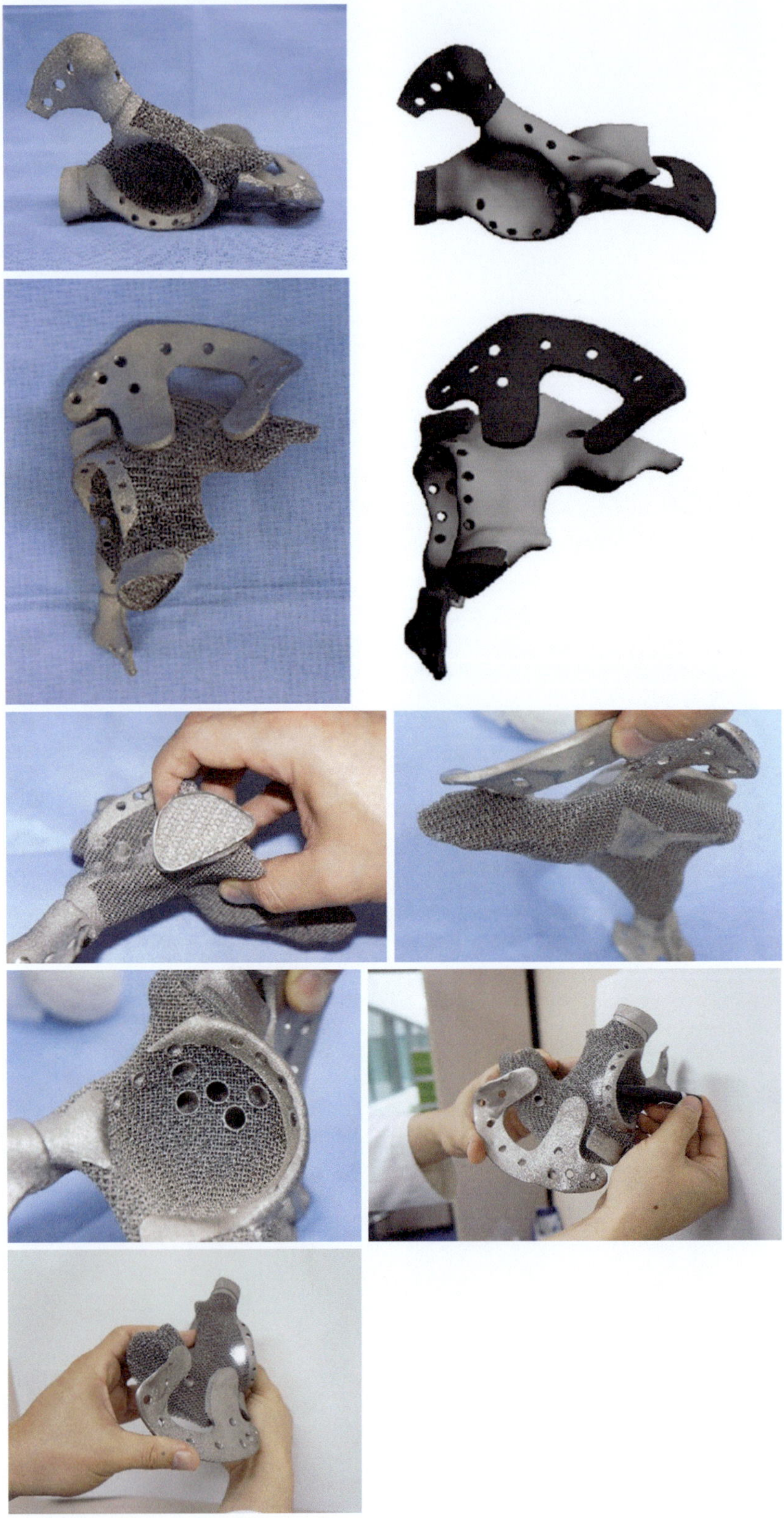

Fig. 2.11 (continued)

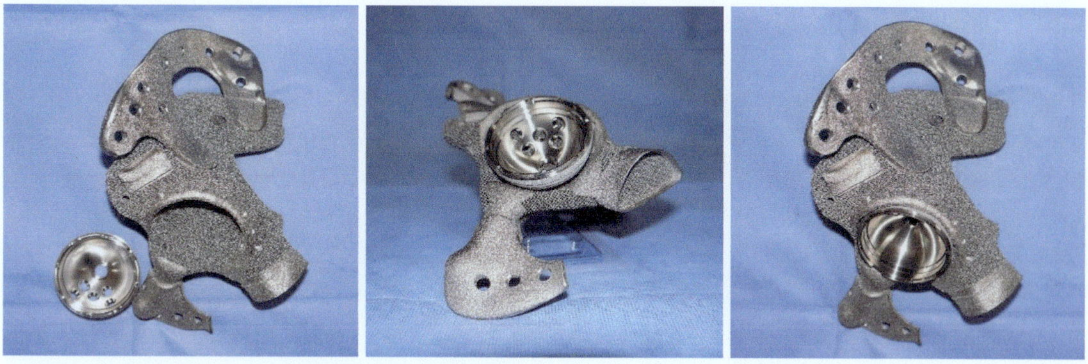

Fig. 2.12 Printed implant combined with total hip joint acetabular metal cup

2.5 Operation

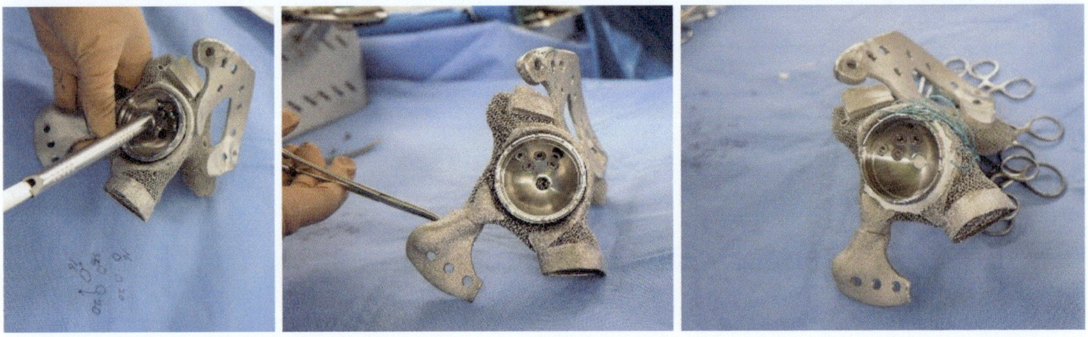

Fig. 2.13 Intraoperative photograph: acetabular cup conjugate with bone cement and original cup screws at the extra-operative field during the operative approach

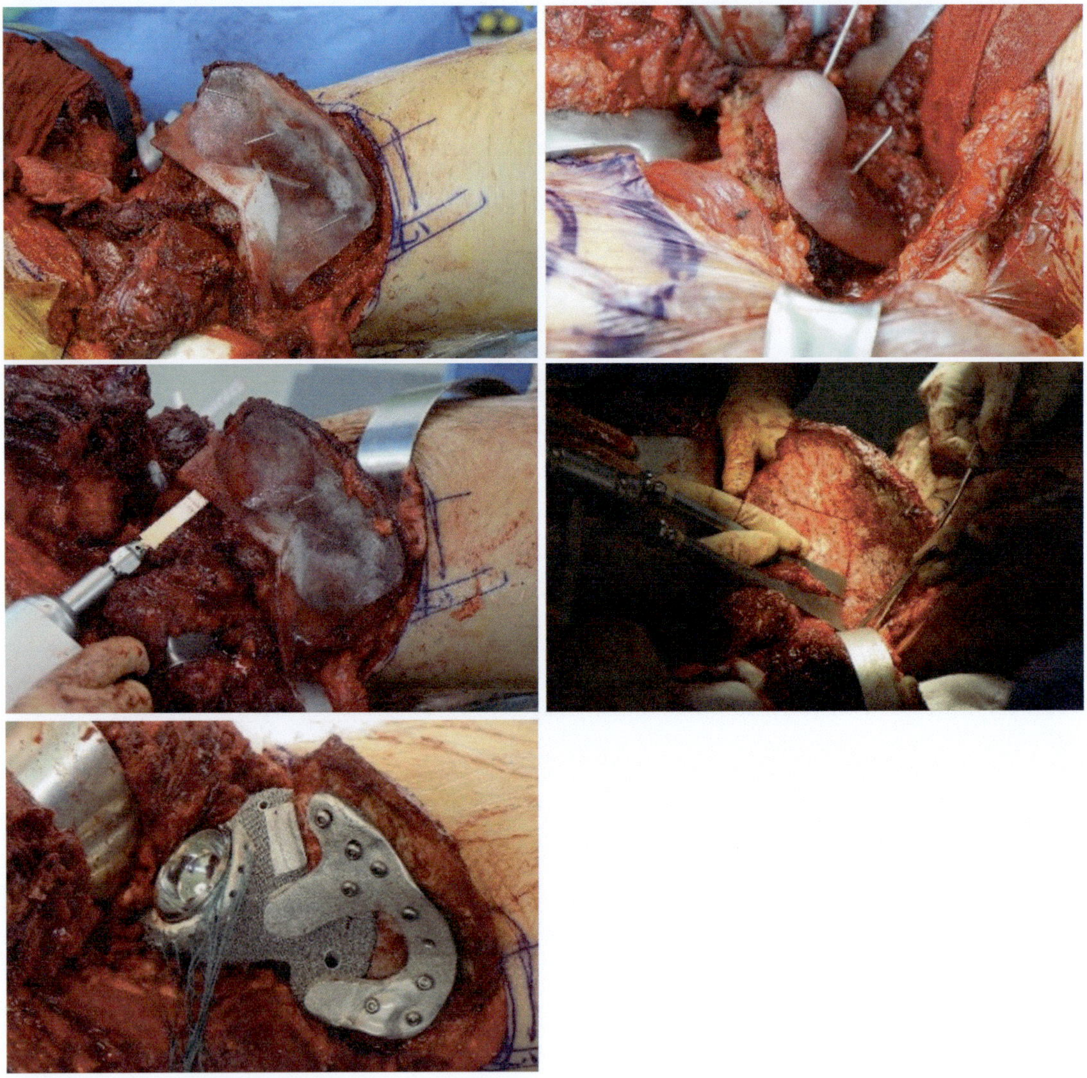

Fig. 2.14 Intraoperative photographs

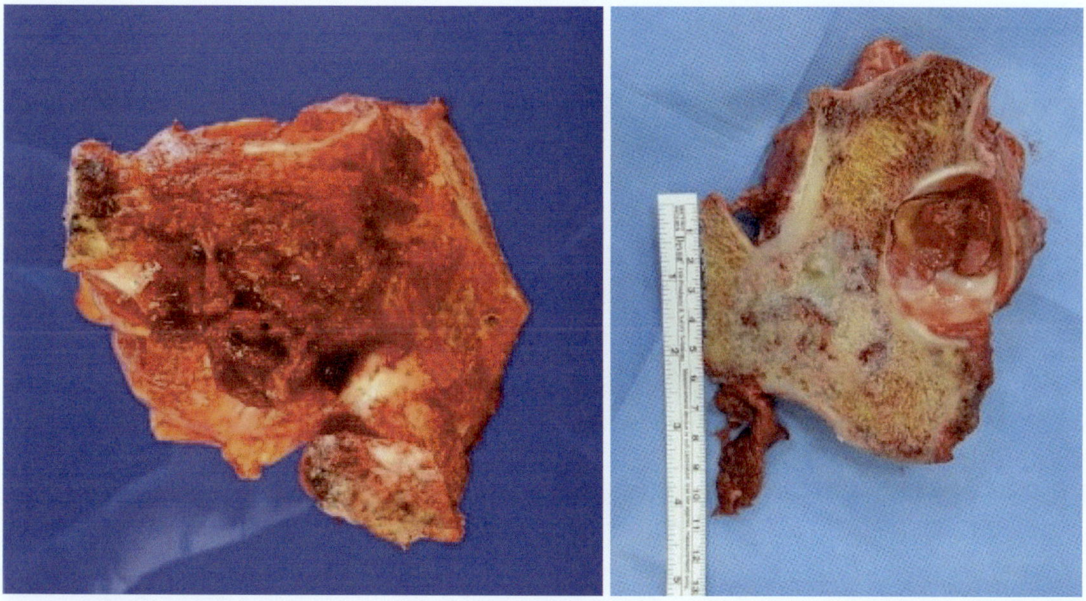

Fig. 2.15 Resected tumor

2.6 Postoperative Images

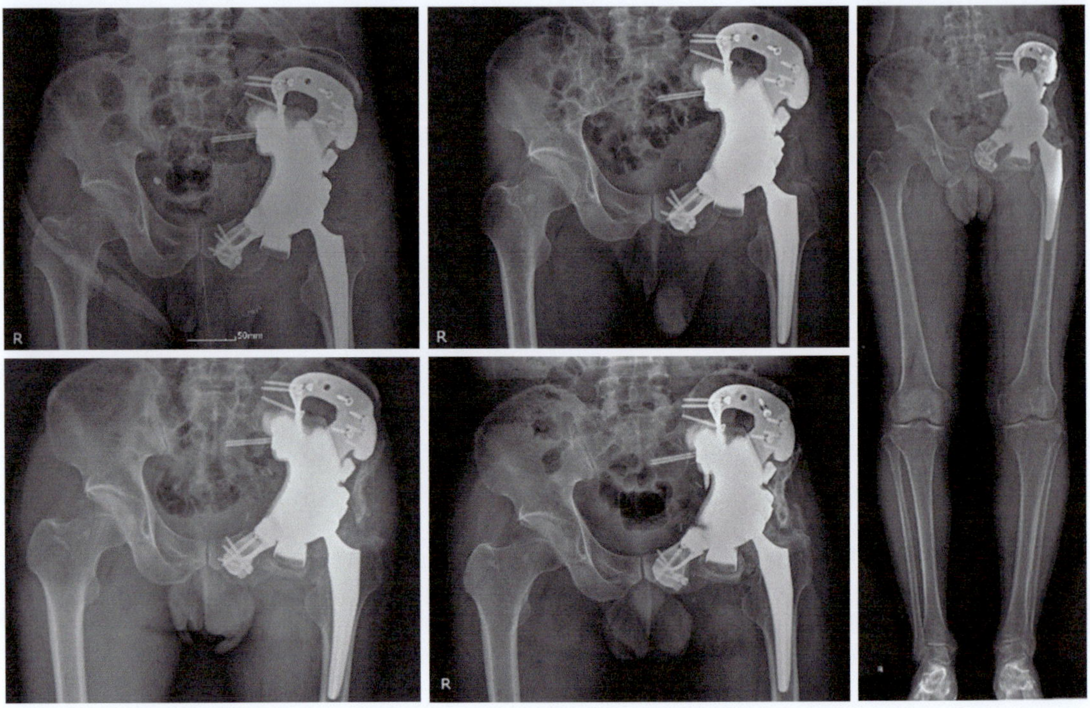

Fig. 2.16 Postoperative X-ray images: asymptomatic ossification around the hip joint at follow-up

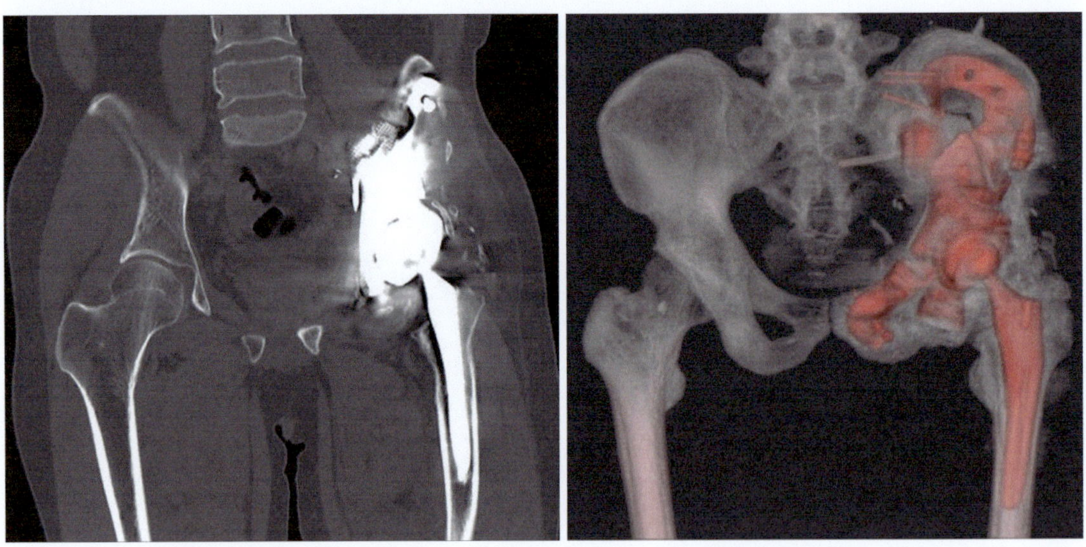

Fig. 2.17 Postoperative CT images

3 Patient Case 3: Mesh-Style Body Without Ischium

3.1 Patient Case 3

Age/sex	51/male
Location/site	Pelvis/right
Diagnosis	Osteosarcoma
Preoperative symptom	Limping gait with cane
Preoperative pain score	Resting 3/Activity 6
BMI (height/weight)	27.02 (172.6/80.5)
Past history	Visit after incisional biopsy
Present illness	Preoperative two times chemotherapy

3.2 Preoperative Images

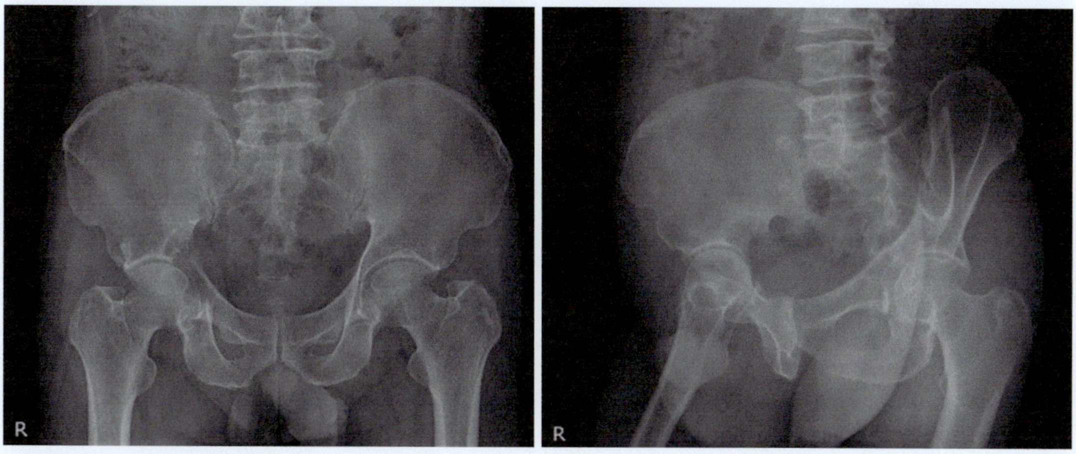

Fig. 3.1 Preoperative X-ray images

H.-G. Kang, *Clinical Atlas of 3D Printing Bone Reconstruction*,
https://doi.org/10.1007/978-981-16-2043-0_3

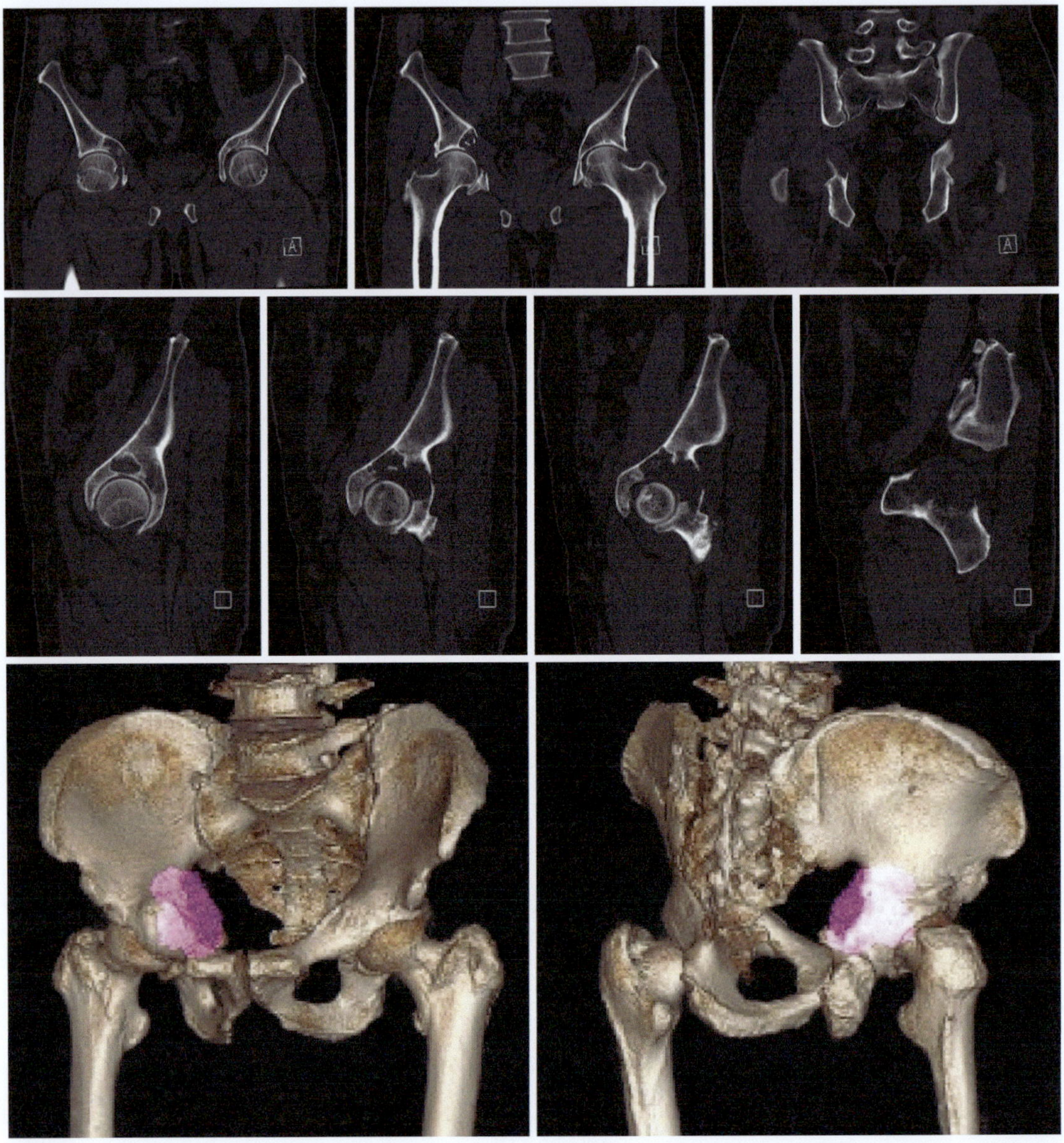

Fig. 3.2 Preoperative CT images

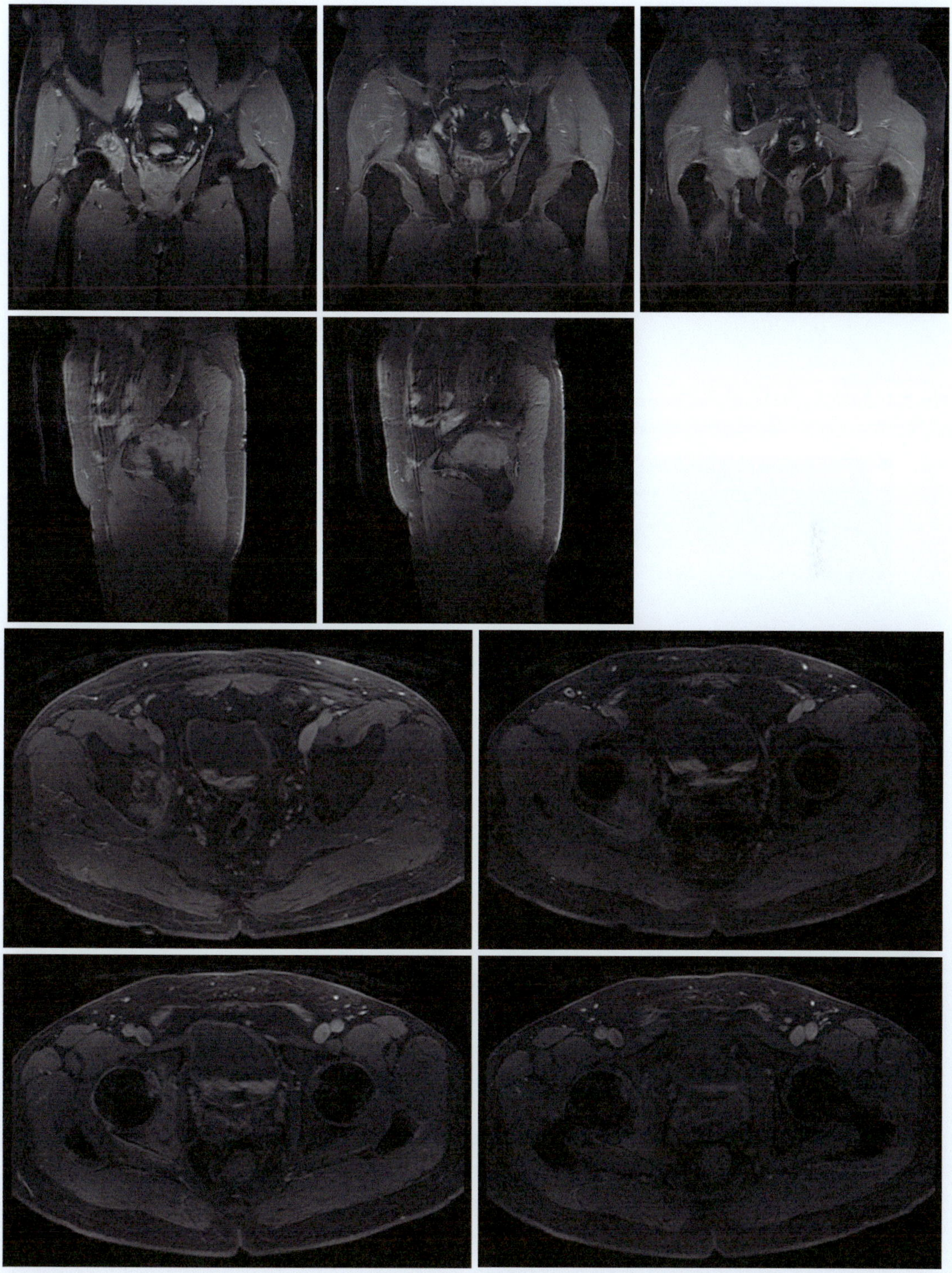

Fig. 3.3 Preoperative MRI images

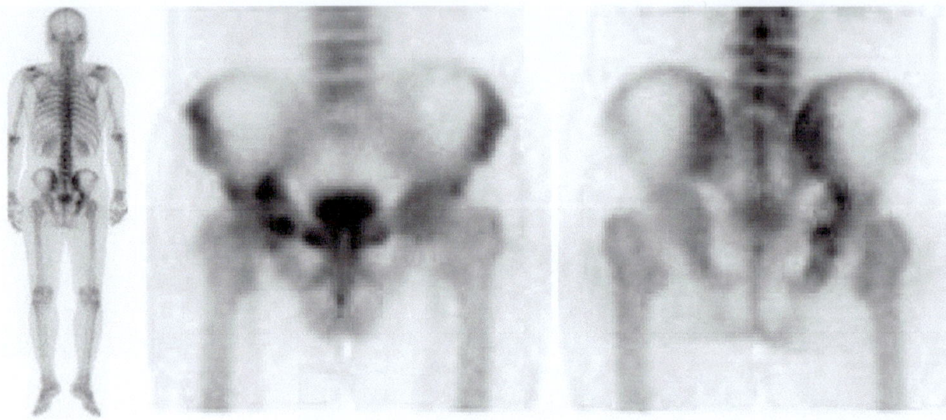

Fig. 3.4 Preoperative bone scan images

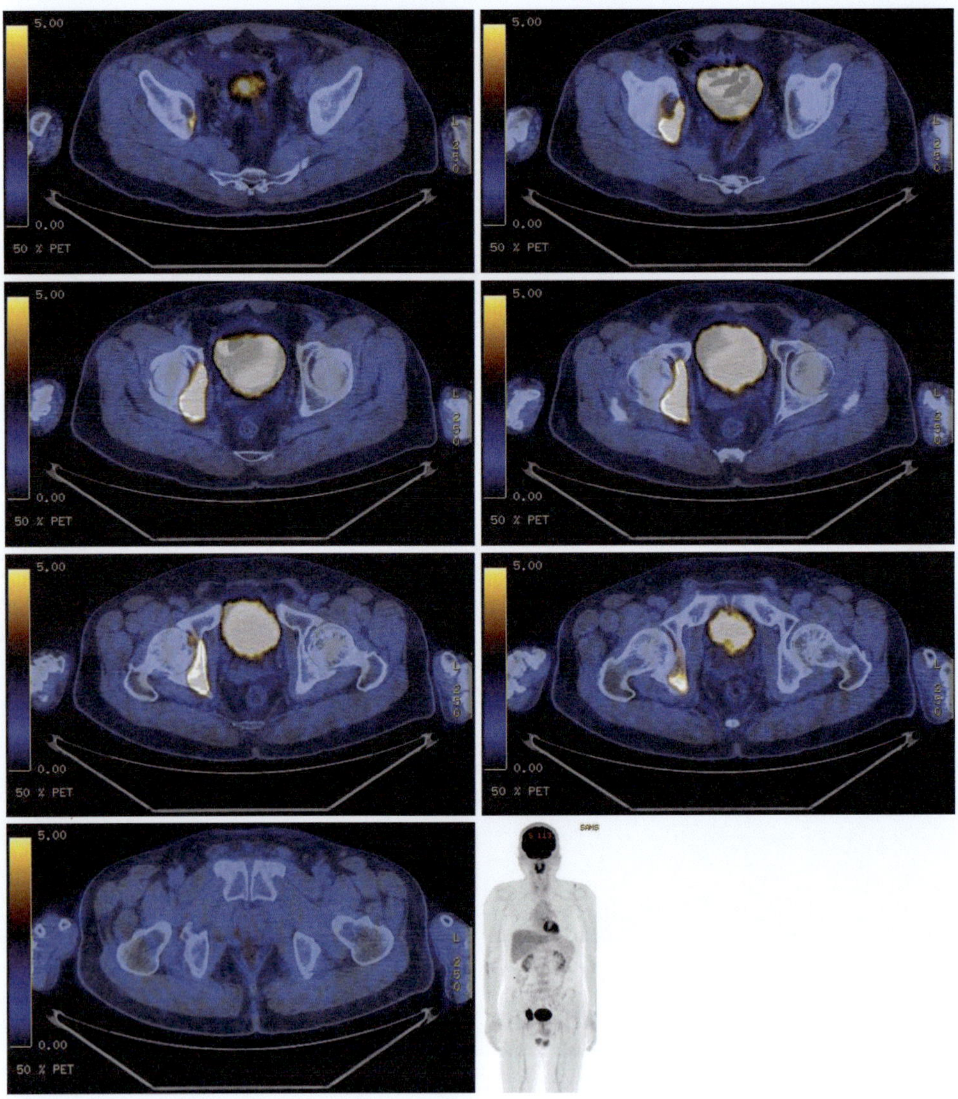

Fig. 3.5 Preoperative PET-CT images

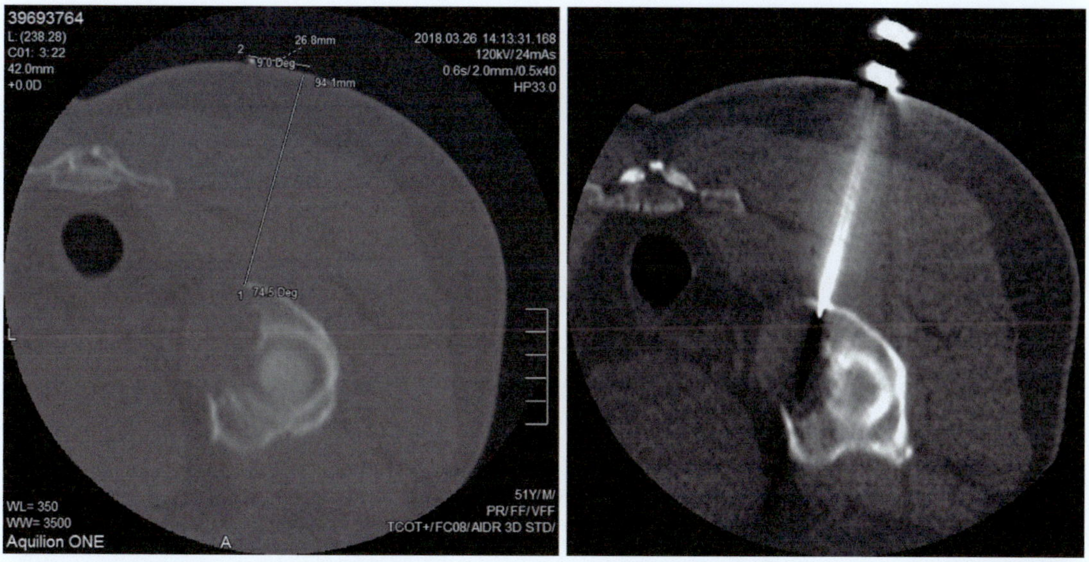

Fig. 3.6 CT guided needle biopsy

3.3 Planning of Surgery

3D printed pelvis, Mesh body

- Pubic ramus is reconstruction
- No ischium

3.4 Design and Fabrication

- Implant measurement
- Implant weight (g): 352 size (mm): 194

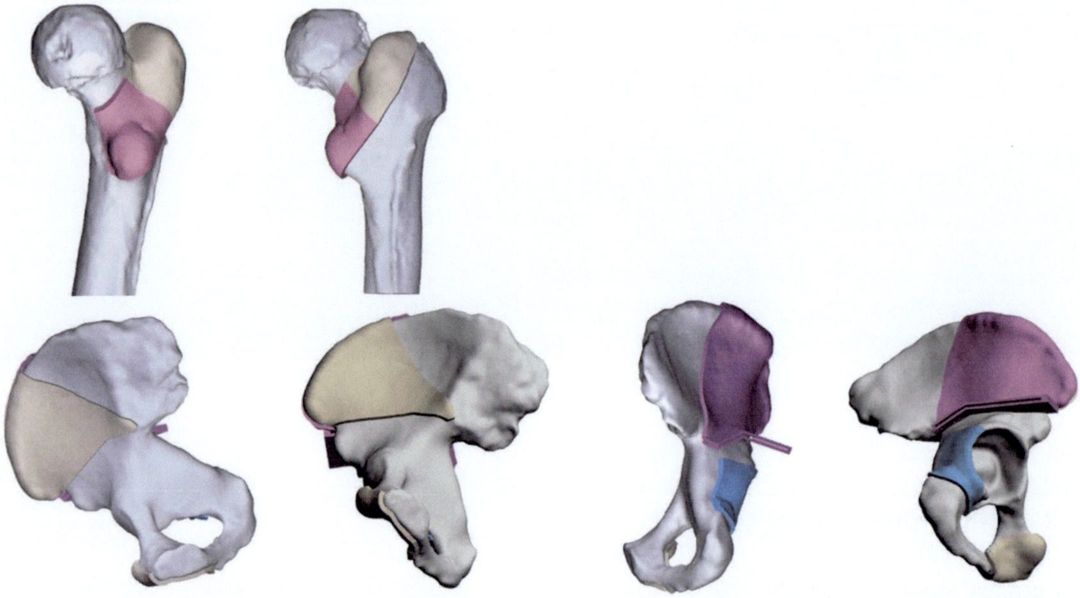

Fig. 3.7 Cutting guide design

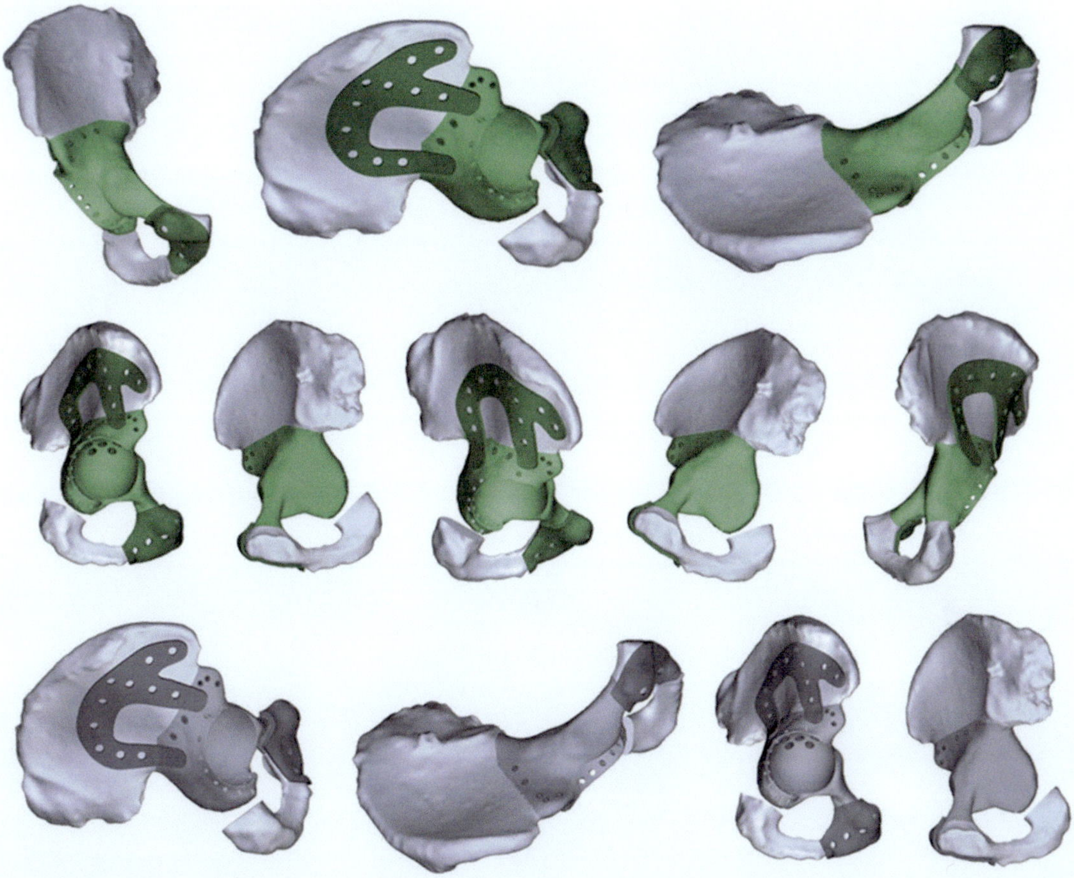

Fig. 3.8 Implant design

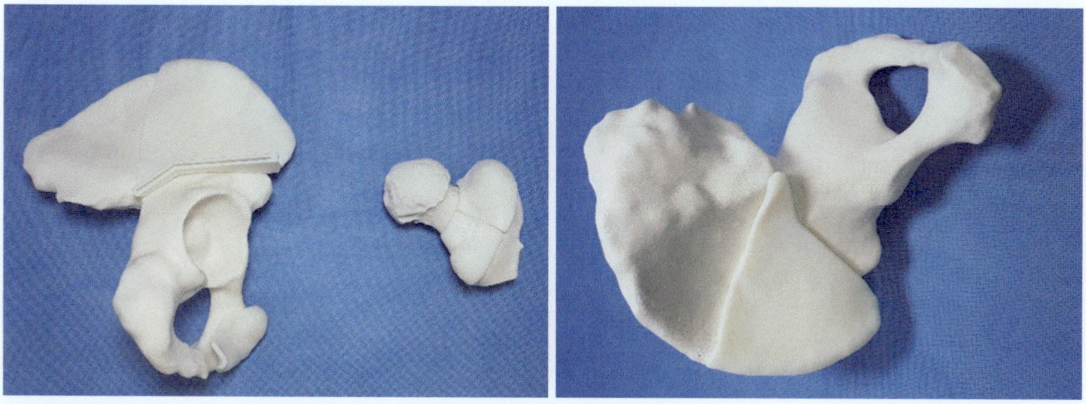

Fig. 3.9 Printed cutting guide

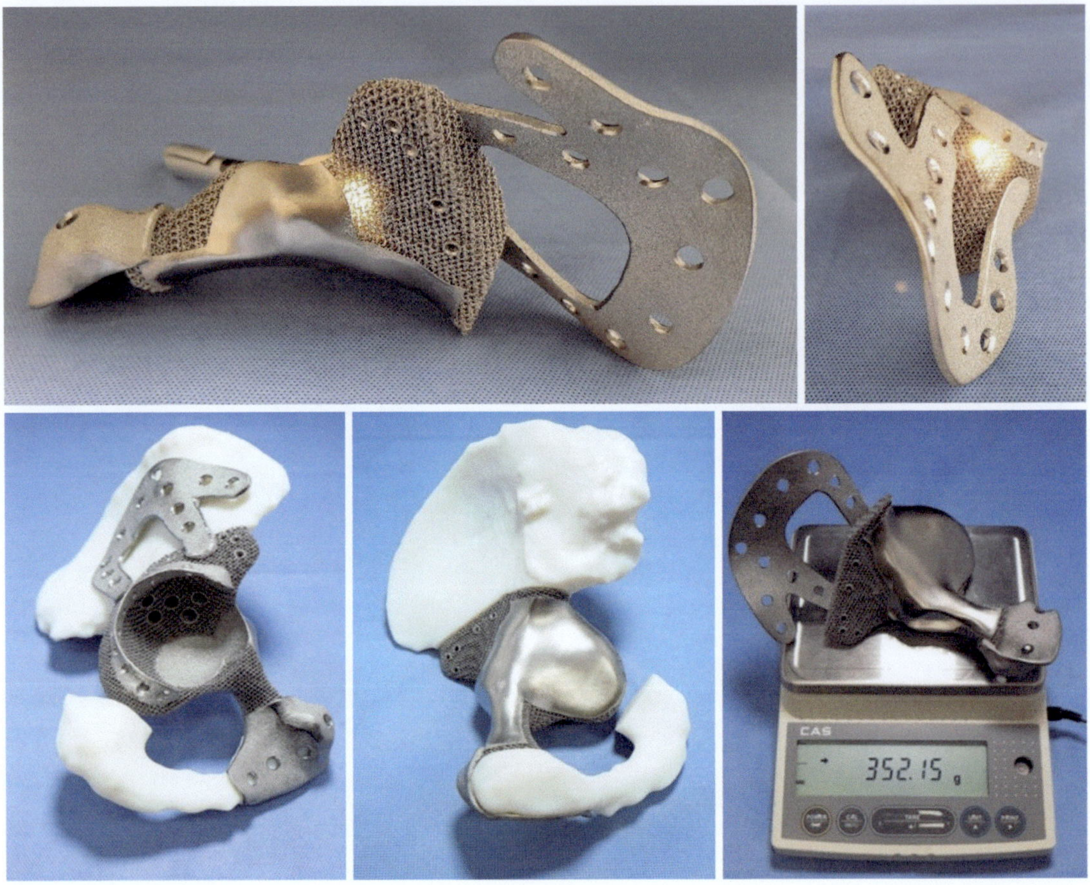

Fig. 3.10 Printed implant

3.5 Operation

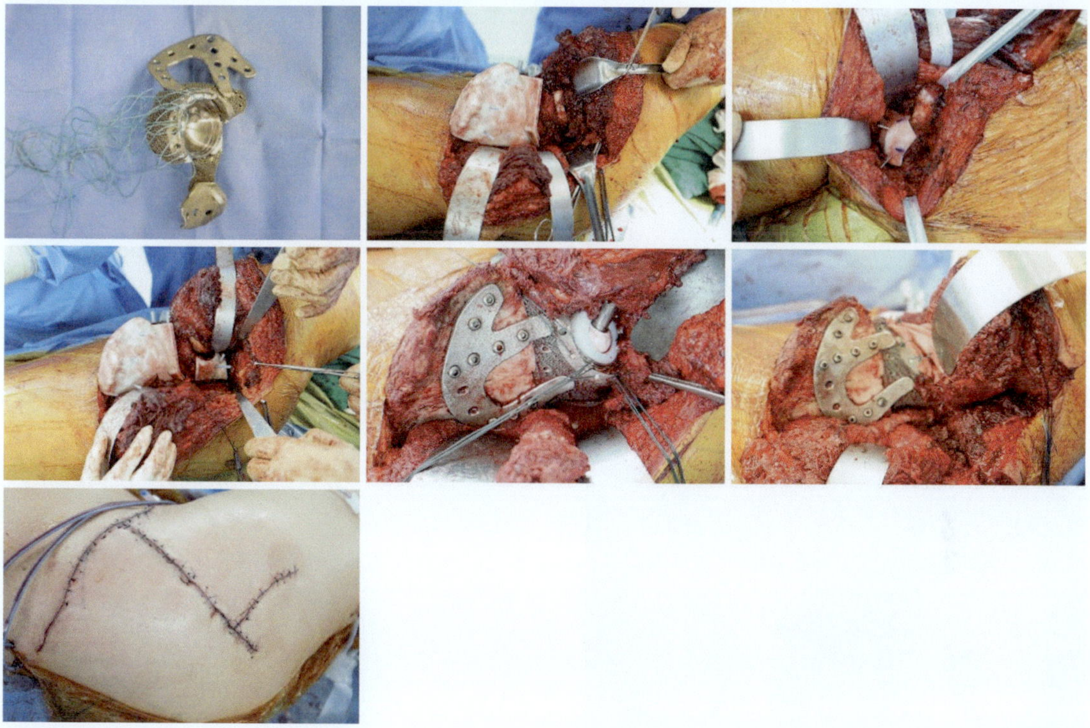

Fig. 3.11 Intraoperative photographs

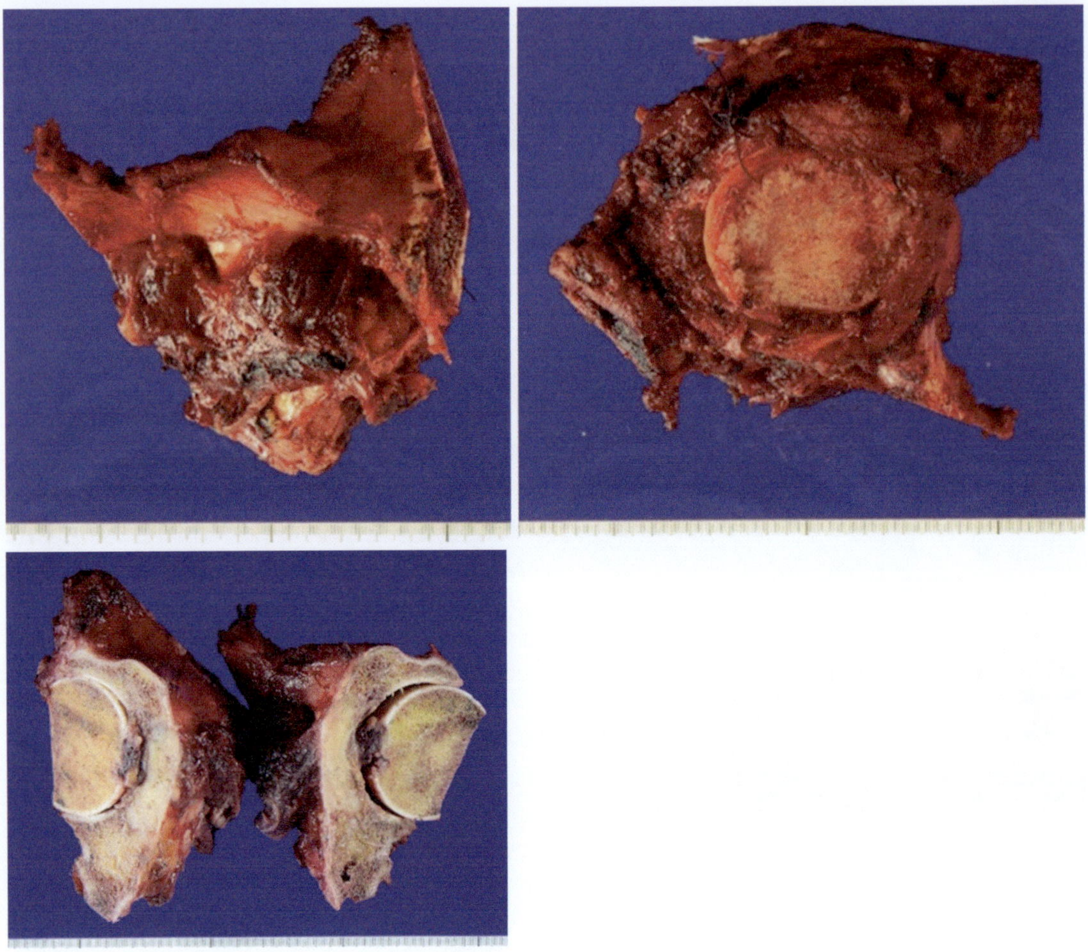

Fig. 3.12 Resected tumor

3.6 Postoperative Images

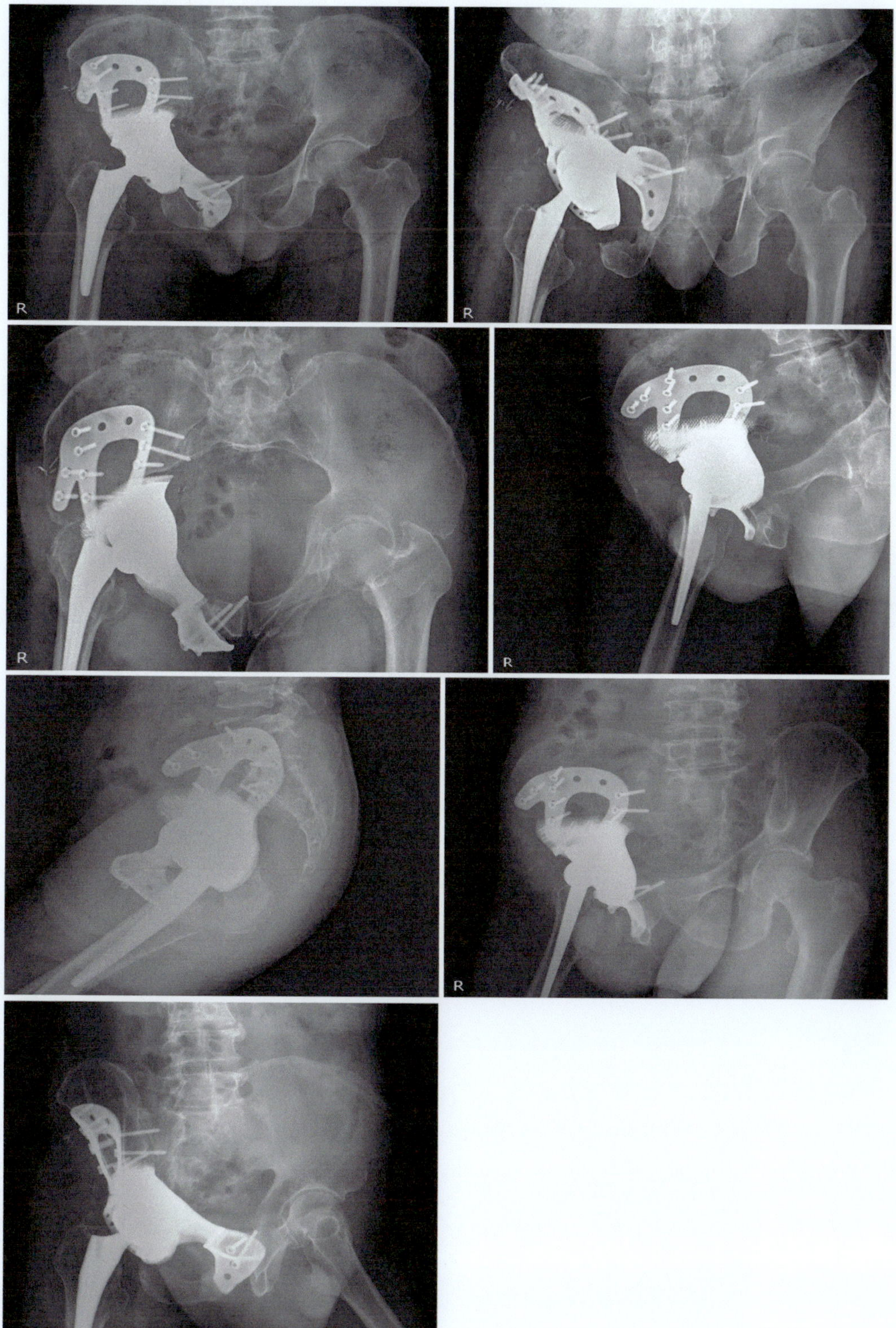

Fig. 3.13 Postoperative X-ray images

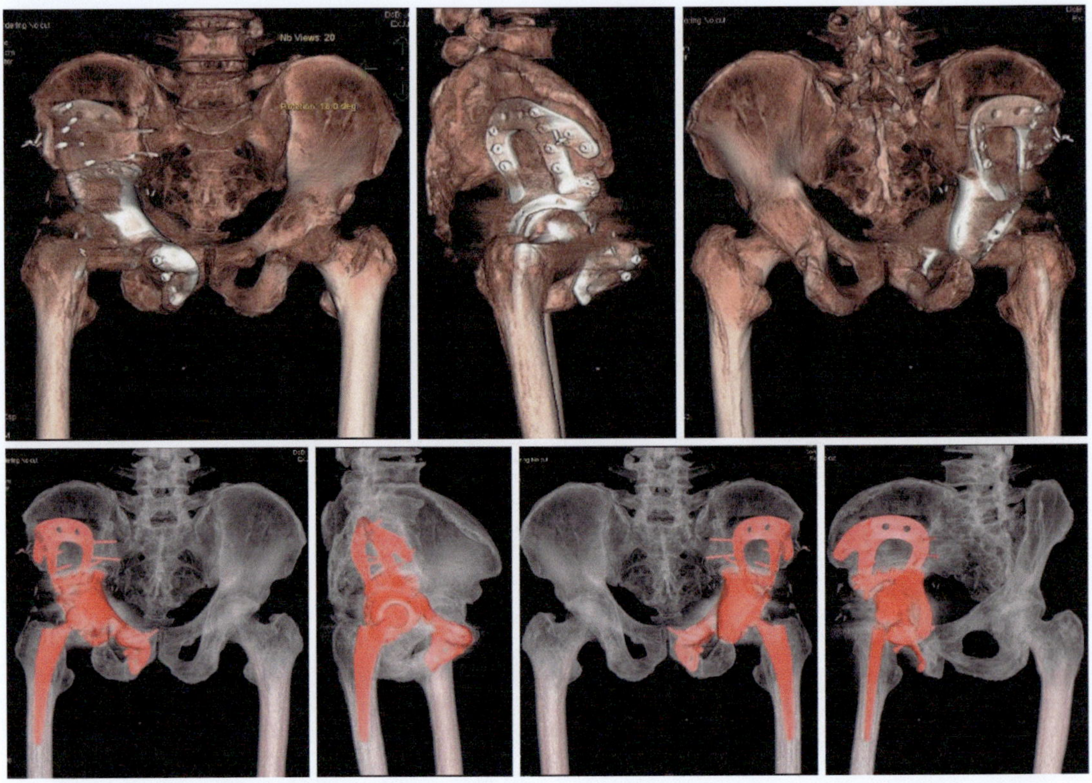

Fig. 3.14 Postoperative CT images

Patient Case 4: Omitting Pubis and Ischium

4

4.1 Patient Case 4

Age/sex	35/female
Location/site	Pelvis/left
Diagnosis	Ewing sarcoma
Preoperative symptom	Antalgic gait
Preoperative pain score	Resting 2/activity 6
BMI (height/weight)	21.96 (170.2/63.6)
Past history	Hip pain management at local clinic for a month
Present illness	Tumor progression after preoperative one-time chemotherapy

H.-G. Kang, *Clinical Atlas of 3D Printing Bone Reconstruction*,
https://doi.org/10.1007/978-981-16-2043-0_4

4.2 Preoperative Images

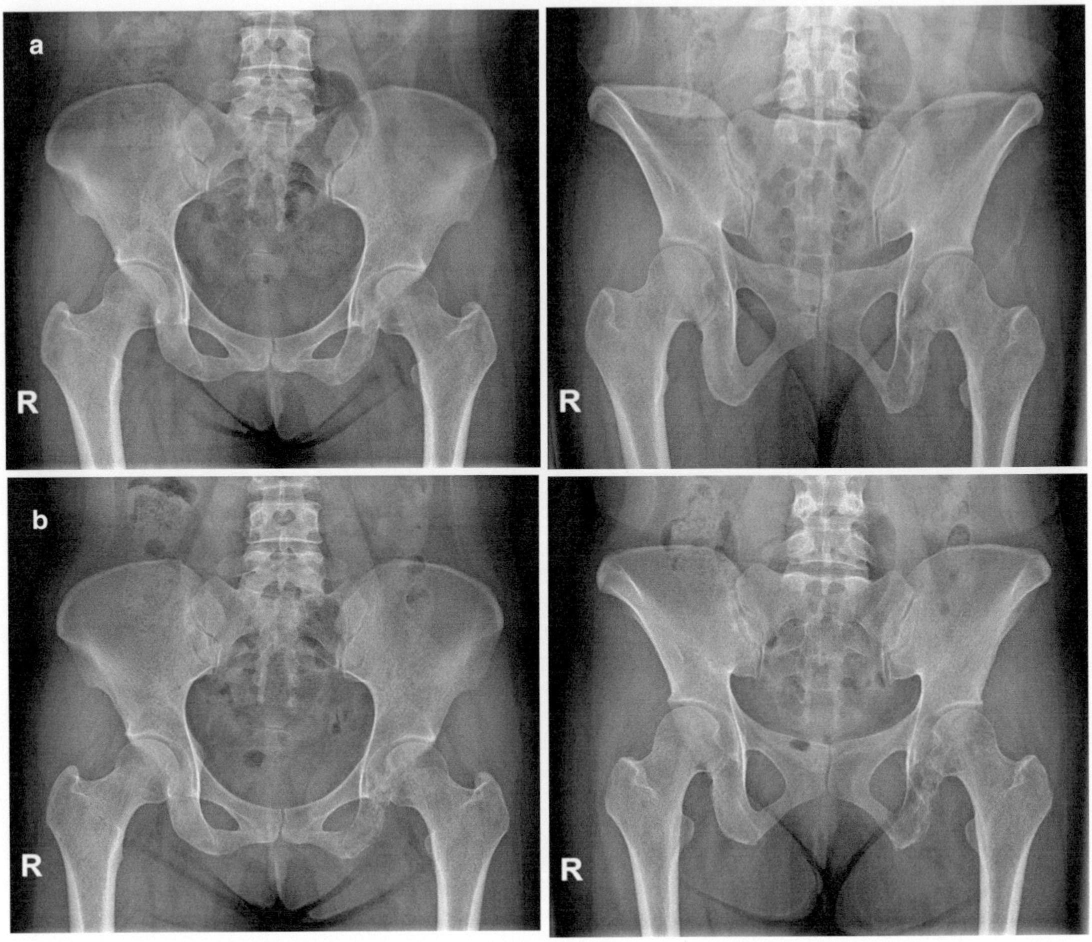

Fig. 4.1 (**a**) Initial X-ray images: pre-chemotherapy, (**b**) preoperative X-ray images: post-chemotherapy

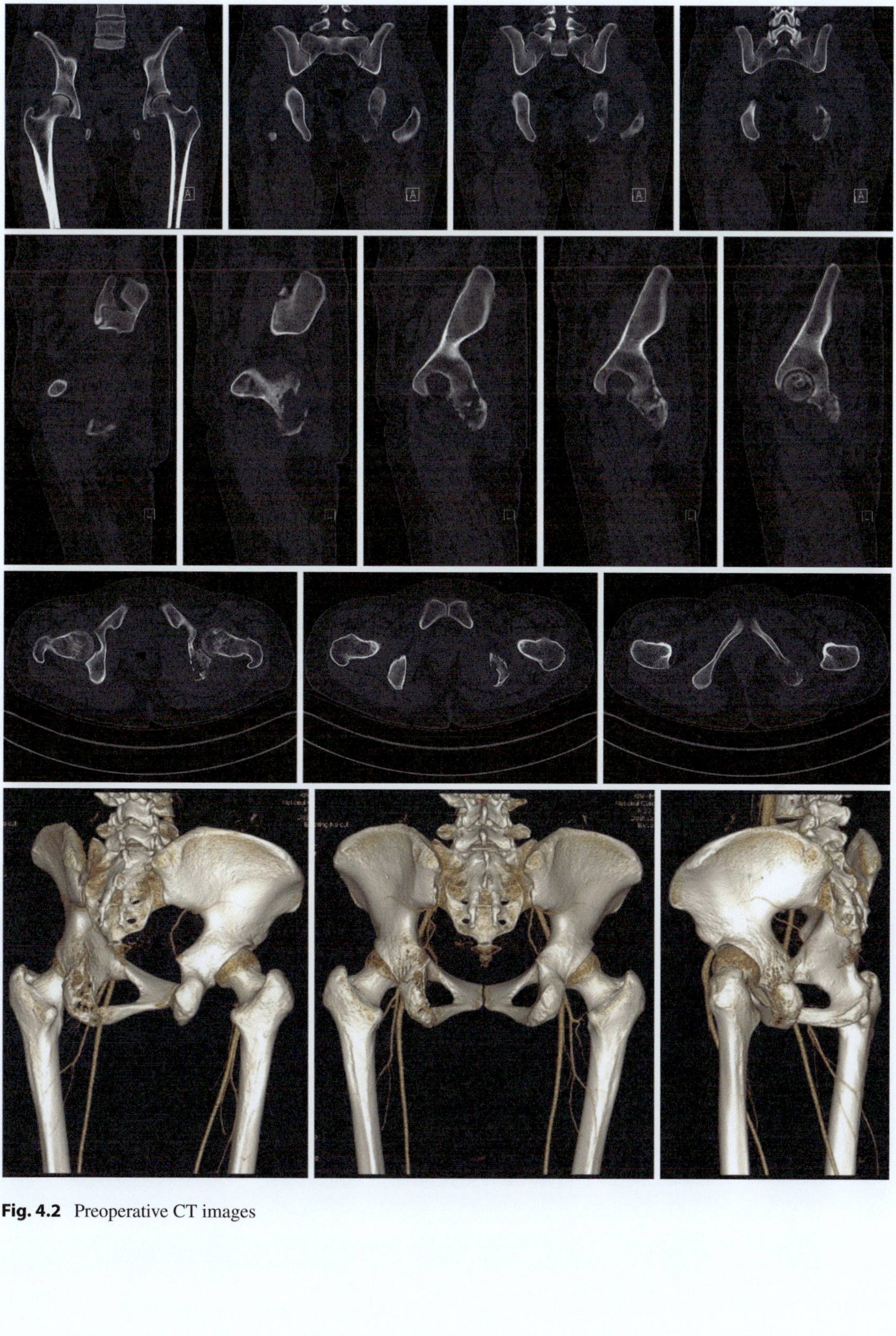

Fig. 4.2 Preoperative CT images

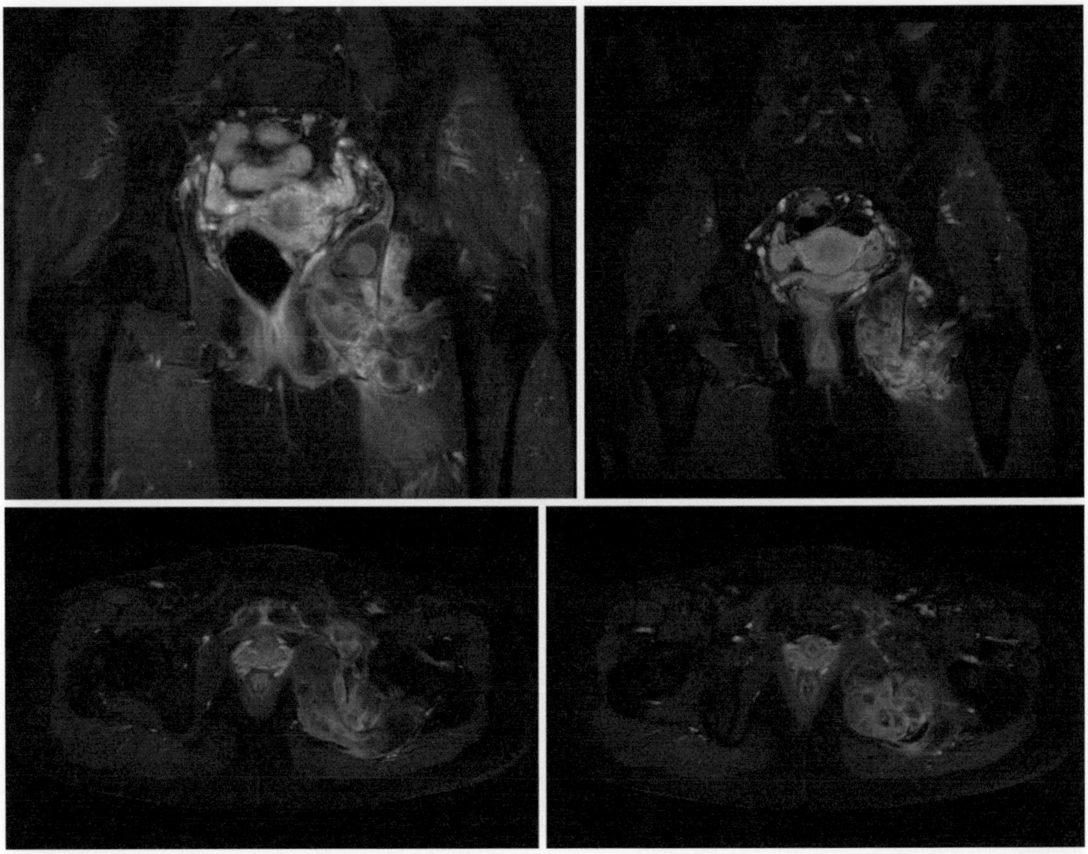

Fig. 4.3 Preoperative MRI images

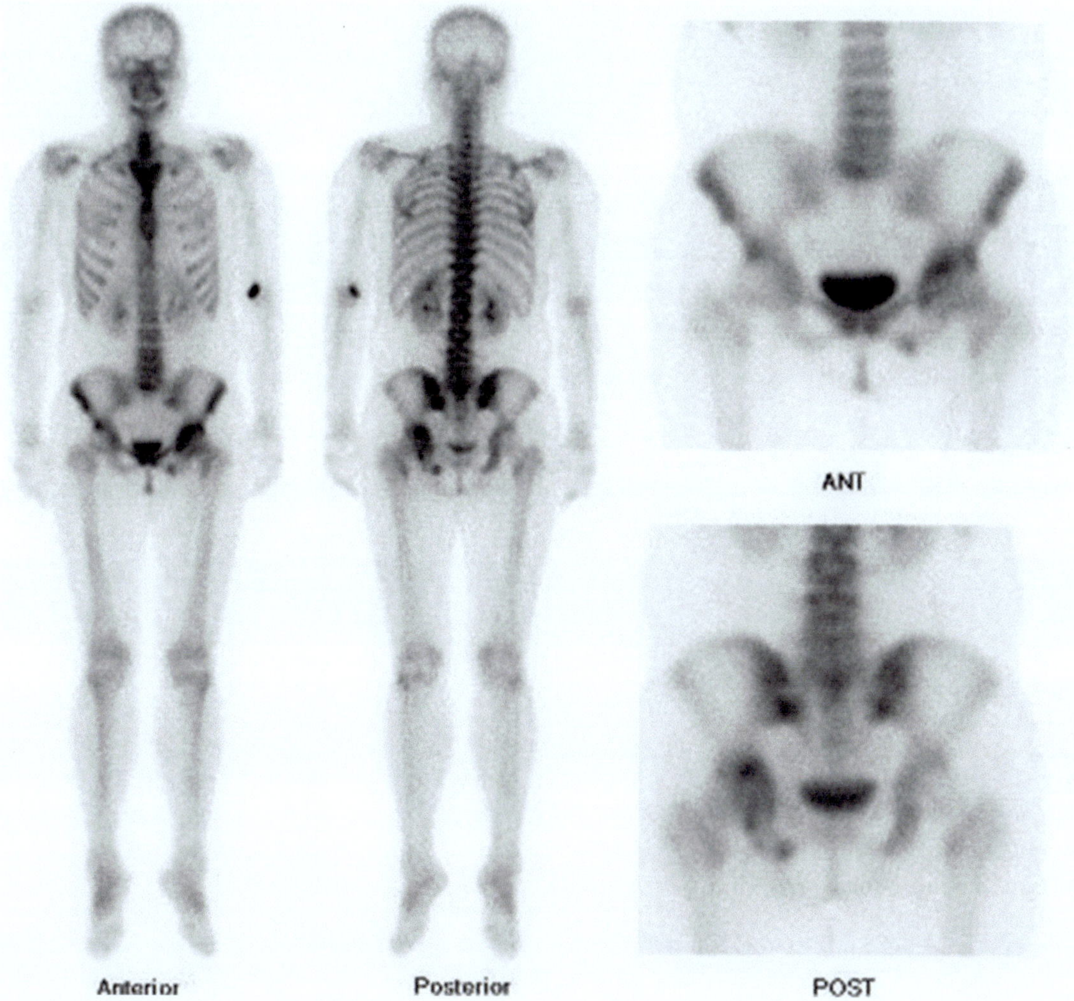

Fig. 4.4 Preoperative bone scan images

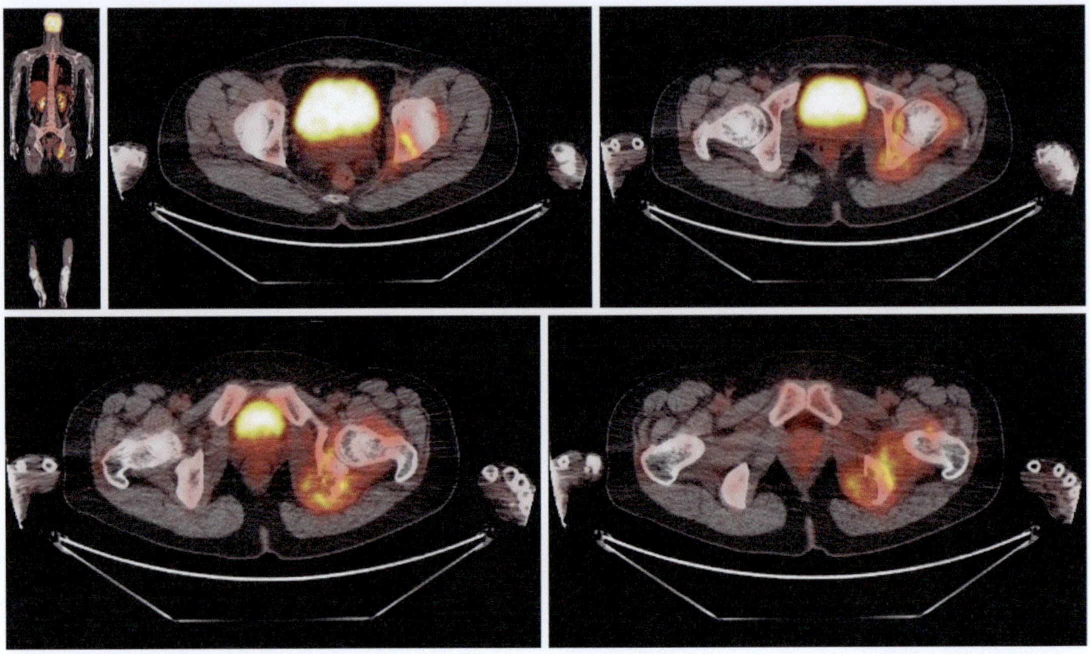

Fig. 4.5 Preoperative PET-CT images

4.3 Planning of Surgery

- Resection at symphysis pubis
- Bone cutting at iliac bone
- 3D printed pelvis
- No pubic and ischium

4.4 Design and Fabrication

- Implant measurement
- Implant weight (g): 462
- Size (mm): 136

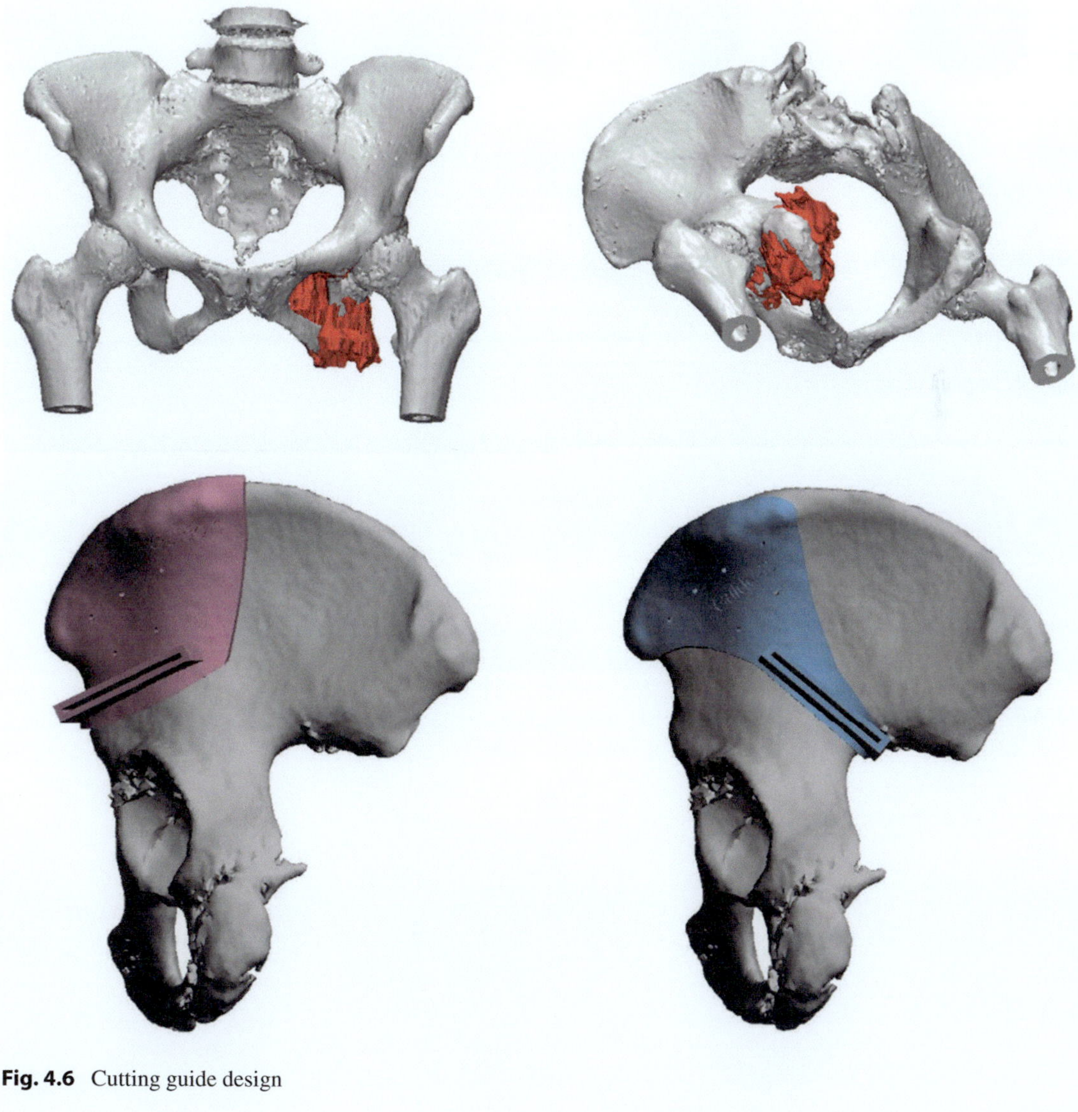

Fig. 4.6 Cutting guide design

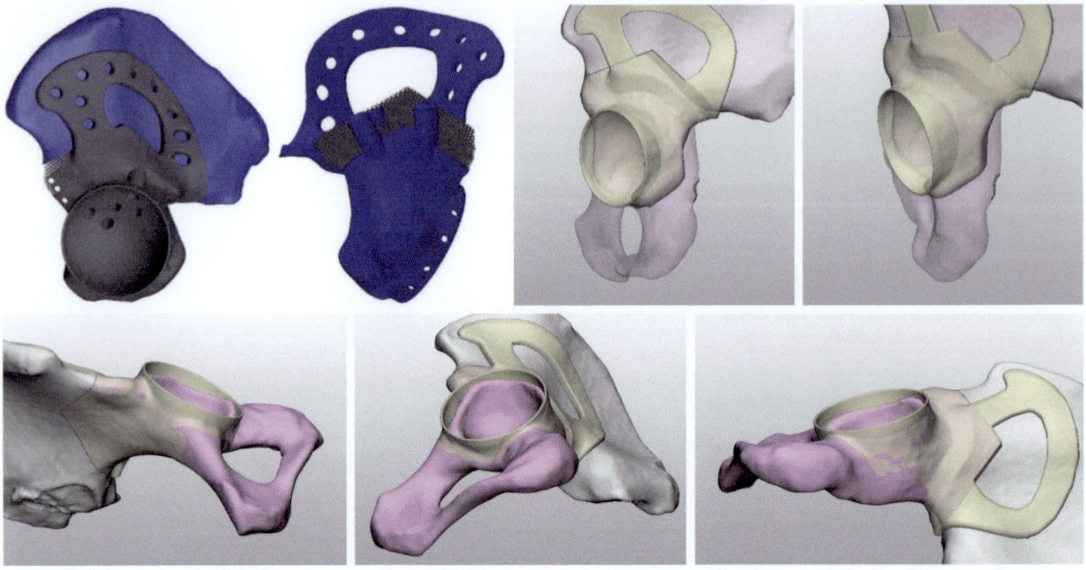

Fig. 4.7 Implant design

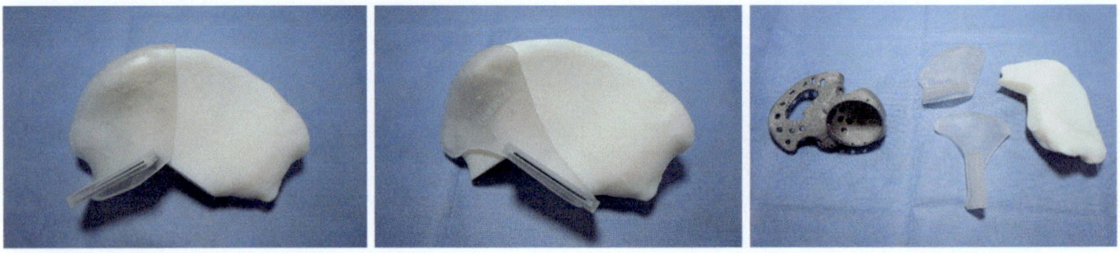

Fig. 4.8 Printed cutting guide

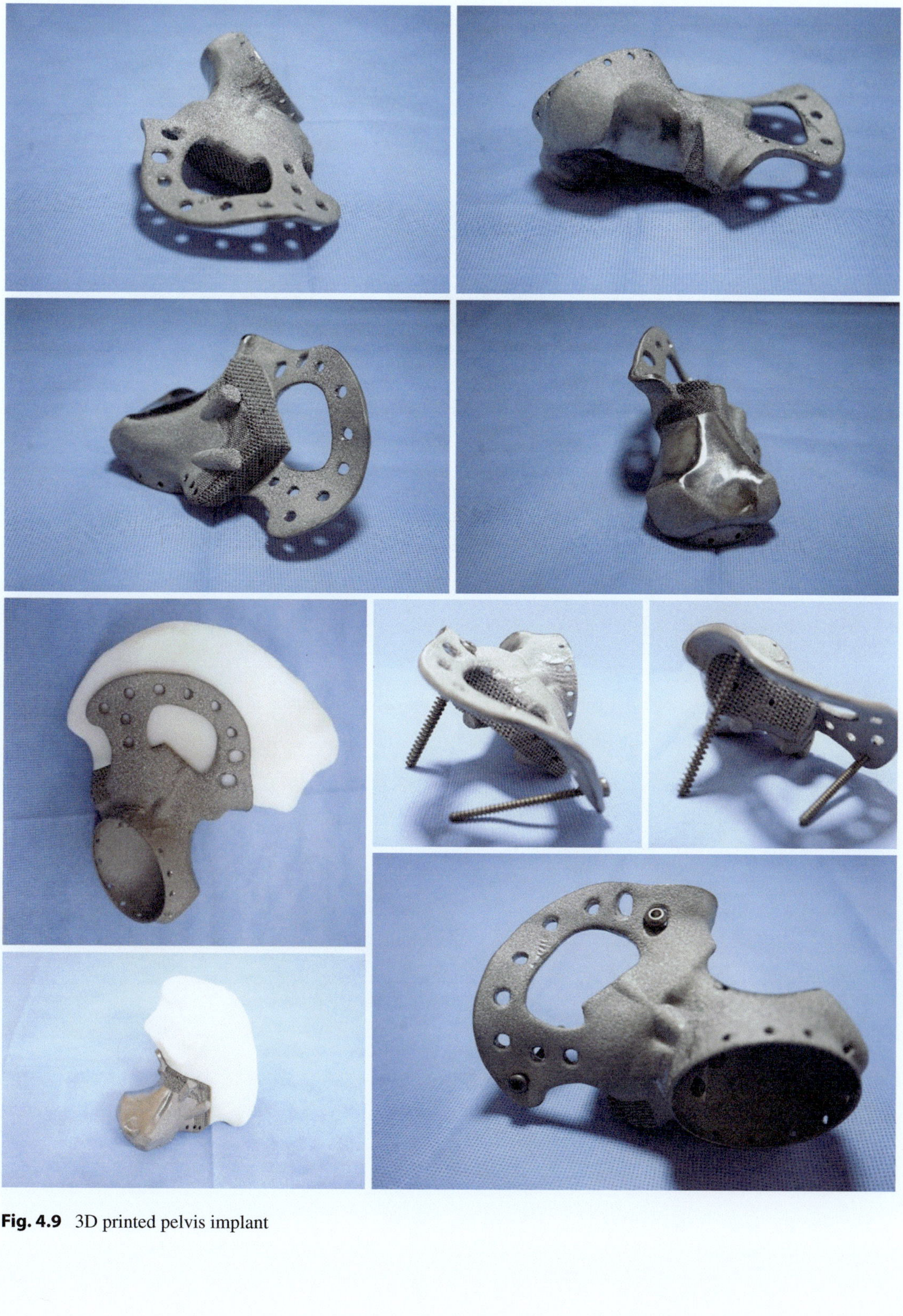

Fig. 4.9 3D printed pelvis implant

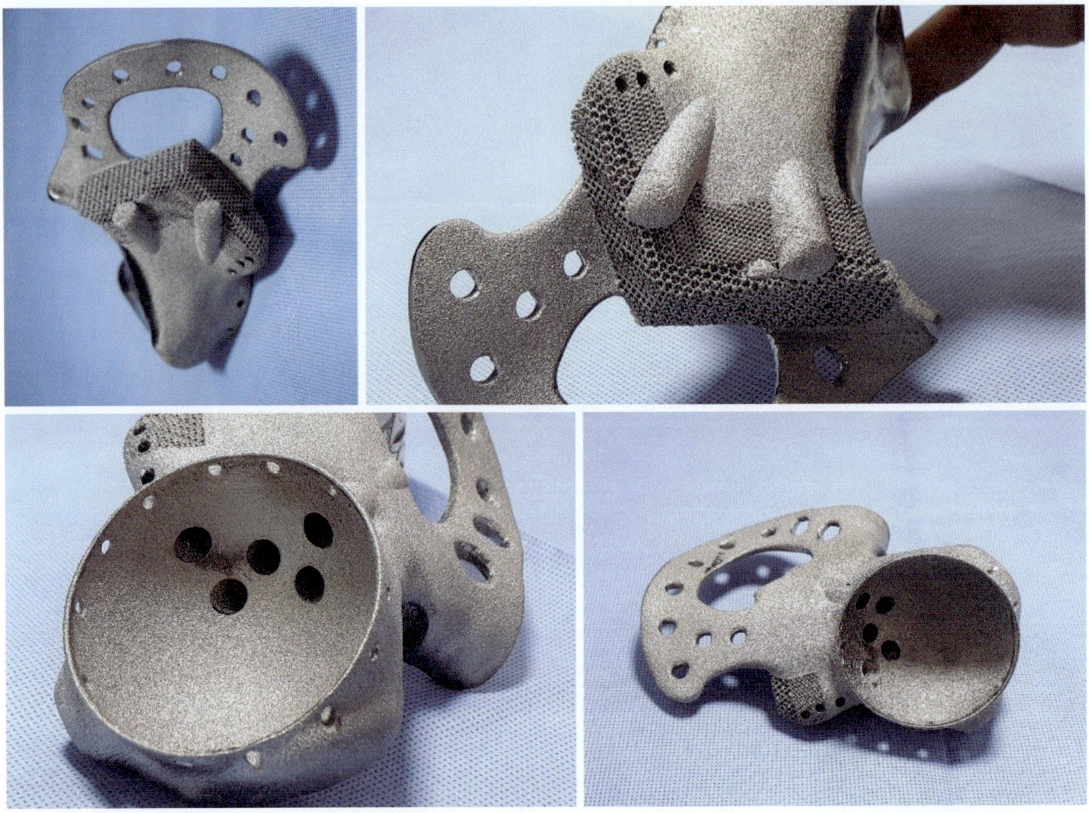

Fig. 4.10 Acetabular cup screw holes deepening with ridges for easy combination of total hip cup without screw cut trimming

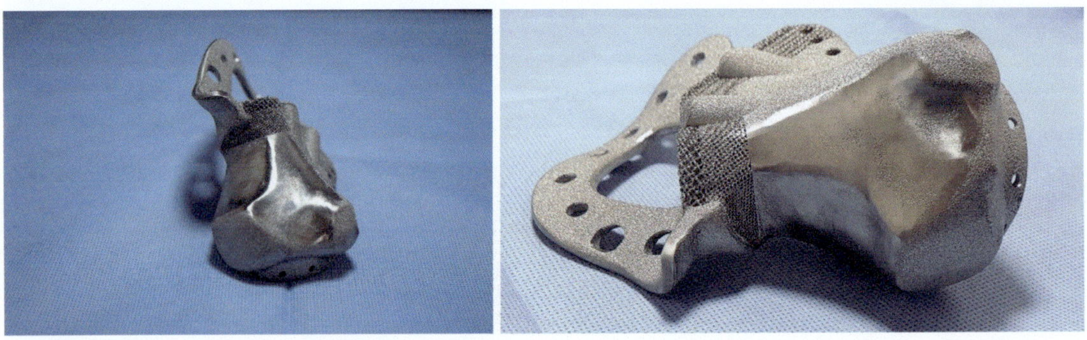

Fig. 4.11 Omitting the pubis and ischium

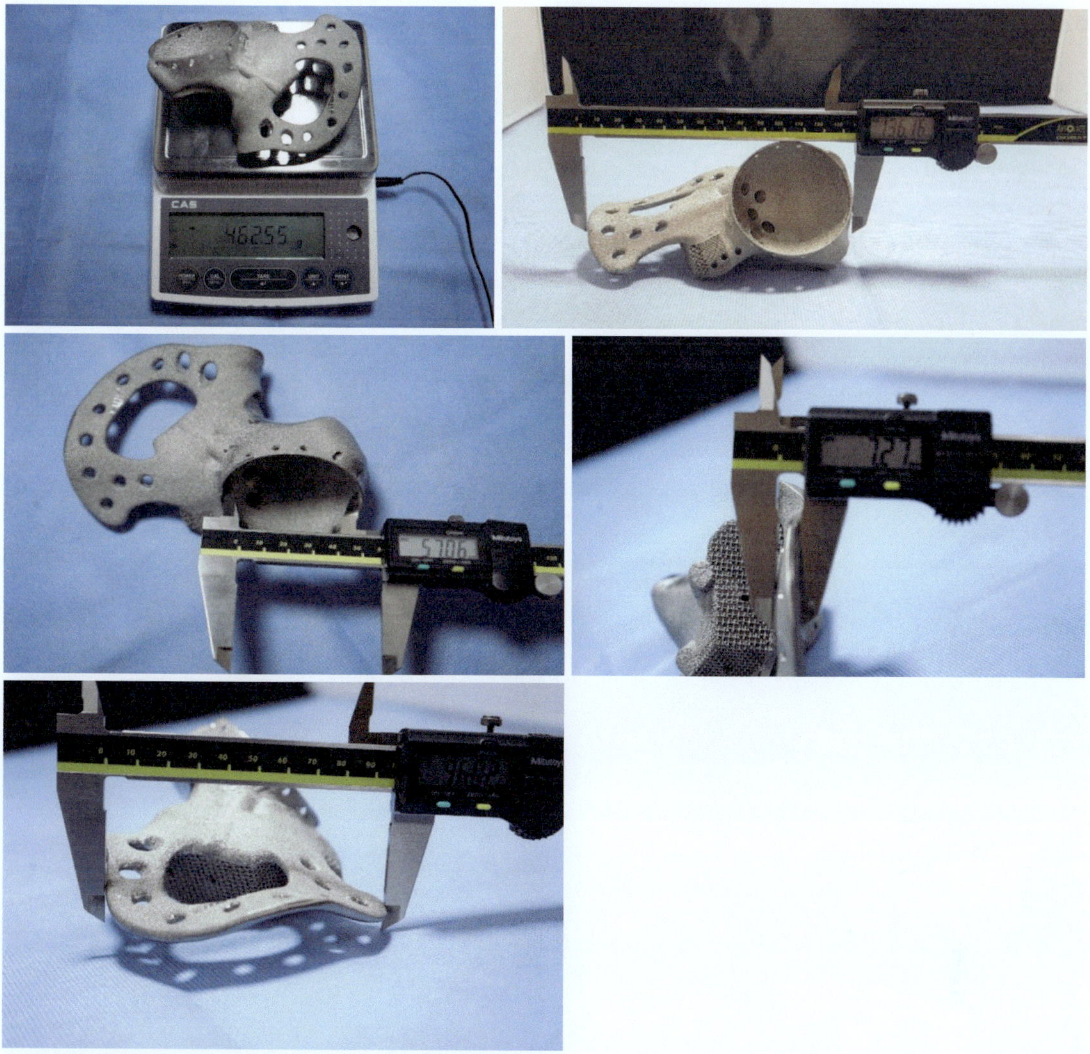

Fig. 4.12 Measurement of 3D printed implant

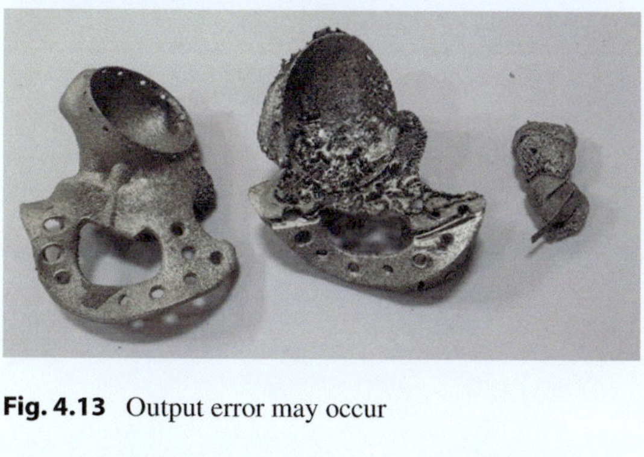

Fig. 4.13 Output error may occur

4.5 Operation

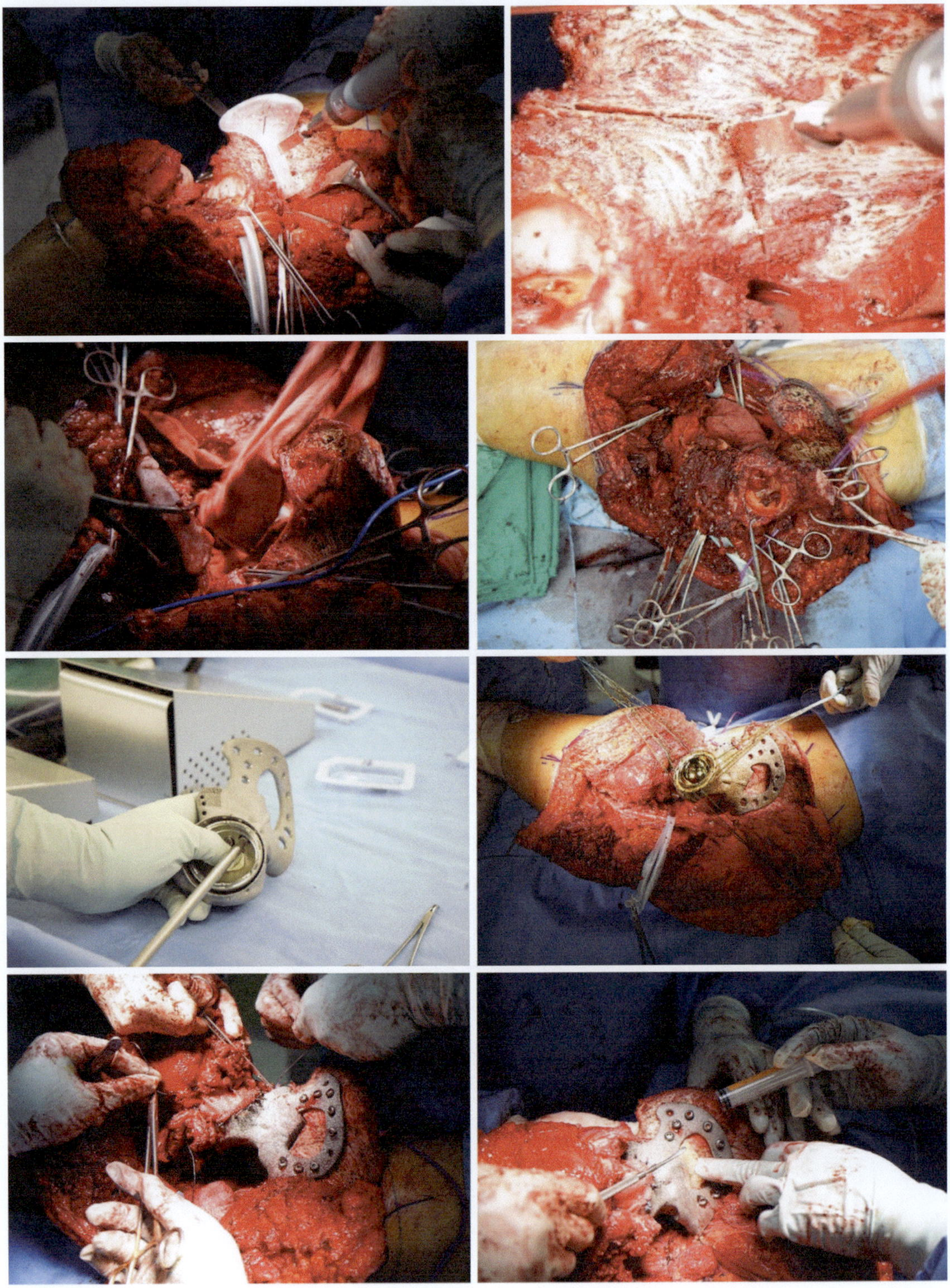

Fig. 4.14 Intraoperative photographs

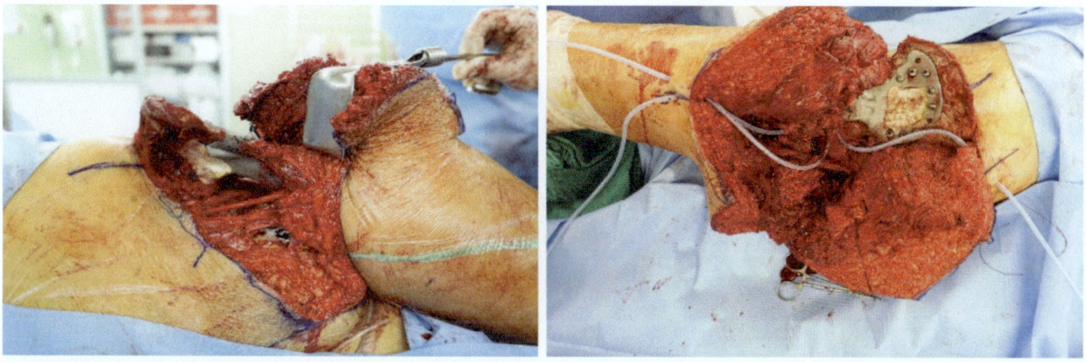

Fig. 4.14 (continued)

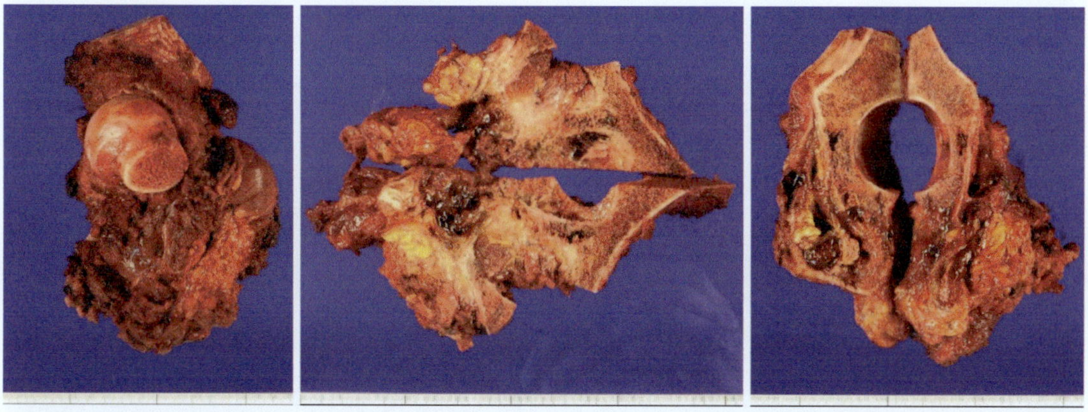

Fig. 4.15 Resected tumor

4.6 Postoperative Images

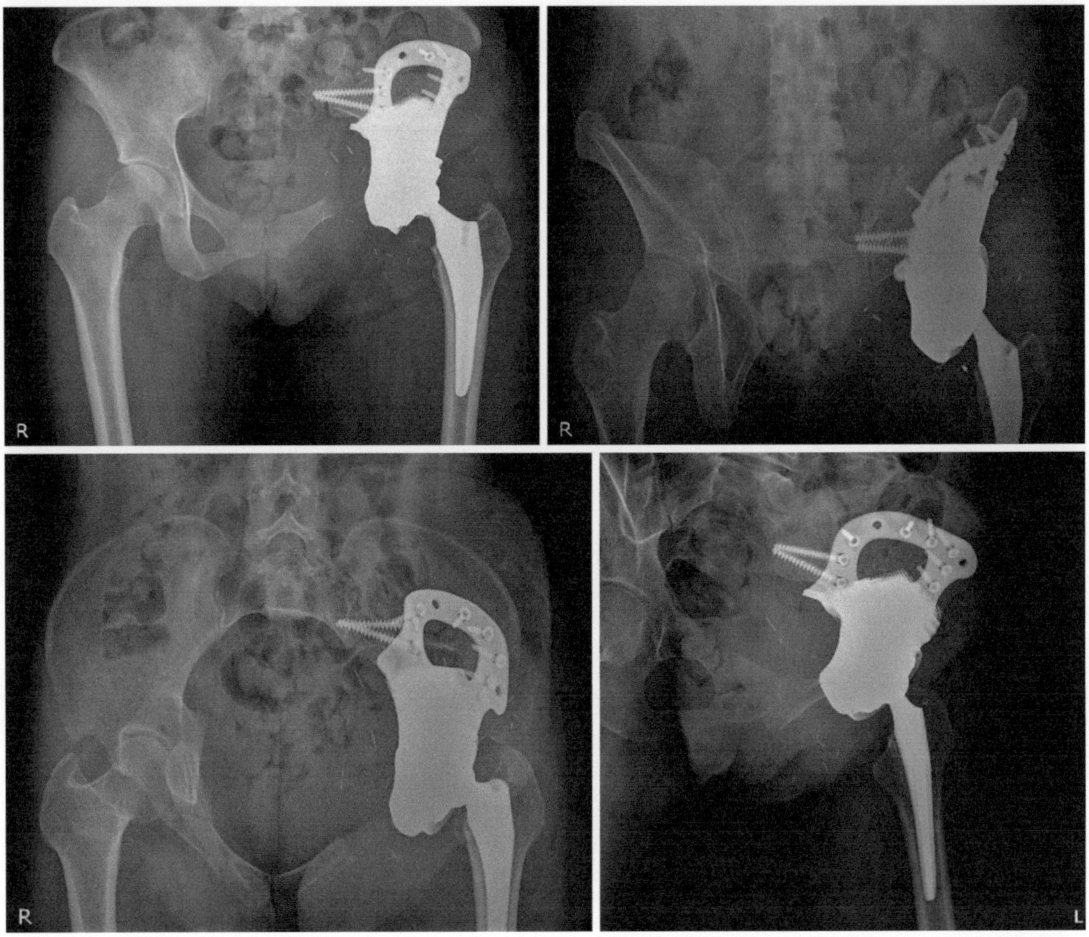

Fig. 4.16 Postoperative X-ray images

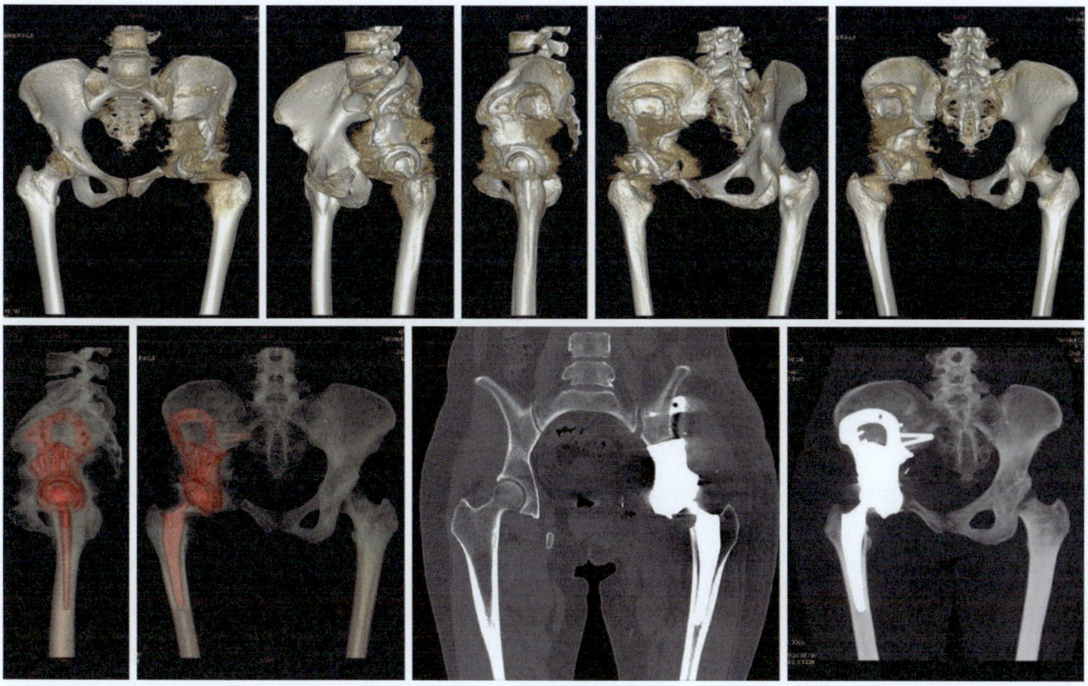

Fig. 4.17 Postoperative CT images

5 Patient Case 5: Iliac Wing

5.1 Patient Case 5

Age/sex	26/female
Location/site	Pelvis/right
Diagnosis	Chondrosarcoma, grade 2
Preoperative symptom	Right buttock pain
Preoperative pain score	Resting 2/activity 5
BMI (height/weight)	20.84 (156.5/60.4)
Past history	Hip pain for 6 months
Present illness	Found at a health checkup for her first job as a nurse

5.2 Preoperative Images

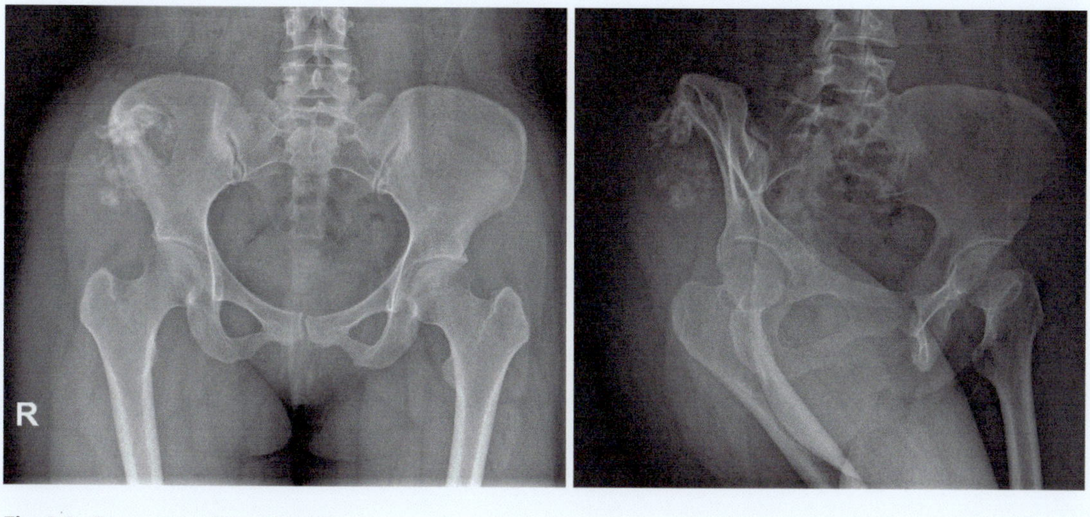

Fig. 5.1 Preoperative X-ray images

H.-G. Kang, *Clinical Atlas of 3D Printing Bone Reconstruction*,
https://doi.org/10.1007/978-981-16-2043-0_5

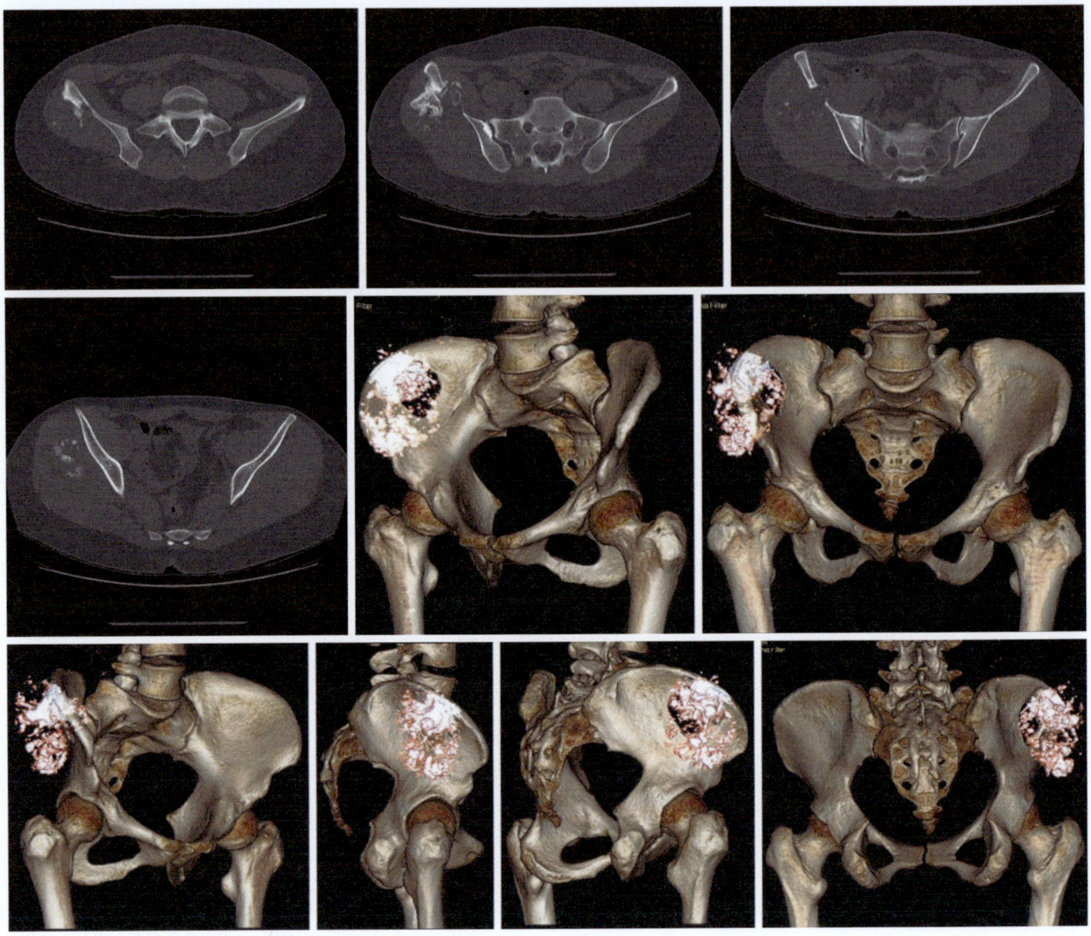

Fig. 5.2 Preoperative CT images

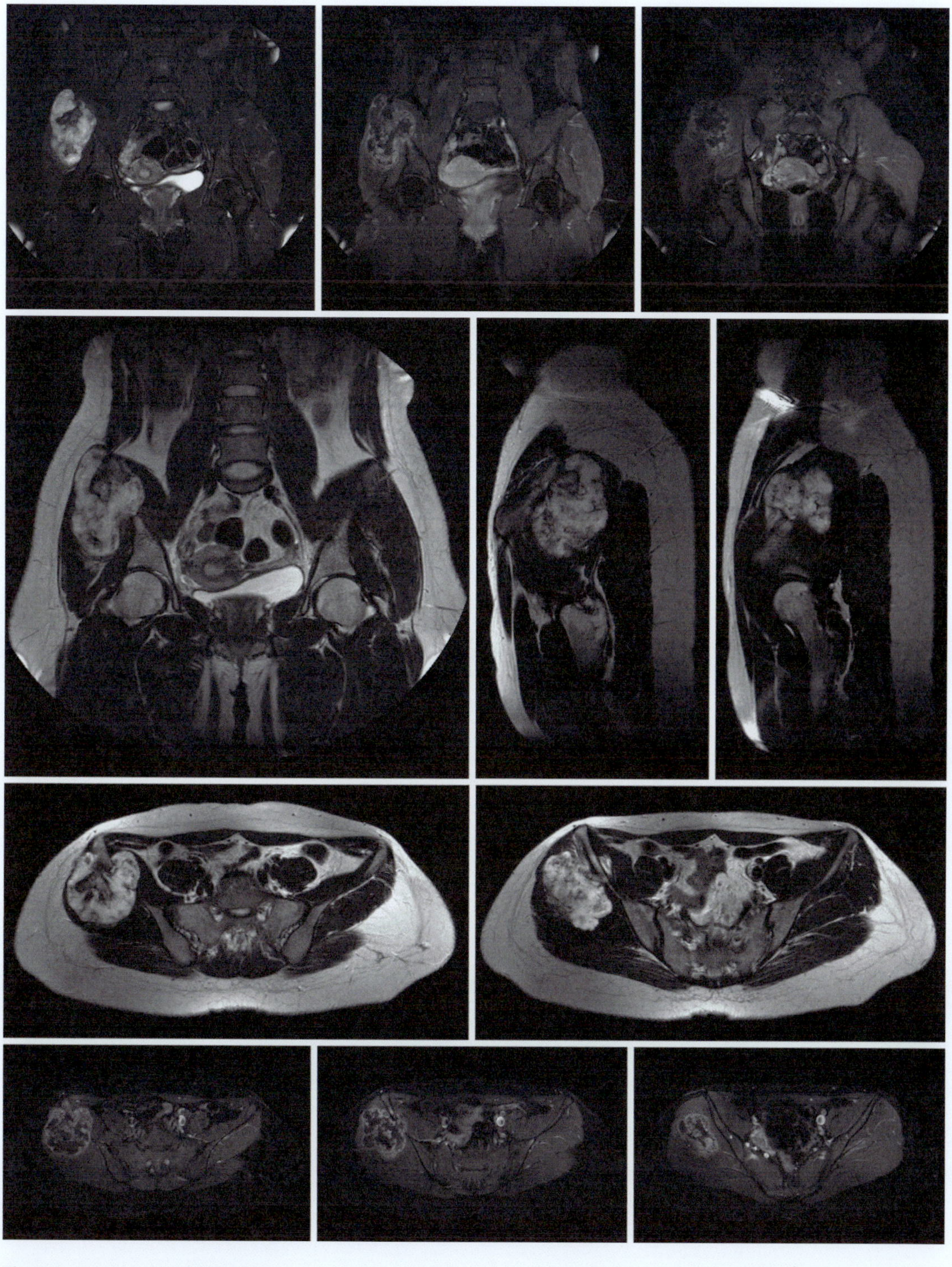

Fig. 5.3 Preoperative MRI images

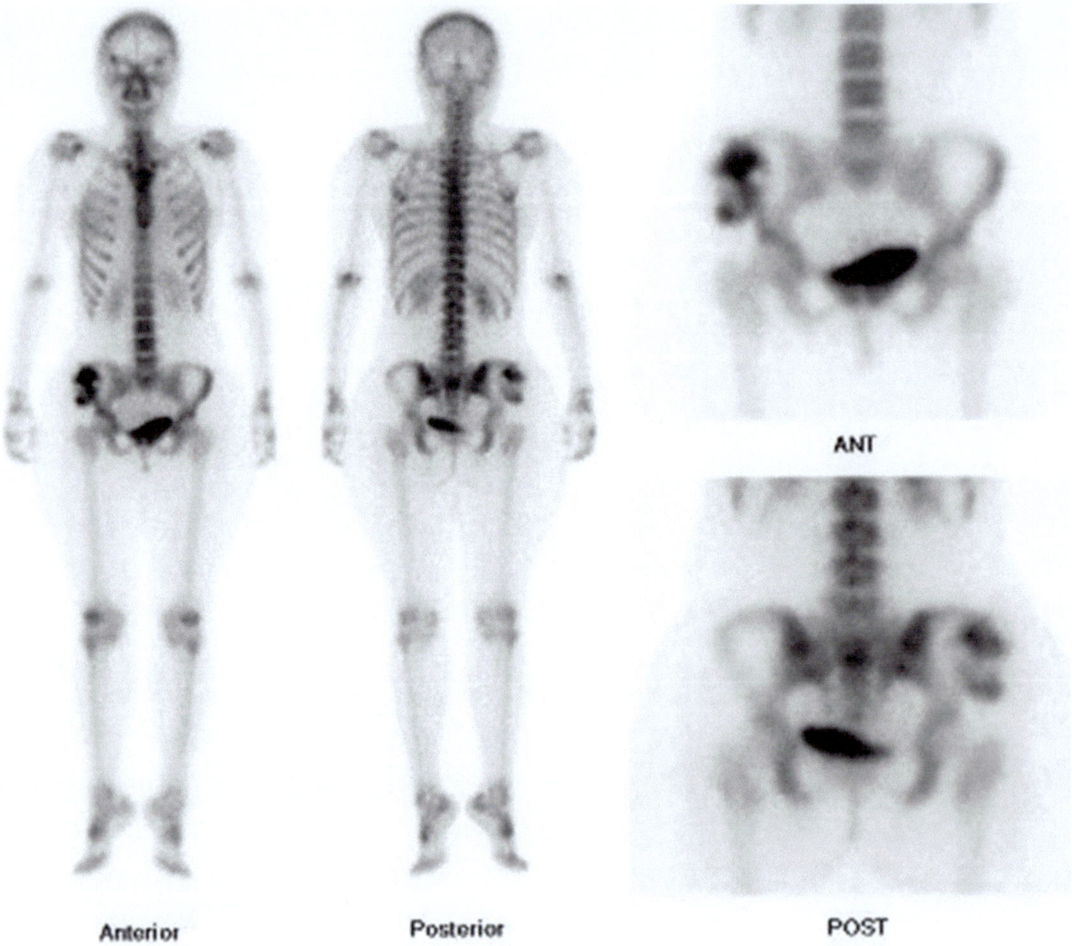

Fig. 5.4 Preoperative bone scan images

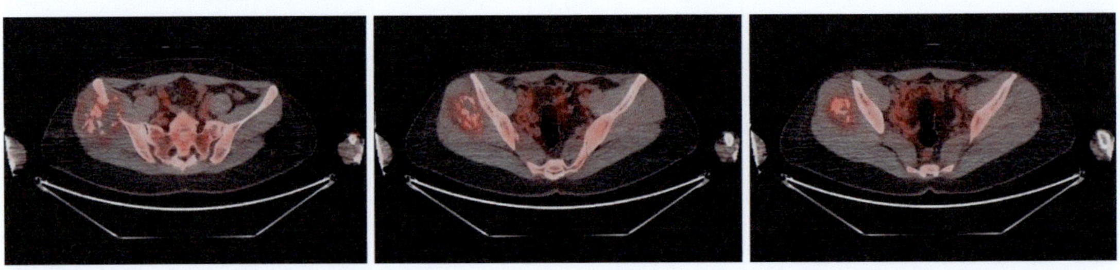

Fig. 5.5 Preoperative PET-CT images

5.3 Planning of Surgery

Iliac bone resection
3D printed iliac wing implant

5.4 Design and Fabrication

- Implant measurement
- Implant weight (g): 40
- Size (mm): 89

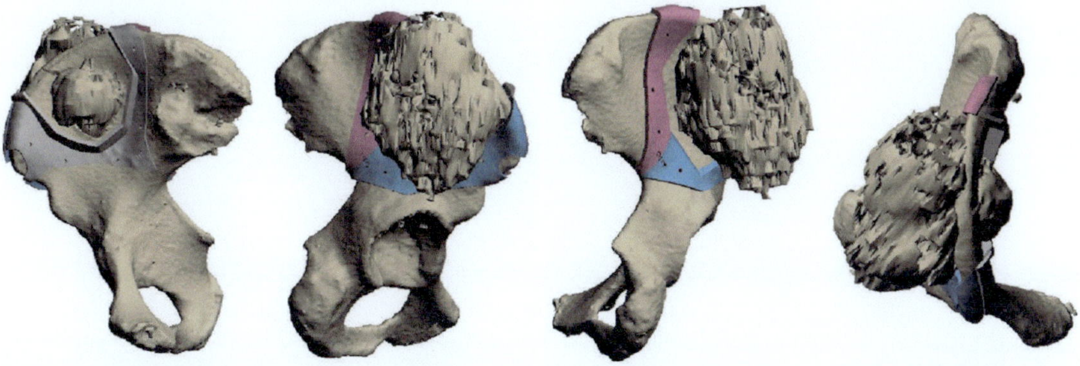

Fig. 5.6 Cutting guide design

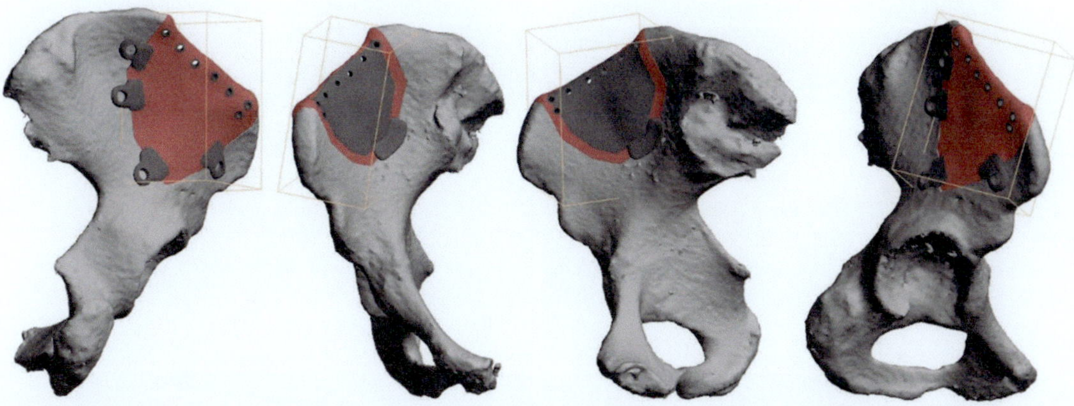

Fig. 5.7 Implant design

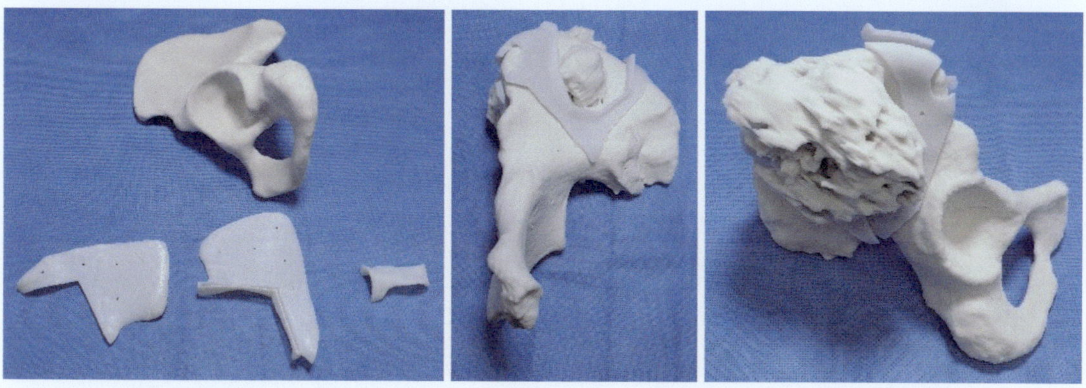

Fig. 5.8 Printed cutting guide

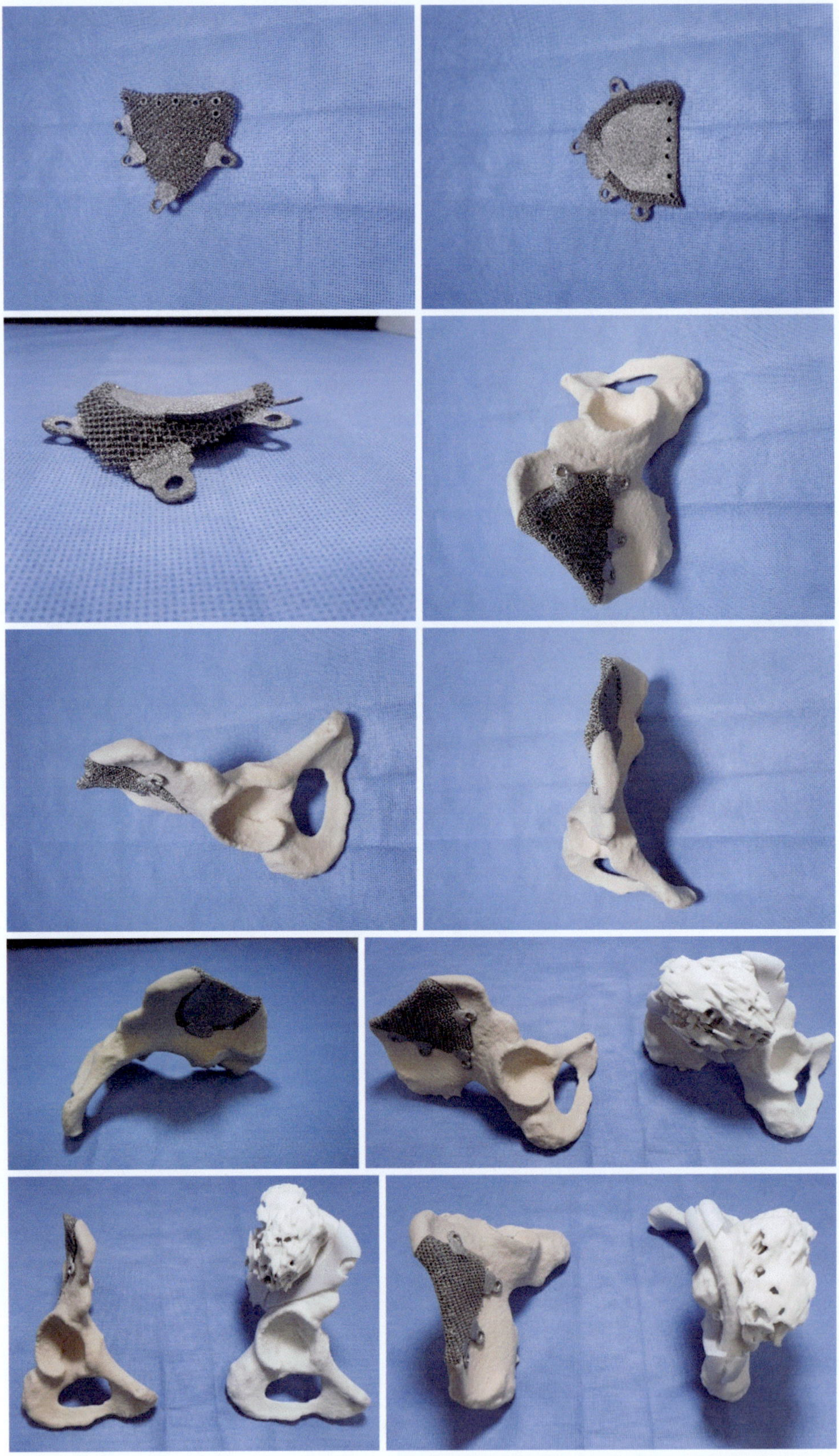

Fig. 5.9 Printed implant: reduce iliac crest bump to prevent skin irritation

5.5 Operation

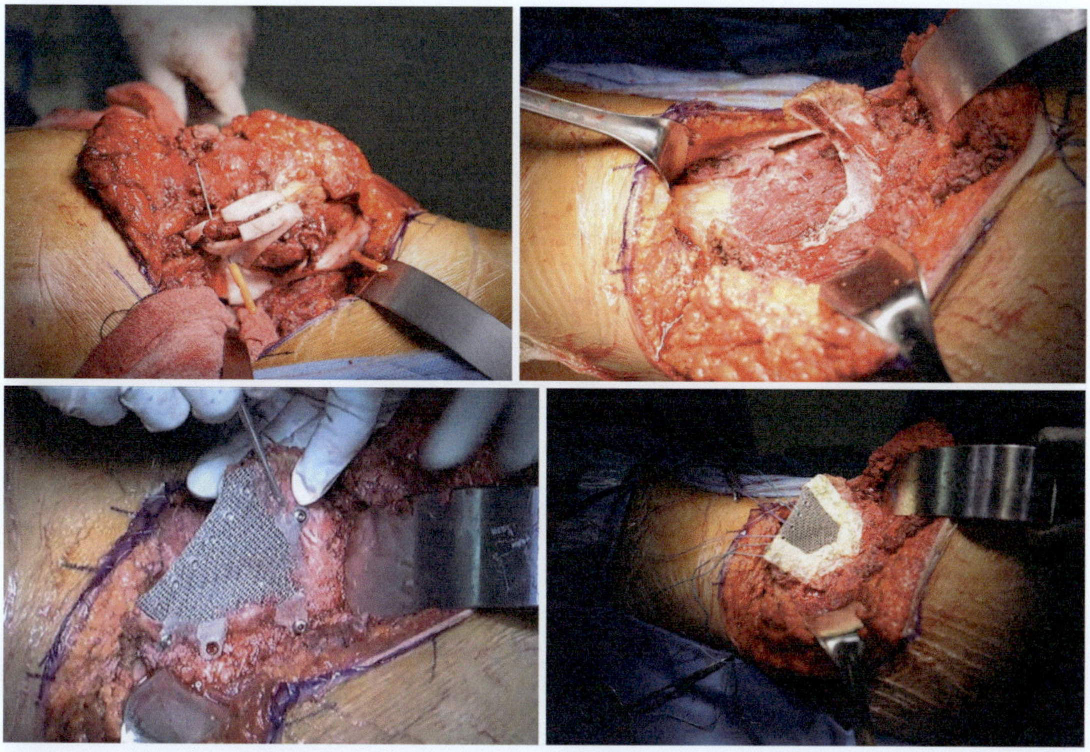

Fig. 5.10 Intraoperative photographs

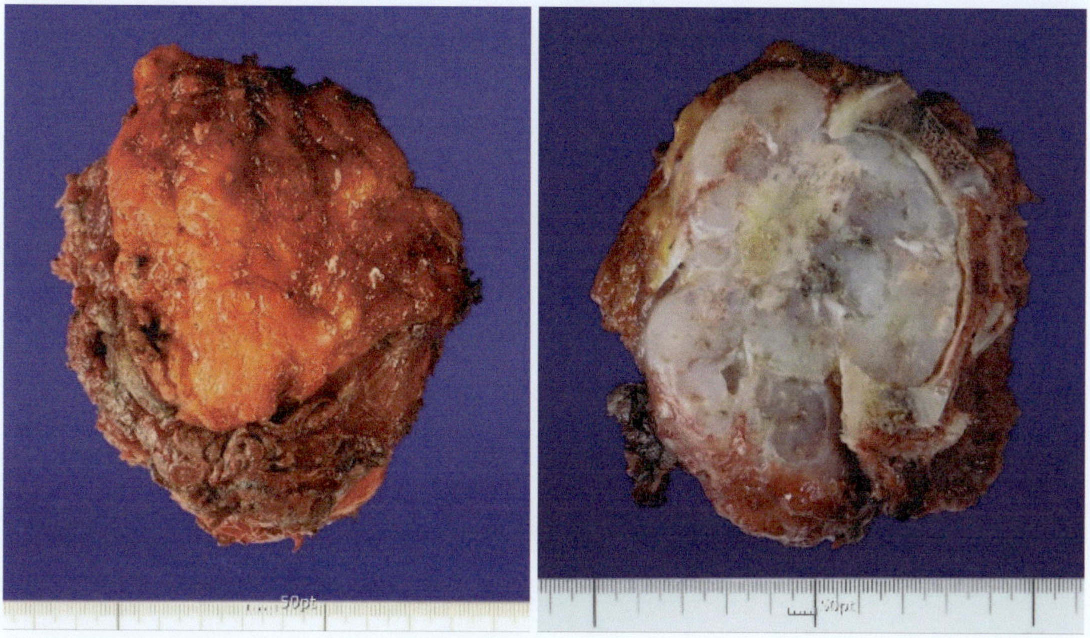

Fig. 5.11 Resected tumor

5.6 Postoperative Images

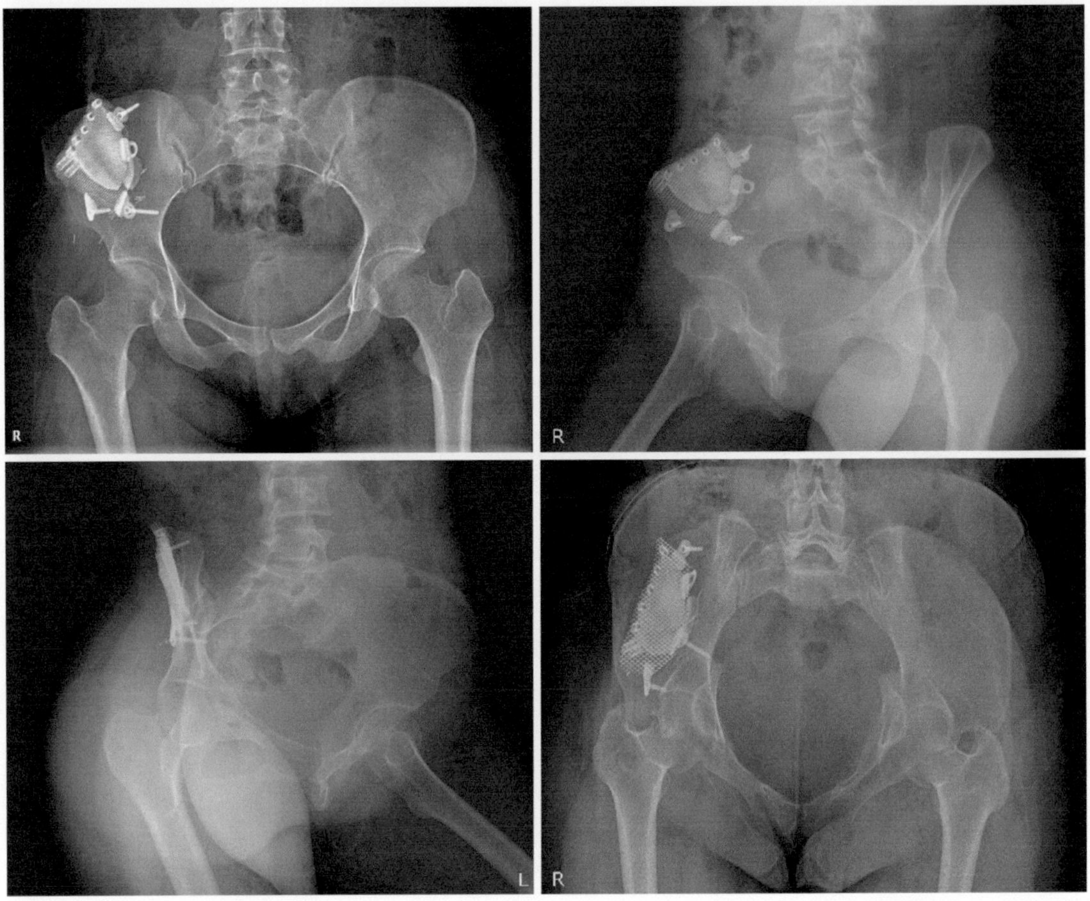

Fig. 5.12 Postoperative X-ray images

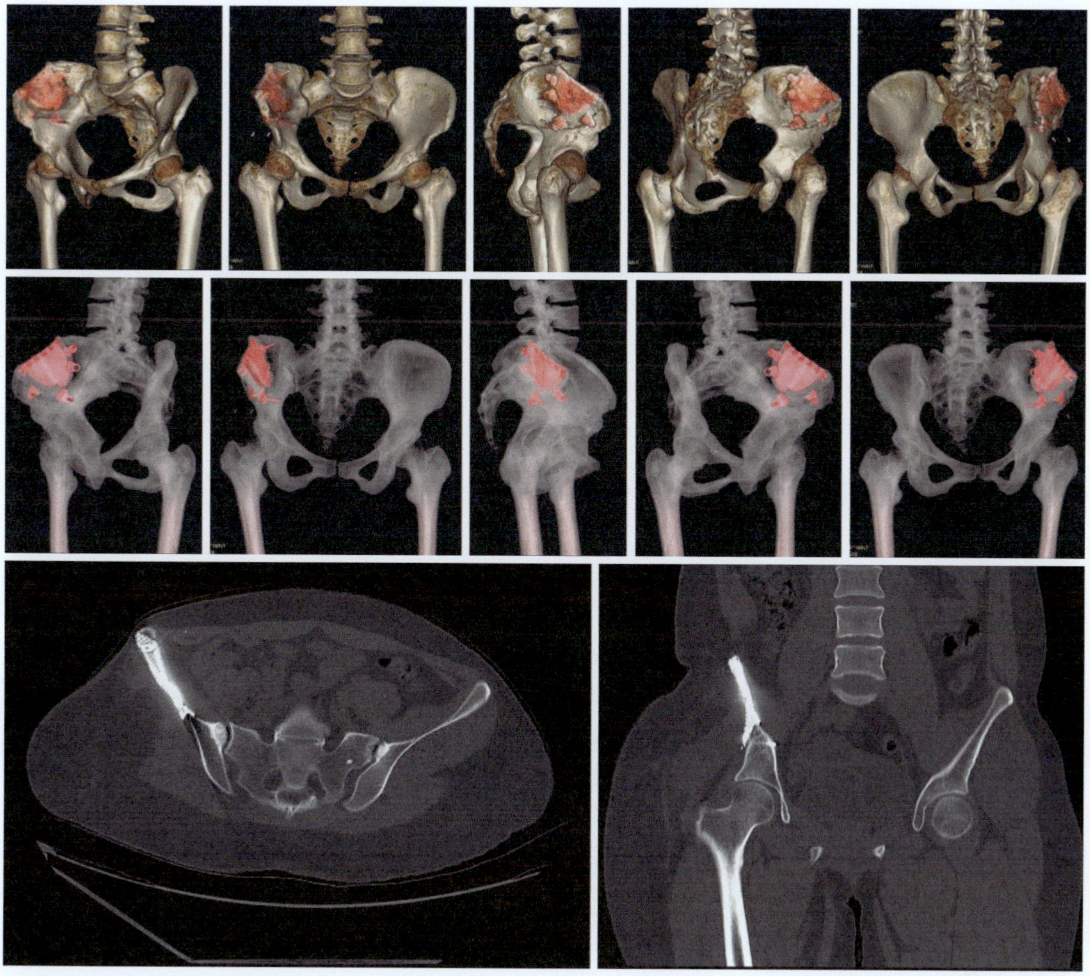

Fig. 5.13 Postoperative CT images

Patient Case 6: Iliac Spacer with Cavitary Resection

6

6.1 Patient Case 6

Age/sex	56/male
Location/site	Pelvis/right
Diagnosis	Gastrointestinal stromal tumor (GIST) Solitary bone metastasis
Preoperative symptom	Antalgic gait
Preoperative pain score	Resting 2/activity 5
BMI (height/weight)	20.55 (169.3/58.9)
Past history	GIST in the liver diagnosed 5 years ago
Present illness	Partial hepatectomy and Gleevec medication for 3 years Accidentally found on abdominal CT follow-up

H.-G. Kang, *Clinical Atlas of 3D Printing Bone Reconstruction*,
https://doi.org/10.1007/978-981-16-2043-0_6

6.2 Preoperative Images

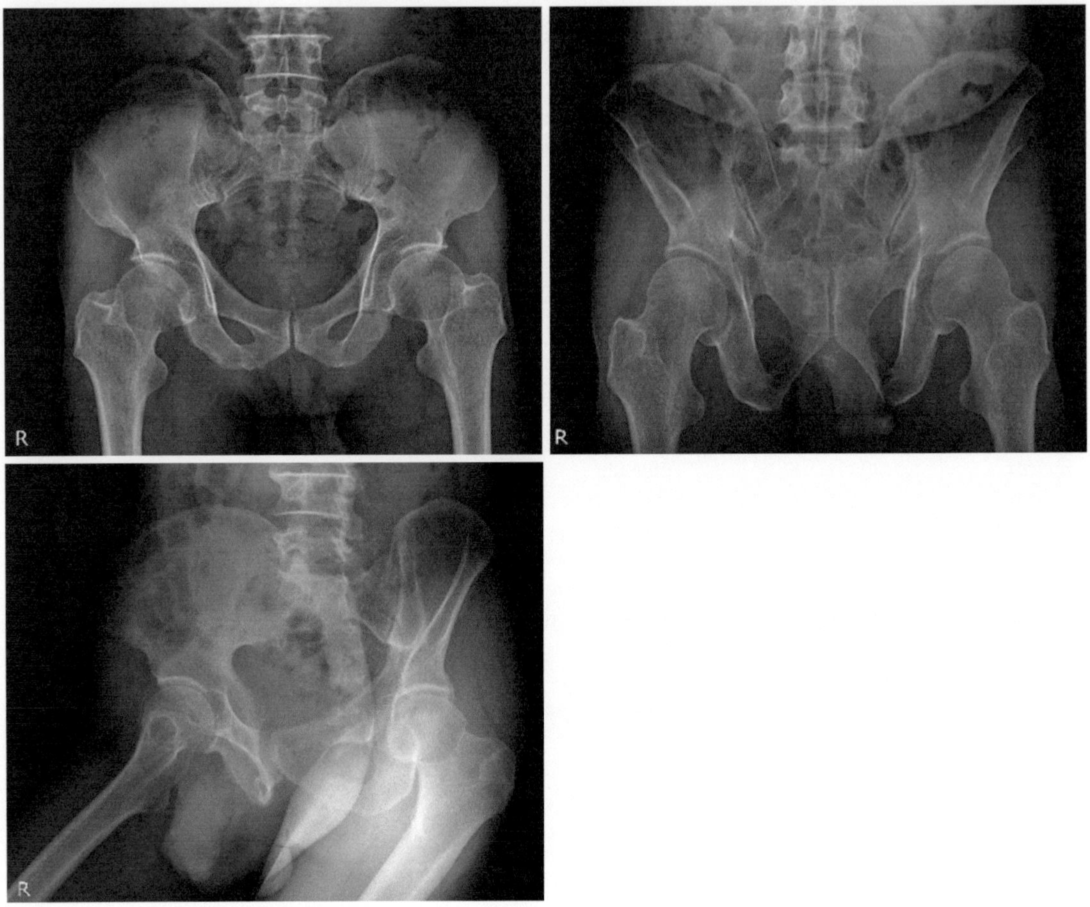

Fig. 6.1 Preoperative X-ray images

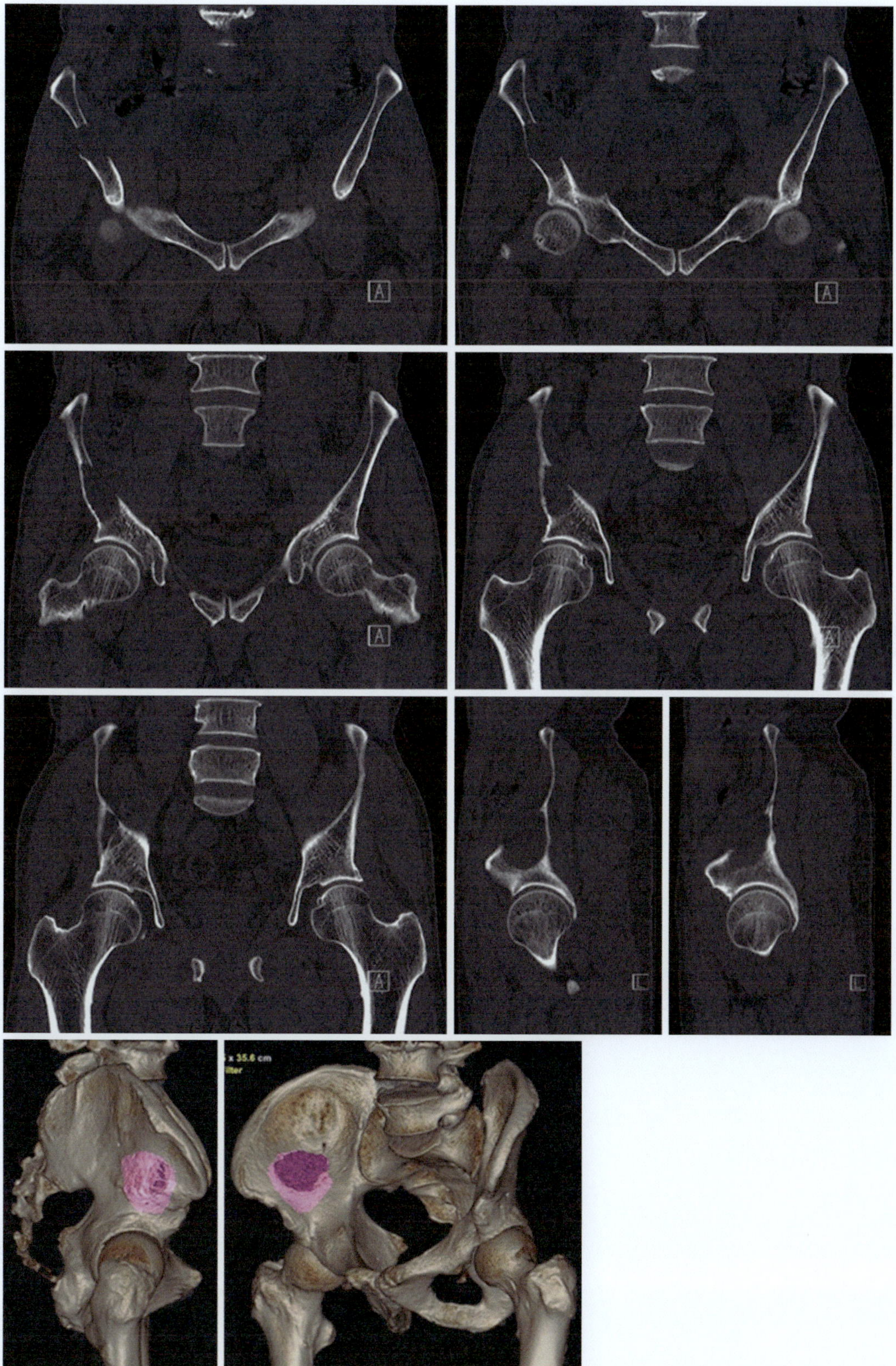

Fig. 6.2 Preoperative CT images

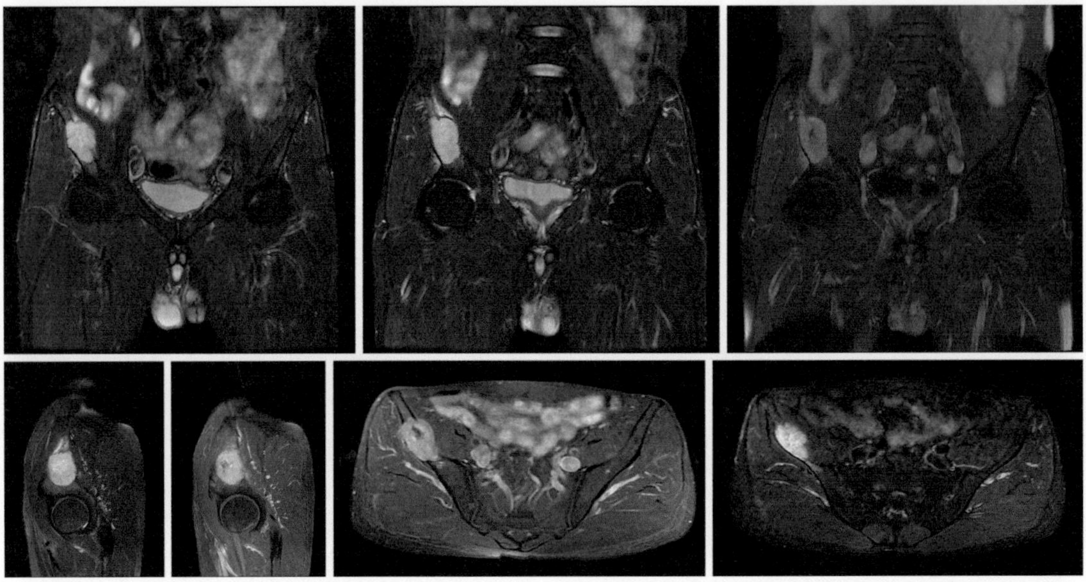

Fig. 6.3 Preoperative MRI images

Fig. 6.4 Preoperative bone scan images

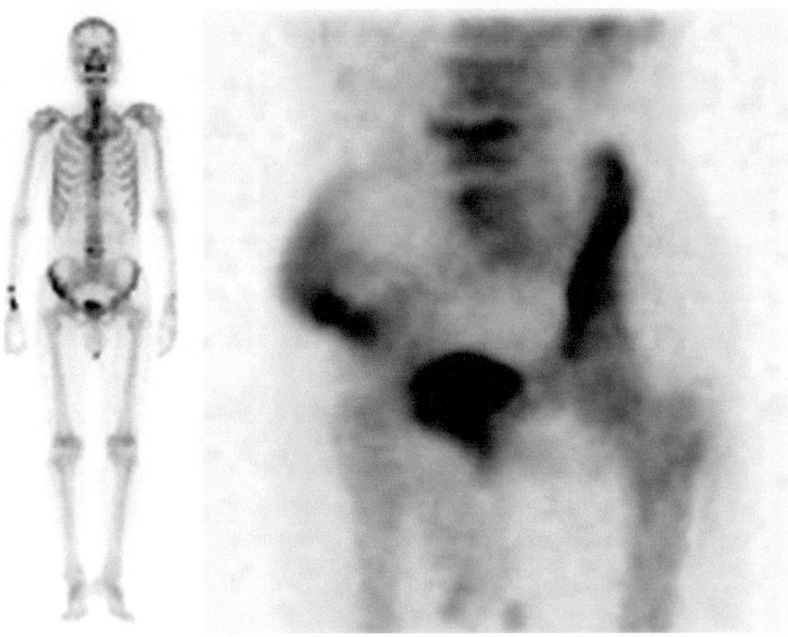

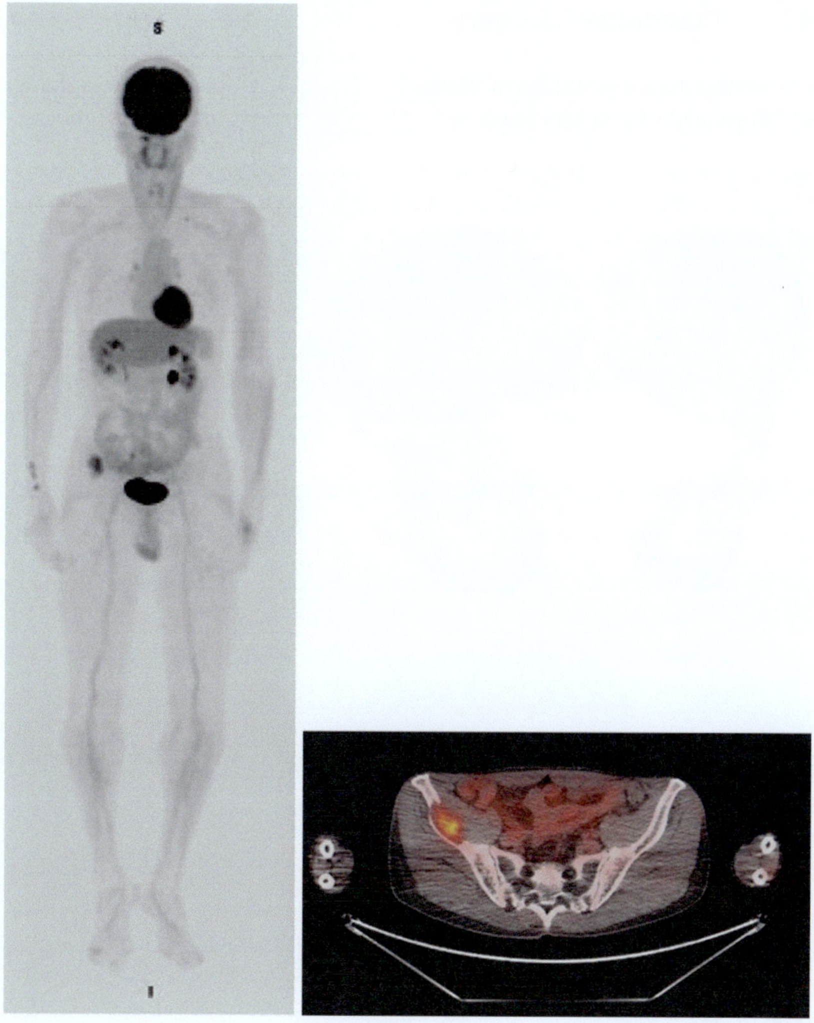

Fig. 6.5 Preoperative PET-CT images

6.3 Planning of Surgery

- Cavitary tumor resection of ilium
- 3D printed iliac spacer implant

6.4 Design and Fabrication

- Implant measurement
- Implant weight (g): 19.22
- Size (mm): 70

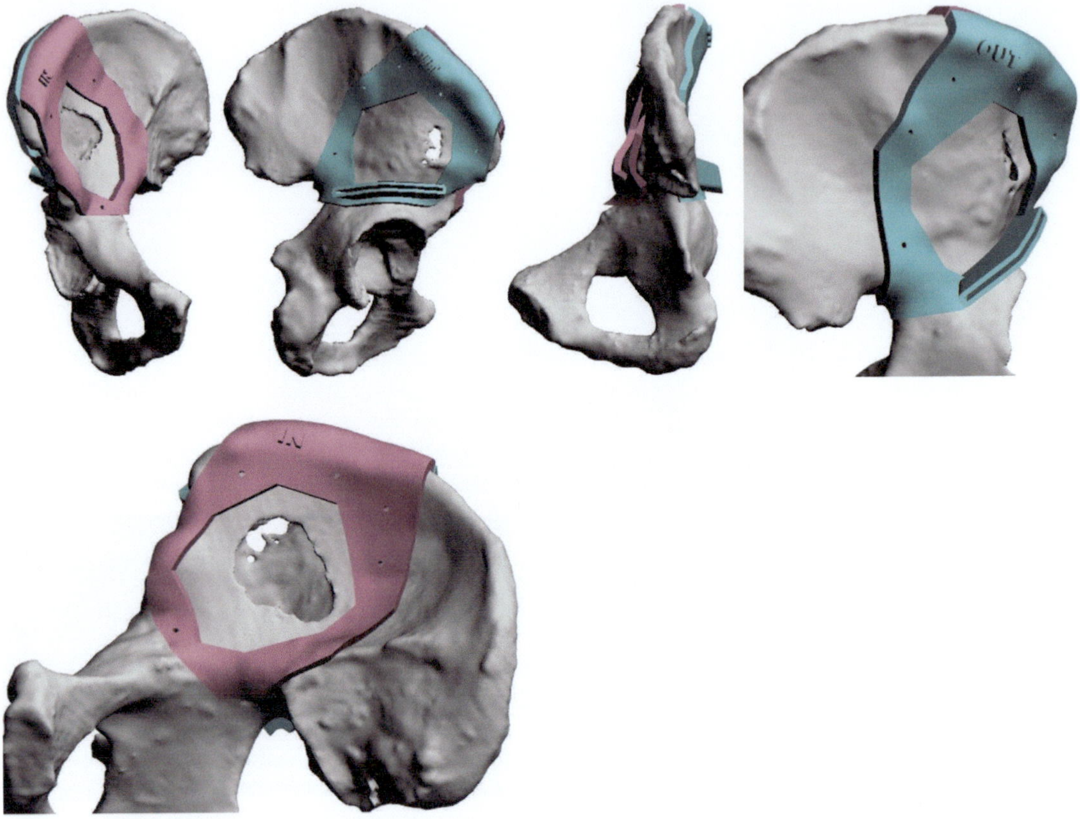

Fig. 6.6 Cutting guide design

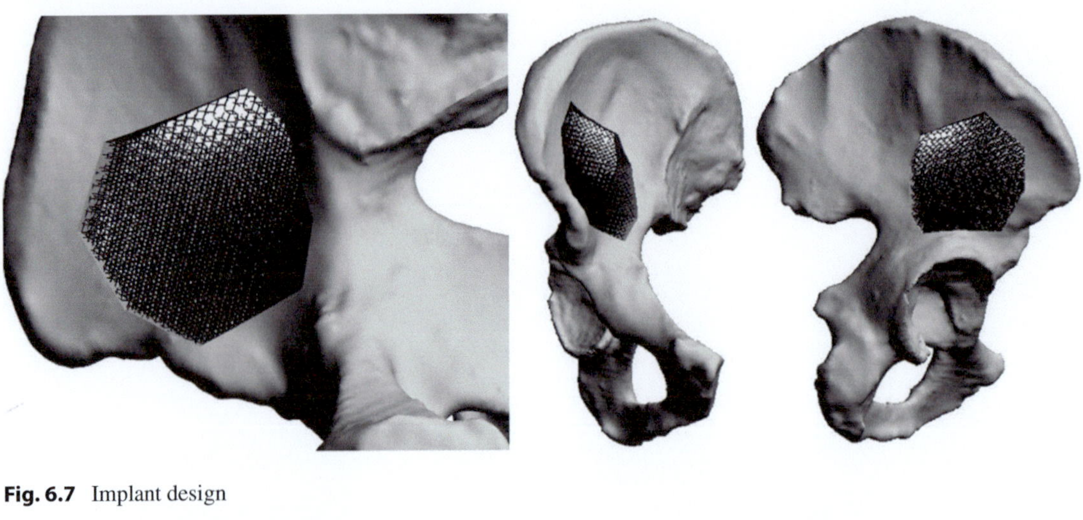

Fig. 6.7 Implant design

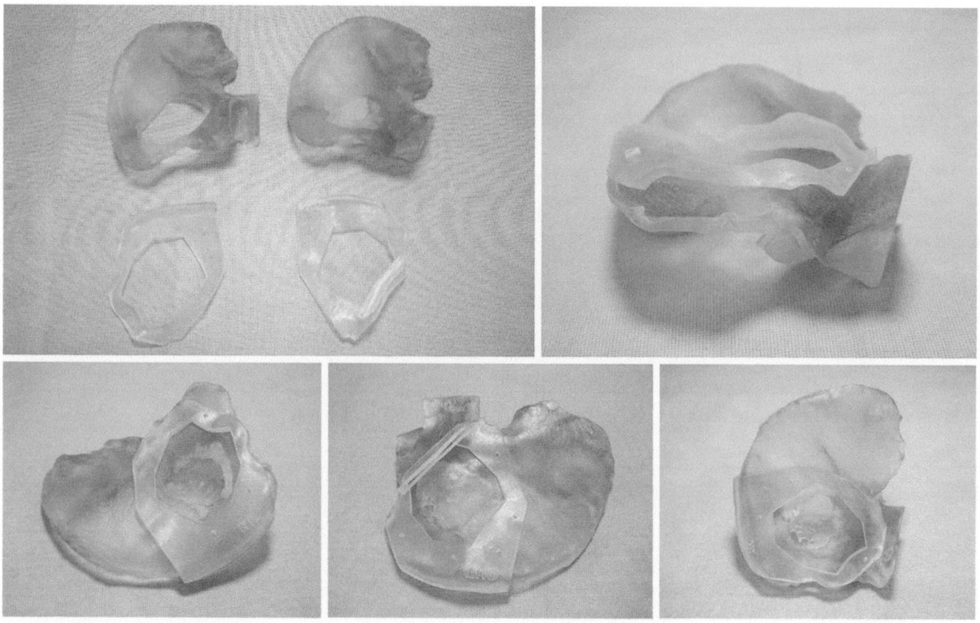

Fig. 6.8 Printed cutting guide

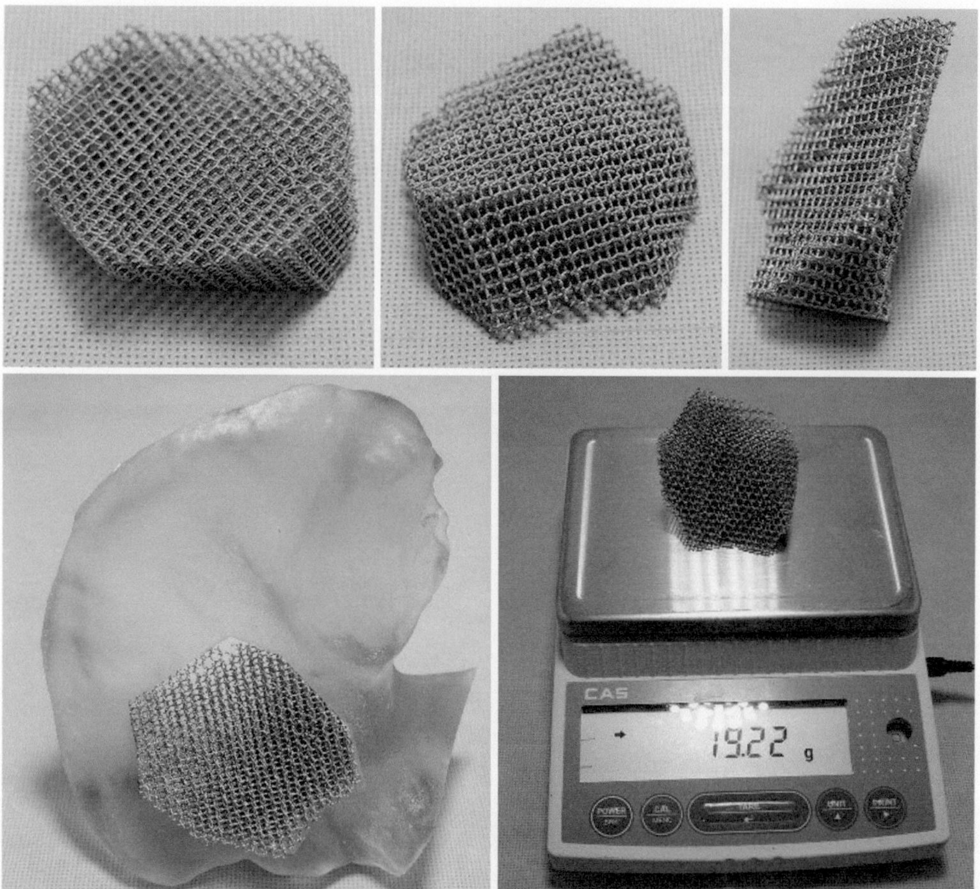

Fig. 6.9 Printed Implant: whole mesh style without connecting plate

6.5 Operation

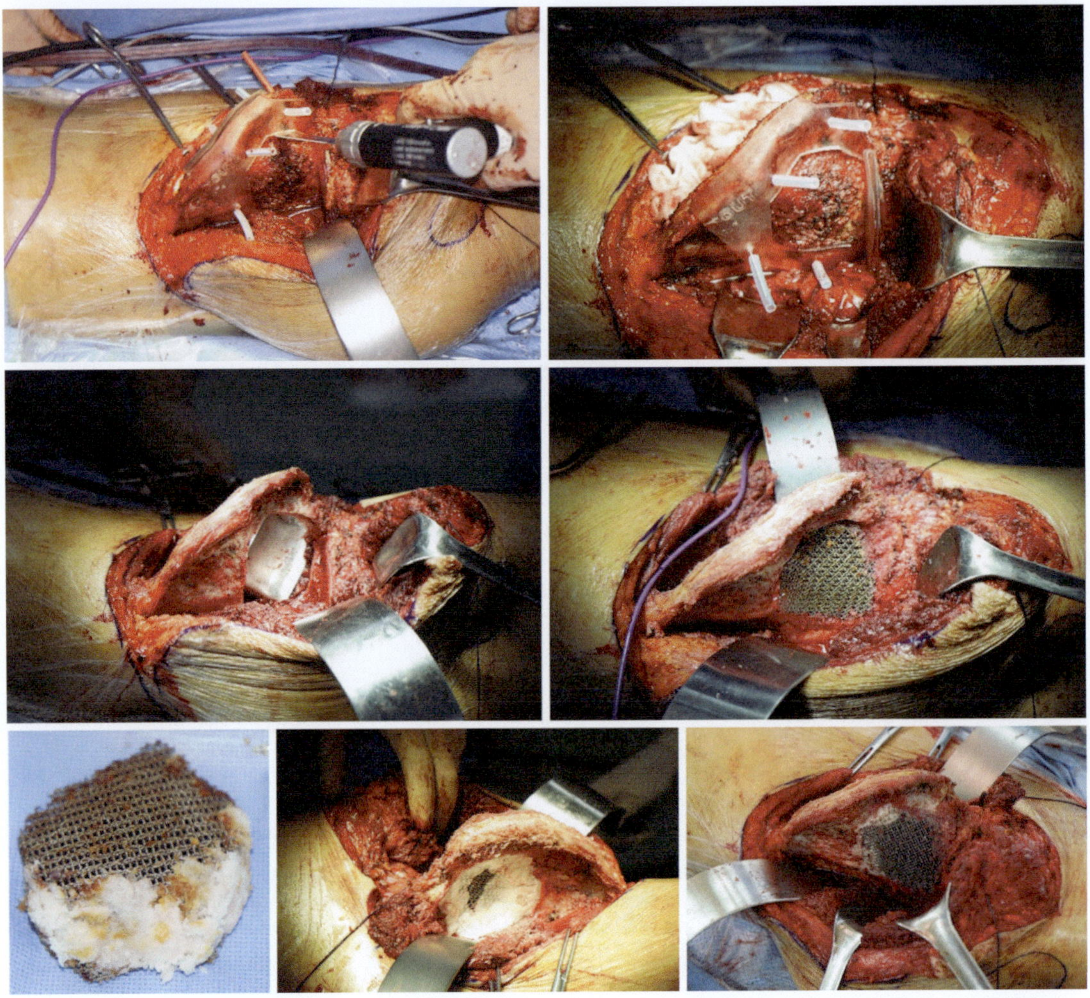

Fig. 6.10 Intraoperative photographs: demineralized bone matrix (DBM) attaching to the bone contact surface and connecting to the surrounding bone using calcium bone substitutes

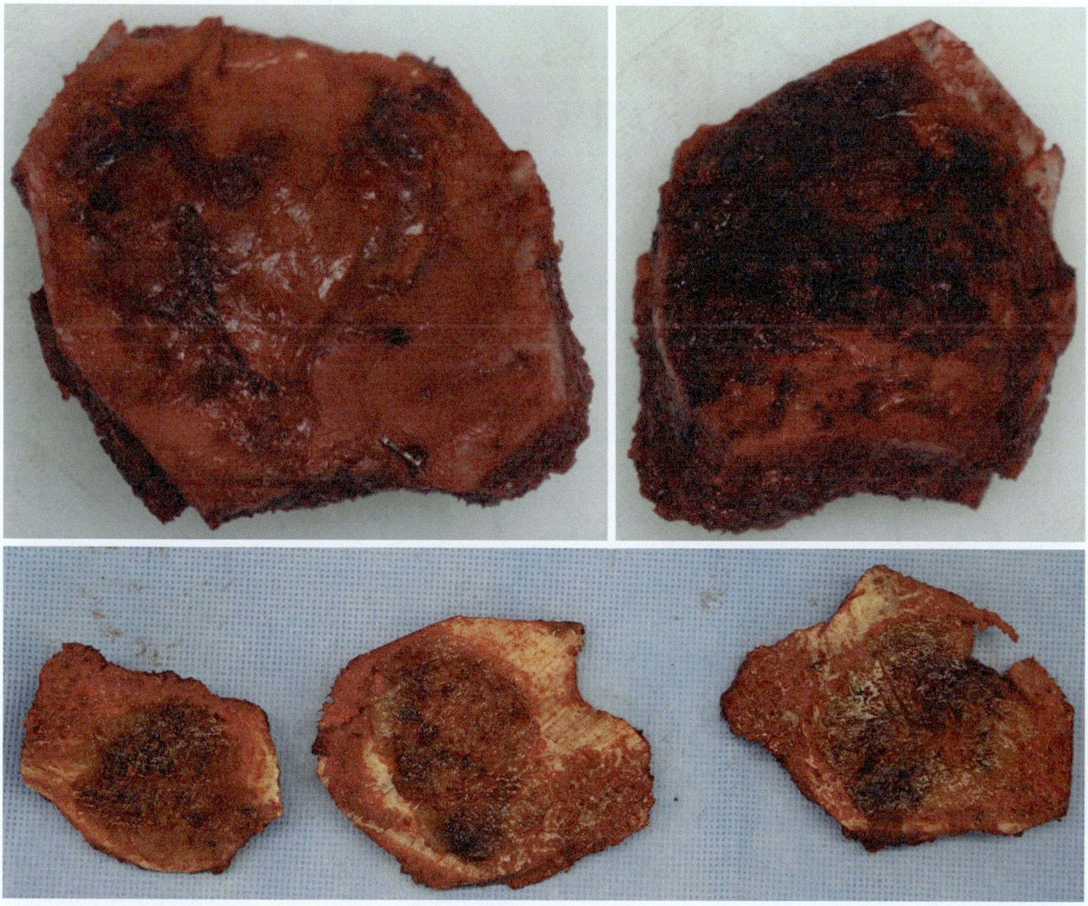

Fig. 6.11 Resected tumor

6.6 Postoperative Images

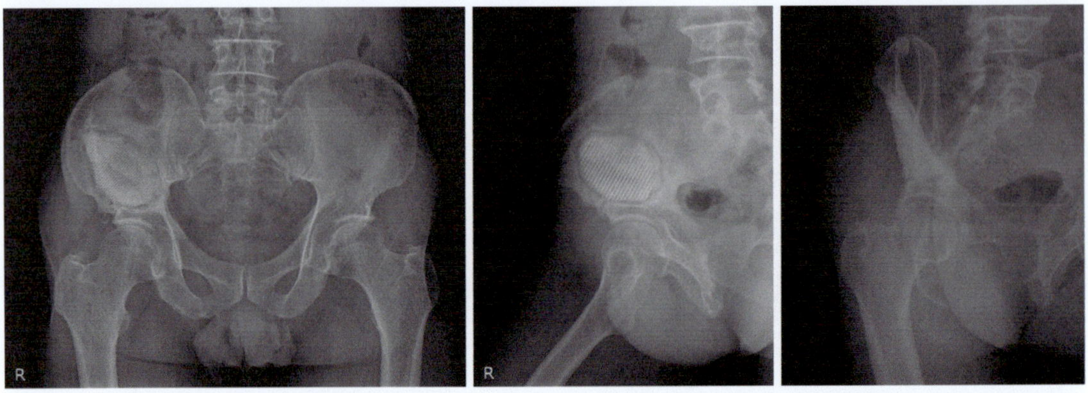

Fig. 6.12 Postoperative X-ray images

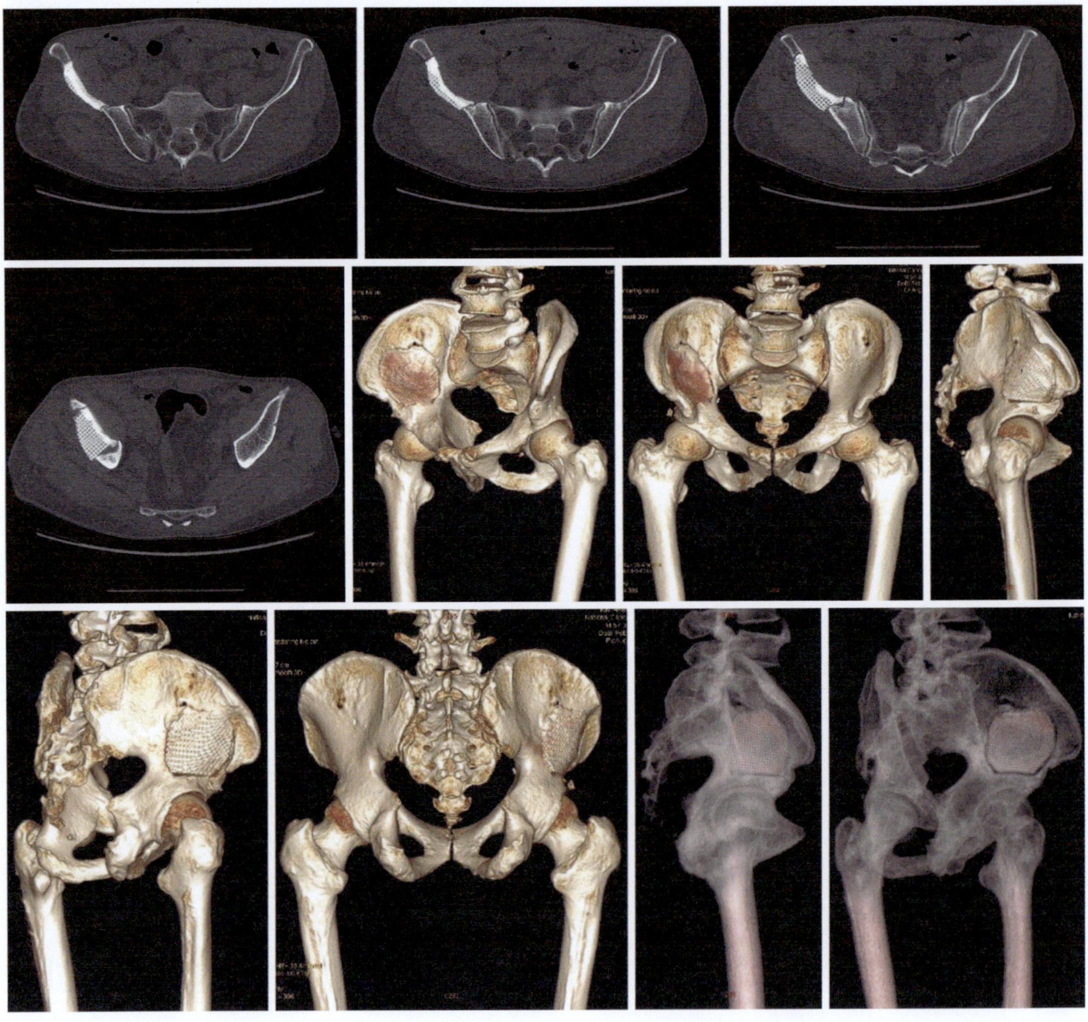

Fig. 6.13 Postoperative CT images

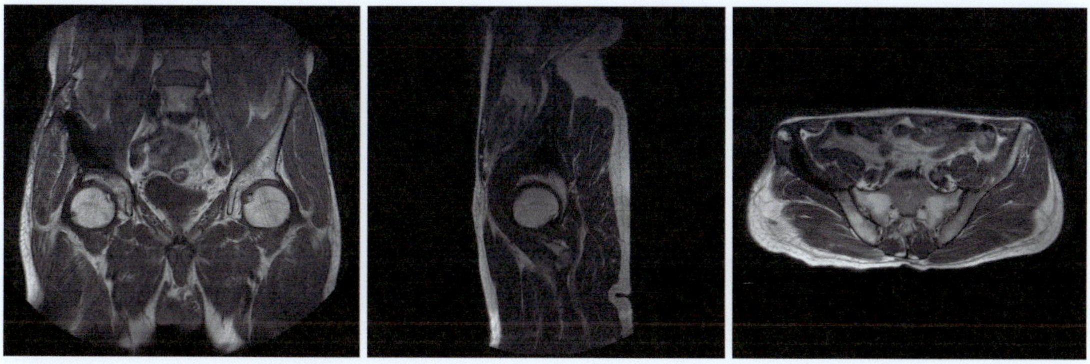

Fig. 6.14 Postoperative MRI images

7 Patient Case 7: Acetabular Subchondral Block

7.1 Patient Case 7

Age/sex	37/female
Location/site	Pelvis/right
Diagnosis	Osteosarcoma Solitary bone metastasis
Preoperative symptom	Right hip pain
Preoperative pain score	Resting 0/activity 4
BMI (height/weight)	18.83 (159.0/47.6)
Past history	Osteosarcoma, T11 Total spondylectomy and reconstruction at 13 months ago Postoperative radiation therapy and chemotherapy
Present illness	Abnormal finding on the follow-up PET-CT Incisional biopsy and confirmed osteosarcoma before patient refer

H.-G. Kang, *Clinical Atlas of 3D Printing Bone Reconstruction*,
https://doi.org/10.1007/978-981-16-2043-0_7

7.2 Preoperative Images

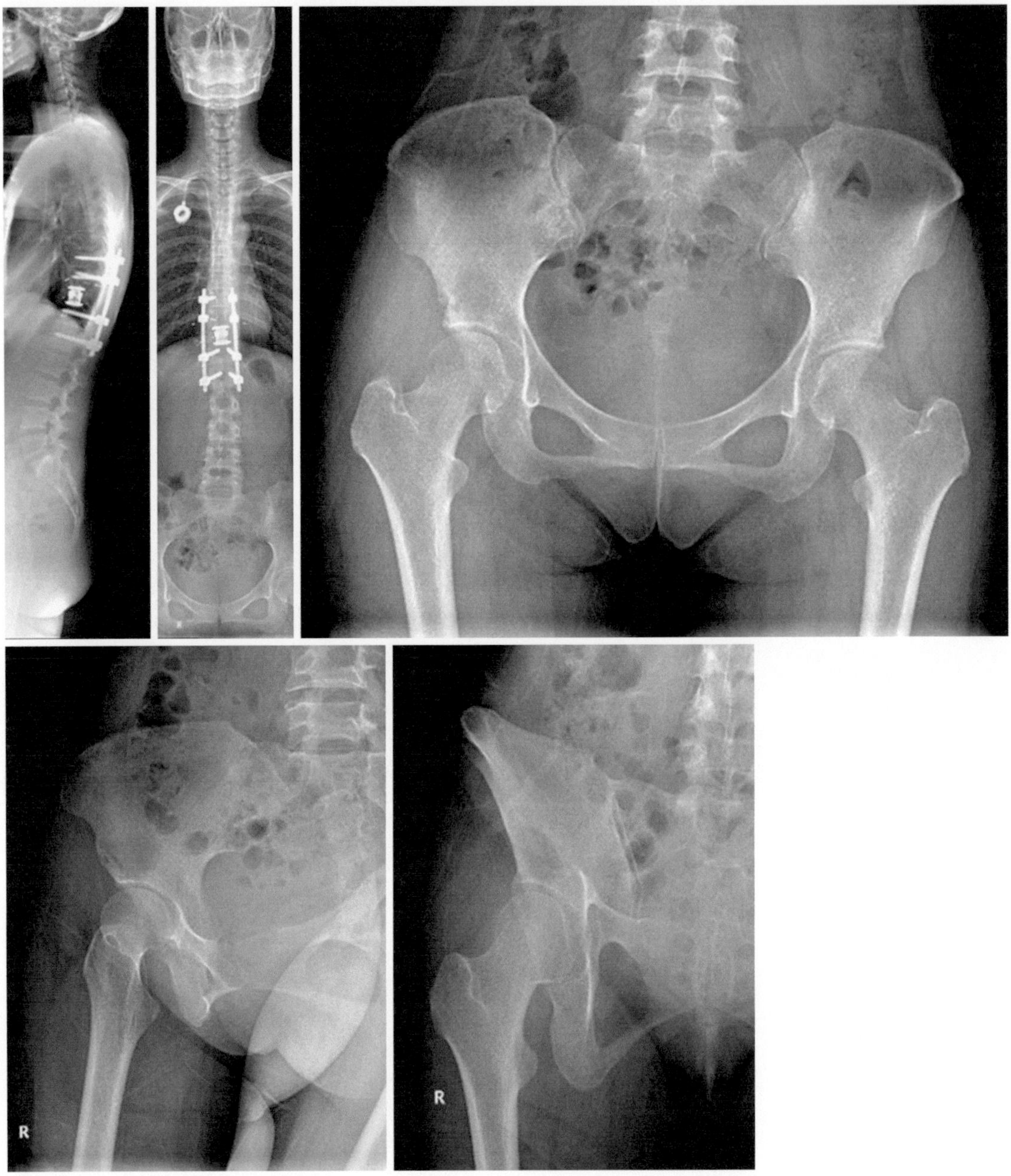

Fig. 7.1 Preoperative X-ray images

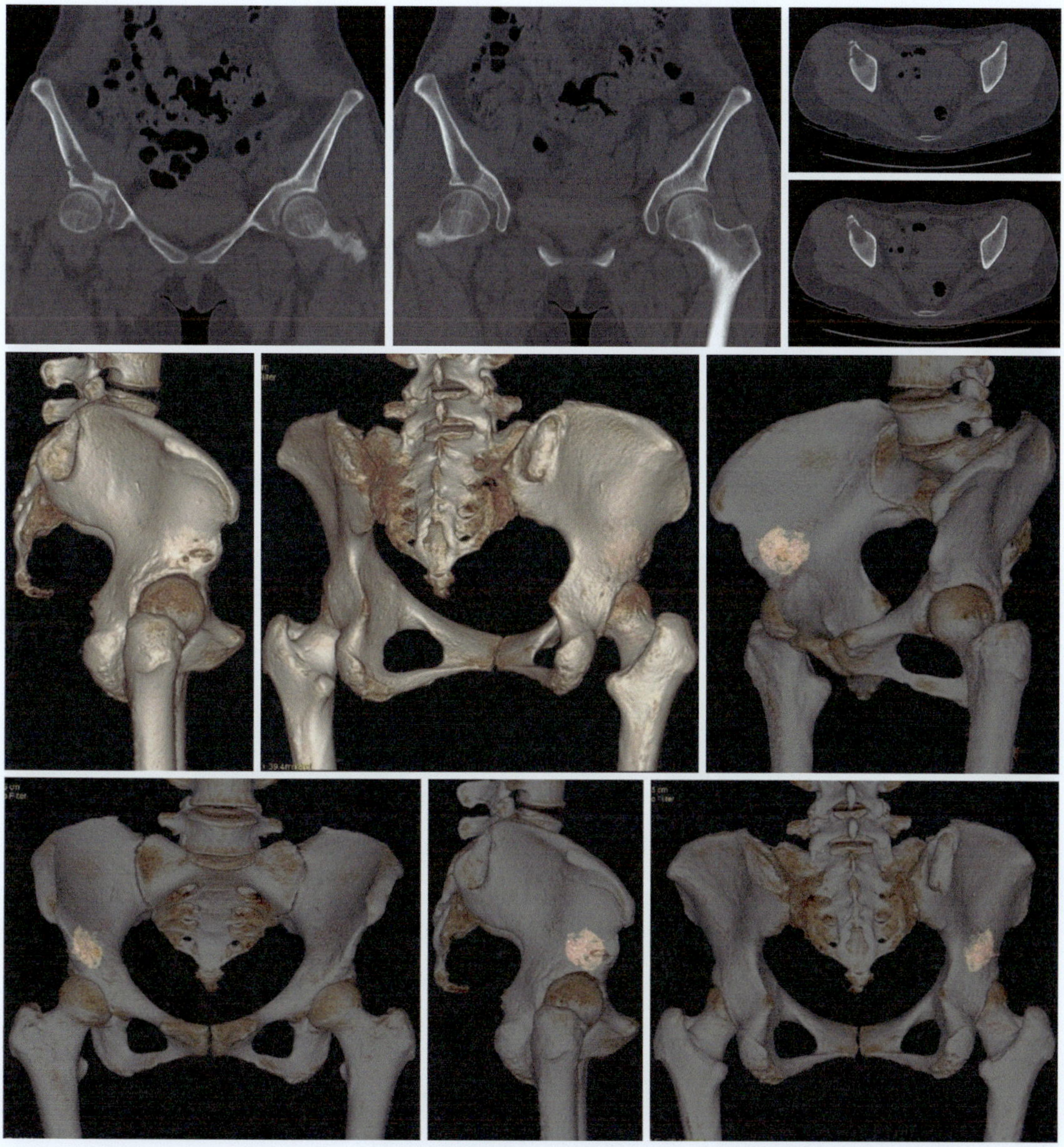

Fig. 7.2 Preoperative CT images

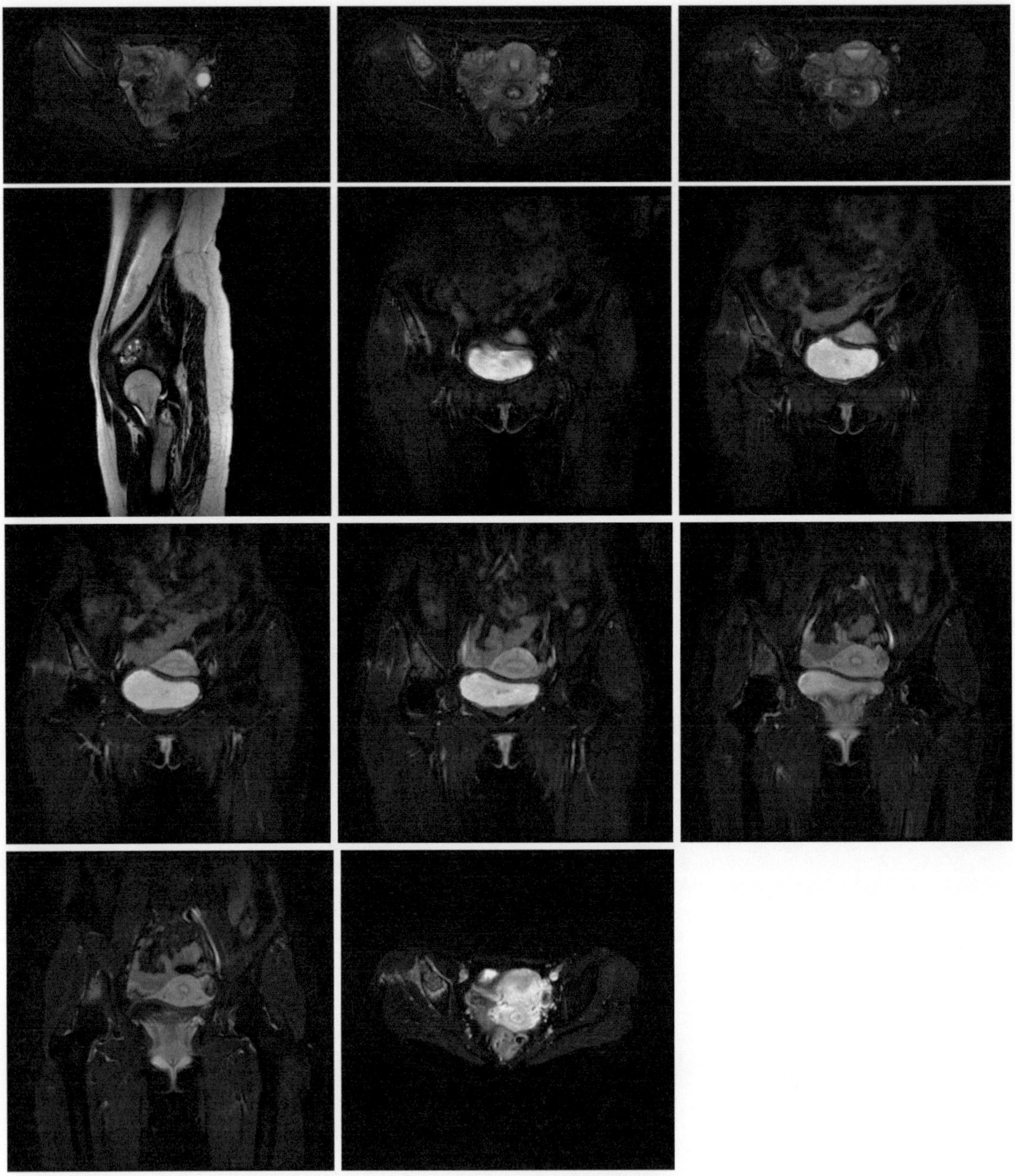

Fig. 7.3 Preoperative MRI images: a transmuscular small incisional biopsy tract was observed

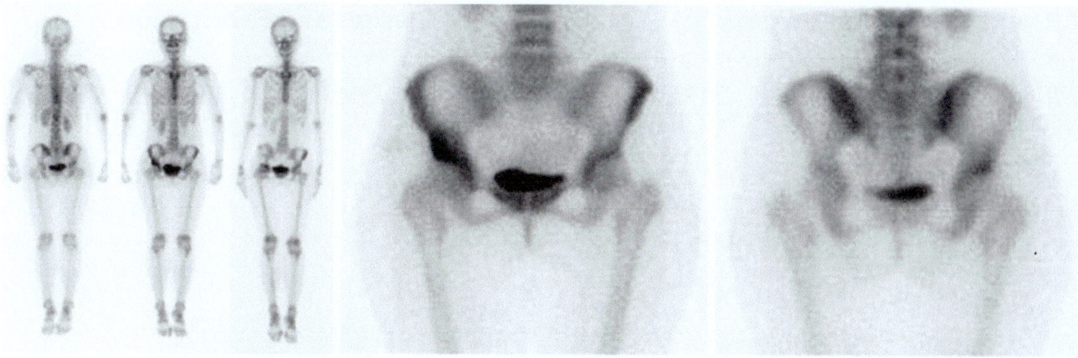

Fig. 7.4 Preoperative Bone scan images

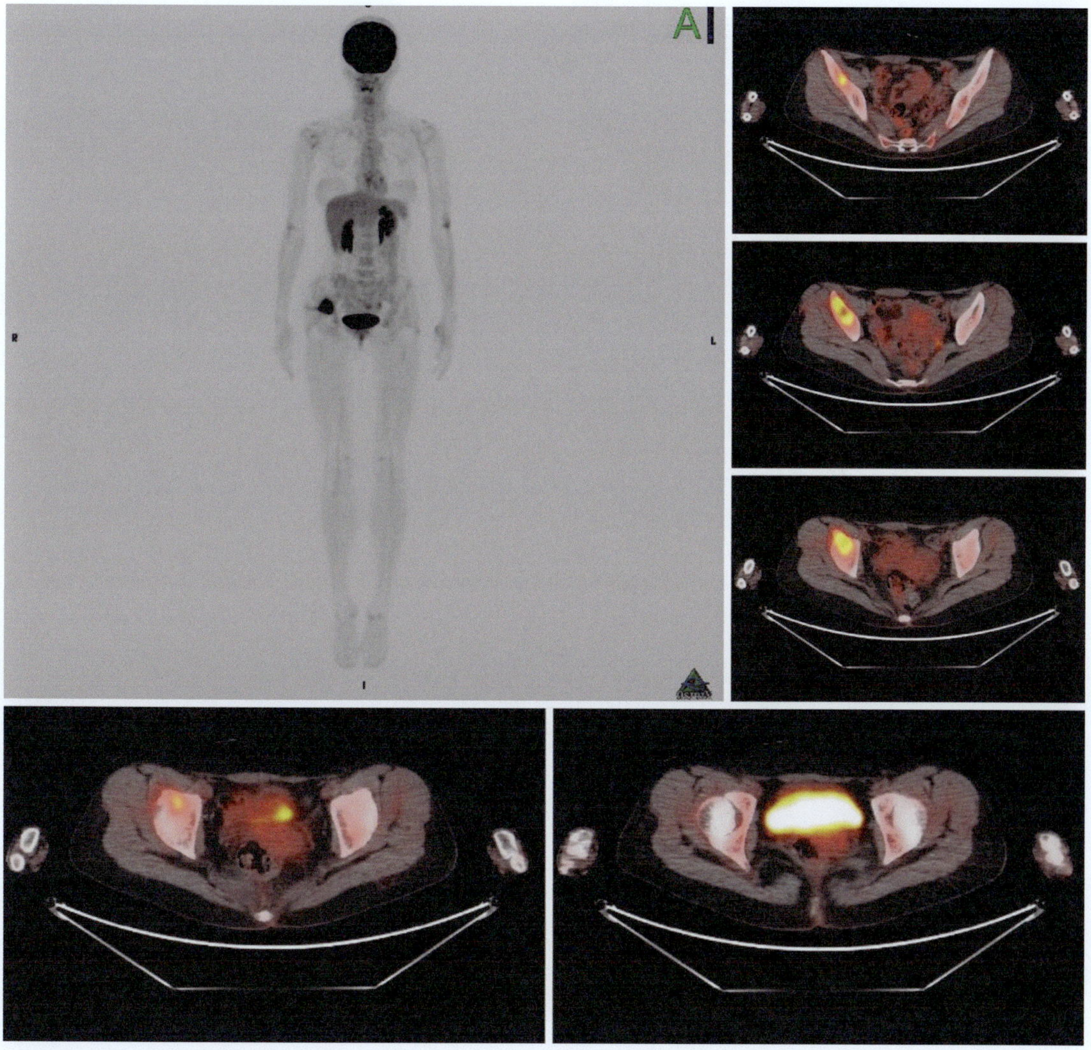

Fig. 7.5 Preoperative PET-CT images

7.3 Planning of Surgery

Hip joint saving resection at subchondral of acetabulum

3D printed acetabular dome spacer implant

No interconnecting plates

7.4 Design and Fabrication

Closed-type guide

- Implant measurement
- Implant weight (g): 7.53
- Size (mm): 55

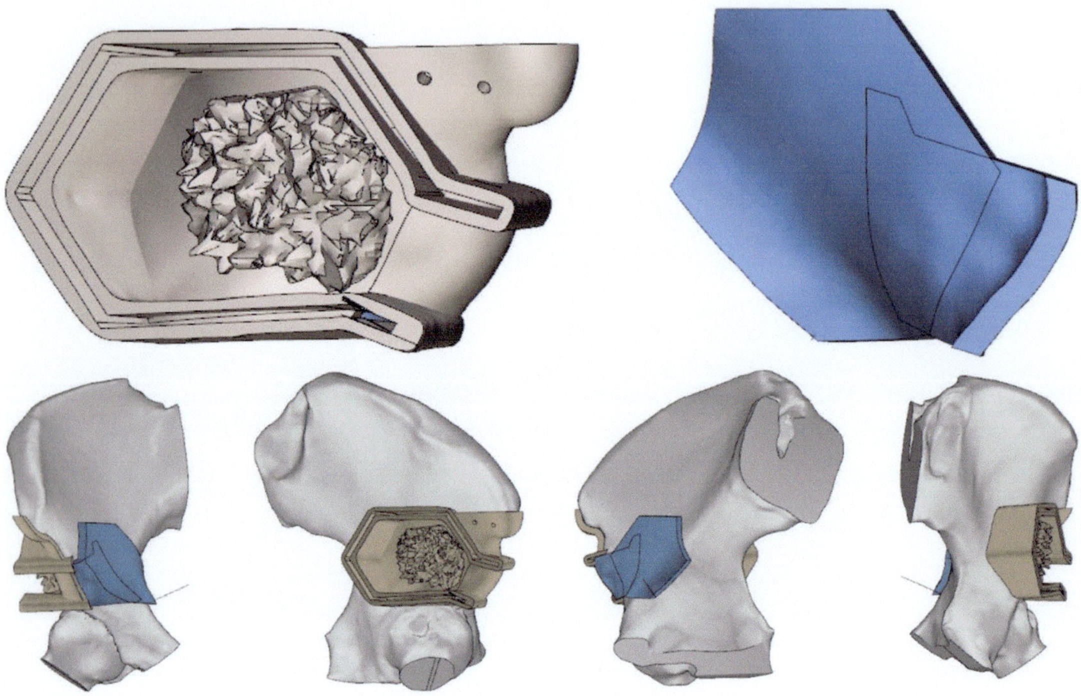

Fig. 7.6 Cutting guide design: tumors can be displayed on the surface of the close-type cutting guide design

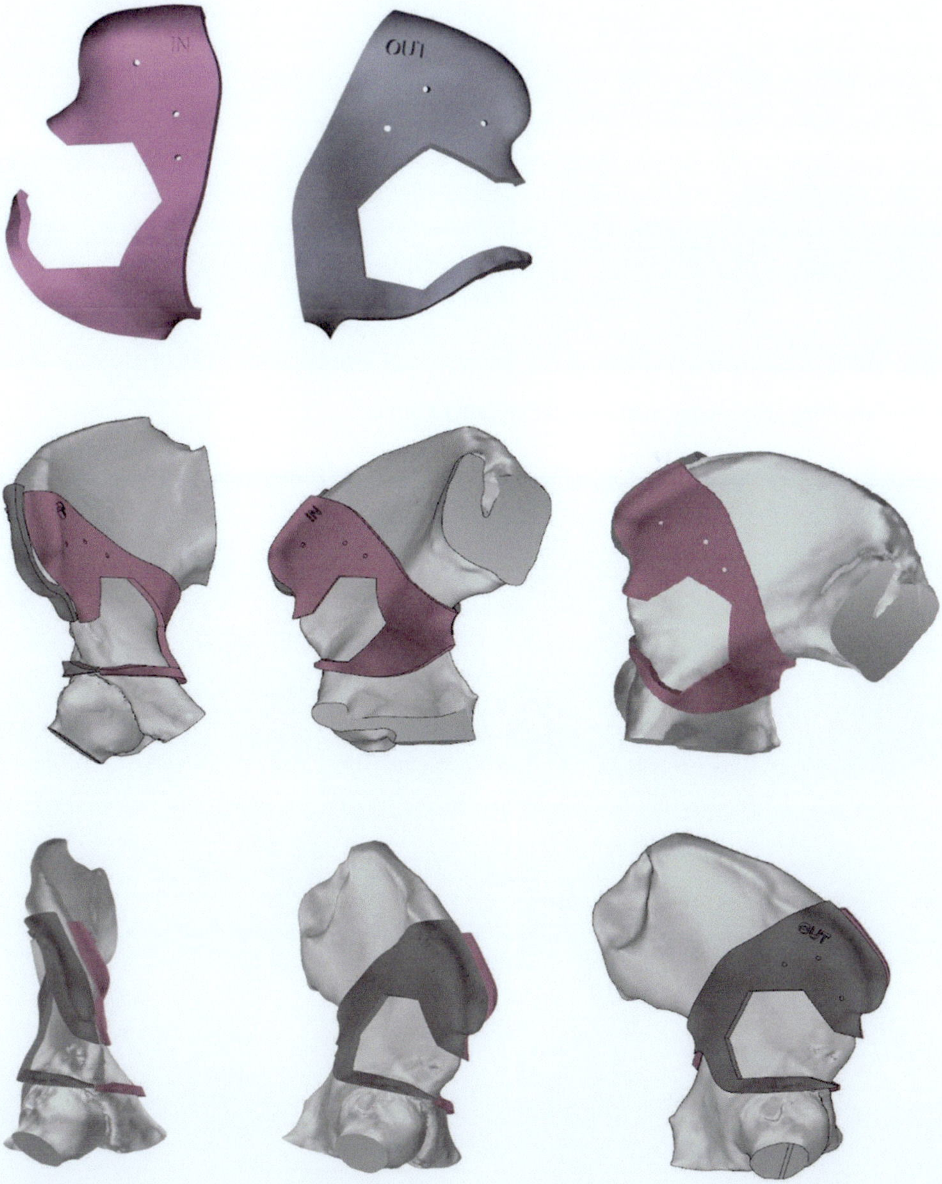

Fig. 7.7 Cutting guide design: open-type cutting design

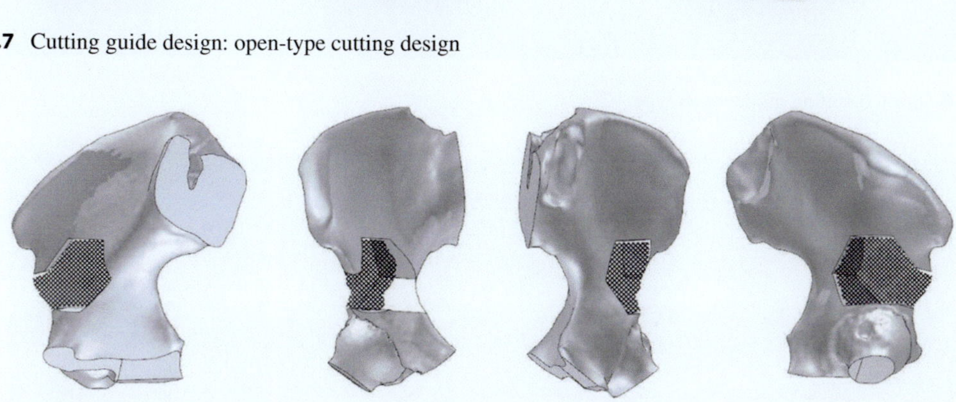

Fig. 7.8 Implant design

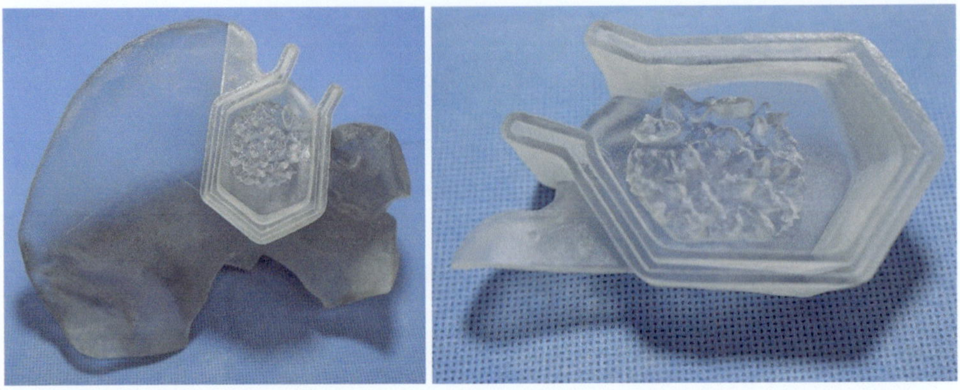

Fig. 7.9 Printed cutting guide: tumor marked on the close-type surface

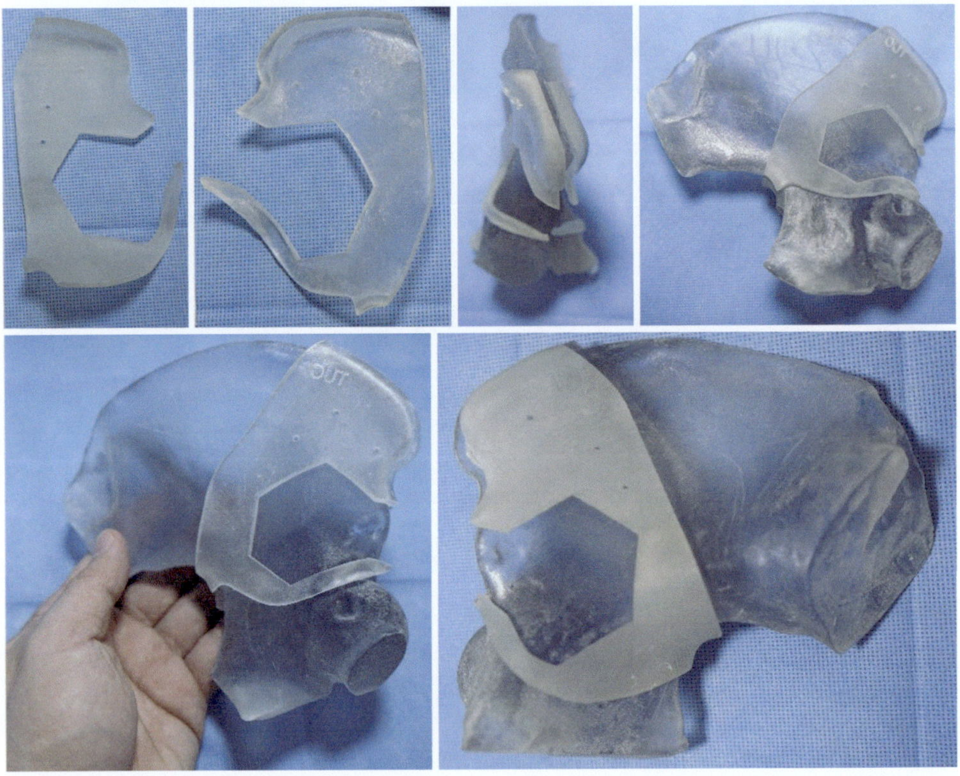

Fig. 7.10 Printed cutting guide: open type

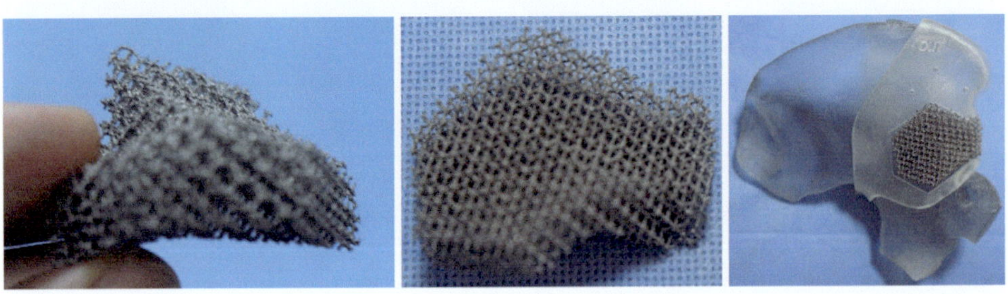

Fig. 7.11 Printed implant

7.5 Operation

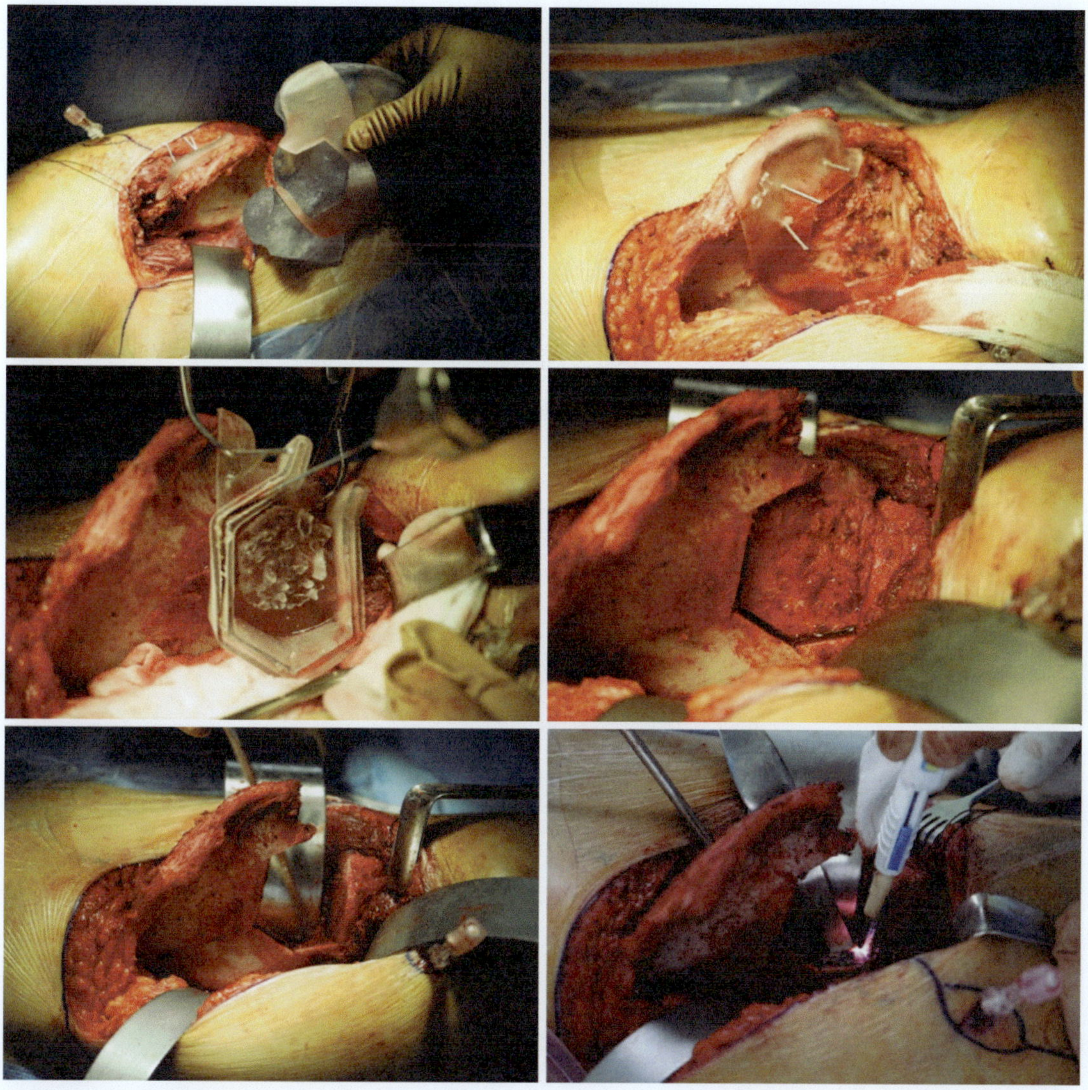

Fig. 7.12 Intraoperative photographs: after marking the biopsy track with a needle, inserting a liquid nitrogen gun nozzle and cryotherapy

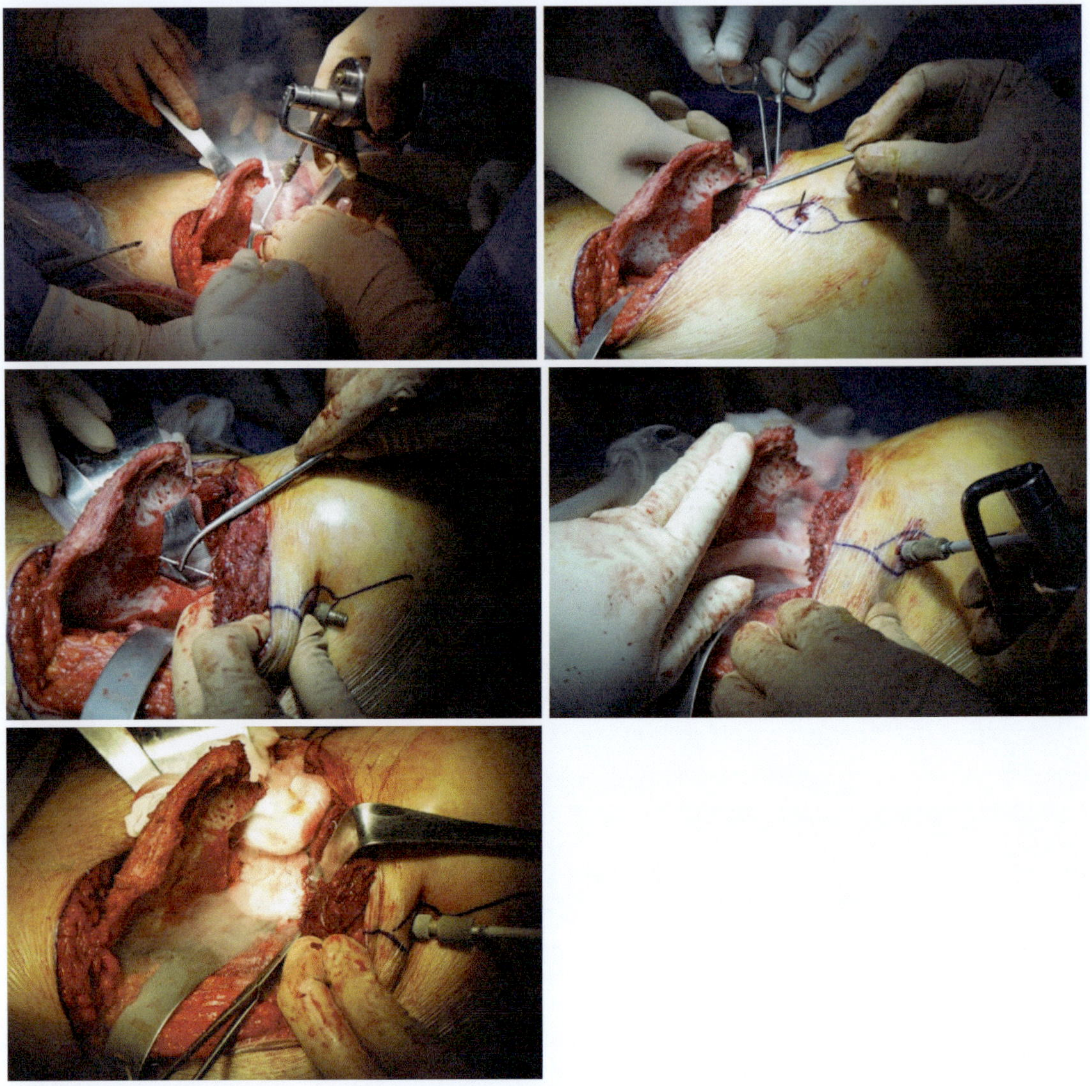

Fig. 7.12 (continued)

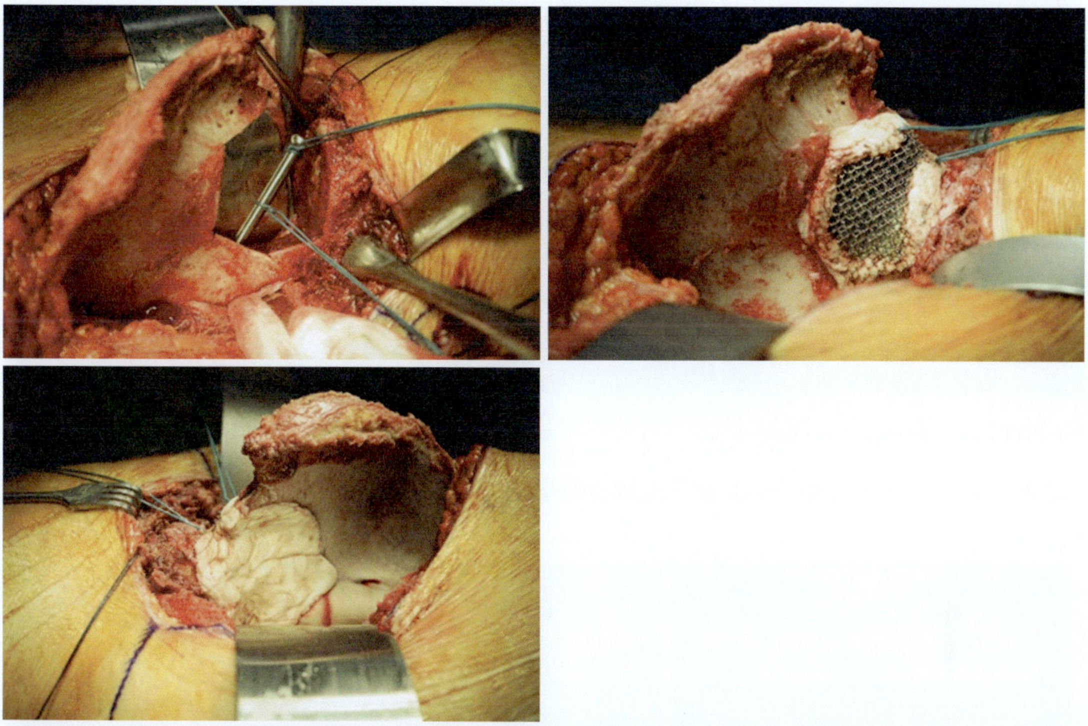

Fig. 7.13 Intraoperative photographs: fixation with a cannulated screw and PMMA bone cement

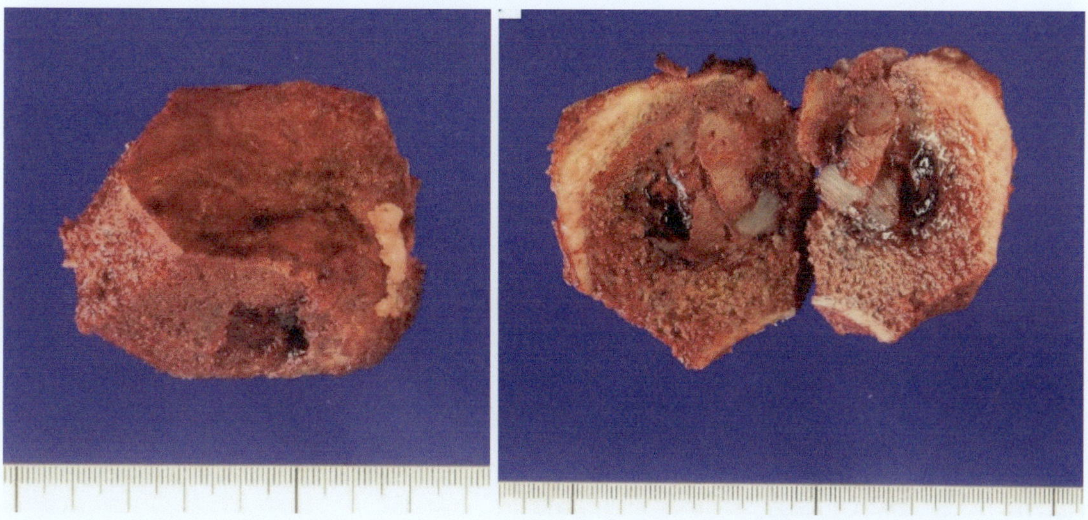

Fig. 7.14 Resected tumor

7.6 Postoperative Images

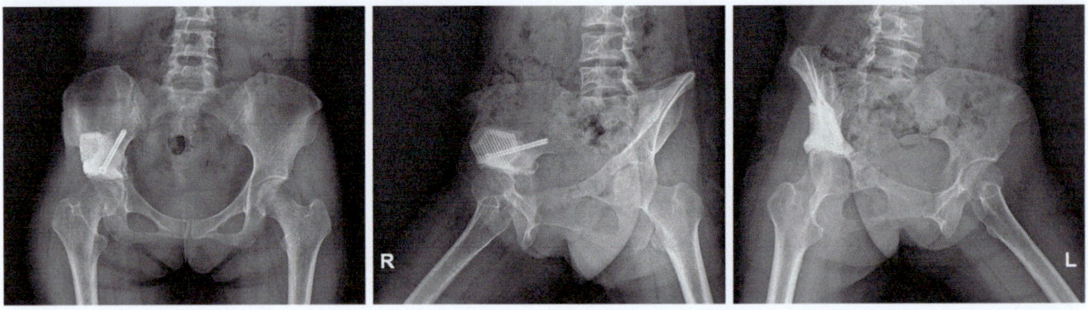

Fig. 7.15 Postoperative X-ray images

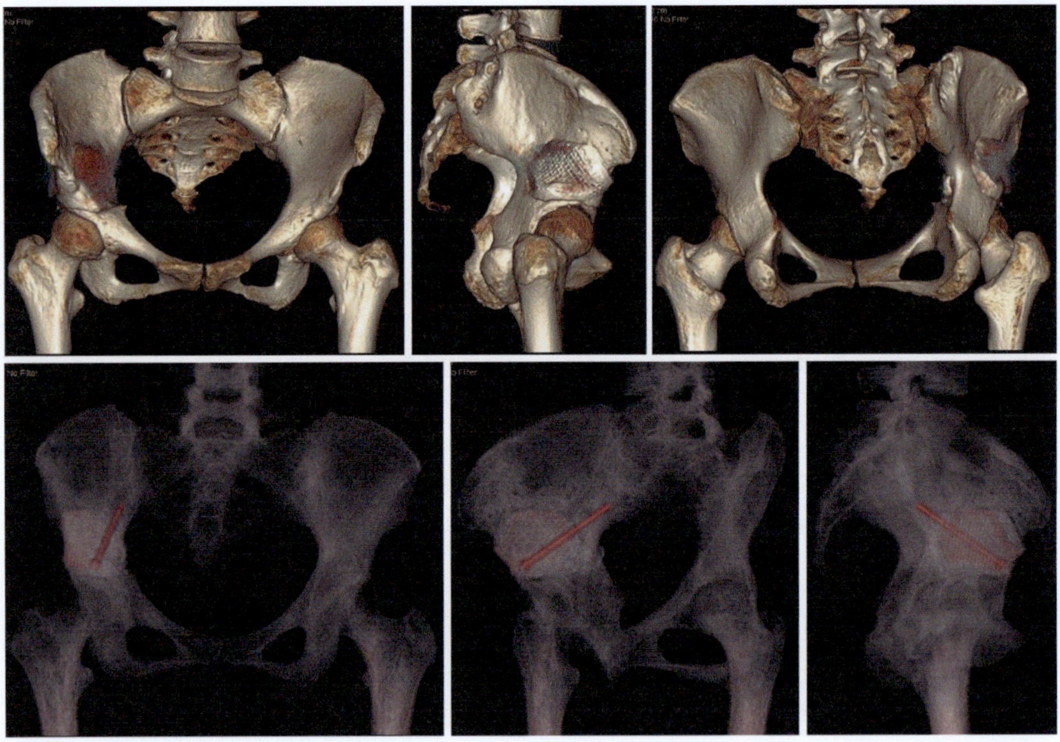

Fig. 7.16 Postoperative CT images

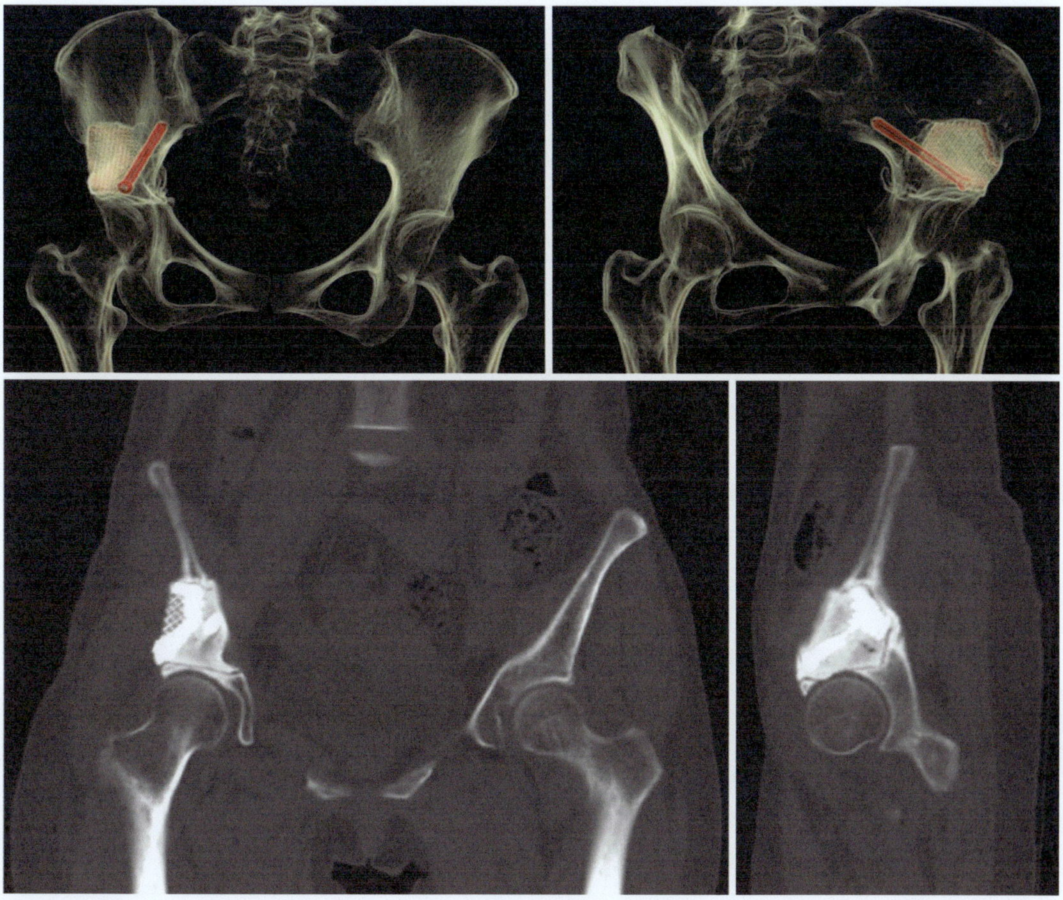

Fig. 7.16 (continued)

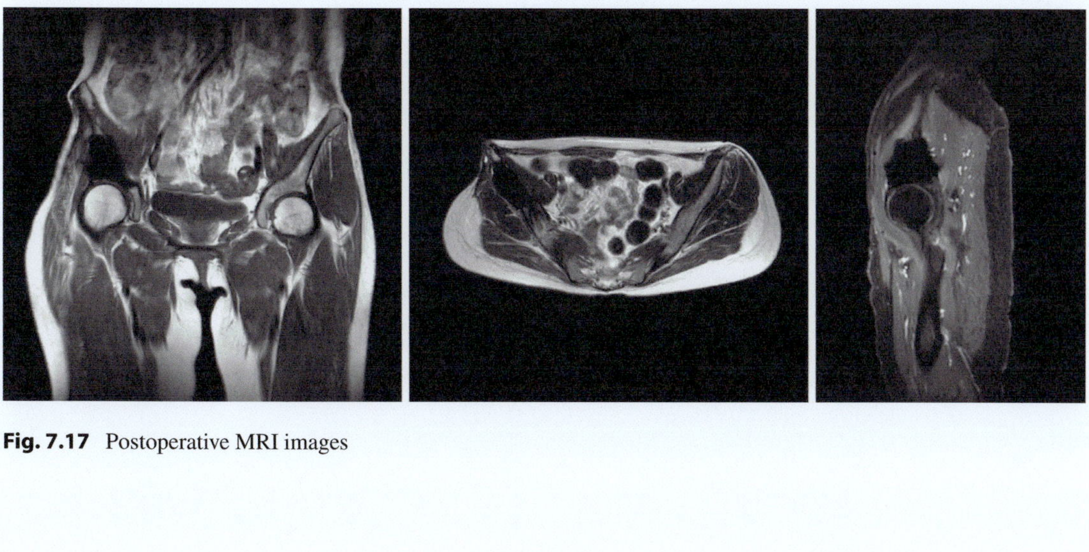

Fig. 7.17 Postoperative MRI images

Patient Case 8: Iliac Acetabular Block and Plate

8

8.1 Patient Case 8

Age/sex	48/female
Location/site	Pelvis/left
Diagnosis	Osteosarcoma, osteoblastic type
Preoperative symptom	Antalgic gait
Preoperative pain score	Resting: 2/activity: 5
BMI (height/weight)	23.55 (152.4/54.7)
Past history	Preoperative diagnosed high grade pleomorphic sarcoma on the sono-guided biopsy
Present illness	Aggravated left hip pain during a month

8.2 Preoperative Images

Fig. 8.1 Preoperative X-ray image

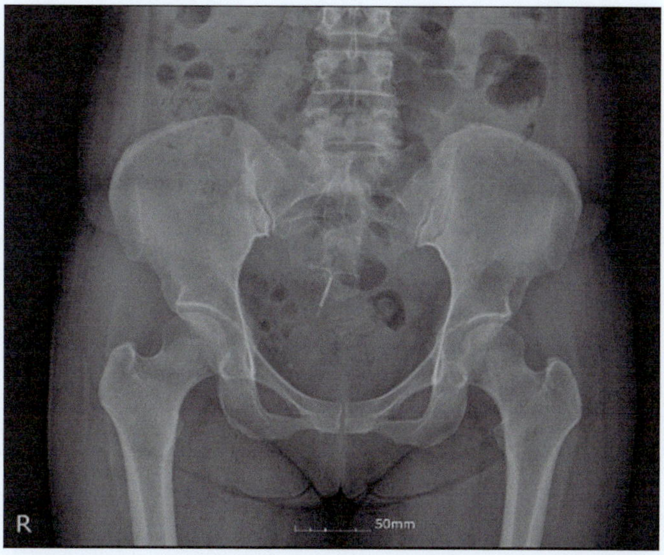

H.-G. Kang, *Clinical Atlas of 3D Printing Bone Reconstruction*,
https://doi.org/10.1007/978-981-16-2043-0_8

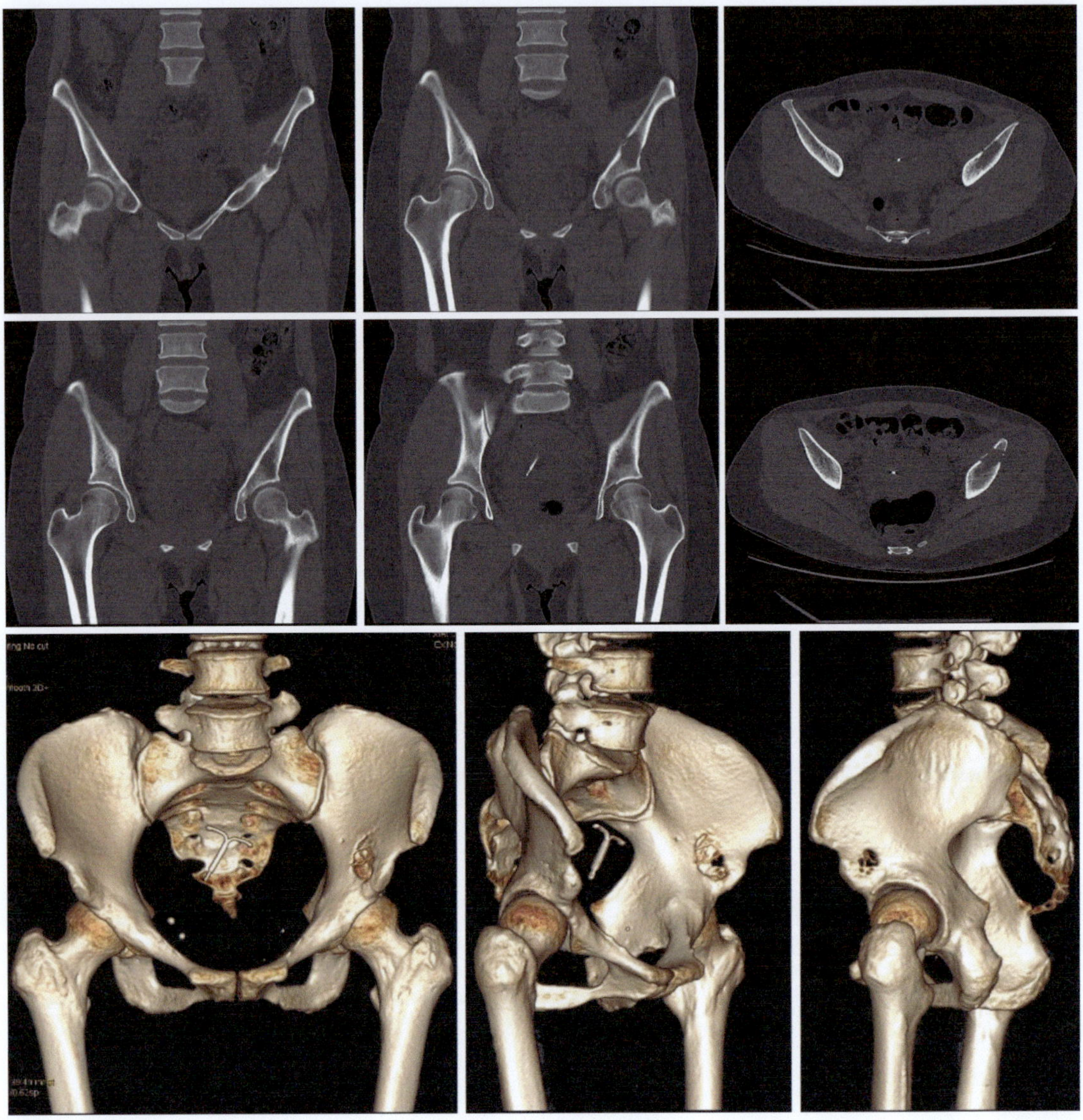

Fig. 8.2 Preoperative CT images

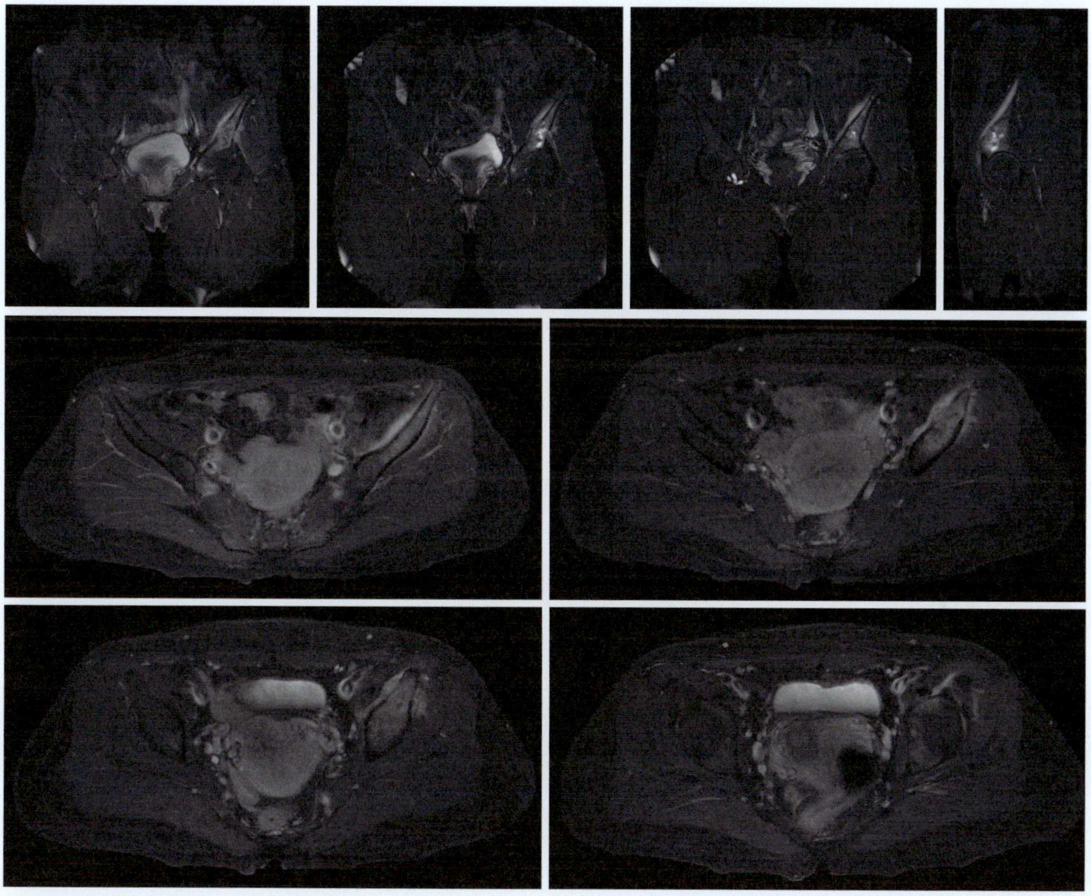

Fig. 8.3 Preoperative MRI images

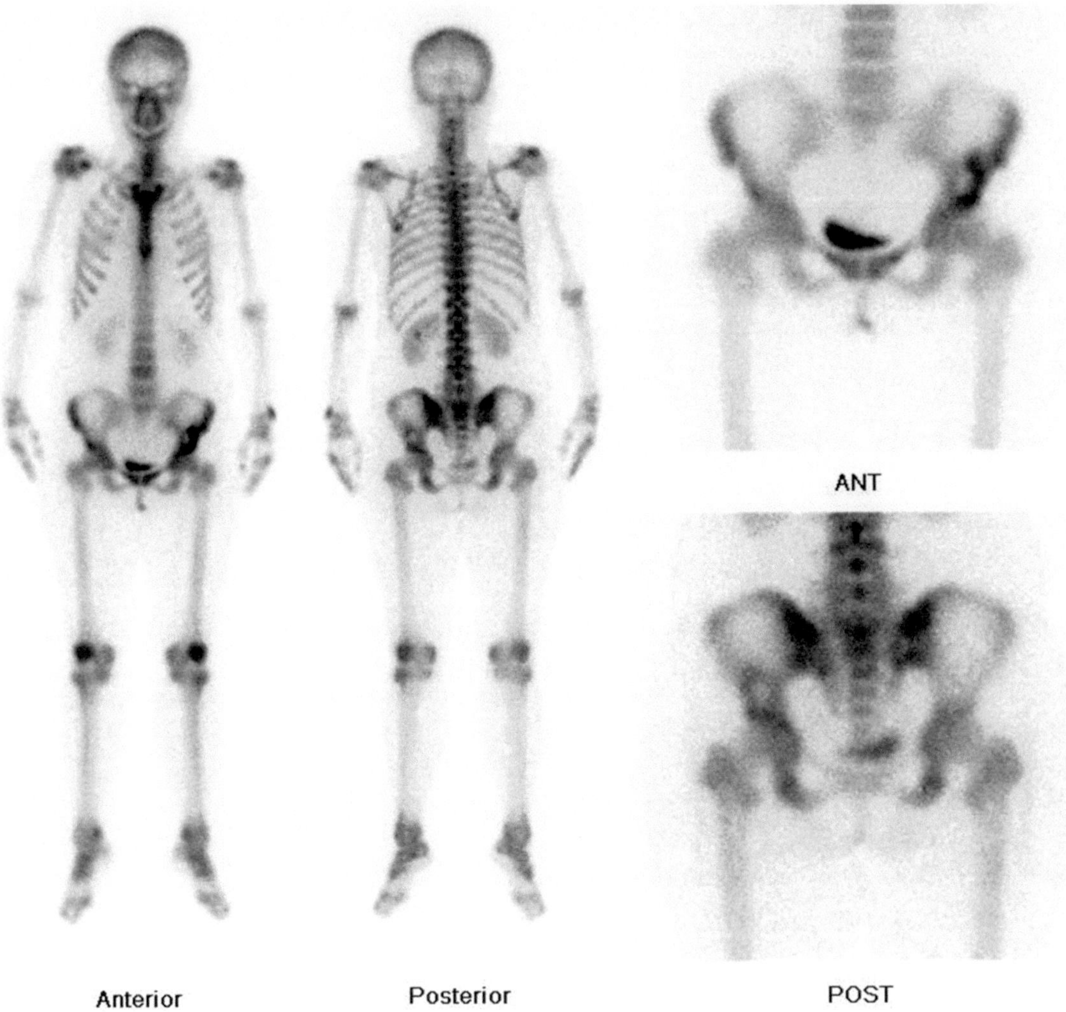

Fig. 8.4 Preoperative bone scan images

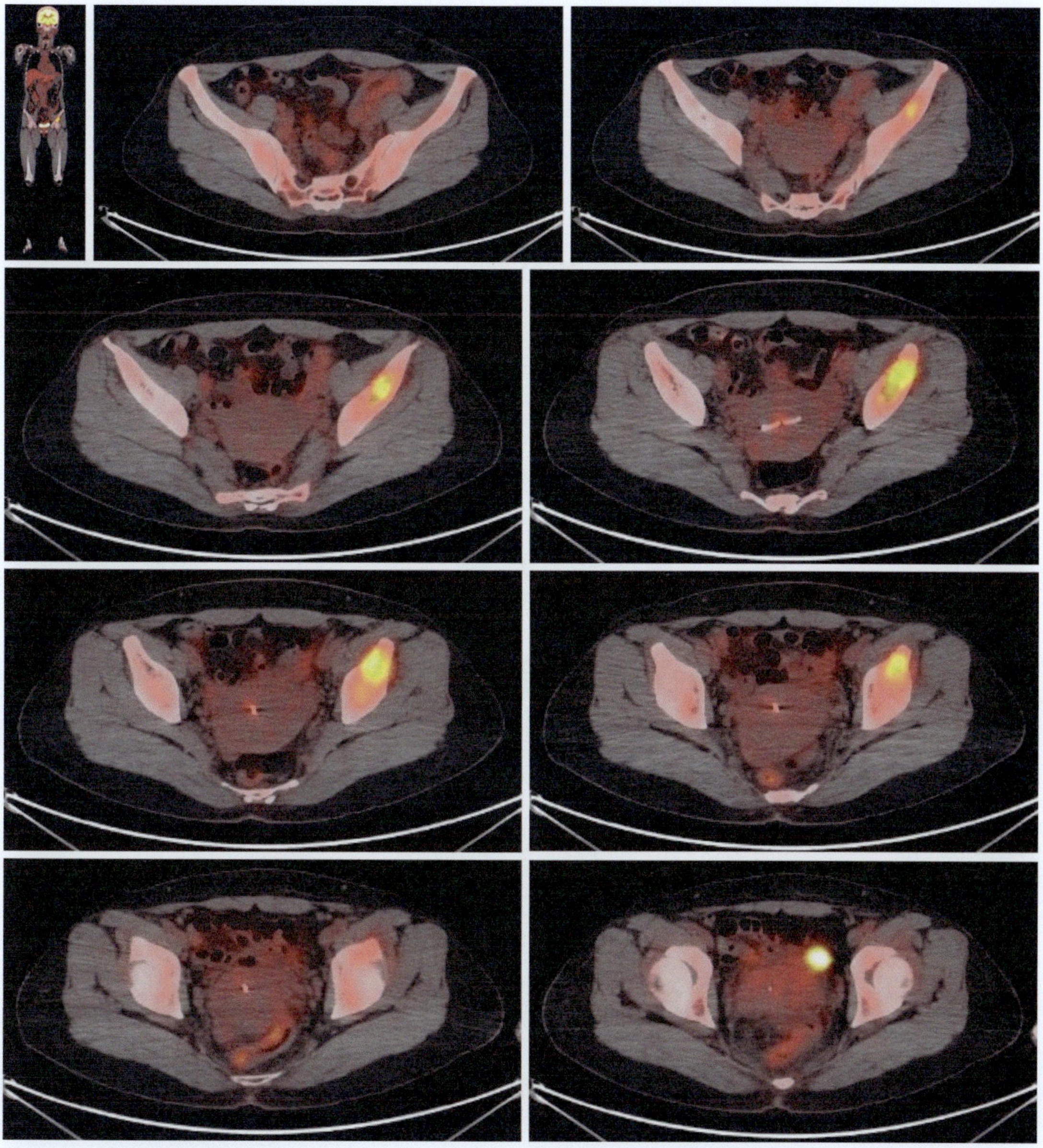

Fig. 8.5 Preoperative PET-CT images

8.3 Planning of Surgery

Hip joint saving resection at subchondral of acetabulum

Intraoperative adjuvant surgery with argon laser and liquid nitrogen gun

3D printed periacetabular iliac spacer implant

Interconnecting plate

8.4 Design and Fabrication

- Implant measurement
- Implant weight (g): 92
- Size (mm): 88

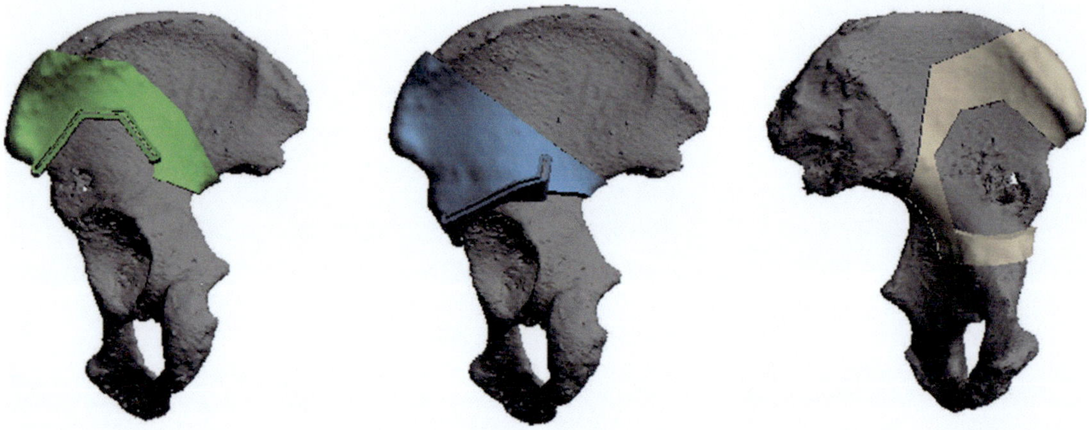

Fig. 8.6 Cutting guide design

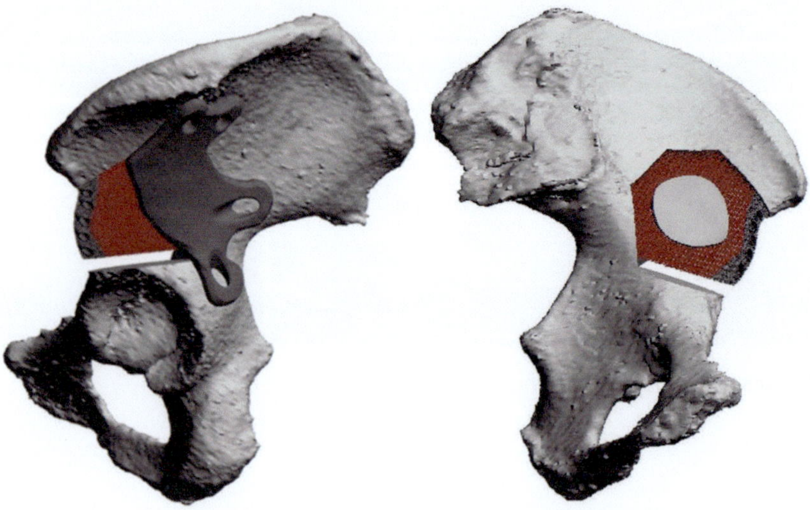

Fig. 8.7 Implant design: space for acetabular cup in future total hip joint arthroplasty

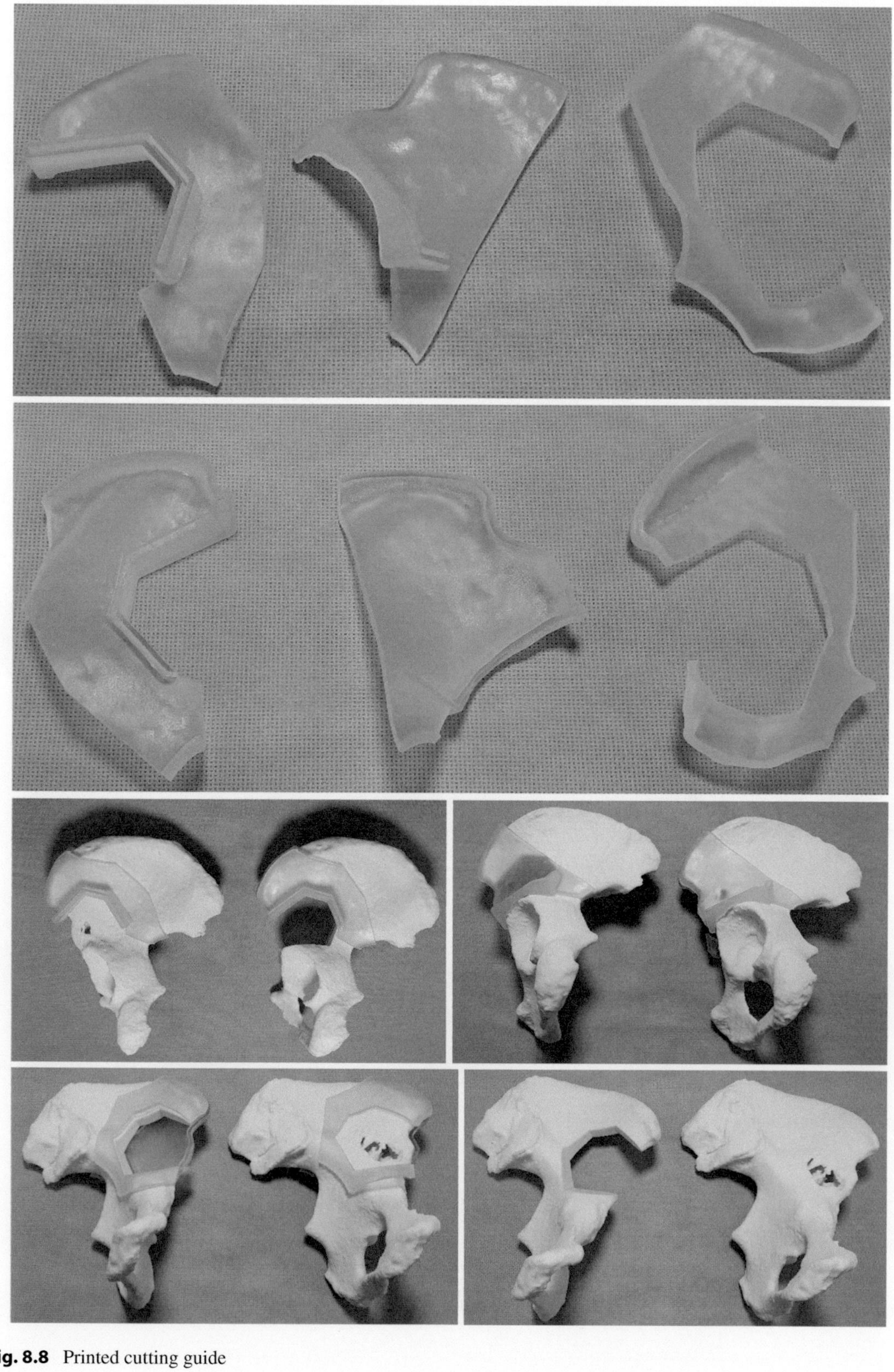

Fig. 8.8 Printed cutting guide

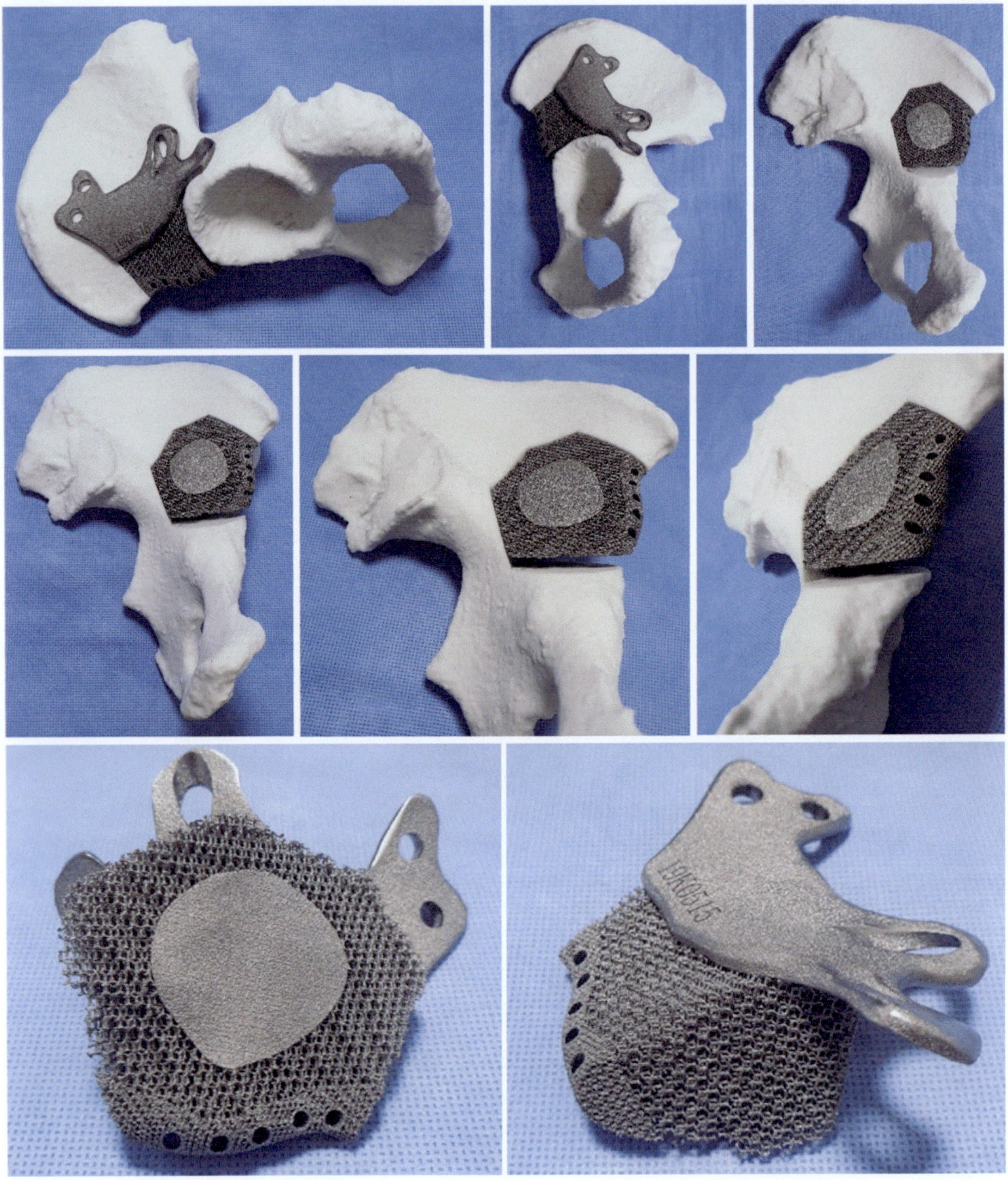

Fig. 8.9 Printed implant

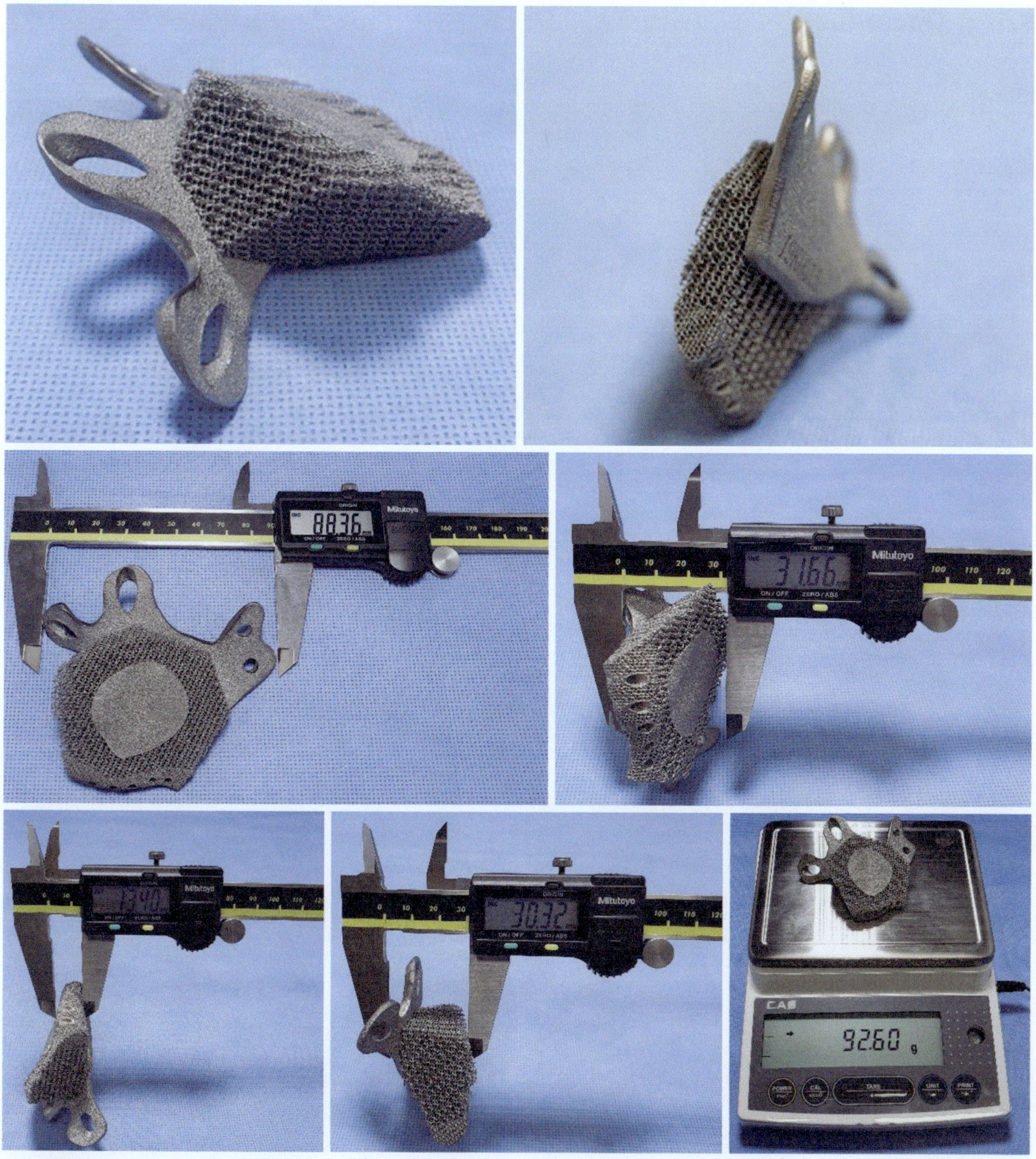

Fig. 8.9 (continued)

8.5 Operation

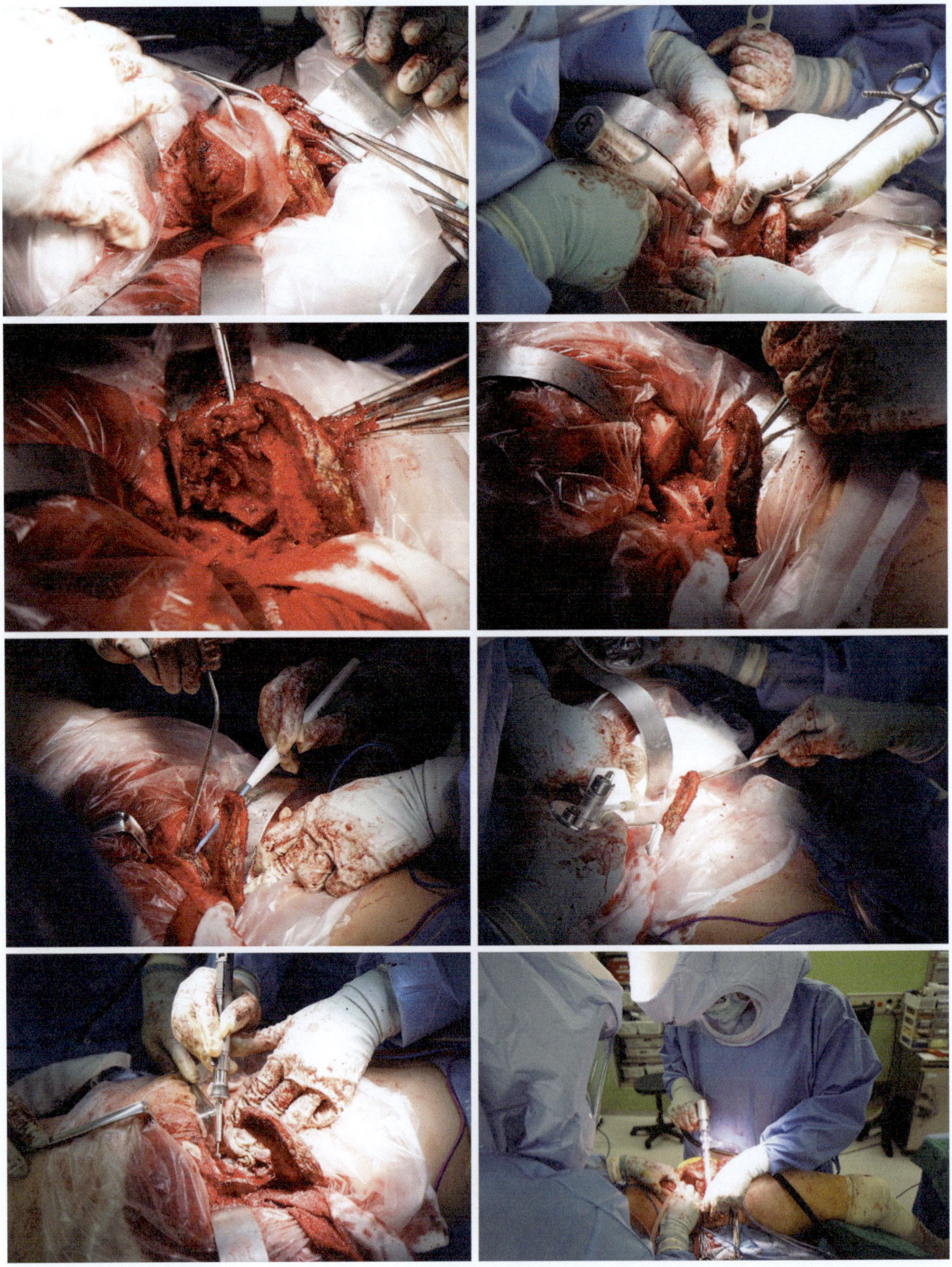

Fig. 8.10 Intraoperative photographs

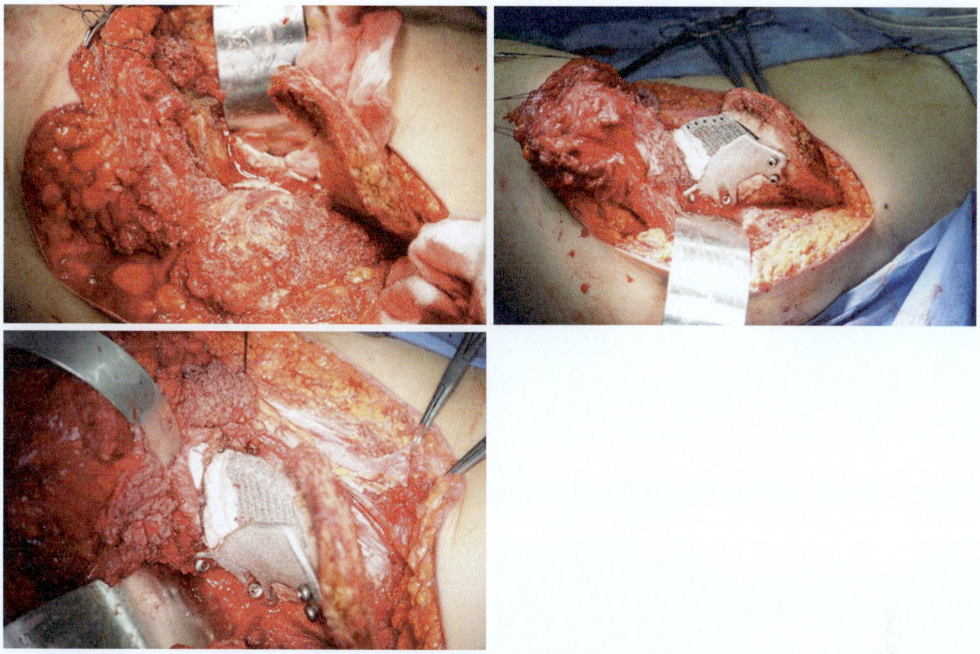

Fig. 8.11 Reinforced with PMMA bone cement of acetabular subchondral space

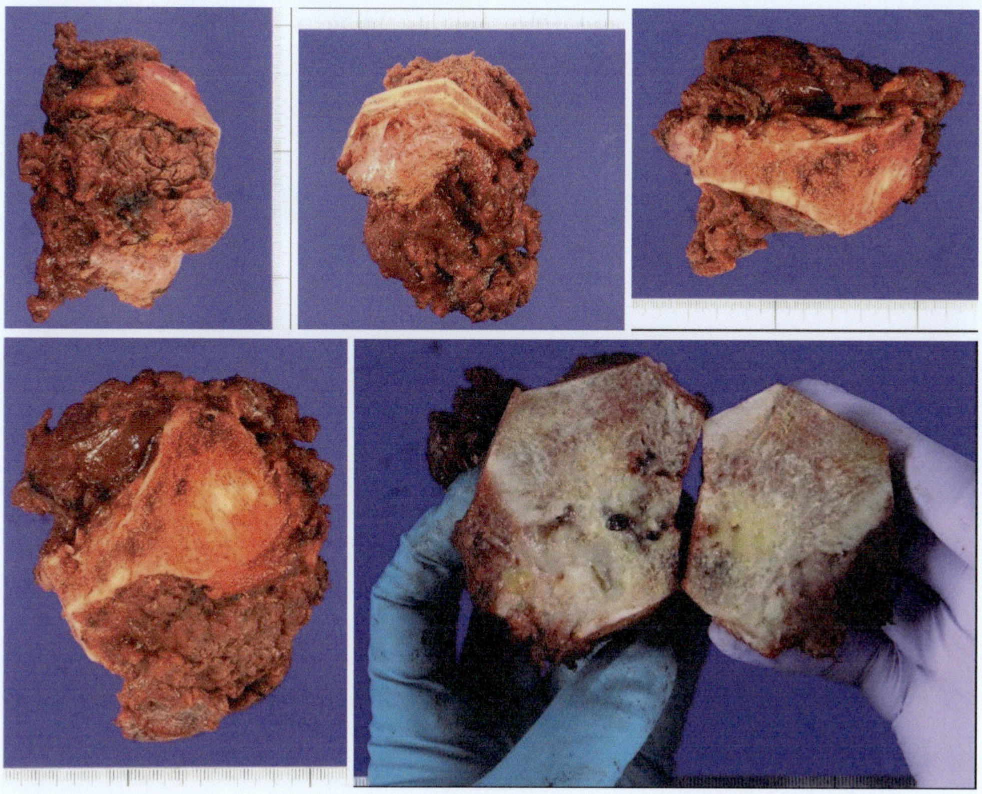

Fig. 8.12 Resected tumor

8.6 Postoperative Images

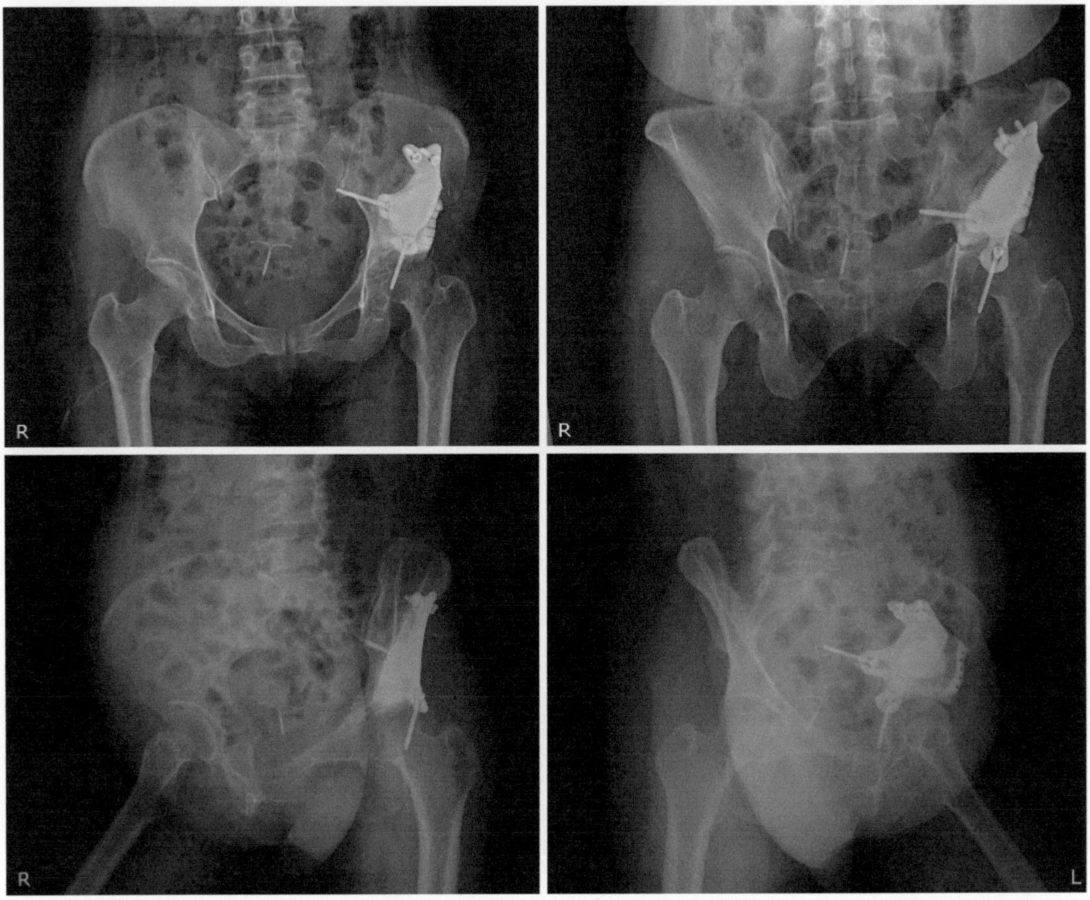

Fig. 8.13 Postoperative X-ray images

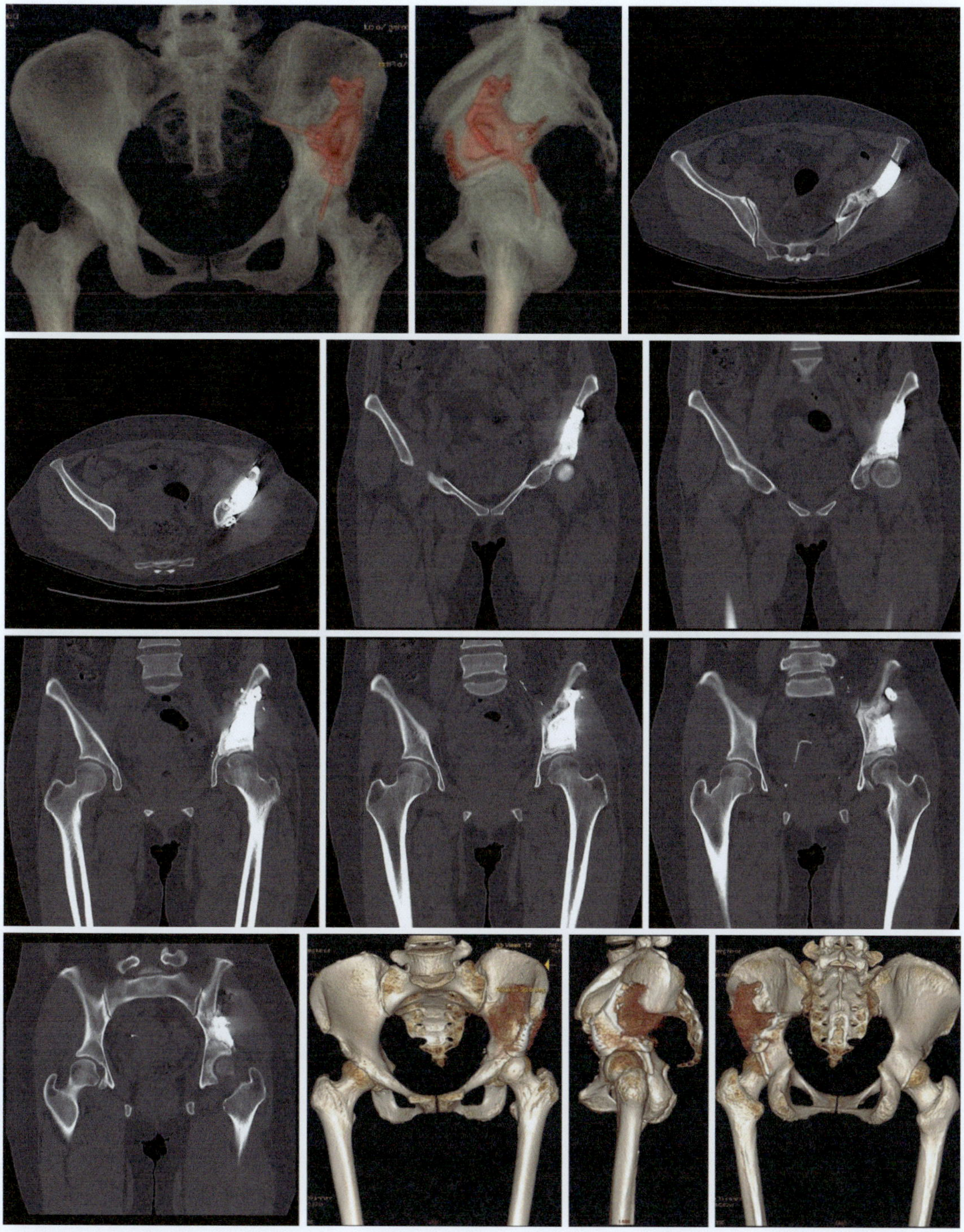

Fig. 8.14 Postoperative CT images

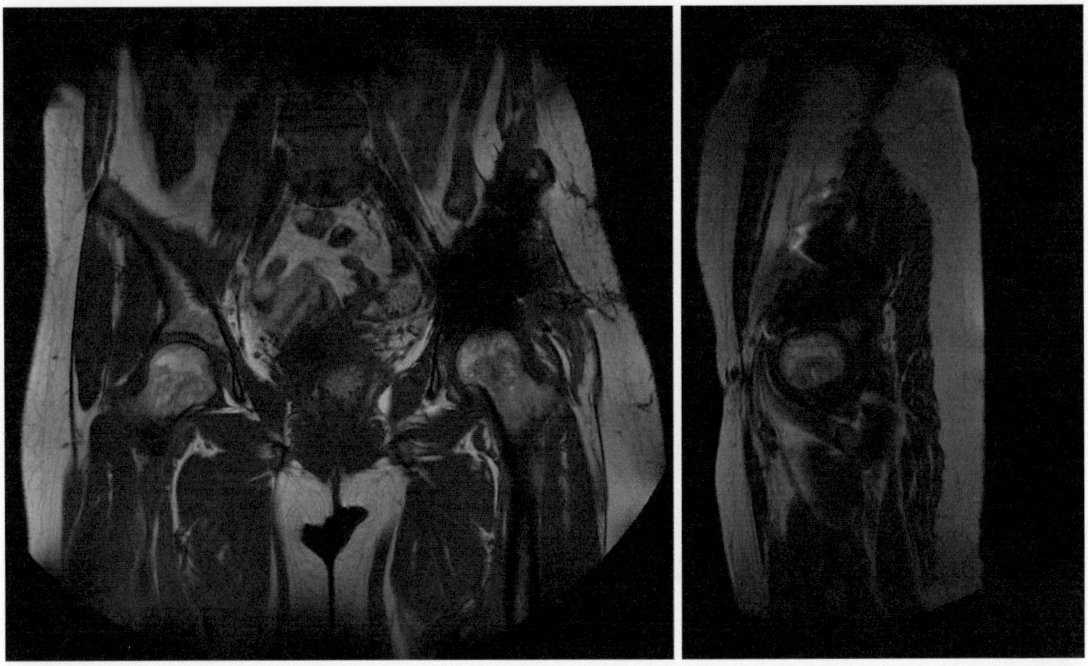

Fig. 8.15 Postoperative MRI images

Patient Case 9: Allograft Bone Shaping Guide

9

9.1 Patient Case 9

Age/sex	57/male
Location/site	Pelvis/right
Diagnosis	Myxoid liposarcoma Solitary bone metastasis
Preoperative symptom	No
Preoperative pain score	Resting: 0/activity: 0
BMI (height/weight)	29.16 (163.7/78.15)
Past history	Wide excision sarcoma of left thigh 5 years ago Chemotherapy and radiation therapy of left thigh Segmental resection of jejunum due to metastasis 2 years ago
Present illness	Right iliac bone lesion found accidentally on abdominal MRI

9.2 Preoperative Images

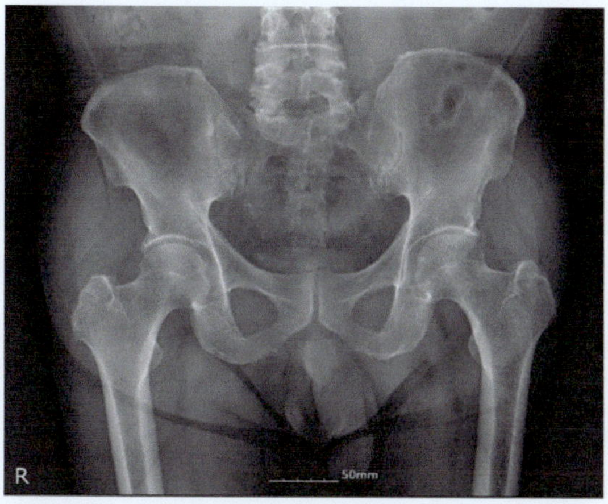

Fig. 9.1 Preoperative X-ray image no observation of tumor

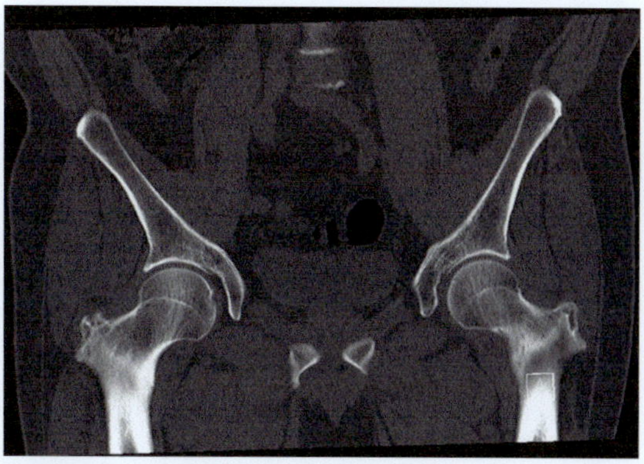

Fig. 9.2 Preoperative CT image: no observation of tumor

H.-G. Kang, *Clinical Atlas of 3D Printing Bone Reconstruction*,
https://doi.org/10.1007/978-981-16-2043-0_9

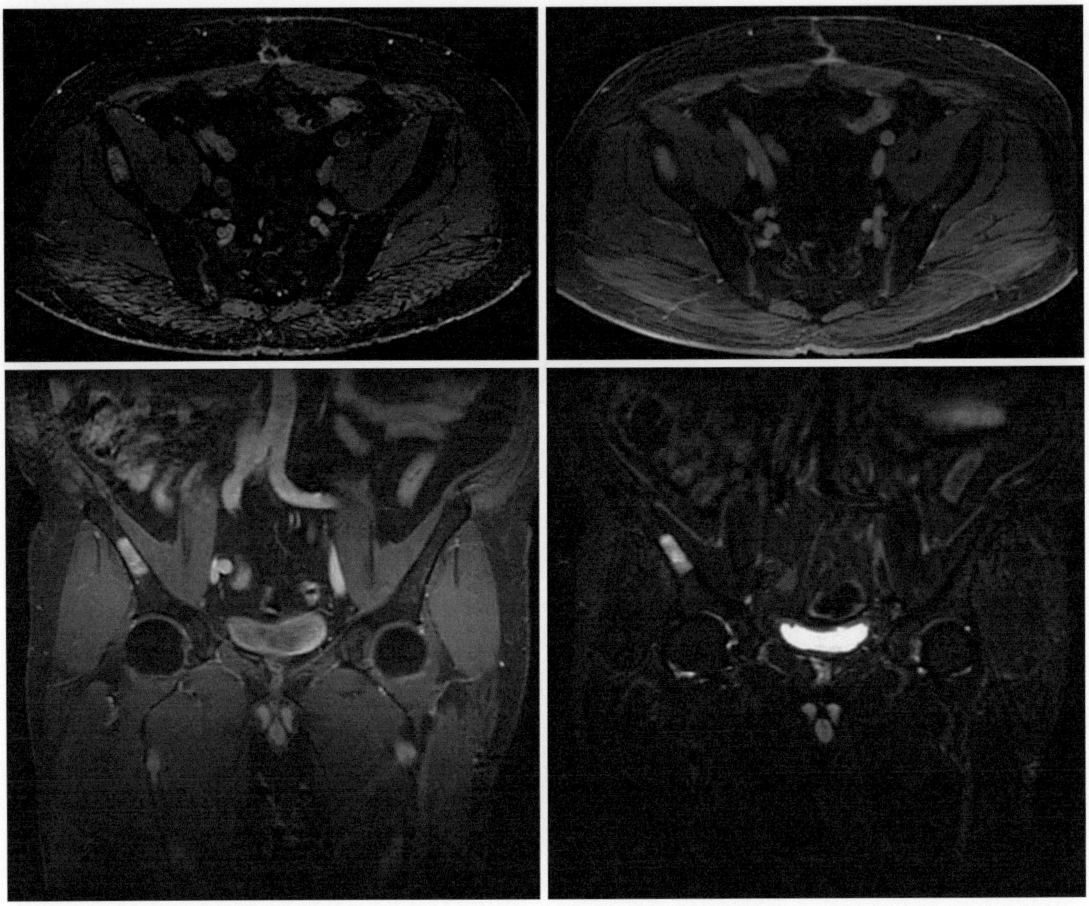

Fig. 9.3 Preoperative MRI images

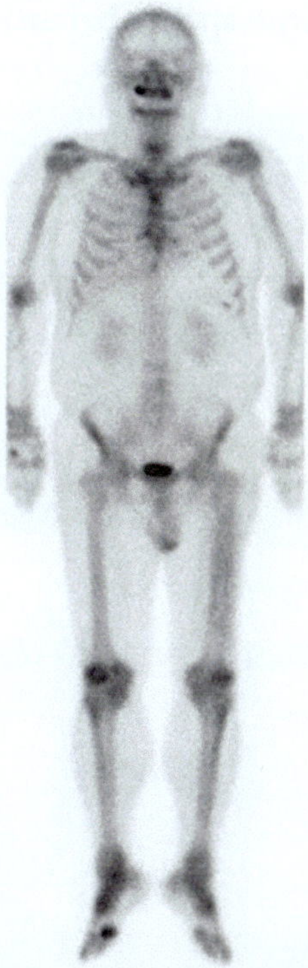

Fig. 9.4 Preoperative bone scan image: no observation of tumor

Fig. 9.5 Preoperative PET-CT image

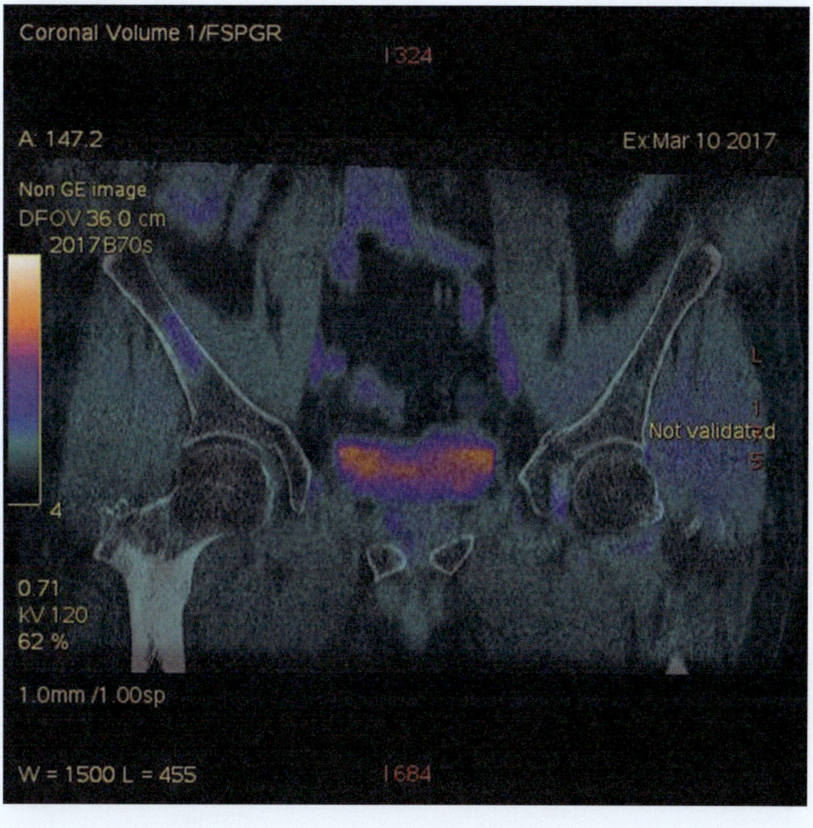

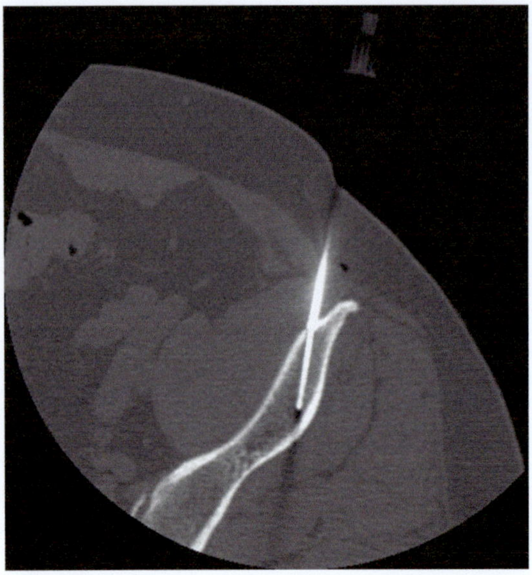

Fig. 9.6 CT guided biopsy under the MRI image reference

9.3 Planning of Surgery

3D-printed iliac tumor resection guide
Cavitary resection
3D-printed allograft bone shaping guide
Allograft bone reconstruction

9.4 Design and Fabrication

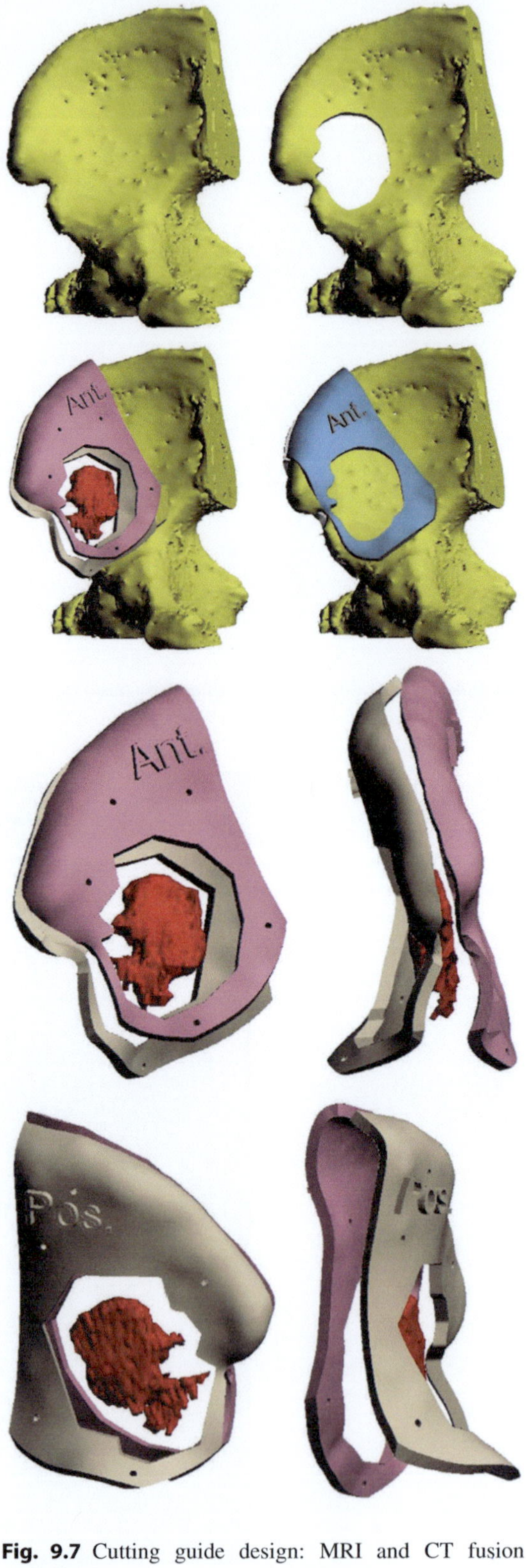

Fig. 9.7 Cutting guide design: MRI and CT fusion modeling

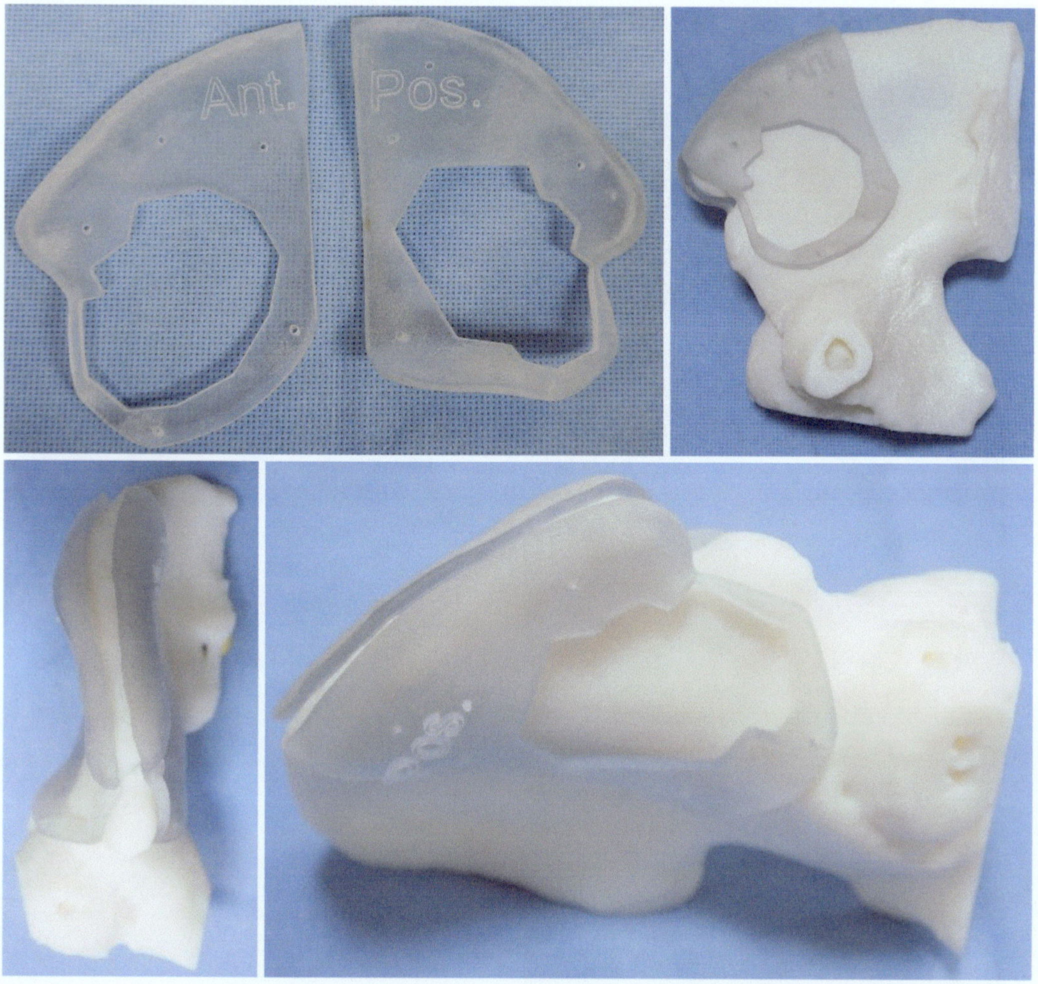

Fig. 9.8 Printed Cutting guide: It is difficult to saw if you make a lot of cutting angles

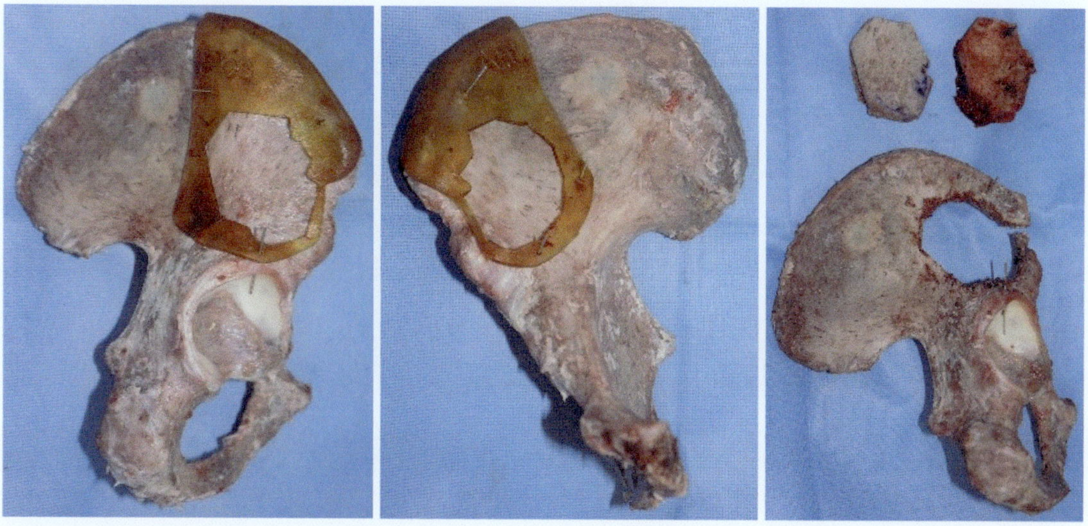

Fig. 9.9 3D-printed allograft bone shaping guide

9.5 Operation

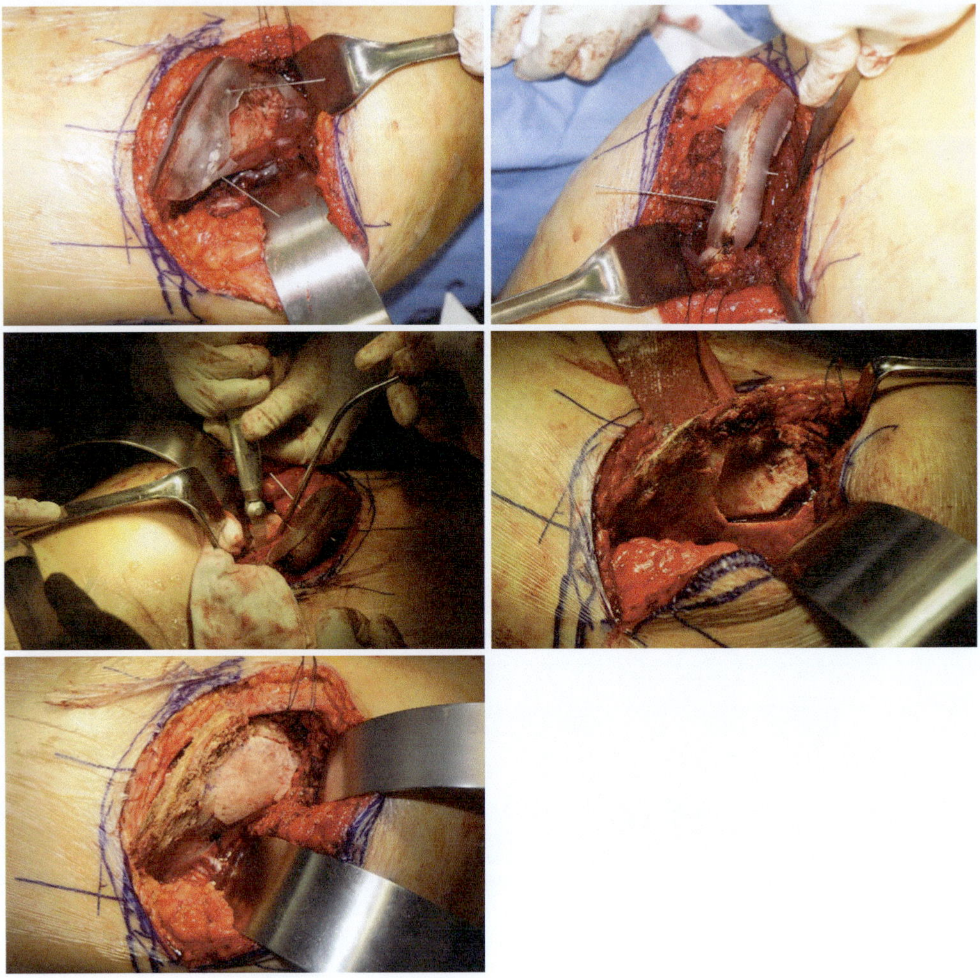

Fig. 9.10 Intraoperative photographs

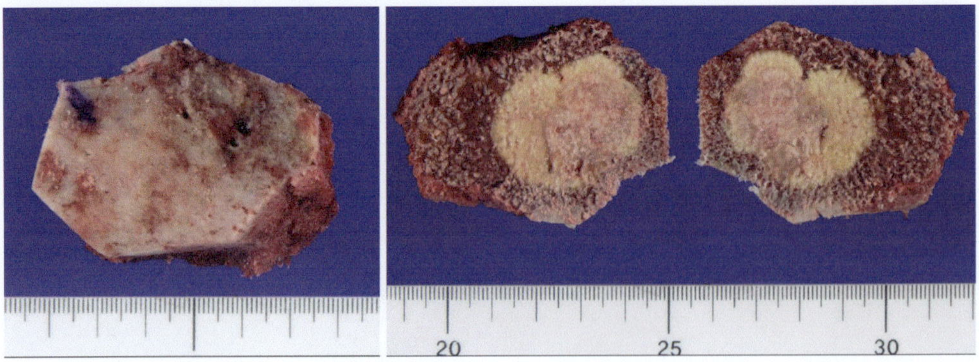

Fig. 9.11 Resected tumor

9.6 Postoperative Images

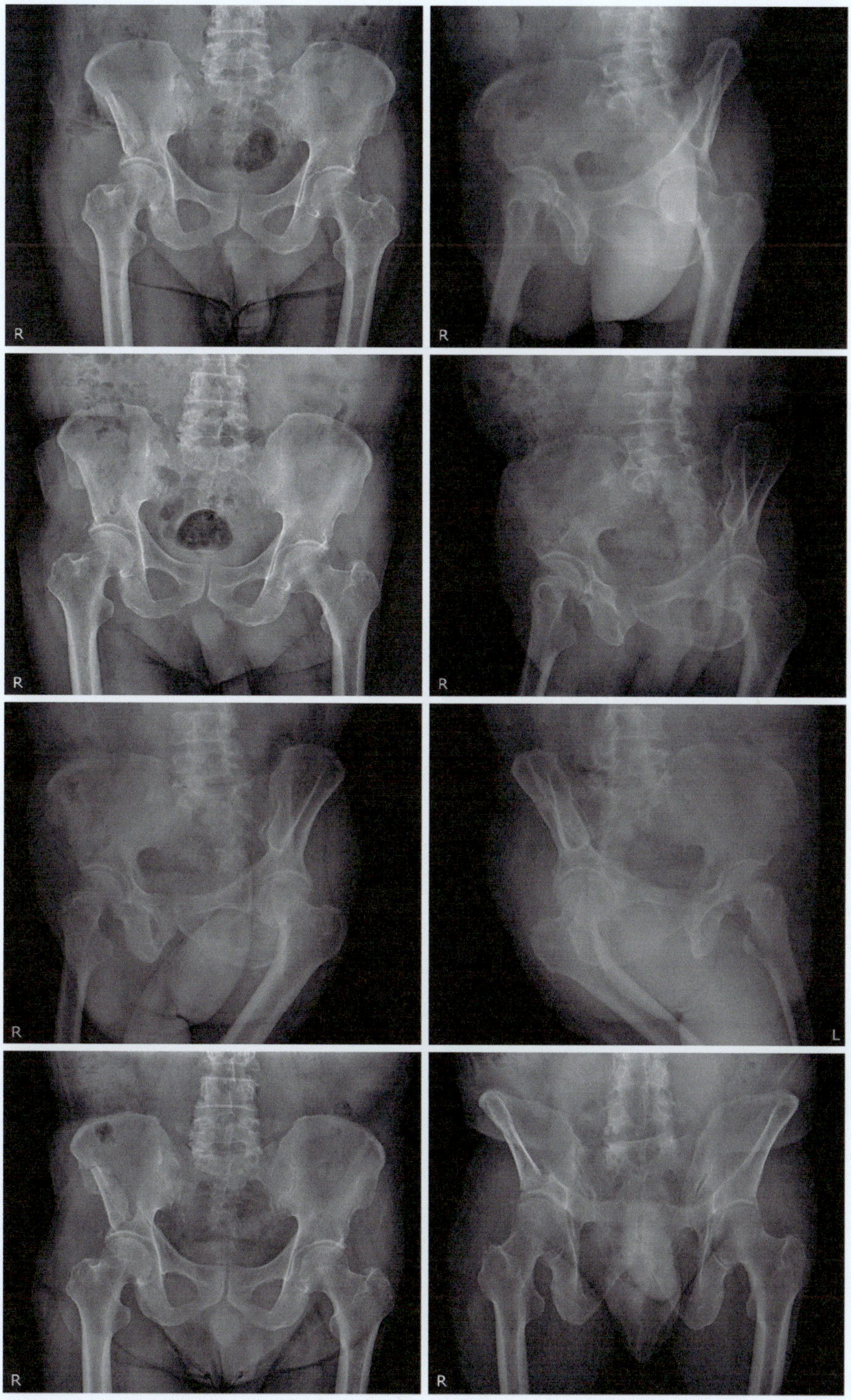

Fig. 9.12 Postoperative X-ray images

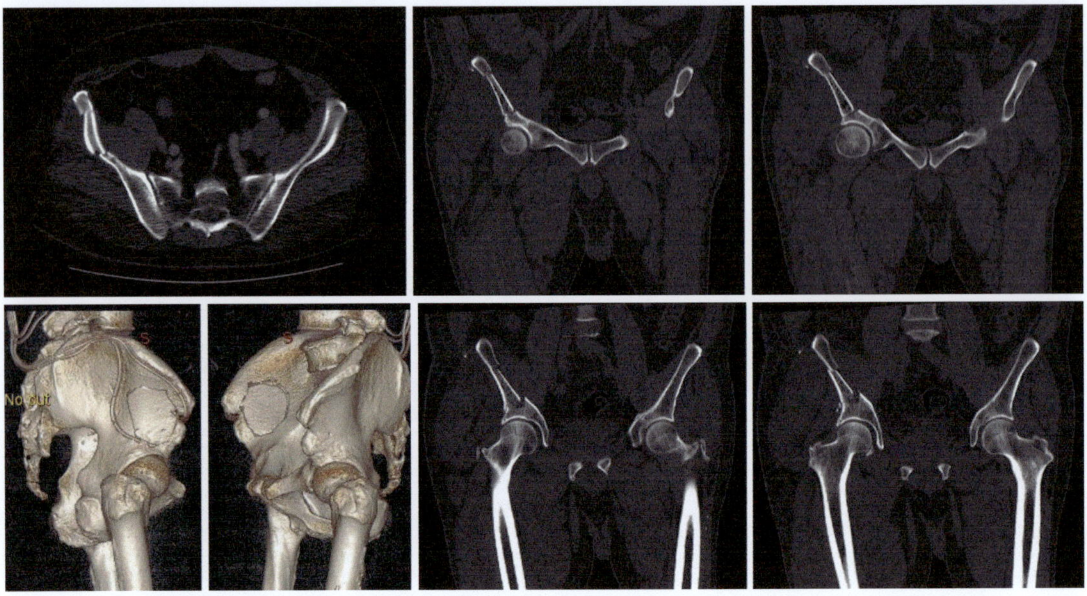

Fig. 9.13 Postoperative CT images

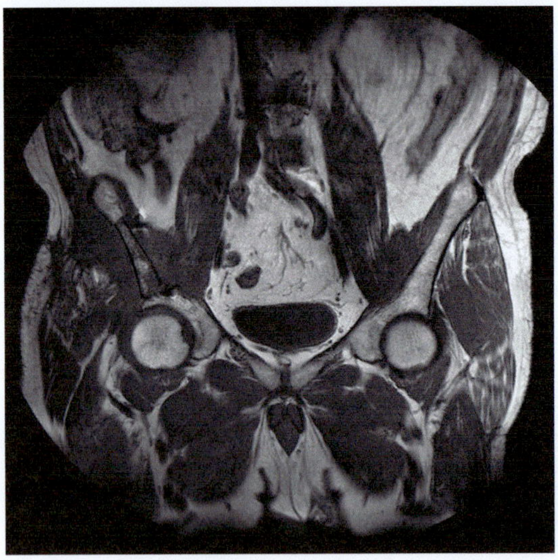

Fig. 9.14 Postoperative MRI image

10 Patient Case 10: Pubis Preventing Genital Deformity and Hernia

10.1 Patient Case 10

Age/sex	56/male
Location/site	Pelvis/right
Diagnosis	Chondrosarcoma, grade 2
Preoperative symptom	Palpable mass right inguinal area
Preoperative pain score	Resting pain 0/Ambulation pain 3
BMI (height/weight)	22.30 (180.7/72.8)
Past history	Taking prostatitis medication
Present illness	Bone tumor found accidentally during examination

10.2 Preoperative Images

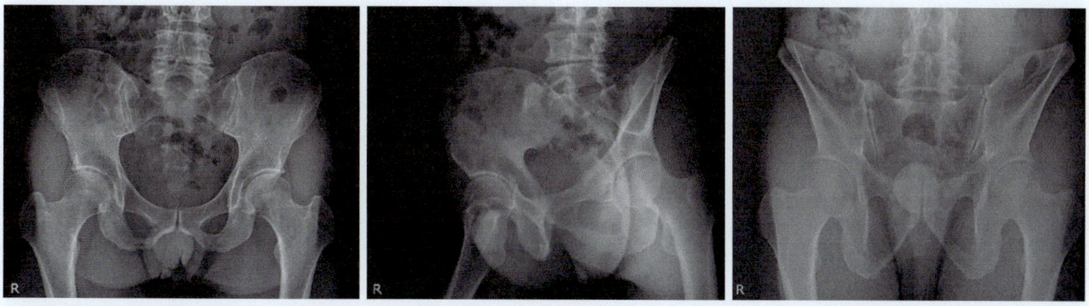

Fig. 10.1 Preoperative X-ray images

H.-G. Kang, *Clinical Atlas of 3D Printing Bone Reconstruction*,
https://doi.org/10.1007/978-981-16-2043-0_10

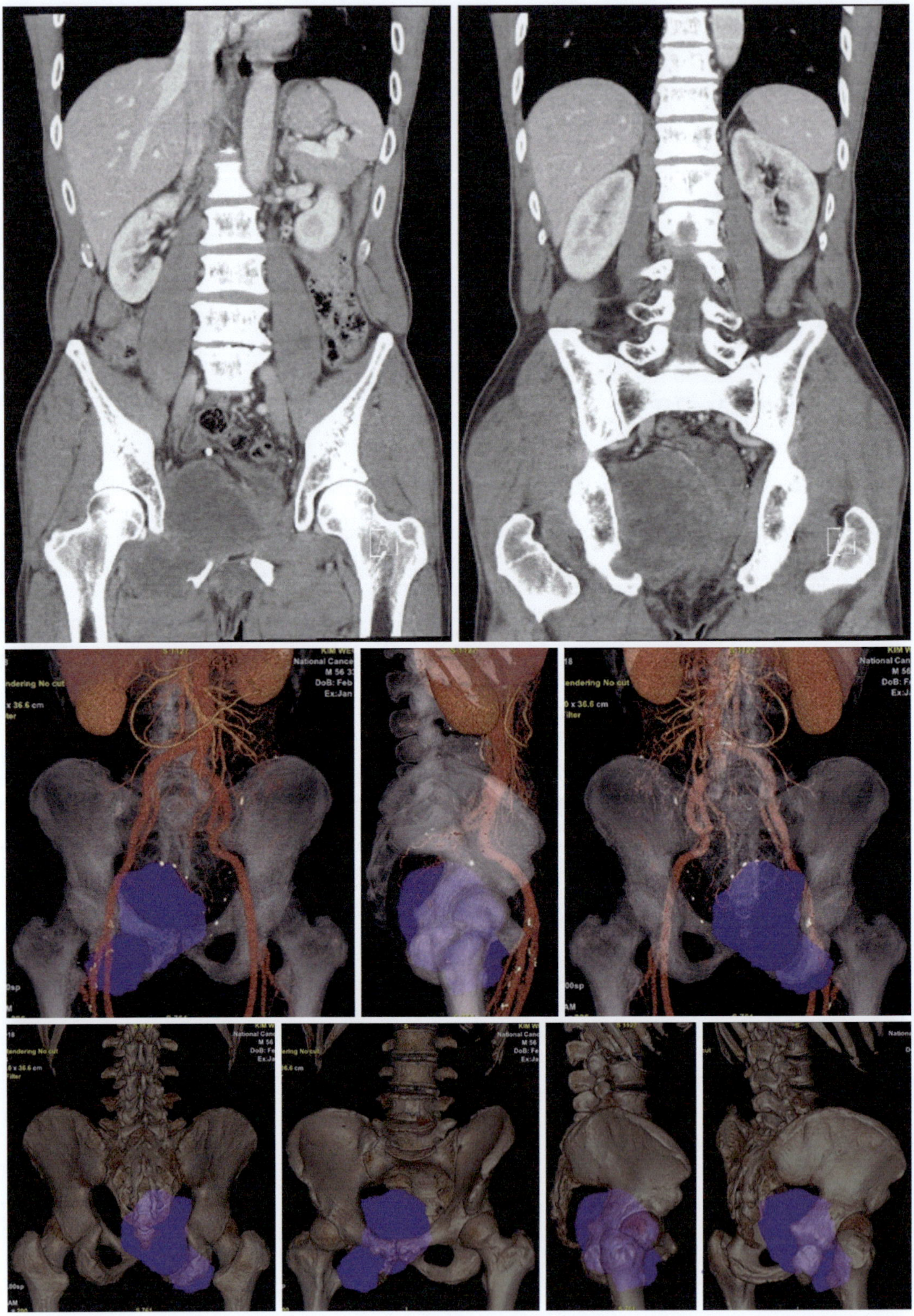

Fig. 10.2 Preoperative CT images

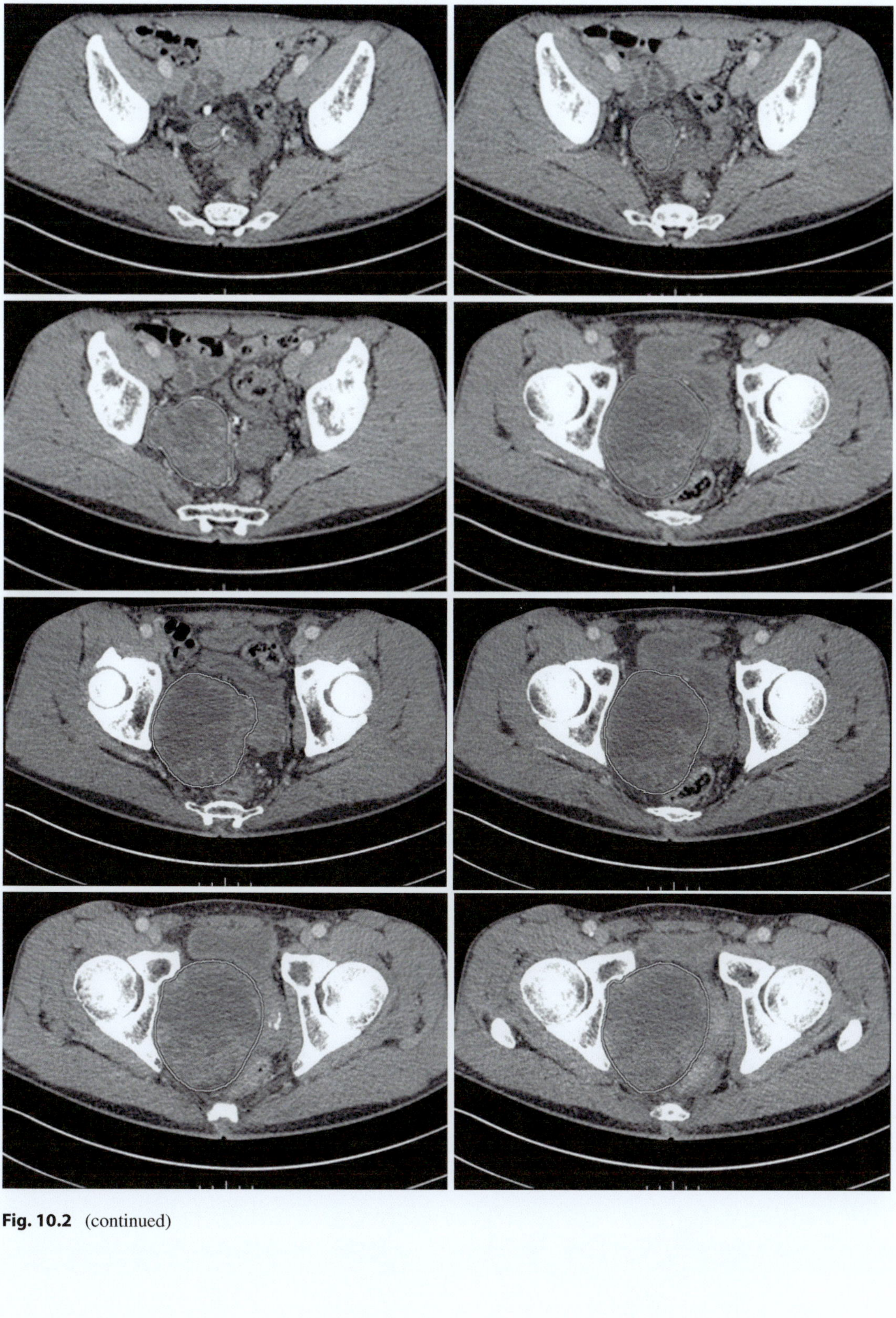

Fig. 10.2 (continued)

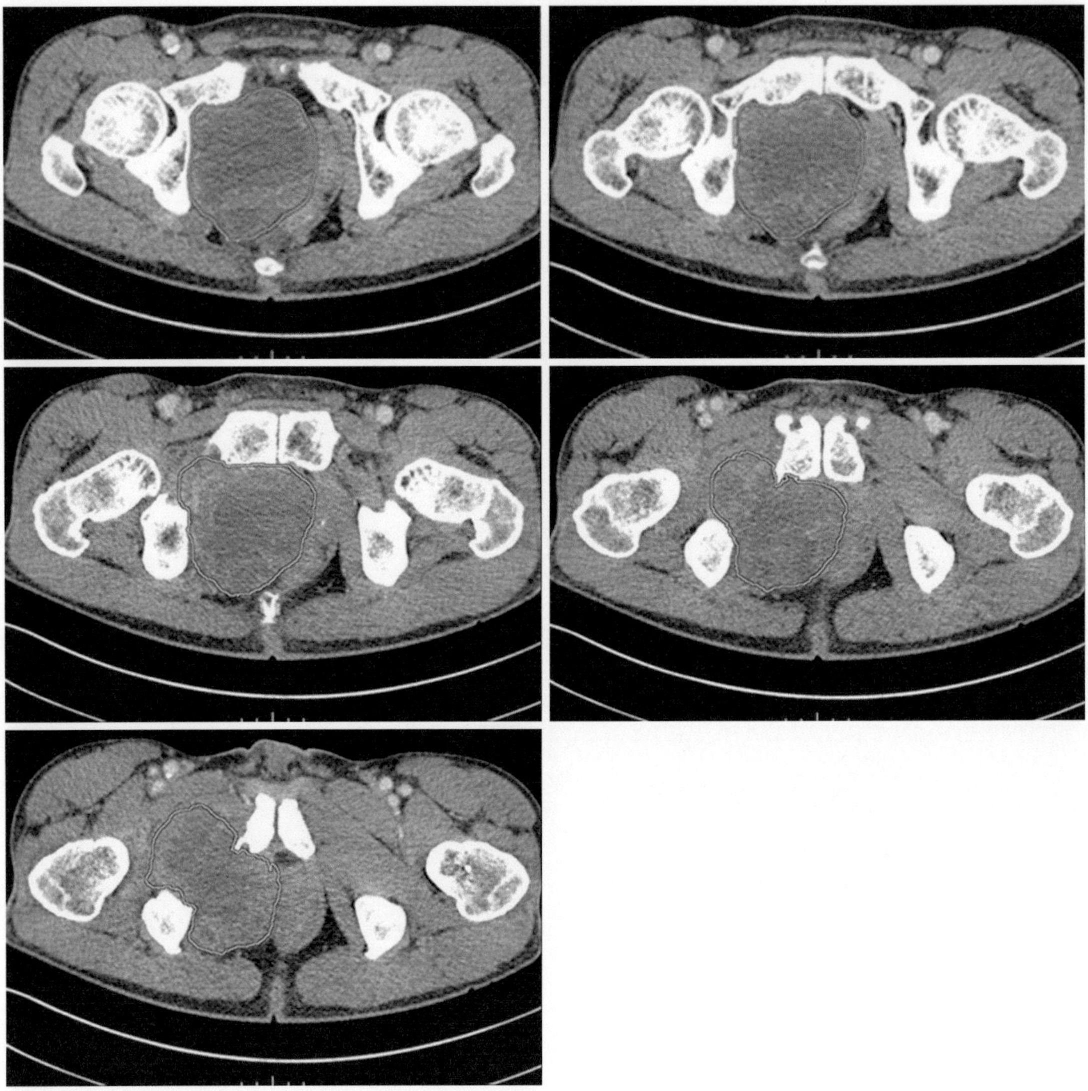

Fig. 10.2 (continued)

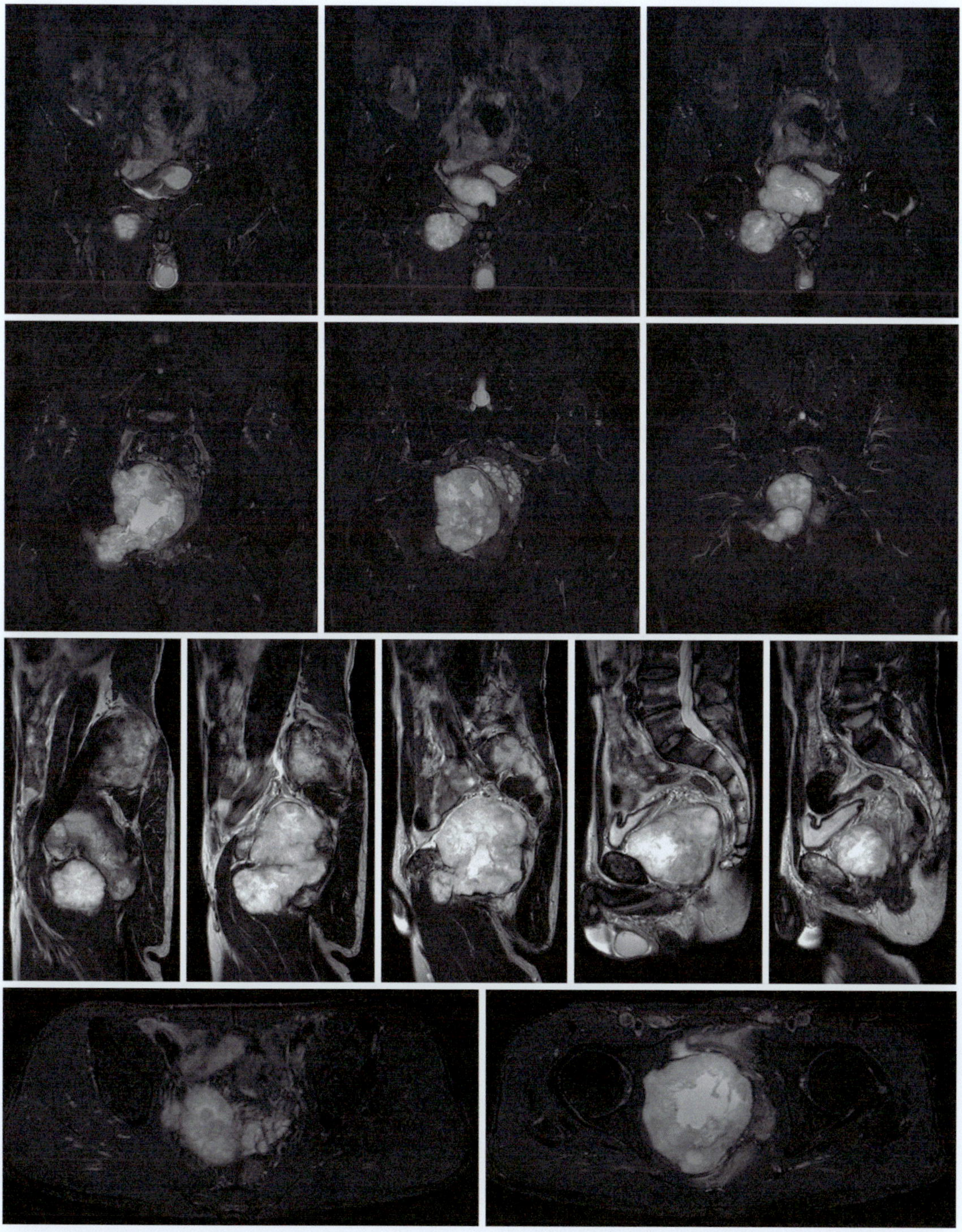

Fig. 10.3 Preoperative MRI images

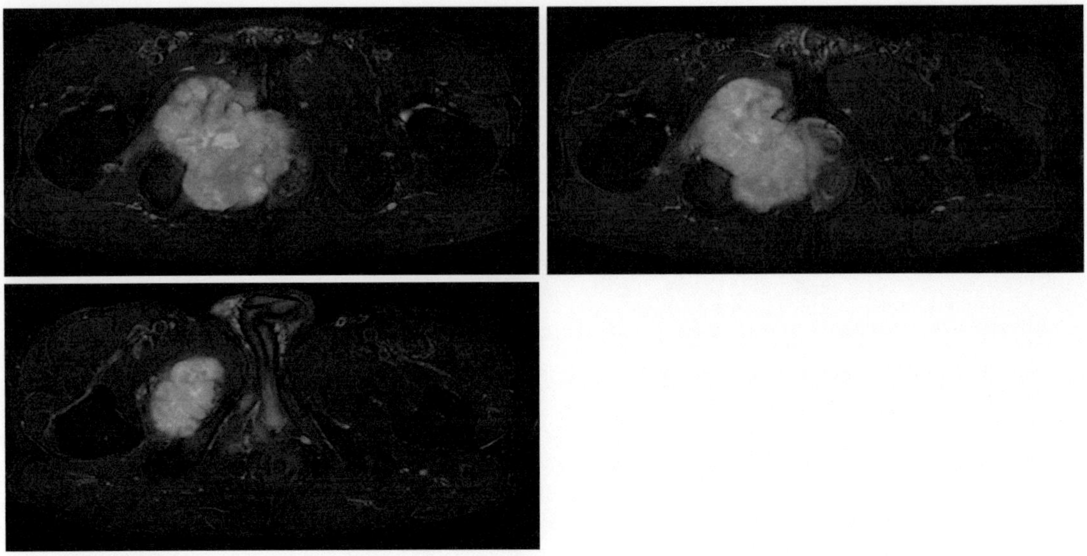

Fig. 10.3 (continued)

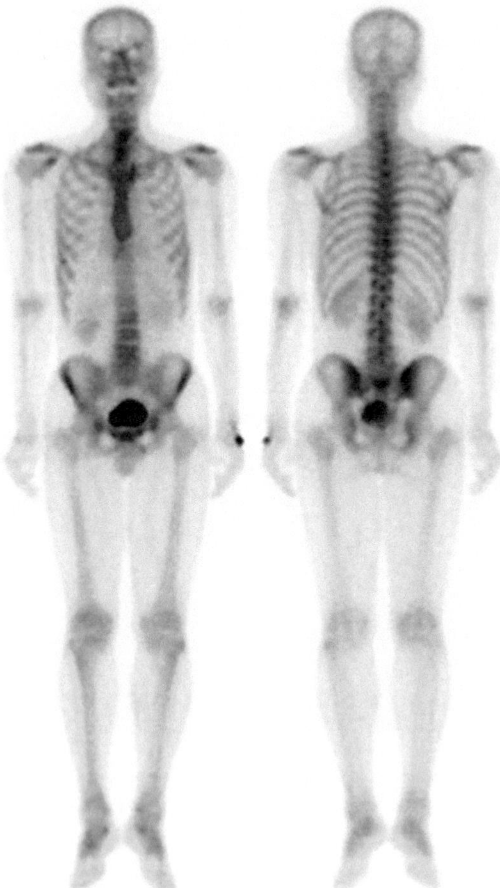

Fig. 10.4 Preoperative bone scan images

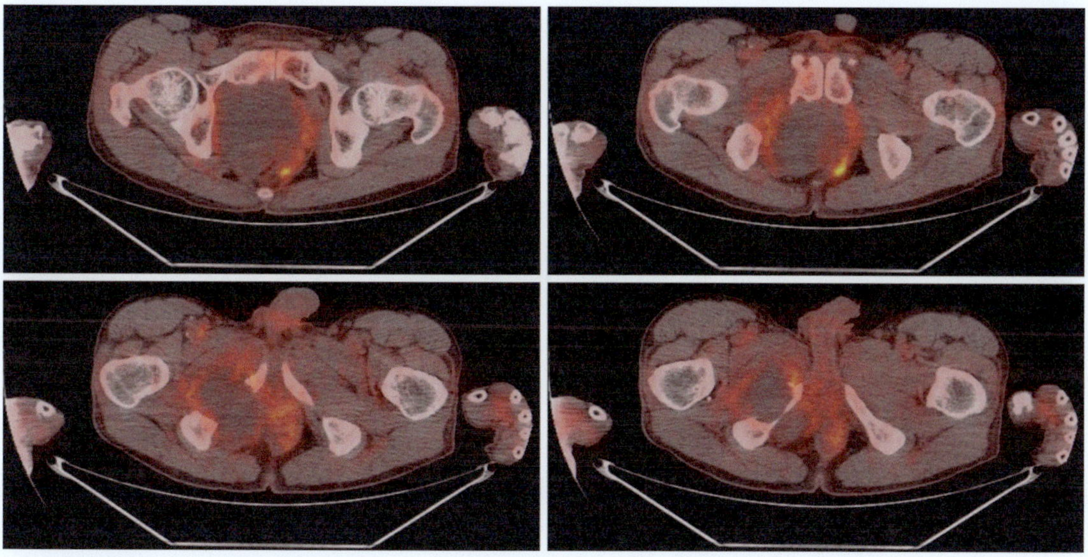

Fig. 10.5 Preoperative PET-CT images

10.3 Planning of Surgery

Hip joint preserving

Pubis resection with 3D printing guide

Ischium resection at ischial tuberosity-free hand cutting

3D printed pubic implant

10.4 Design and Fabrication

- Implant measurement
- Implant weight (g): 153.71
- Size (mm): 113

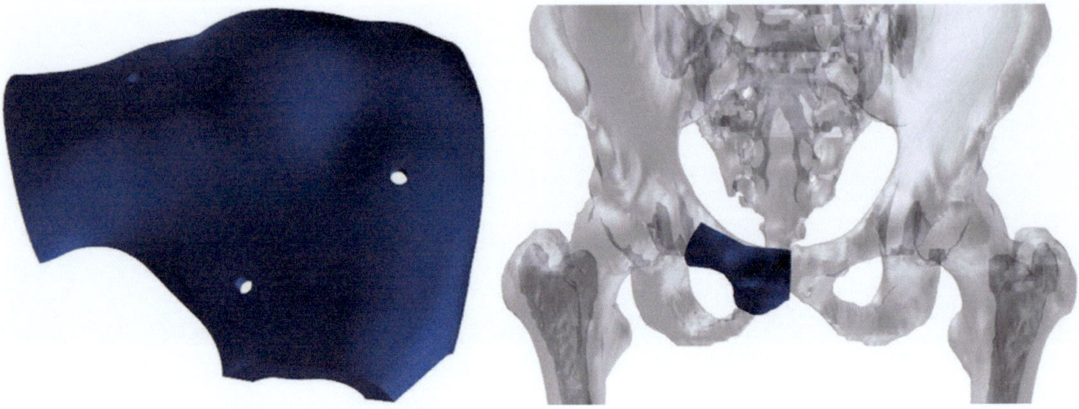

Fig. 10.6 Cutting guide design

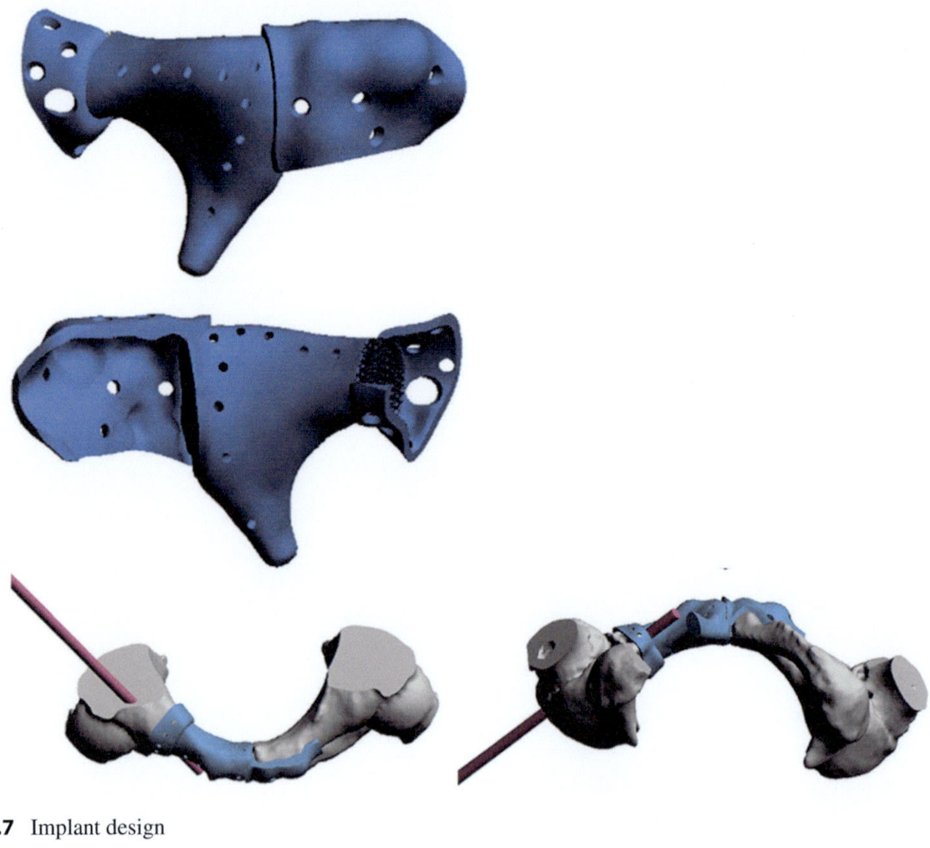

Fig. 10.7 Implant design

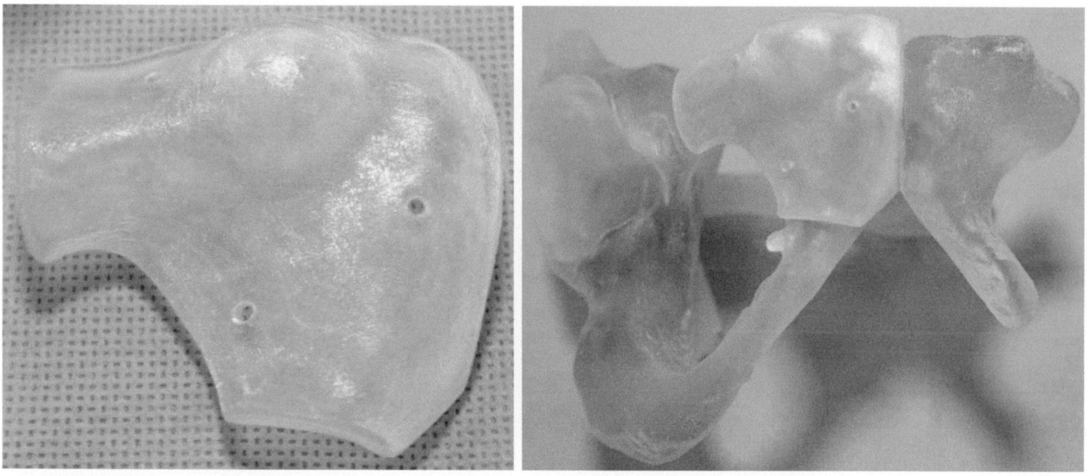

Fig. 10.8 Printed cutting guide

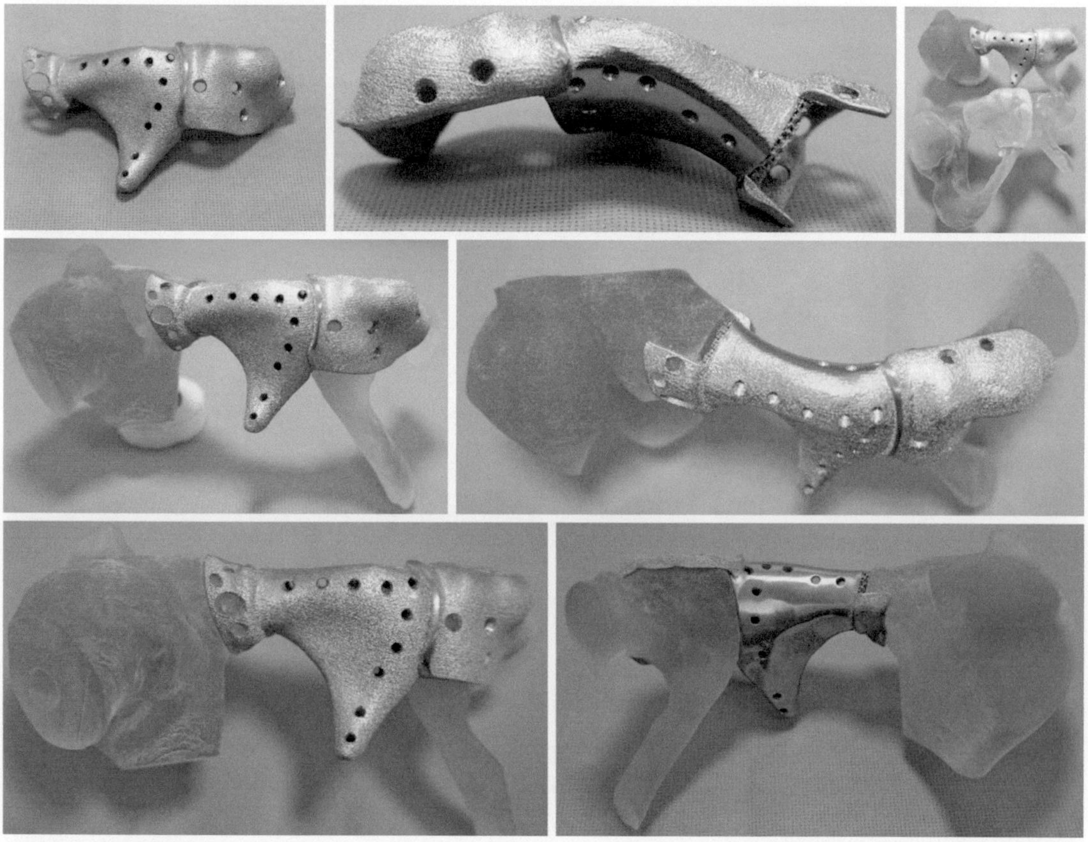

Fig. 10.9 Printed implant

10.5 Operation

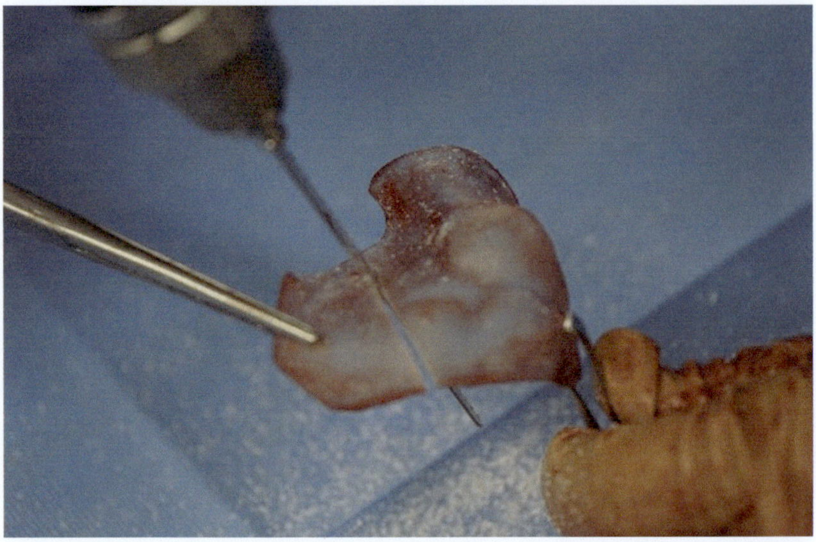

Fig. 10.10 Intra-operative photograph: if the size of the cutting guide is difficult to bone attach, cut it partially

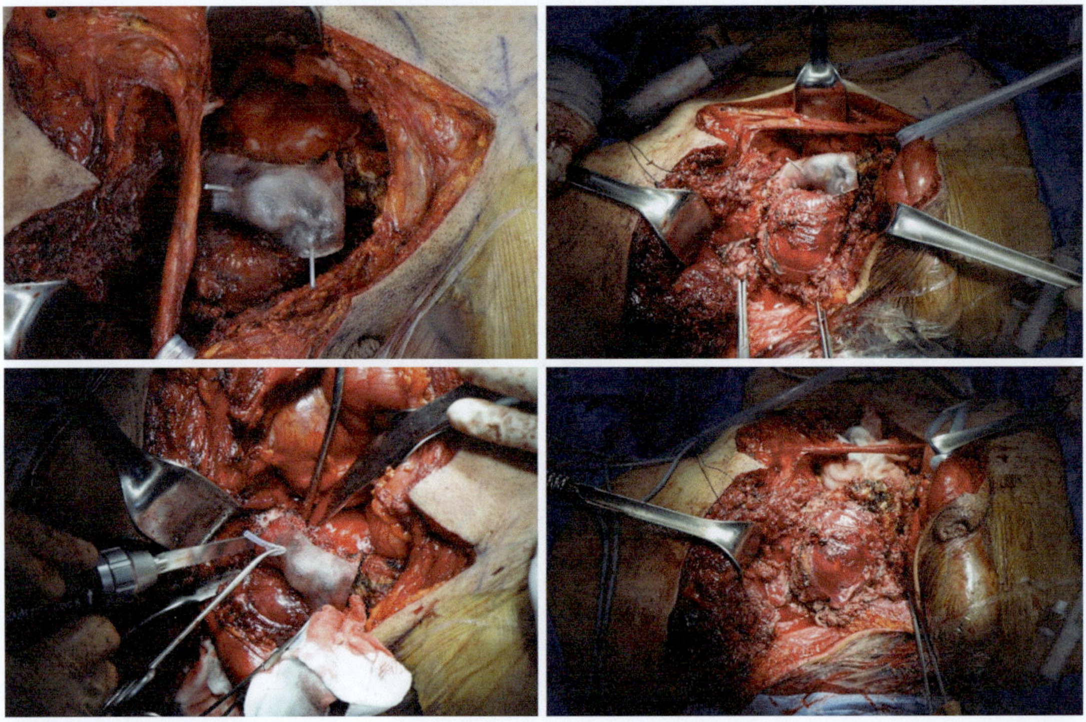

Fig. 10.11 Intraoperative photographs

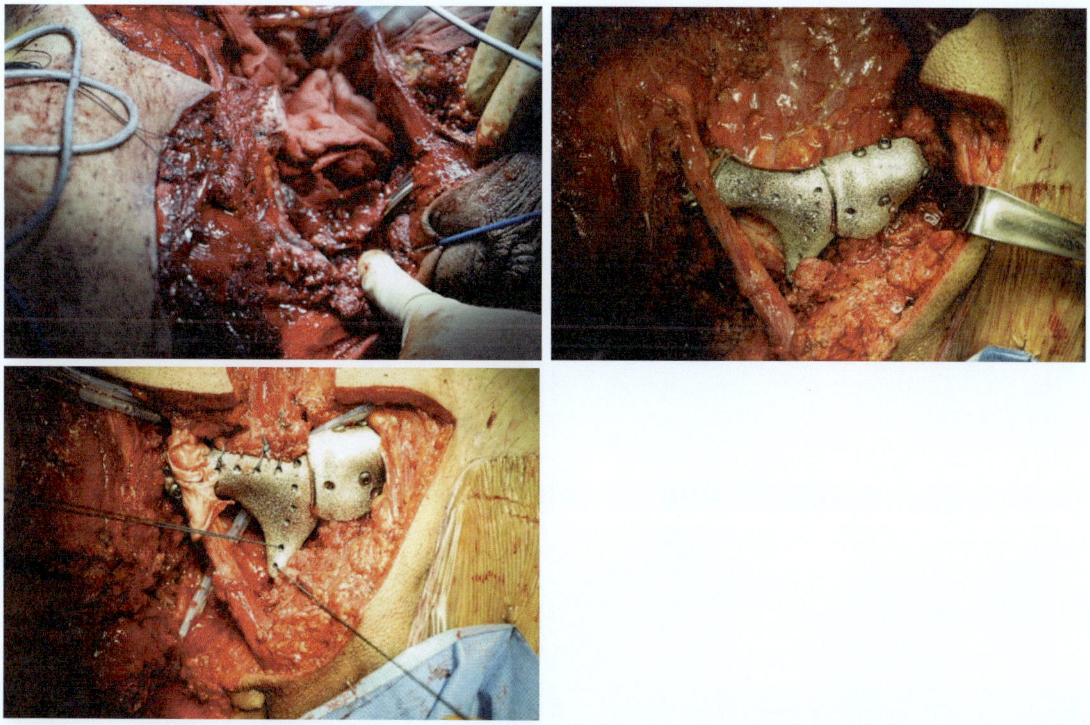

Fig. 10.11 (continued)

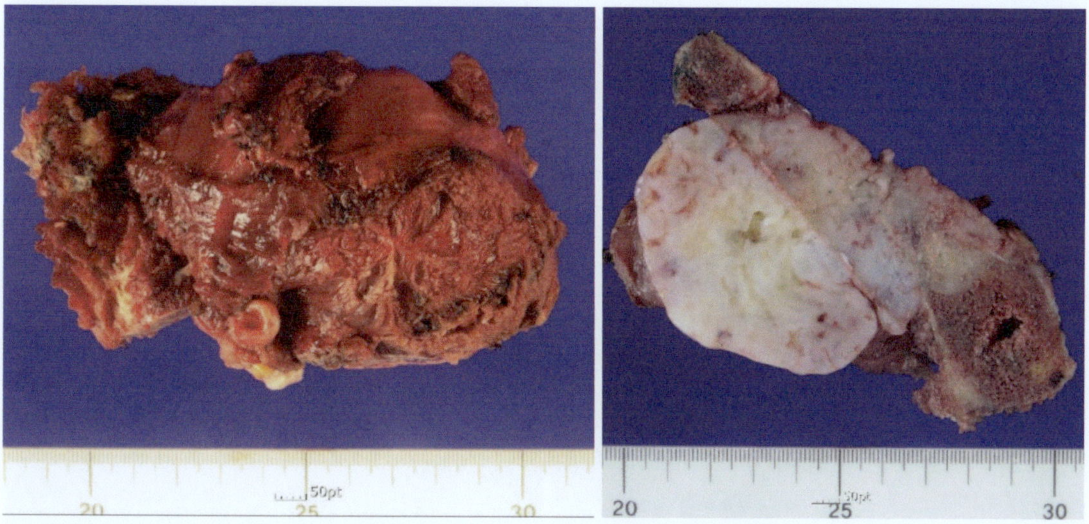

Fig. 10.12 Resected tumor

10.6 Postoperative Images

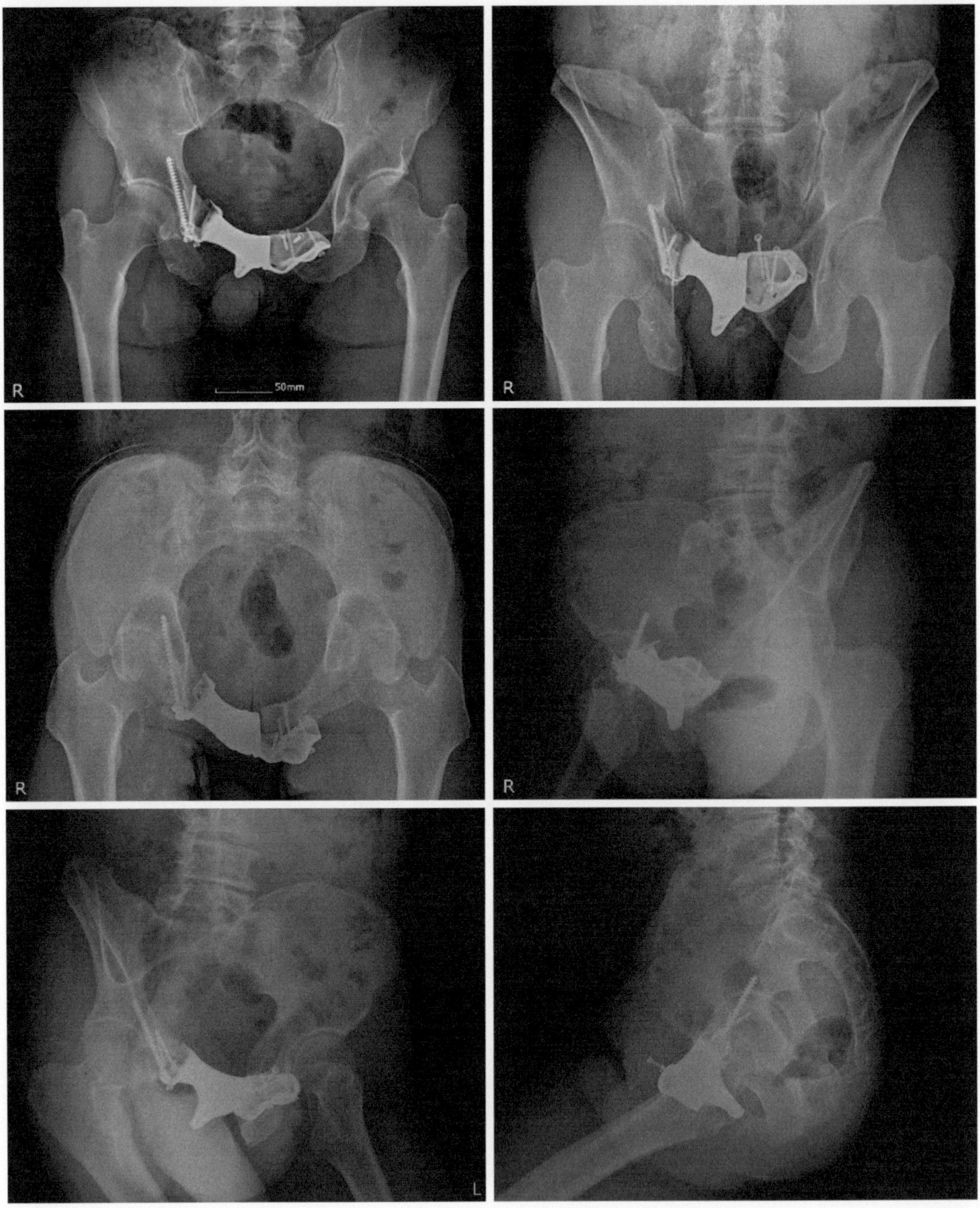

Fig. 10.13 Postoperative X-ray images

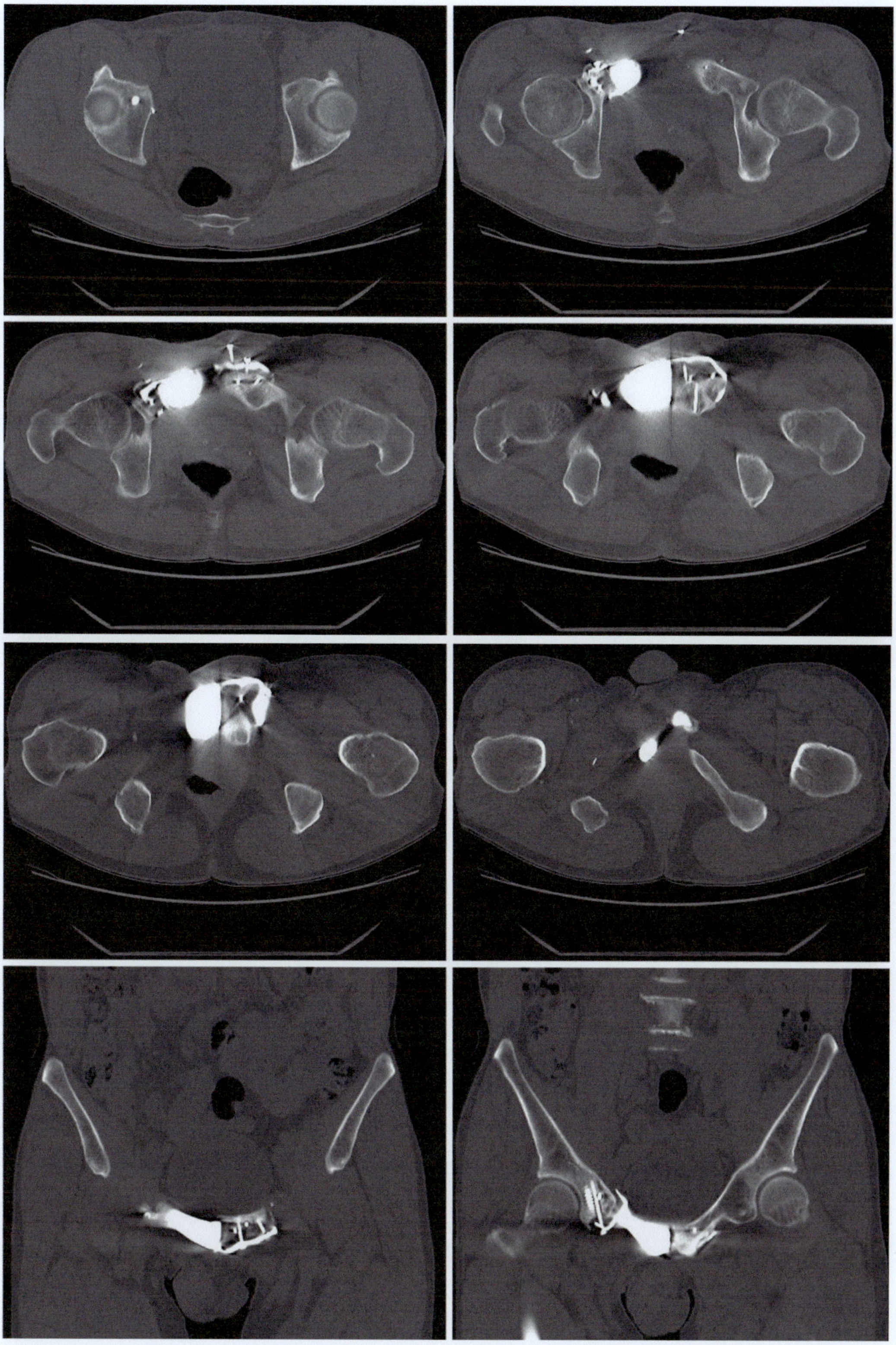

Fig. 10.14 Postoperative CT images

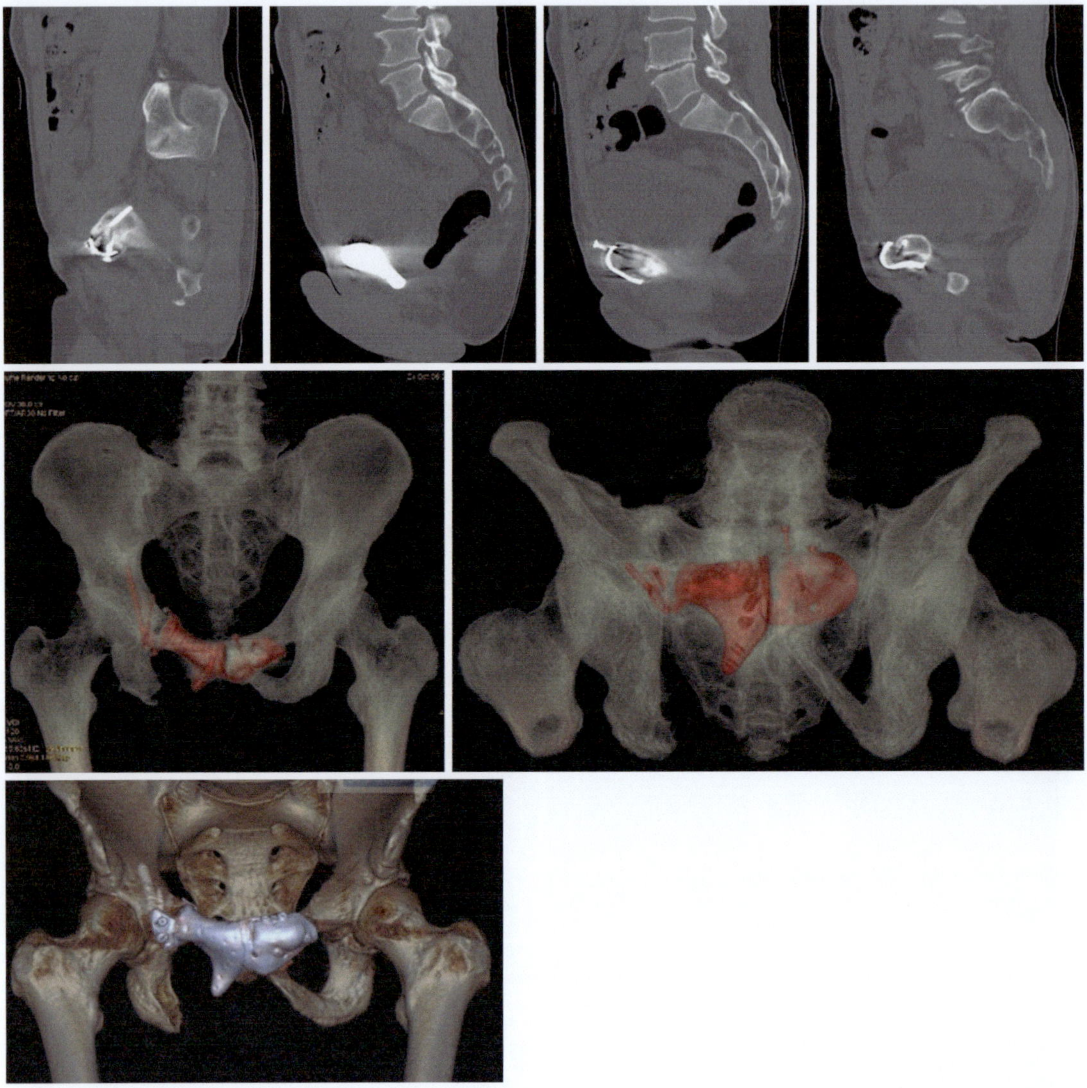

Fig. 10.14 (continued)

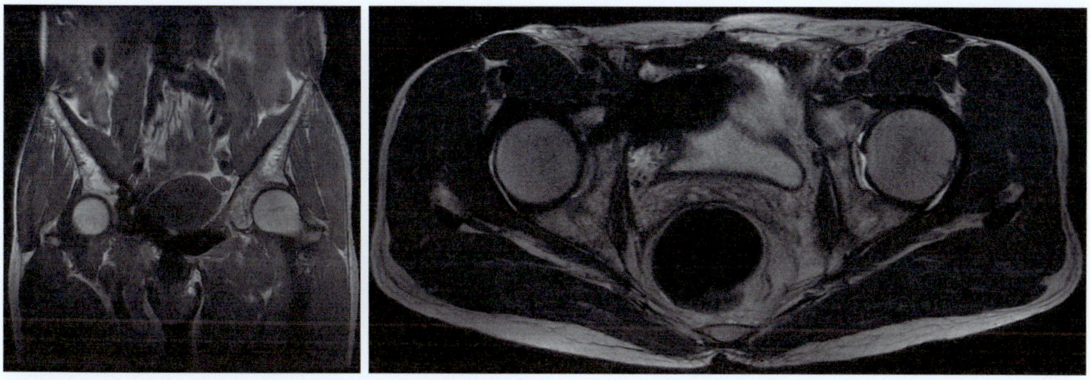

Fig. 10.15 Postoperative MRI images

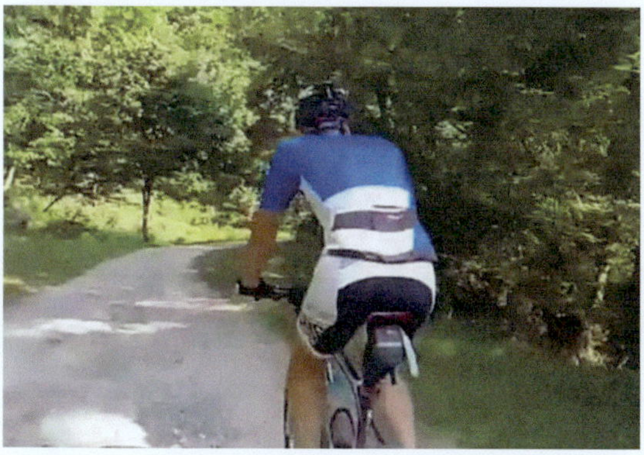

Fig. 10.16 Active sports life

Patient Case 11: Pubis with Acetabular Preservation

11

11.1 Patient Case 11

Age/sex	22/male
Location/site	Pelvis, pubis/left
Diagnosis	Ewing sarcoma
Preoperative symptom	Left inguinal pain
Preoperative pain score	Resting 2/Activity 5
BMI (height/weight)	13.94 (163.6/37.3)
Past history	Ewing sarcoma on right radius 13 years ago Skull bone metastasis 10 years ago Chemotherapy and radiation therapy end 8 years ago Metastasis confirmed by sono-guided biopsy of left pubic tumor
Present illness	Preoperative two times chemotherapy

11.2 Preoperative Images

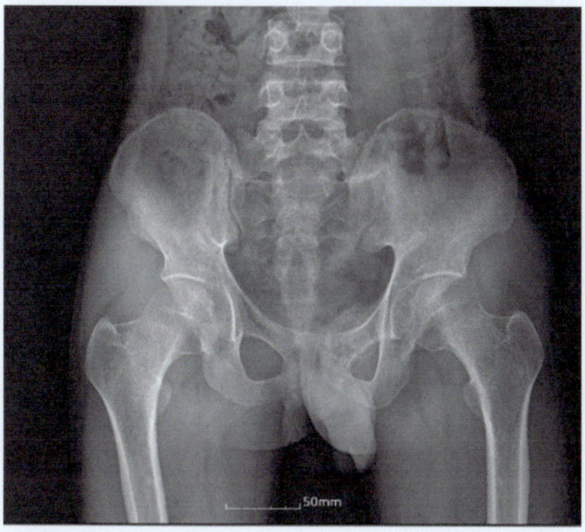

Fig. 11.1 Preoperative X-ray image

H.-G. Kang, *Clinical Atlas of 3D Printing Bone Reconstruction*,
https://doi.org/10.1007/978-981-16-2043-0_11

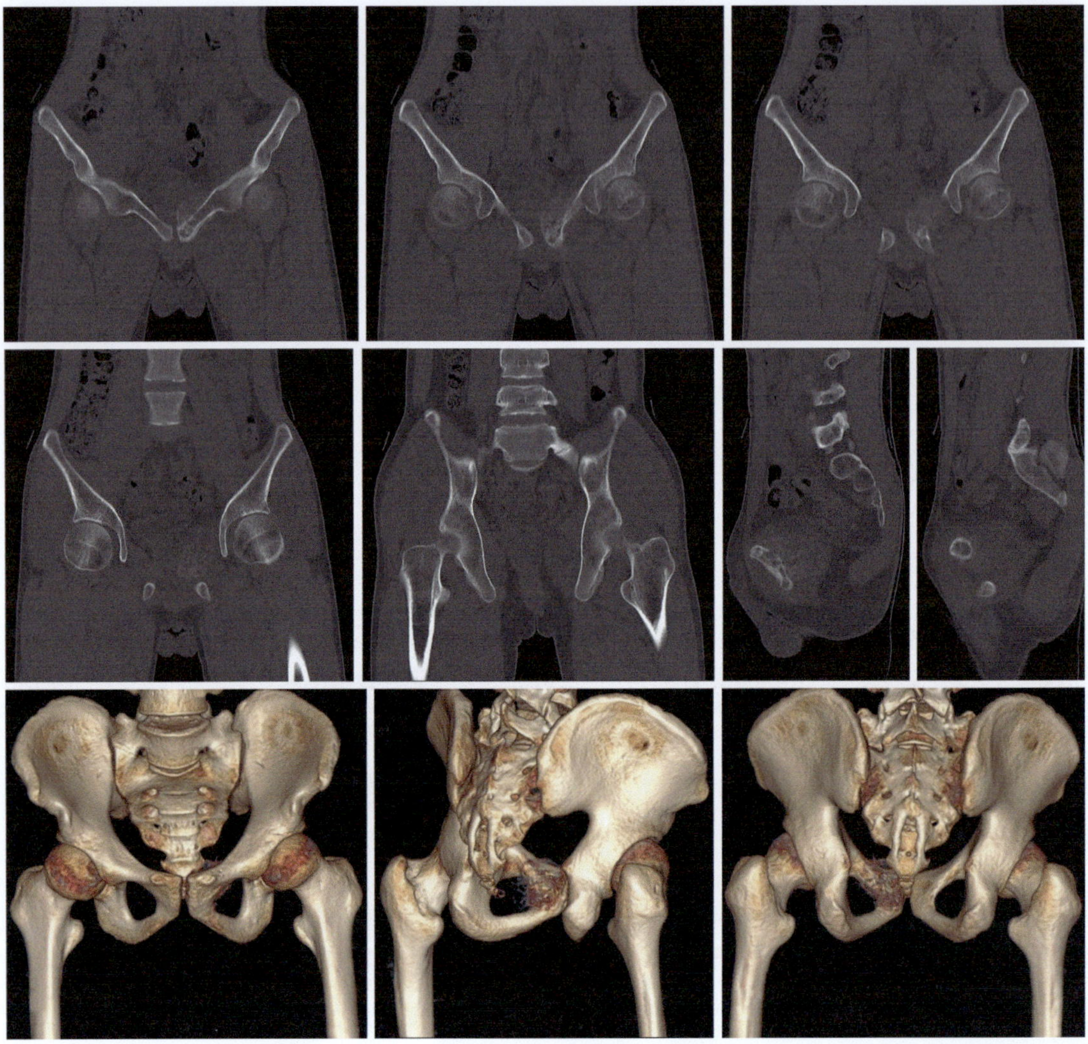

Fig. 11.2 Preoperative CT images

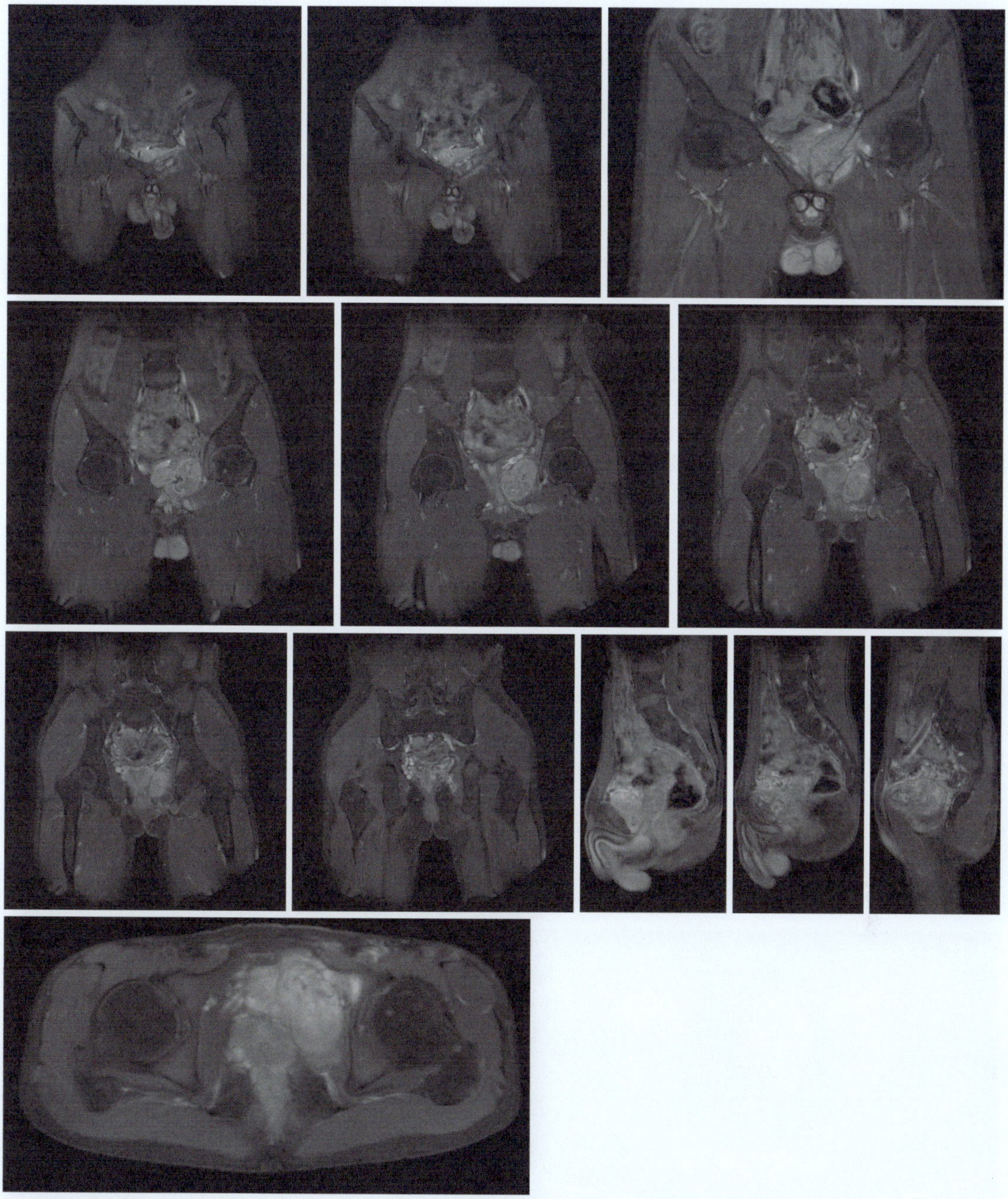

Fig. 11.3 Preoperative MRI images

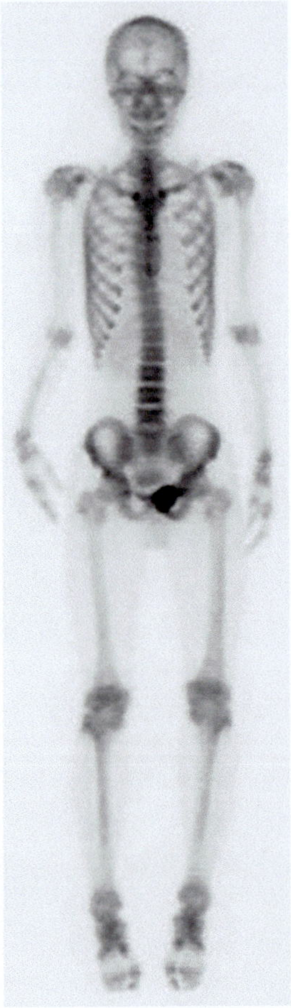

Fig. 11.4 Preoperative bone scan image

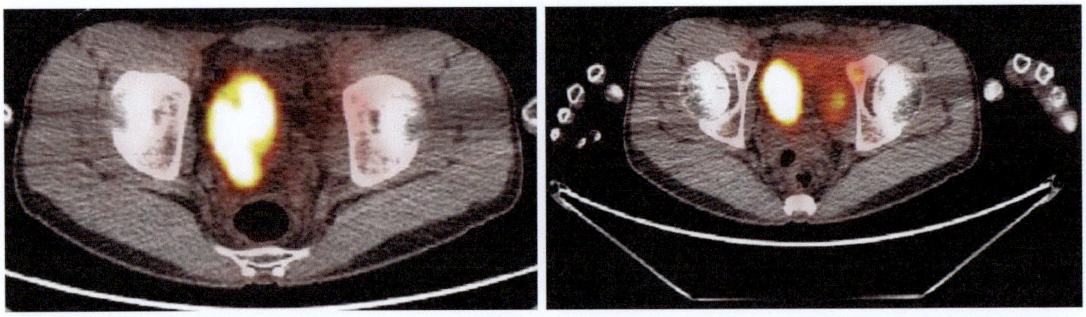

Fig. 11.5 Preoperative PET-CT images: Pre-chemotherapy

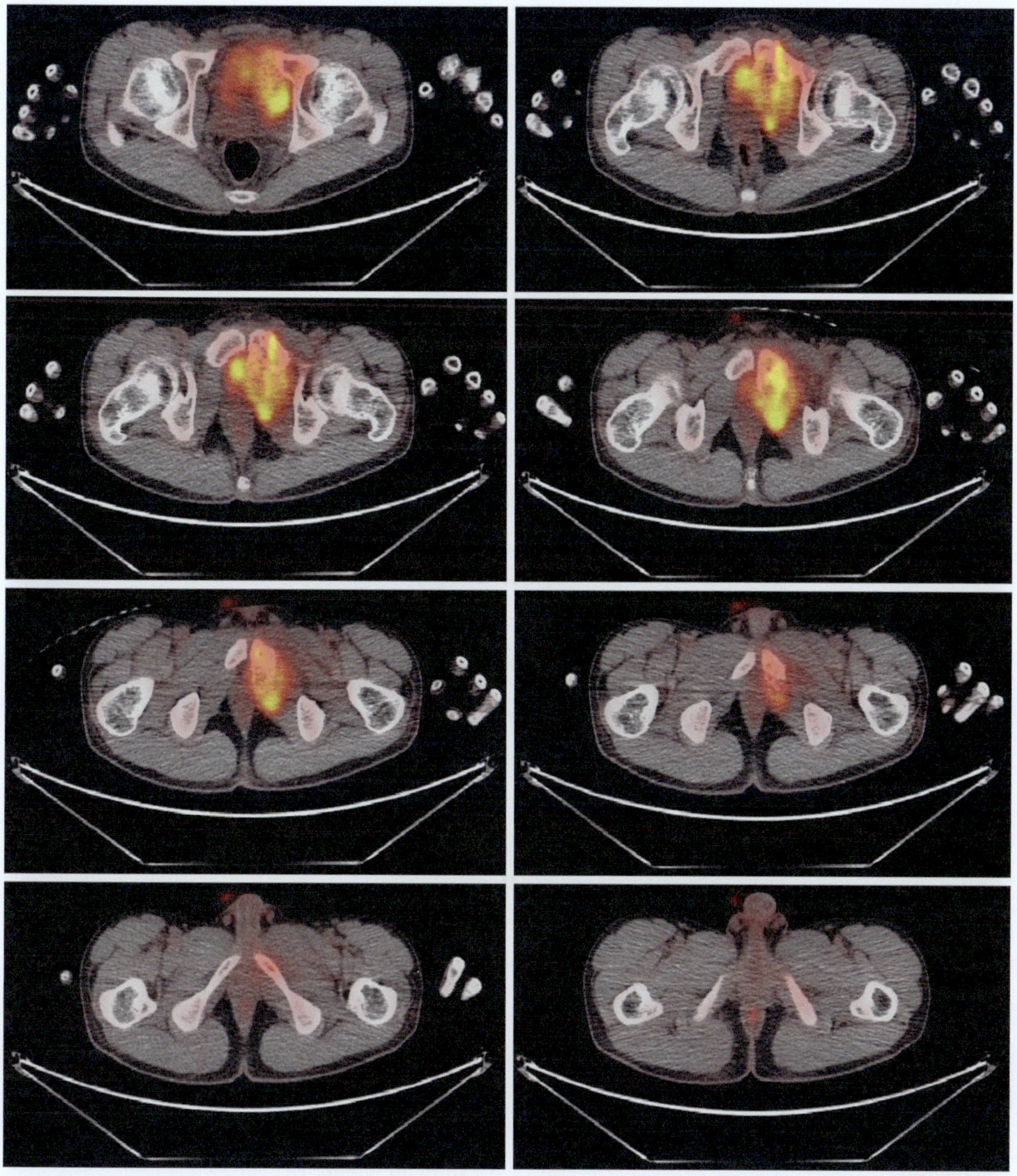

Fig. 11.5 (continued)

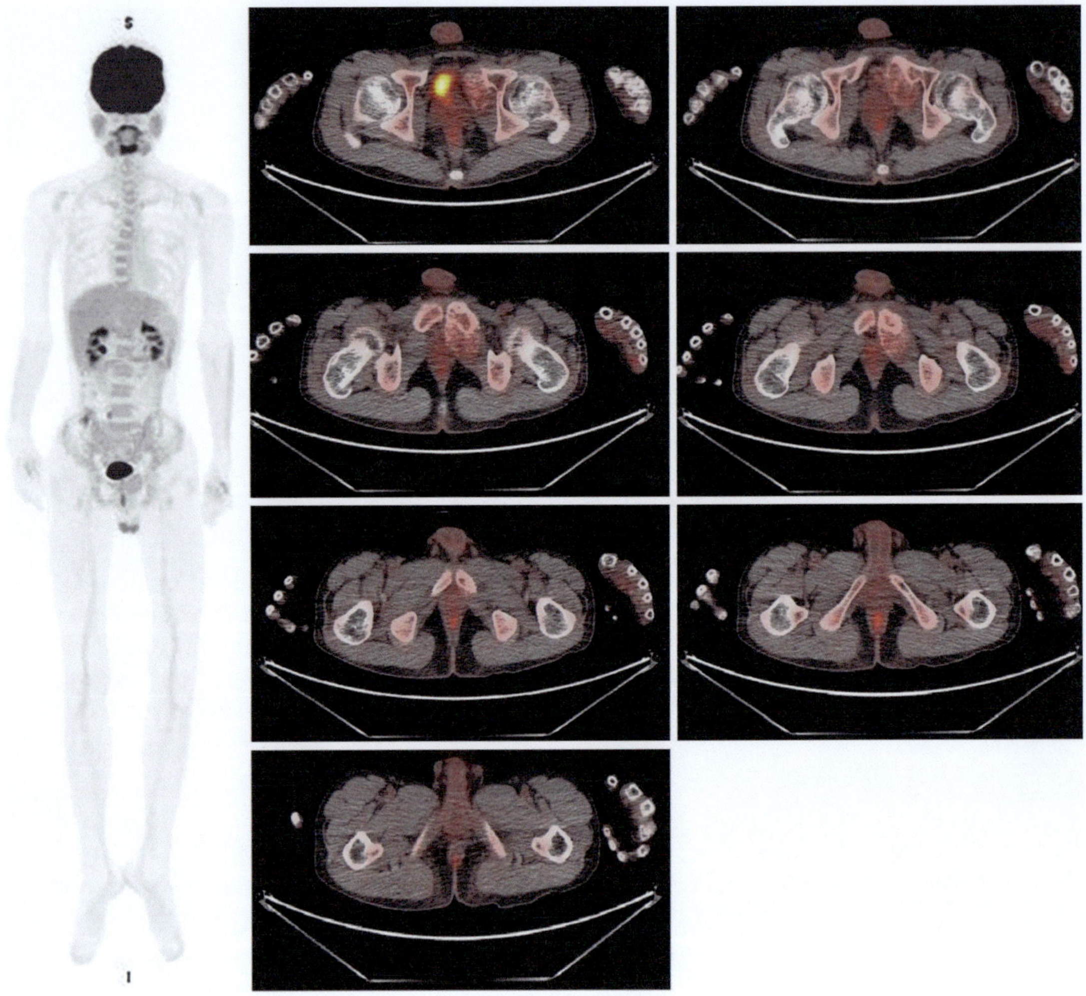

Fig. 11.6 Preoperative PET-CT images: preoperative chemotherapy was effective

11.3 Planning of Surgery

Hip joint saving resection at subchondral of acetabulum

Symphysis pubis cutting

Intraoperative adjuvant surgery with argon laser and liquid nitrogen gun

3D printed pubis implant

11.4 Design and Fabrication

- Implant measurement
- Implant weight (g): 84.82
- Size (mm): 89.21

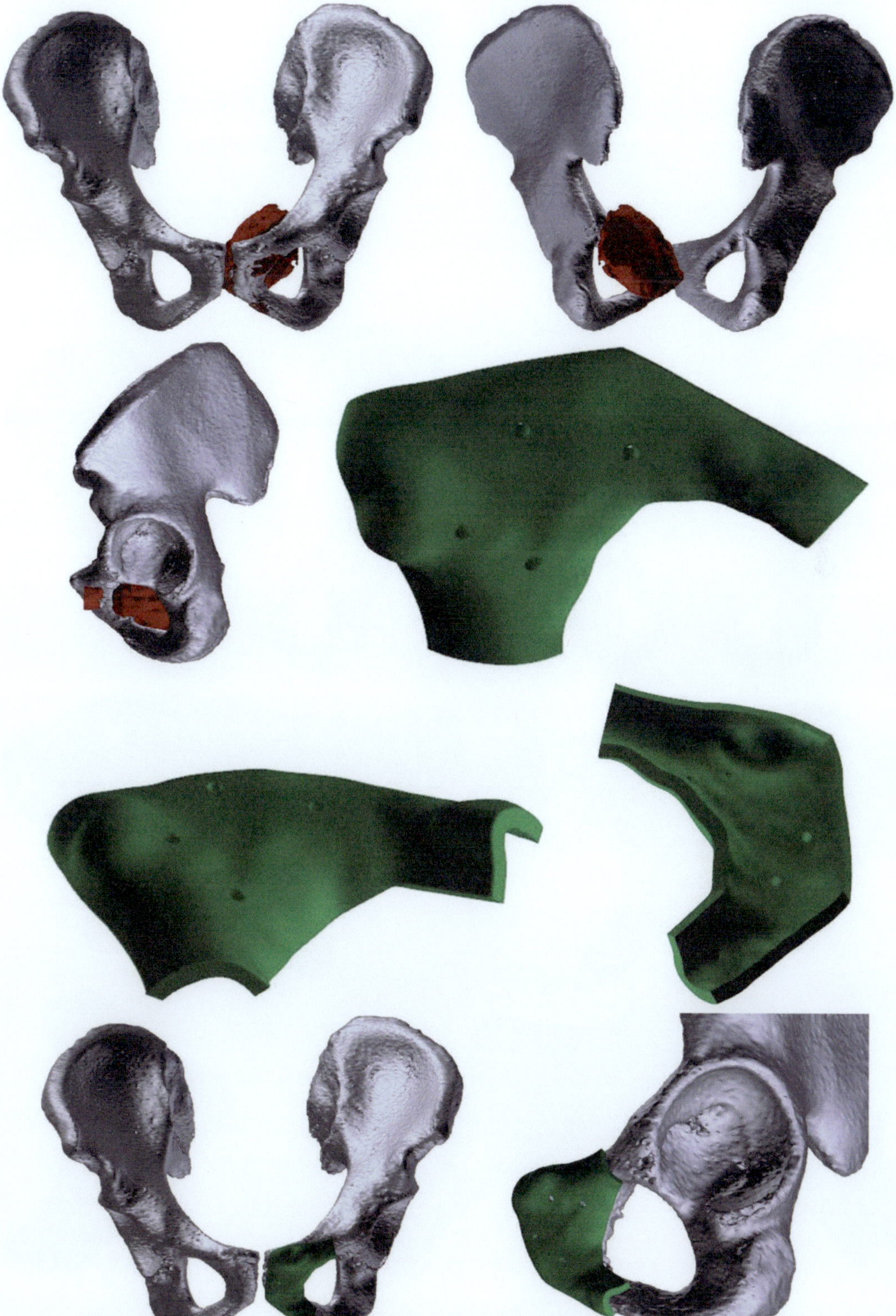

Fig. 11.7 Cutting guide design: modeling is designed with pre-chemotherapy images

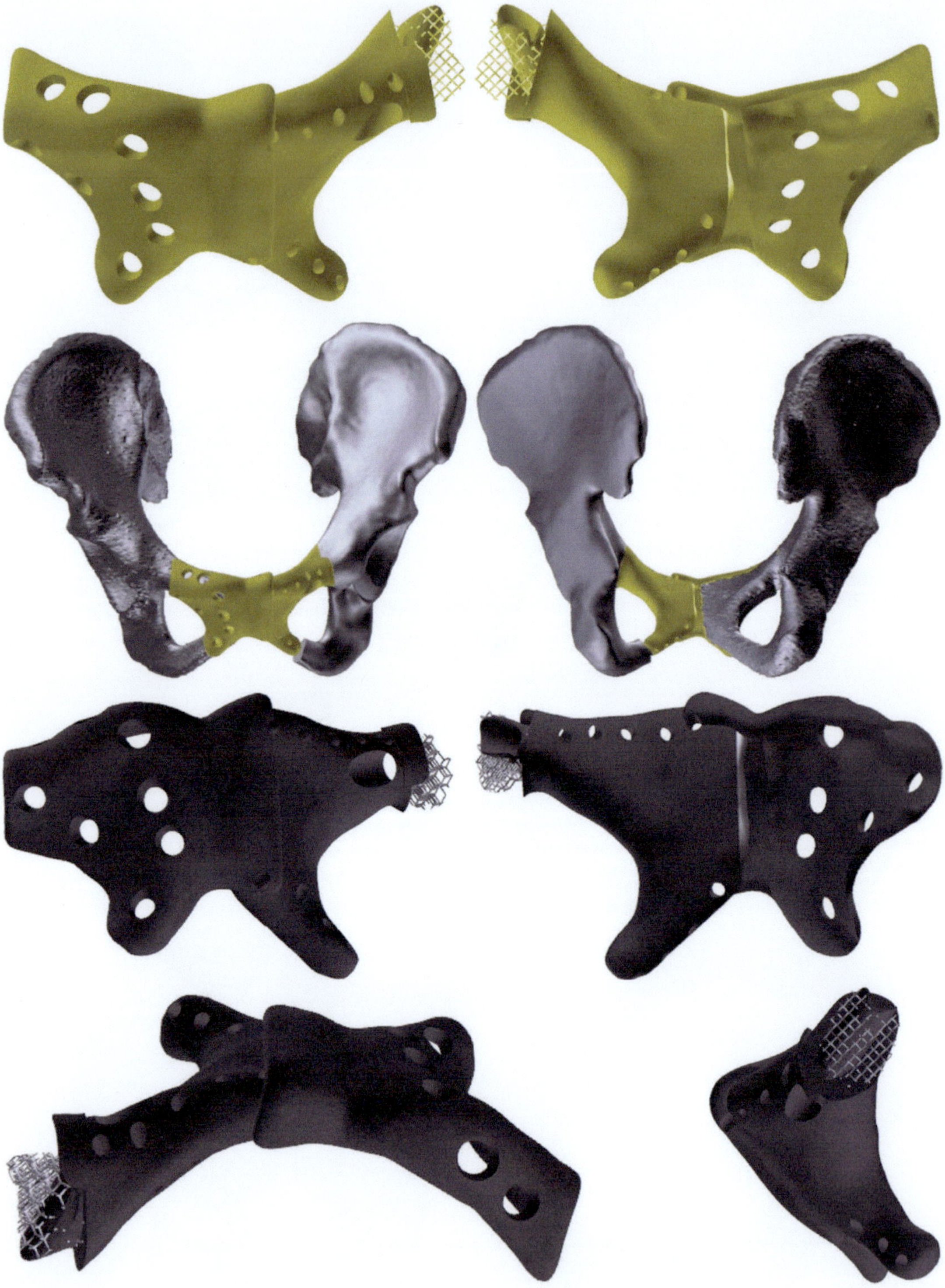

Fig. 11.8 Implant design: make one 6.5 cancellous screw hole, create mesh projection to fix PMMA cement

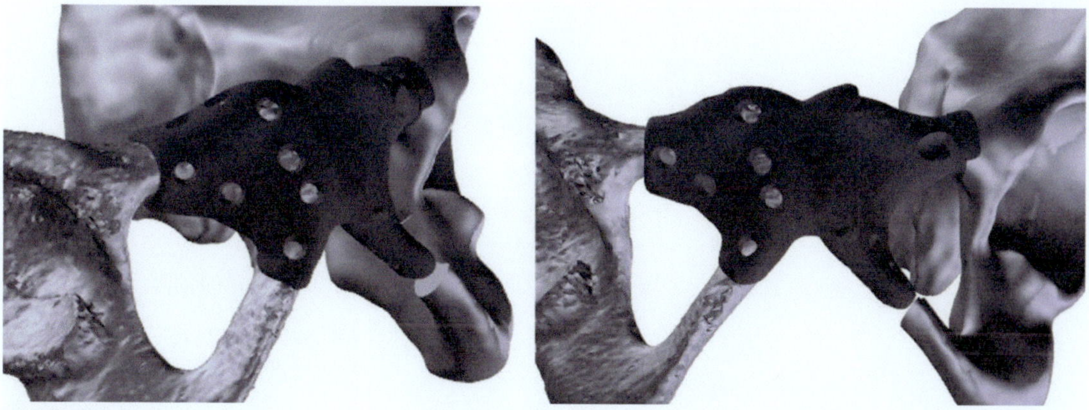

Fig. 11.8 (continued)

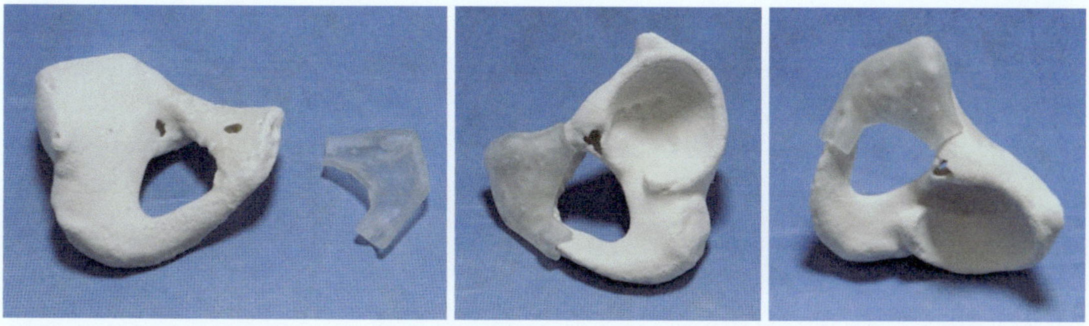

Fig. 11.9 Printed cutting guide

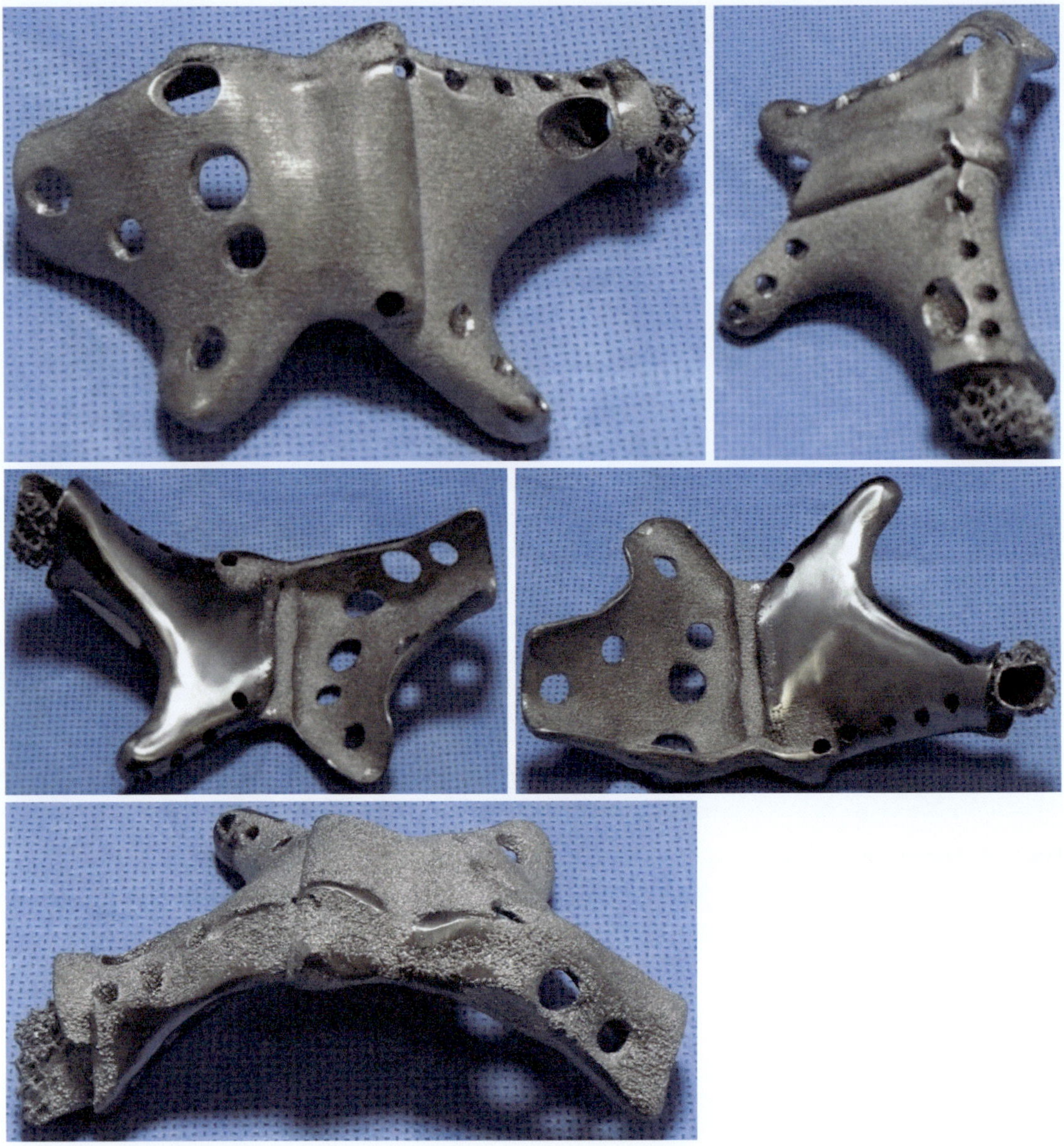

Fig. 11.10 Printed implant

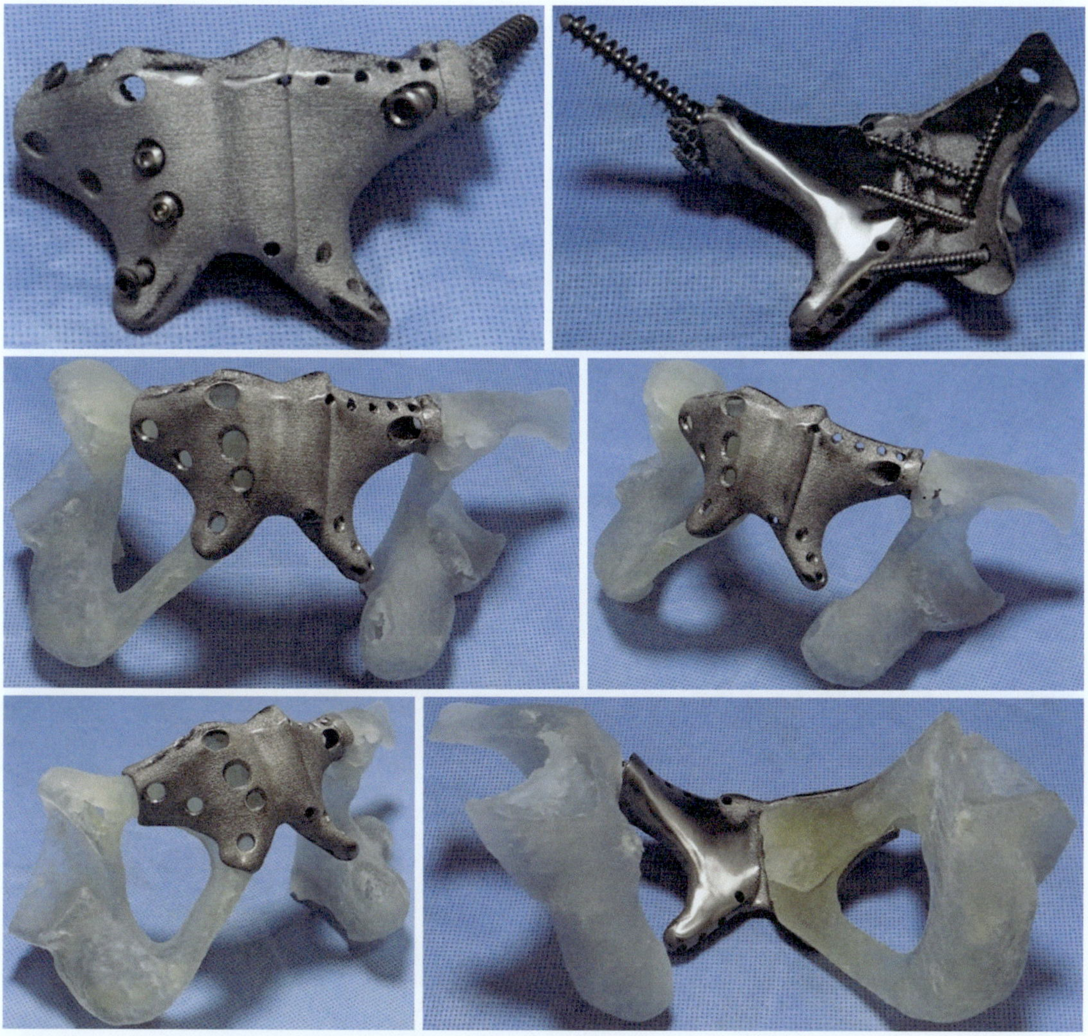

Fig. 11.10 (continued)

11.5 Operation

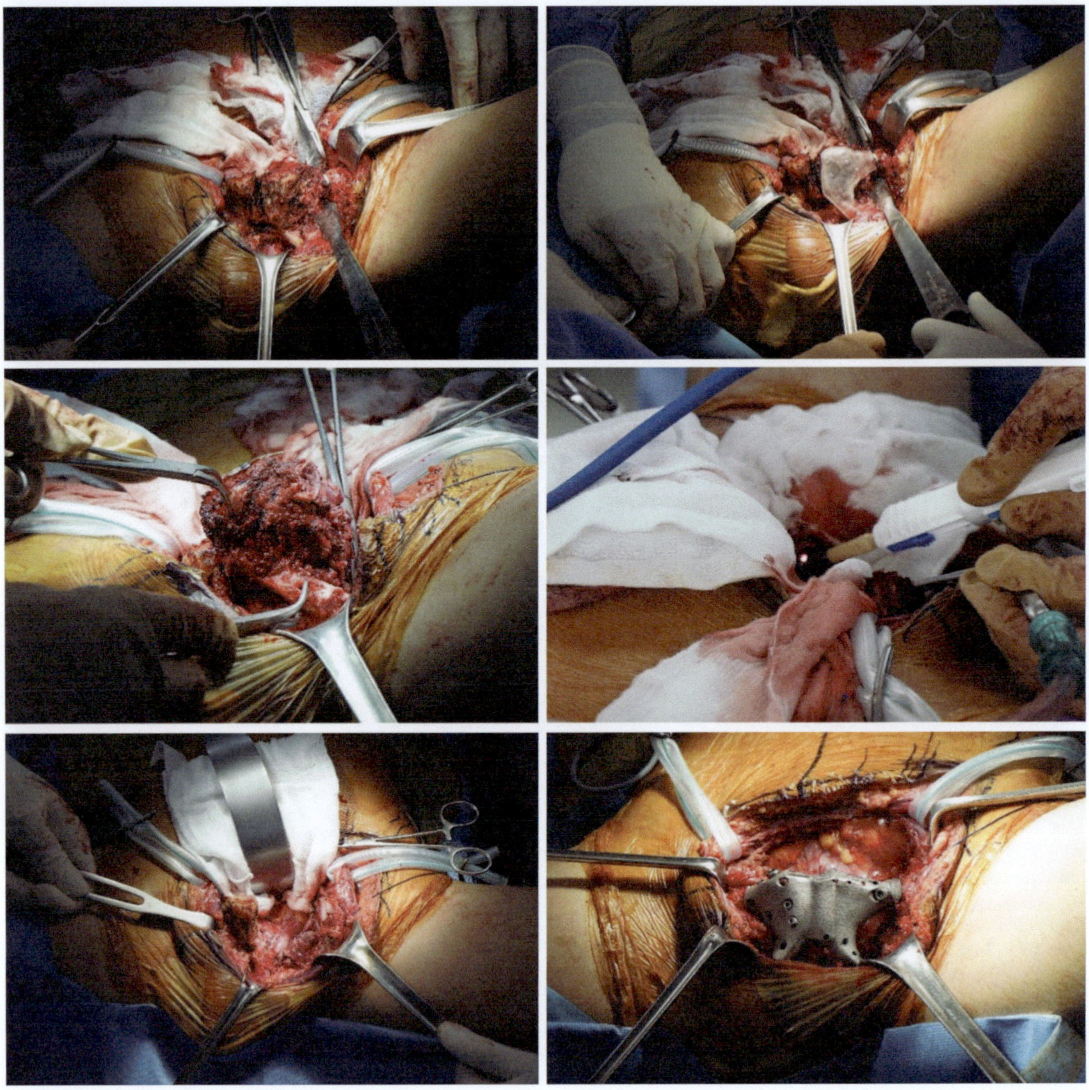

Fig. 11.11 Intraoperative photographs

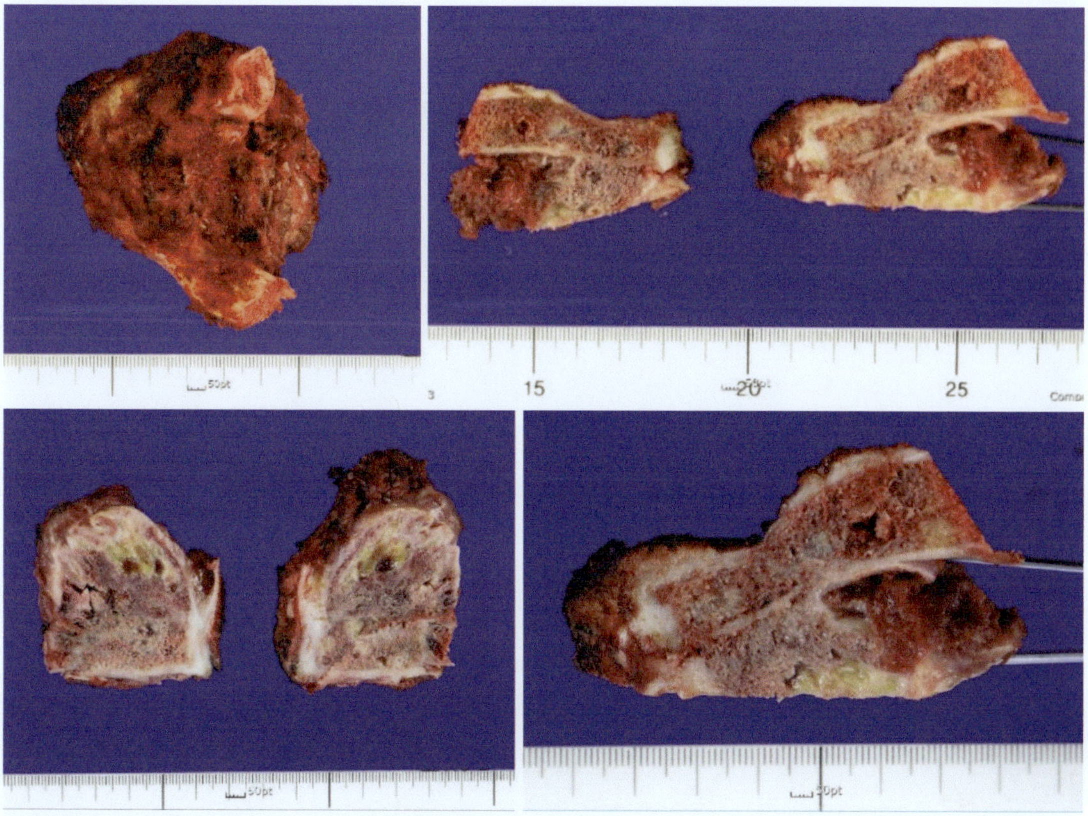

Fig. 11.12 Resected tumor

11.6 Postoperative Images

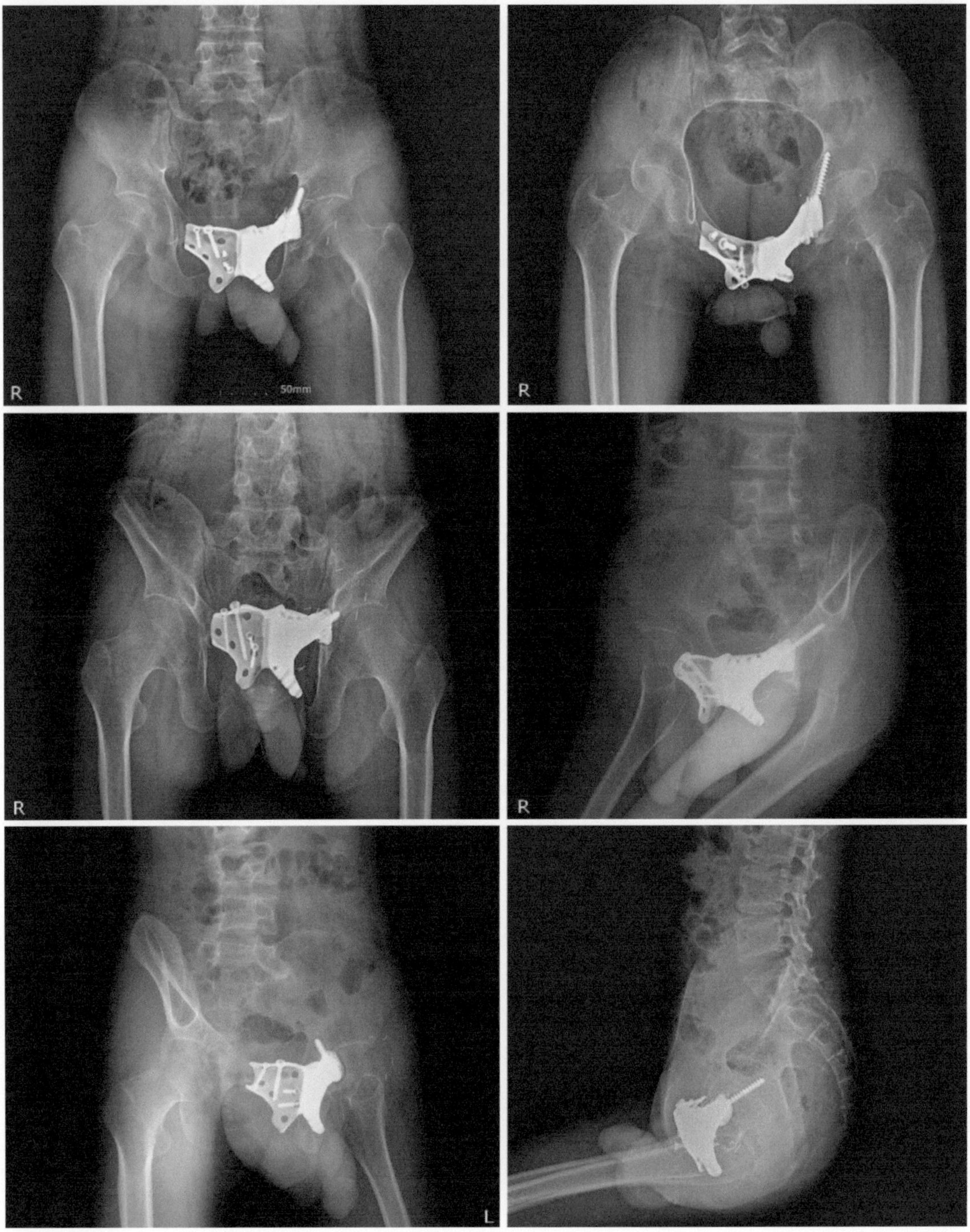

Fig. 11.13 Postoperative X-ray images

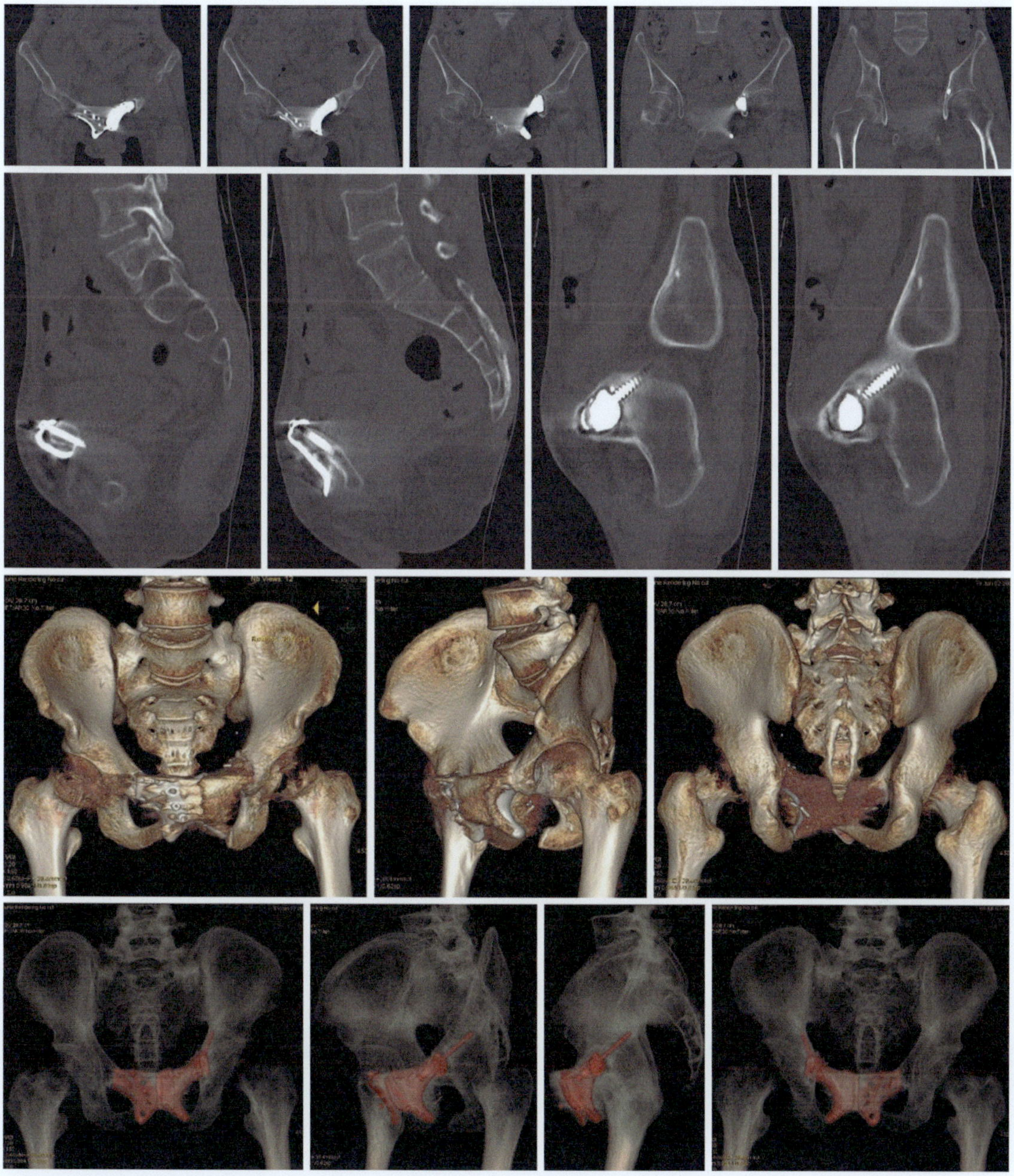

Fig. 11.14 Postoperative CT images

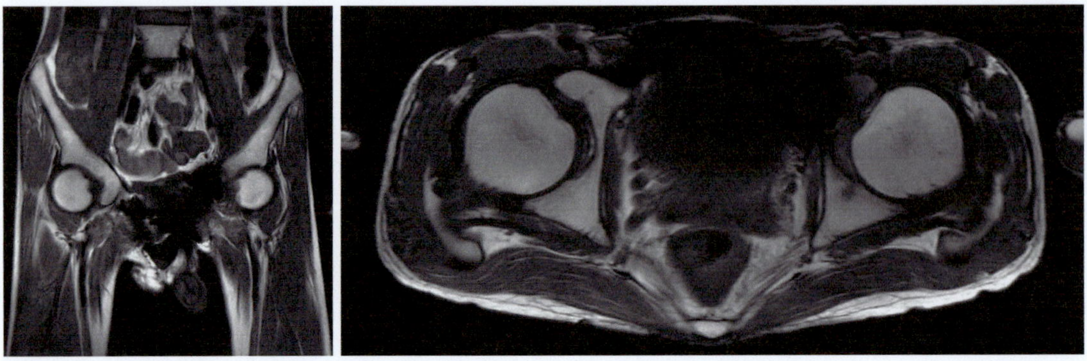

Fig. 11.15 Postoperative MRI images

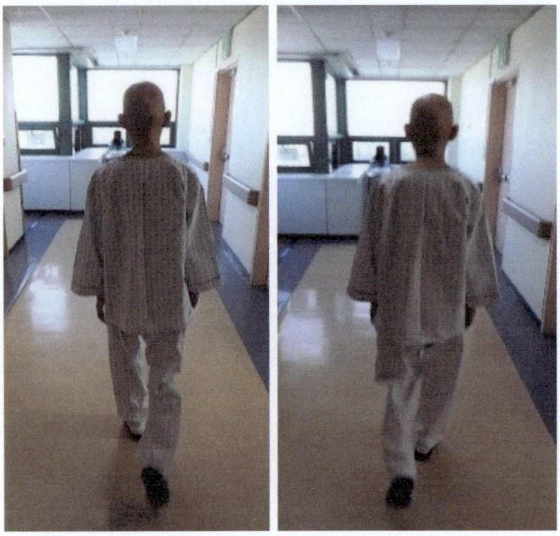

Fig. 11.16 Postoperative walking pictures: normal walking early after surgery

Patient Case 12: Acetabular Reinforcement Cage

12

12.1 Patient Case 12

Age/sex	50/female
Location/site	Pelvis/right
Diagnosis	Acetabular fracture Chronic abscess Sciatic nerve irritation by metal
Preoperative symptom	Bed ridden
Preoperative pain score	Resting 5/Activity 8
Past history	Breast cancer diagnosed 5 years ago Total hip arthroplasty due to bone metastasis 3 years ago Revision surgery due to acetabular loosening 1 year ago Abscess drainage several times
BMI (height/weight)	19.34 (151.5/44.38)
Present illness	Referred for chronic inflammation and pain caused by the acetabular reinforcement cup problem

H.-G. Kang, *Clinical Atlas of 3D Printing Bone Reconstruction*,
https://doi.org/10.1007/978-981-16-2043-0_12

12.2 Preoperative Images

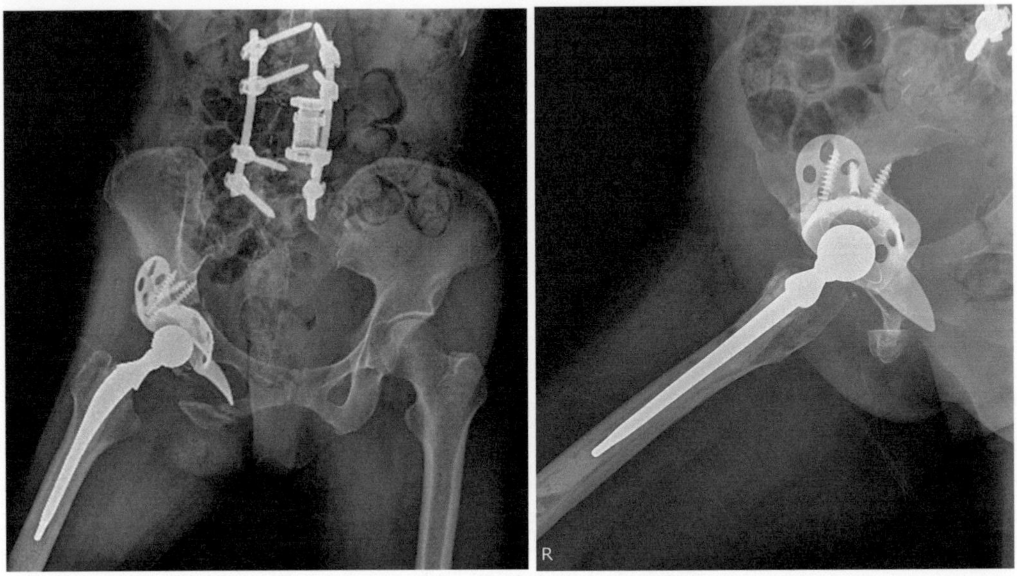

Fig. 12.1 Preoperative X-ray images

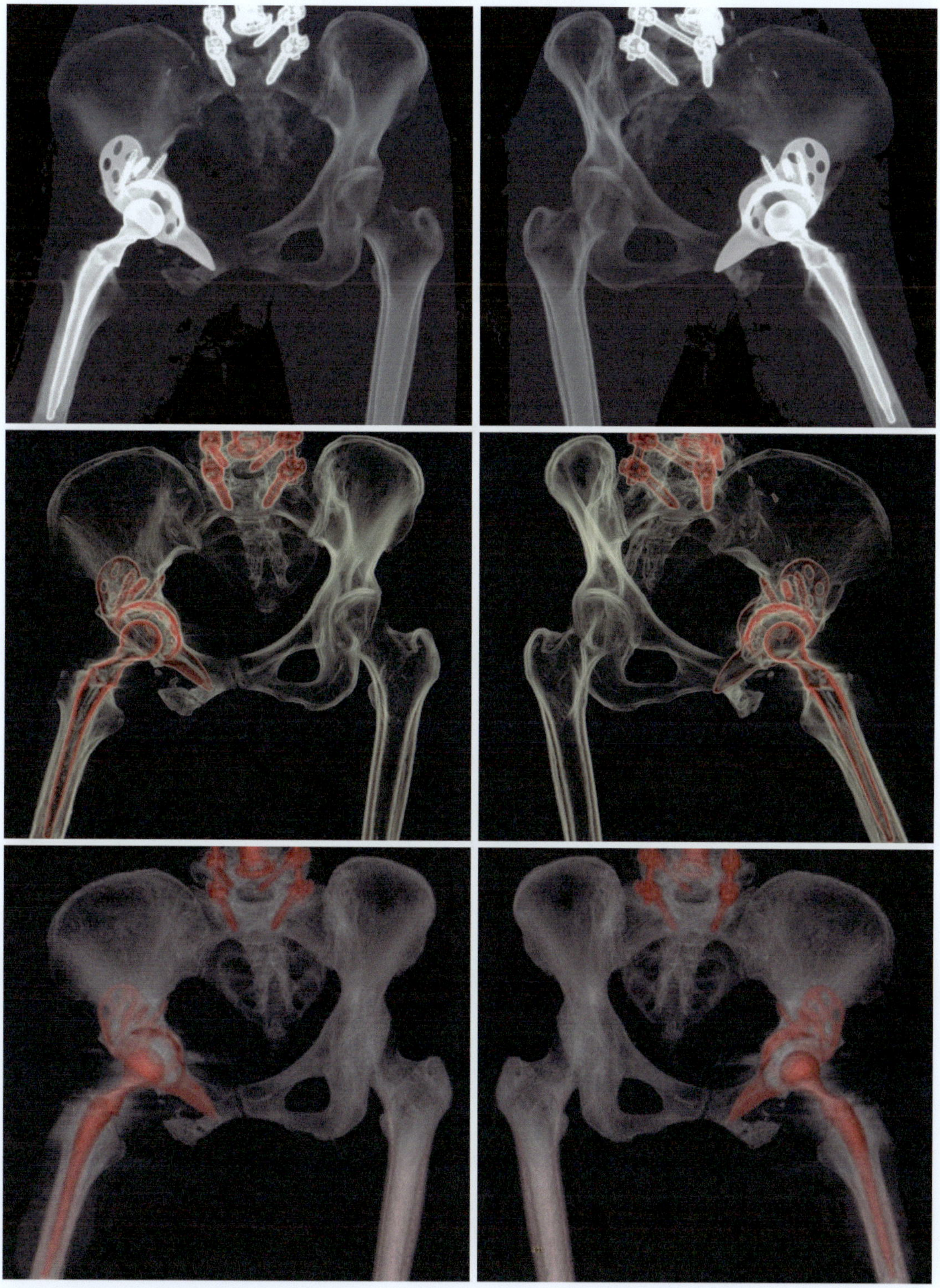

Fig. 12.2 Preoperative CT images

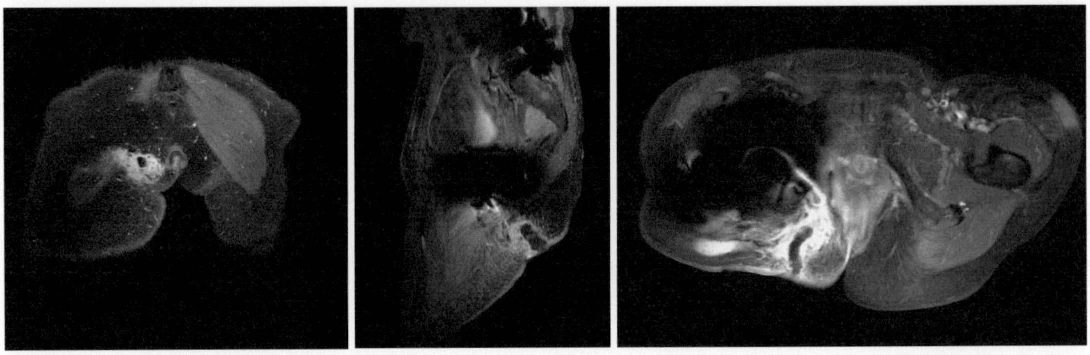

Fig. 12.3 Preoperative MRI images

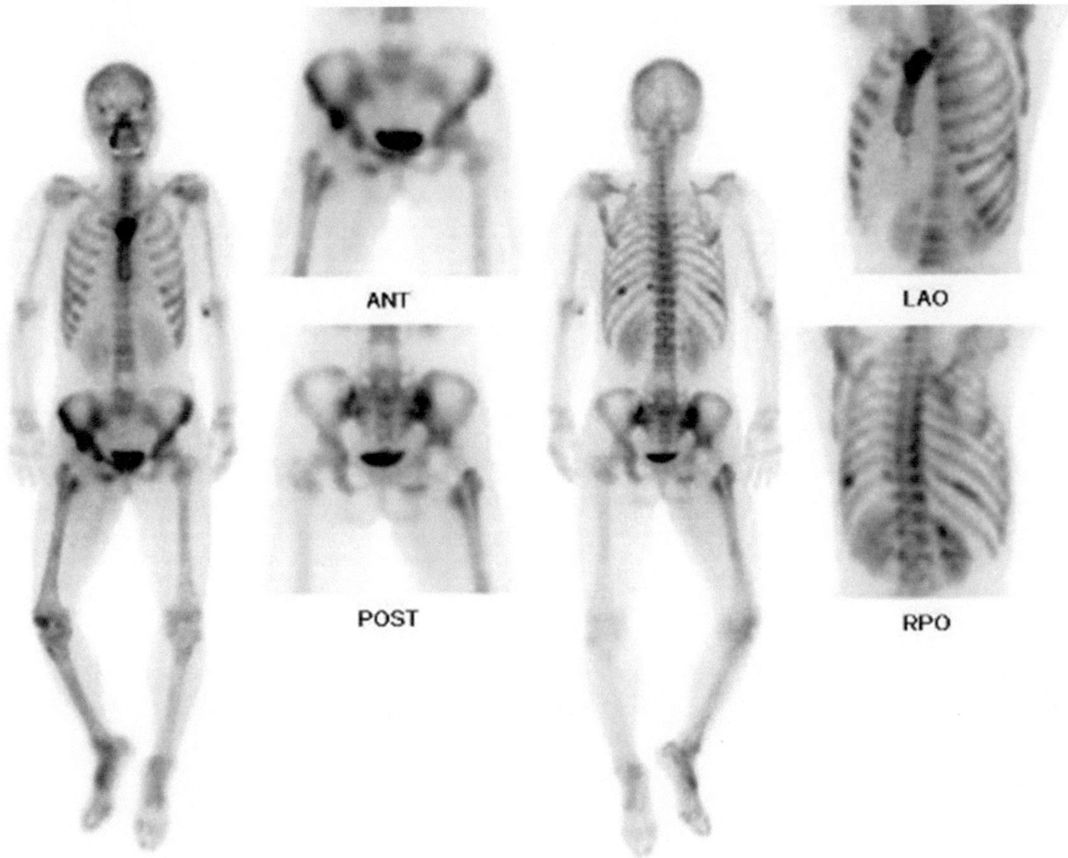

Fig. 12.4 Preoperative bone scan images

12.3 Planning of Surgery

In advanced cancer patients, there is no time for sequential surgery to remove all existing artificial joints to control the infection first, and then rebuild the bone.

Minimal additional metal entry
3D-printed acetabular reinforcement cup
Antibiotic mixed PMMA bone cementing

12.4 Design and Fabrication

- 3D-printed implant fixed to the acetabular with the antibiotic mixed PMMA cement
- The screw fixing area to the ilium is crown shaped and thin.
- Acetabular part is designed with whole mesh.

- Implant measurement
- Implant weight (g): 20.70
- Size (mm): 56.80

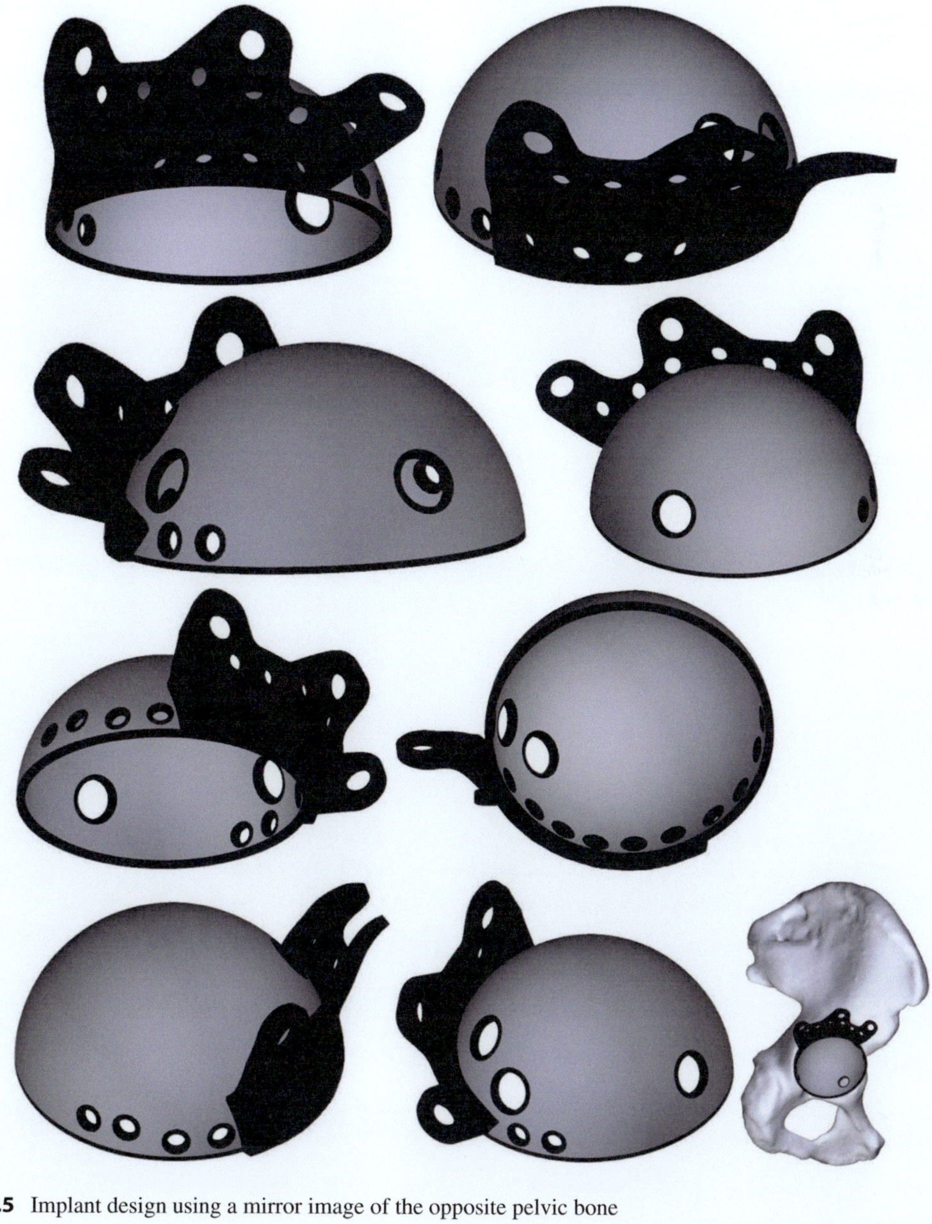

Fig. 12.5 Implant design using a mirror image of the opposite pelvic bone

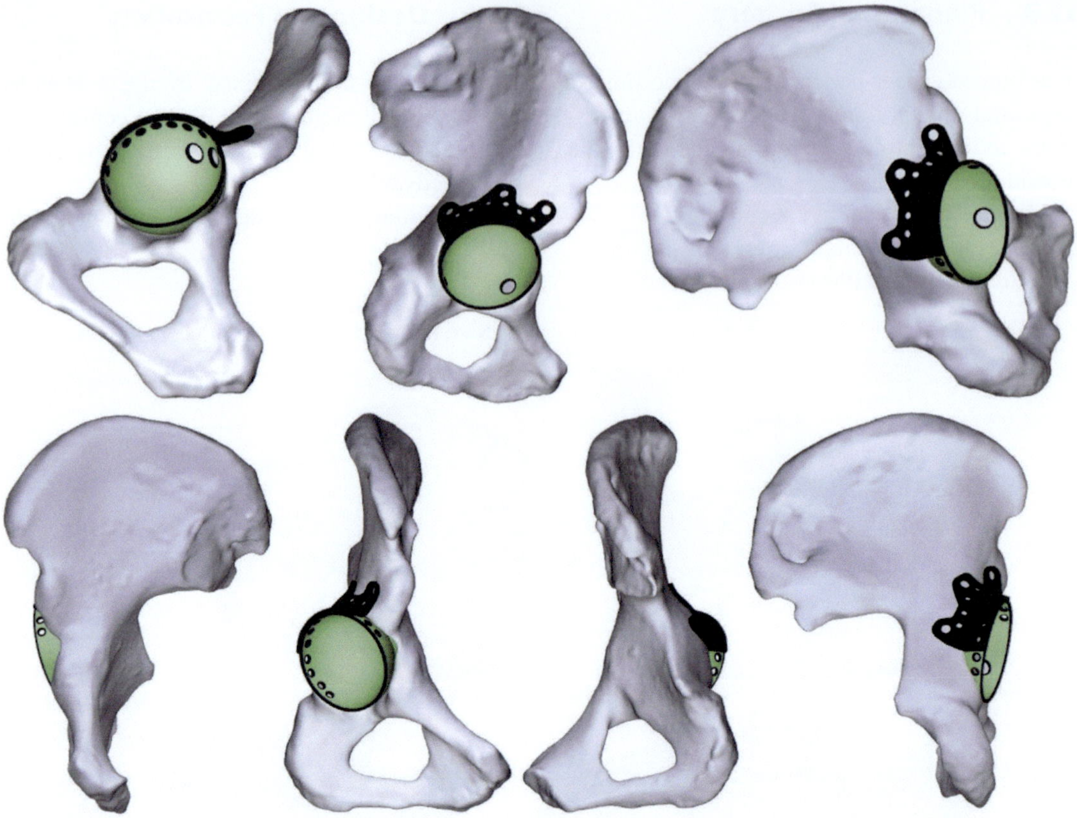

Fig. 12.5 (continued)

Fig. 12.6 Printed bone model: opposite pelvic bone

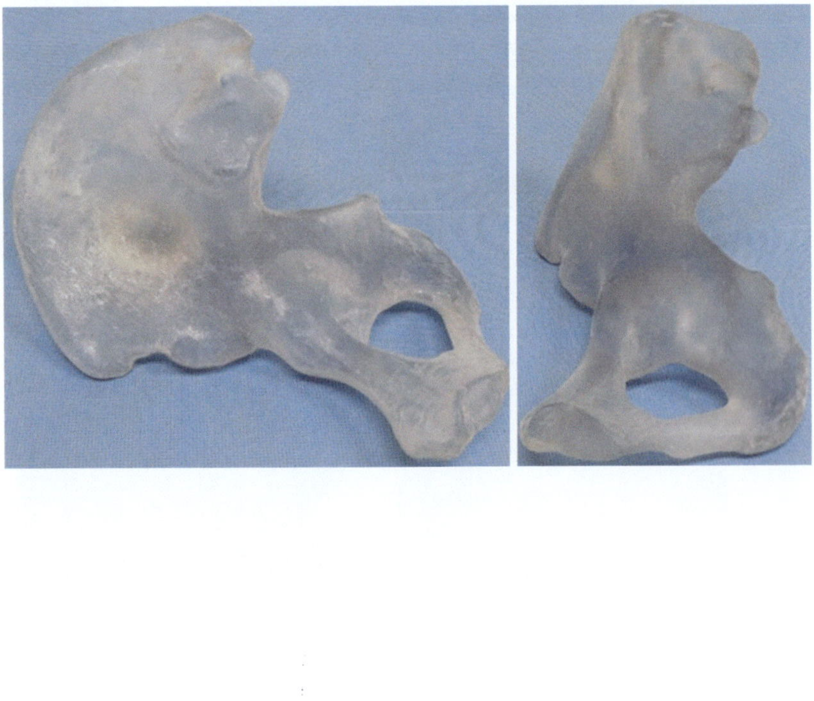

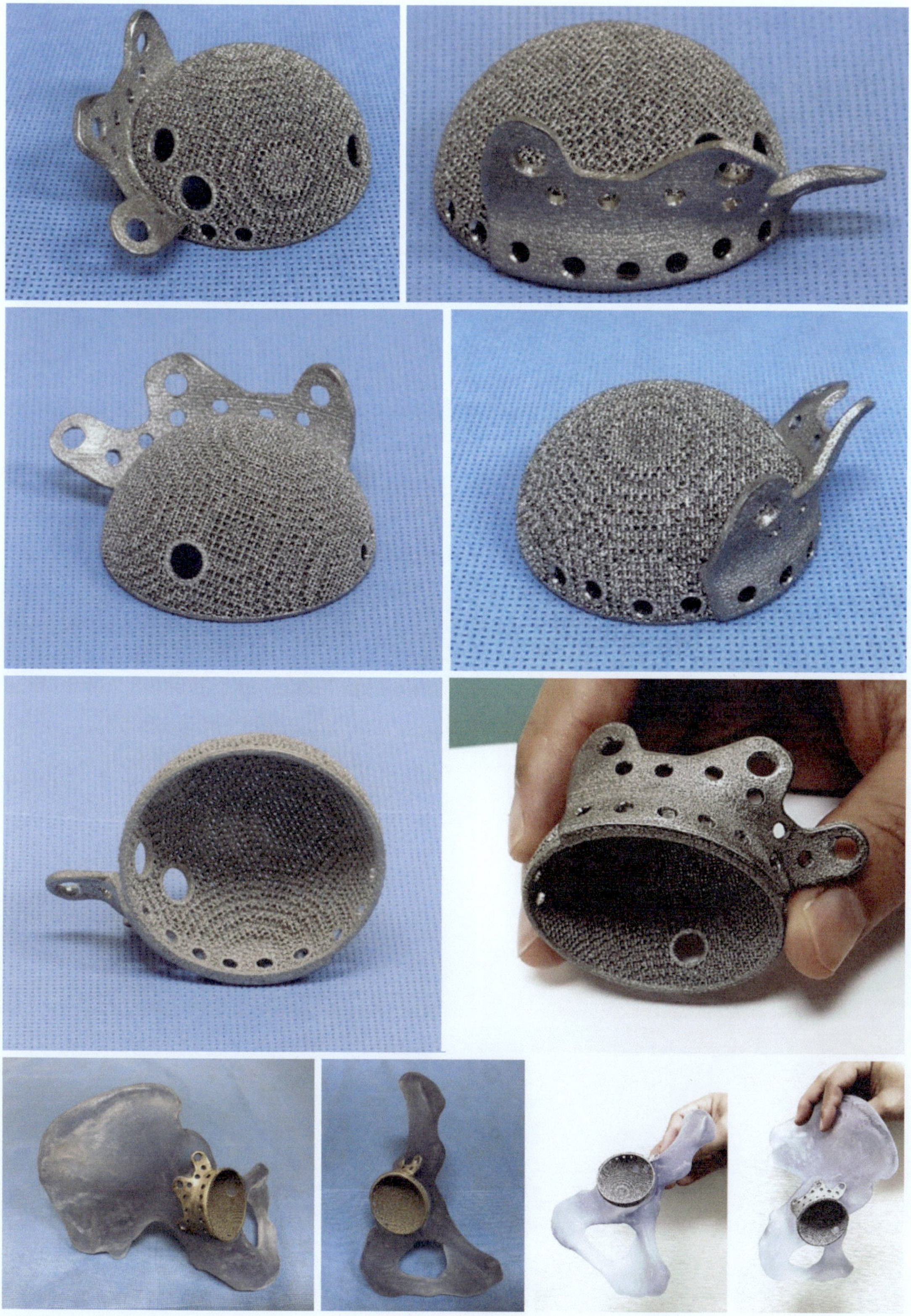

Fig. 12.7 Printed implant

12.5 Operation

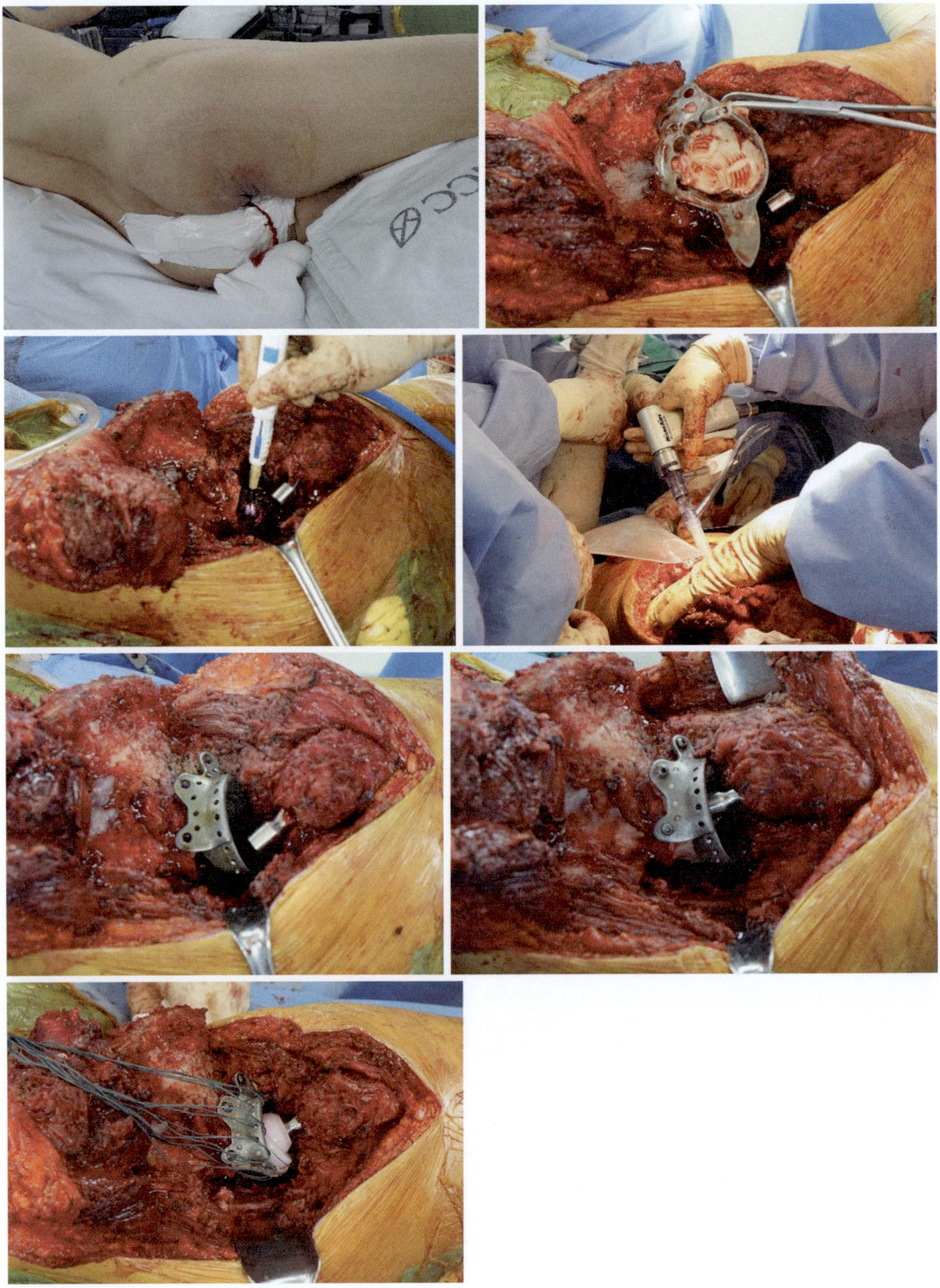

Fig. 12.8 Intraoperative photographs

12.6 Postoperative Images

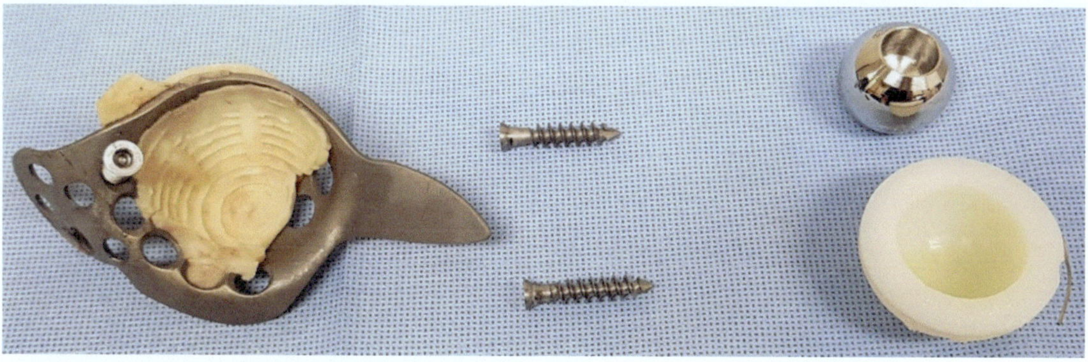

Fig. 12.9 Removed artificial joint components

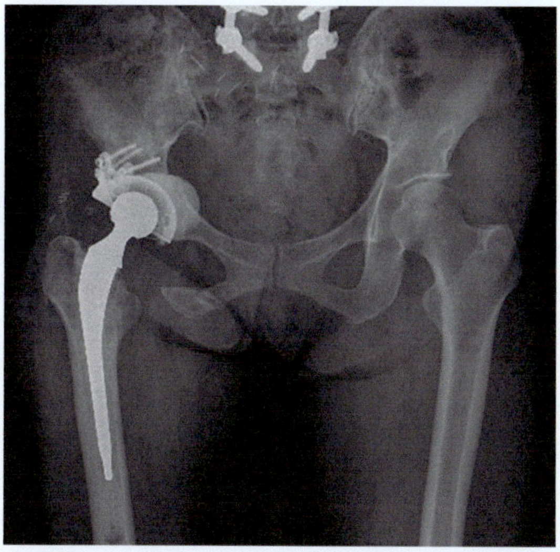

Fig. 12.10 Postoperative X-ray image

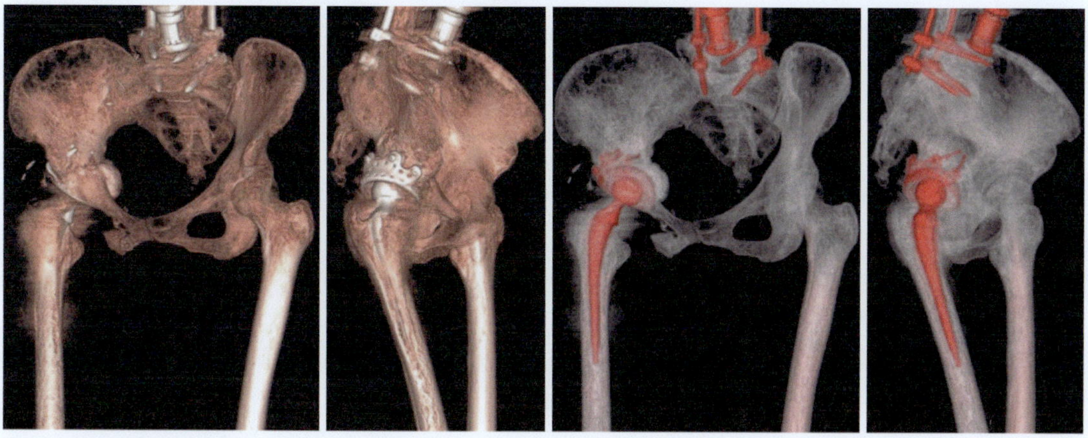

Fig. 12.11 Postoperative CT images

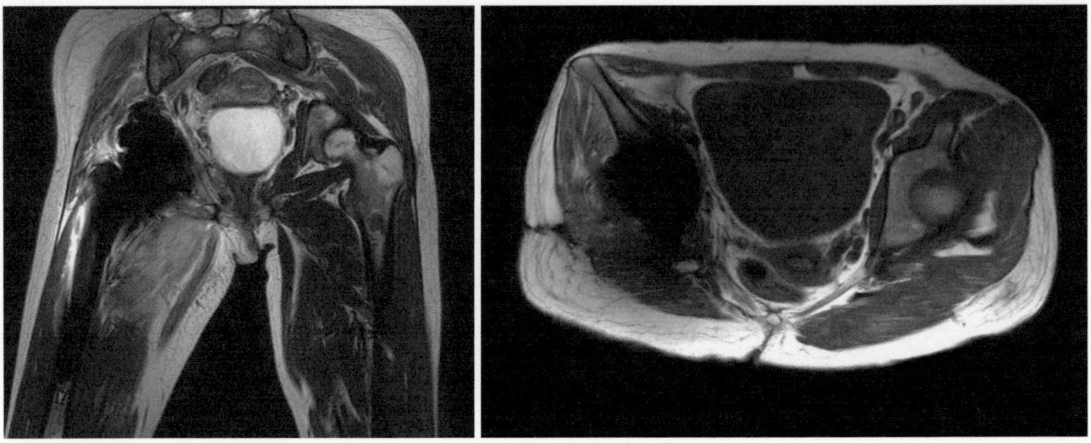

Fig. 12.12 Postoperative MRI images

Patient Case 13: Revision: Failed Allograft Bone Reconstruction

13

13.1 Patient Case 13

Age/sex	47/female
Location/site	Pelvis/right
Diagnosis	Mechanical failure of pelvic reconstruction
Preoperative symptom	Wheelchair ambulation
Preoperative pain score	Resting 3/activity 8
BMI (height/weight)	27.07 (157.8/67.4)
Past history	Chondrosarcoma diagnosis 9 years ago Three times operation at another hospital Allograft reconstruction 4 years ago Deep vein thrombosis femoral vein Common peroneal nerve palsy
Present illness	Progressive allograft destruction and difficulty walking

H.-G. Kang, *Clinical Atlas of 3D Printing Bone Reconstruction*,
https://doi.org/10.1007/978-981-16-2043-0_13

13.2 Preoperative Images

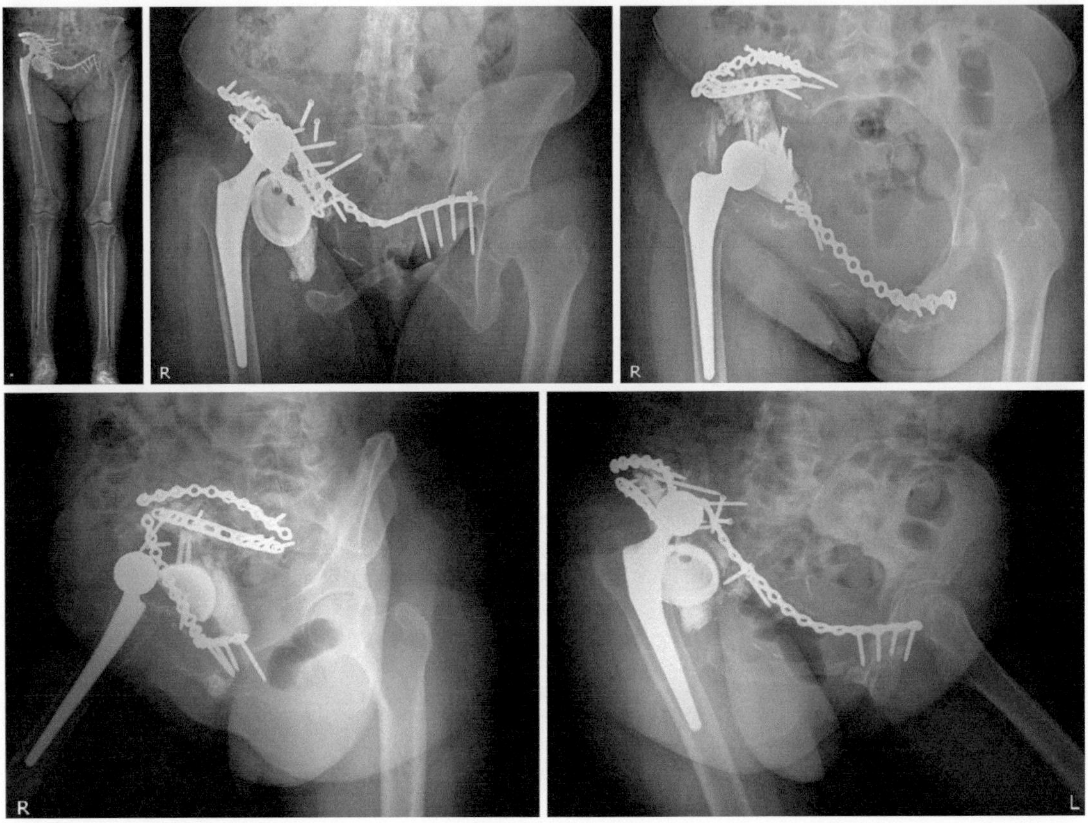

Fig. 13.1 Preoperative X-ray images

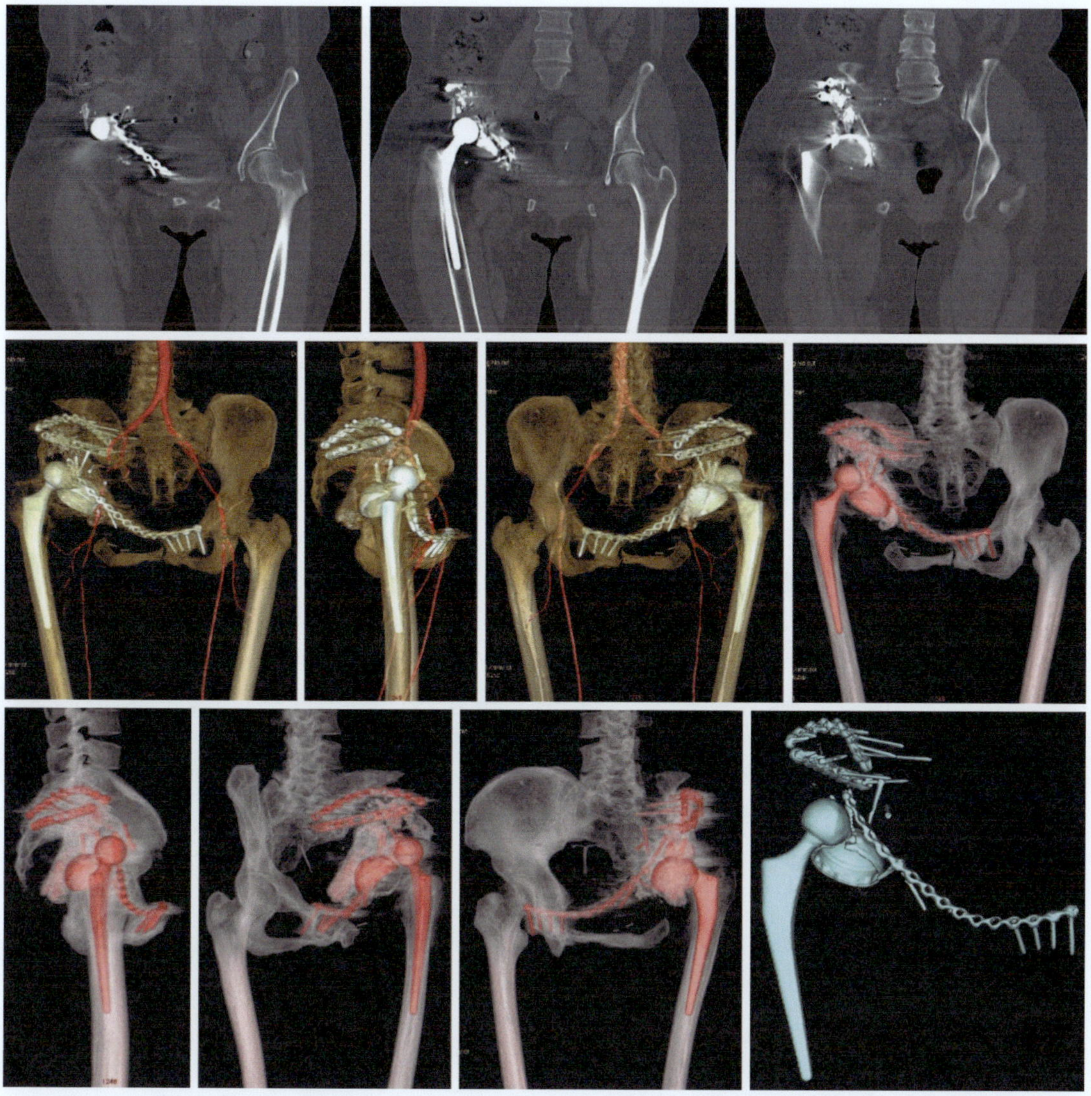

Fig. 13.2 Preoperative CT images

13.3 Planning of Surgery

3D-printed pelvic implant
  Modular pubic implant
  Preserve femoral stem

13.4 Design and Fabrication

- Implant measurement
- Implant weight (g): pelvic acetabulum 480, pubis 108
- Size (mm): pelvic acetabulum 161, pubis 112

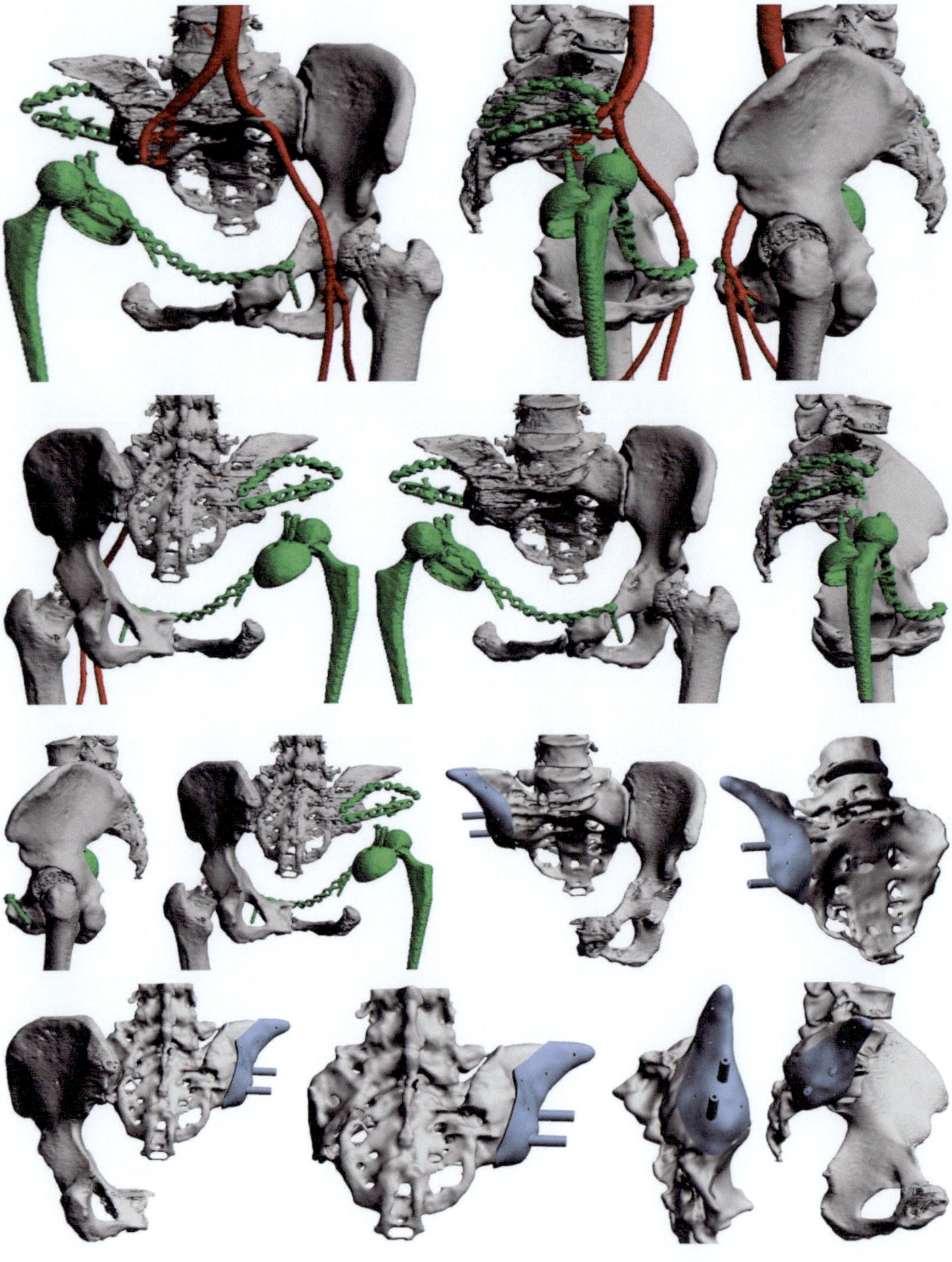

Fig. 13.3 Cutting guide design

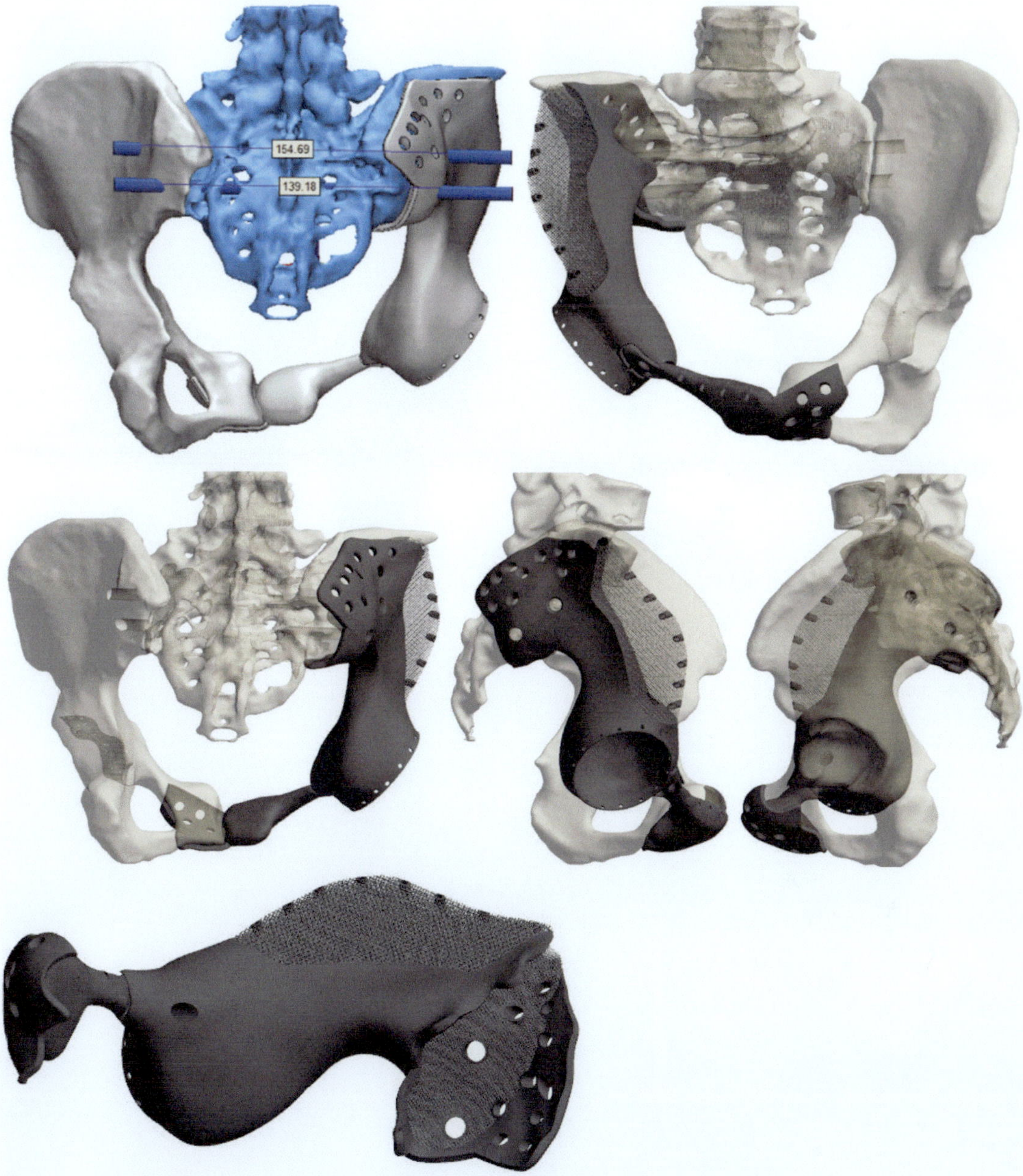

Fig. 13.4 Implant design: make the greater sciatic notch more concave and the iliac crest smaller

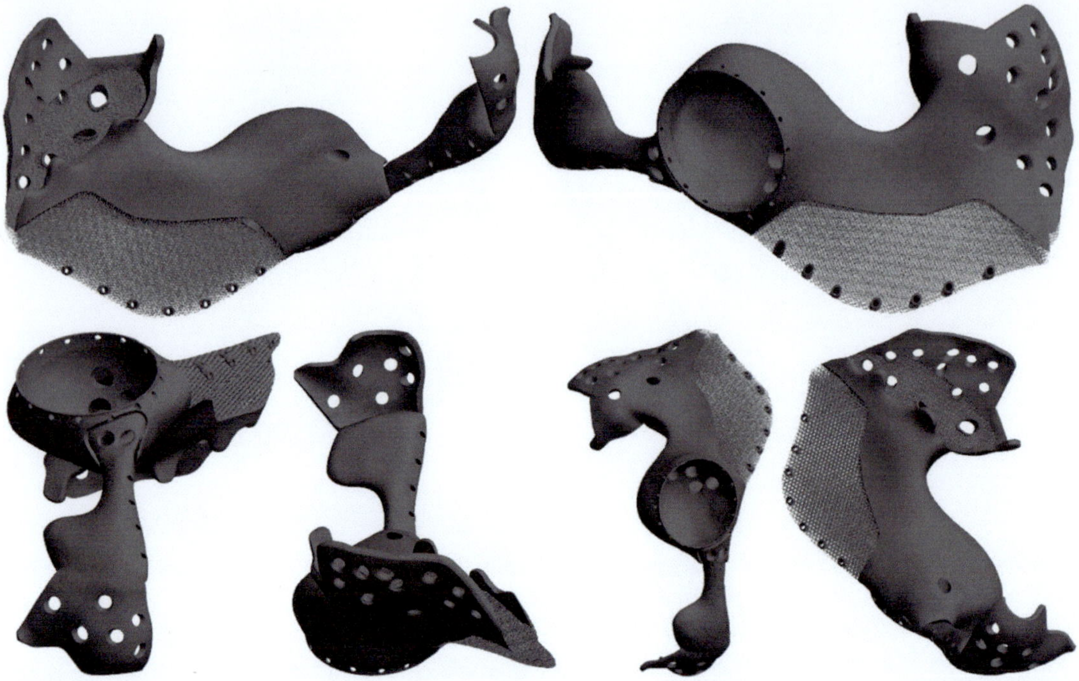

Fig. 13.4 (continued)

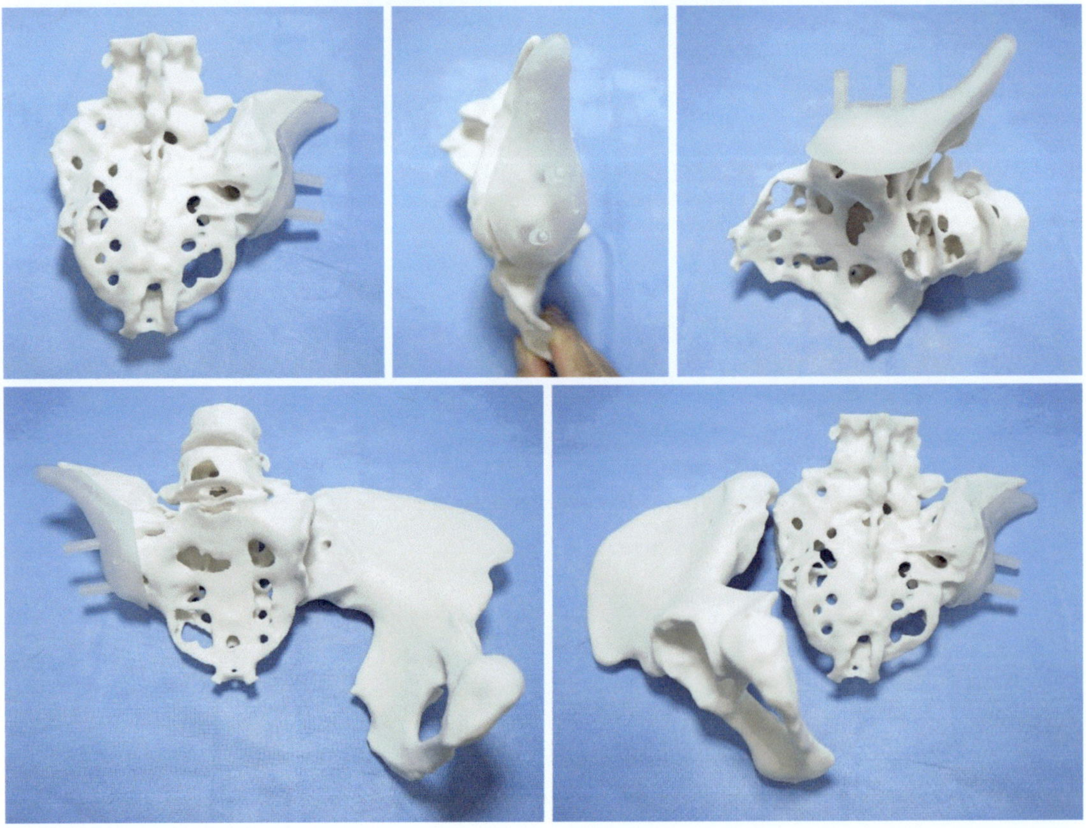

Fig. 13.5 Printed cutting guide

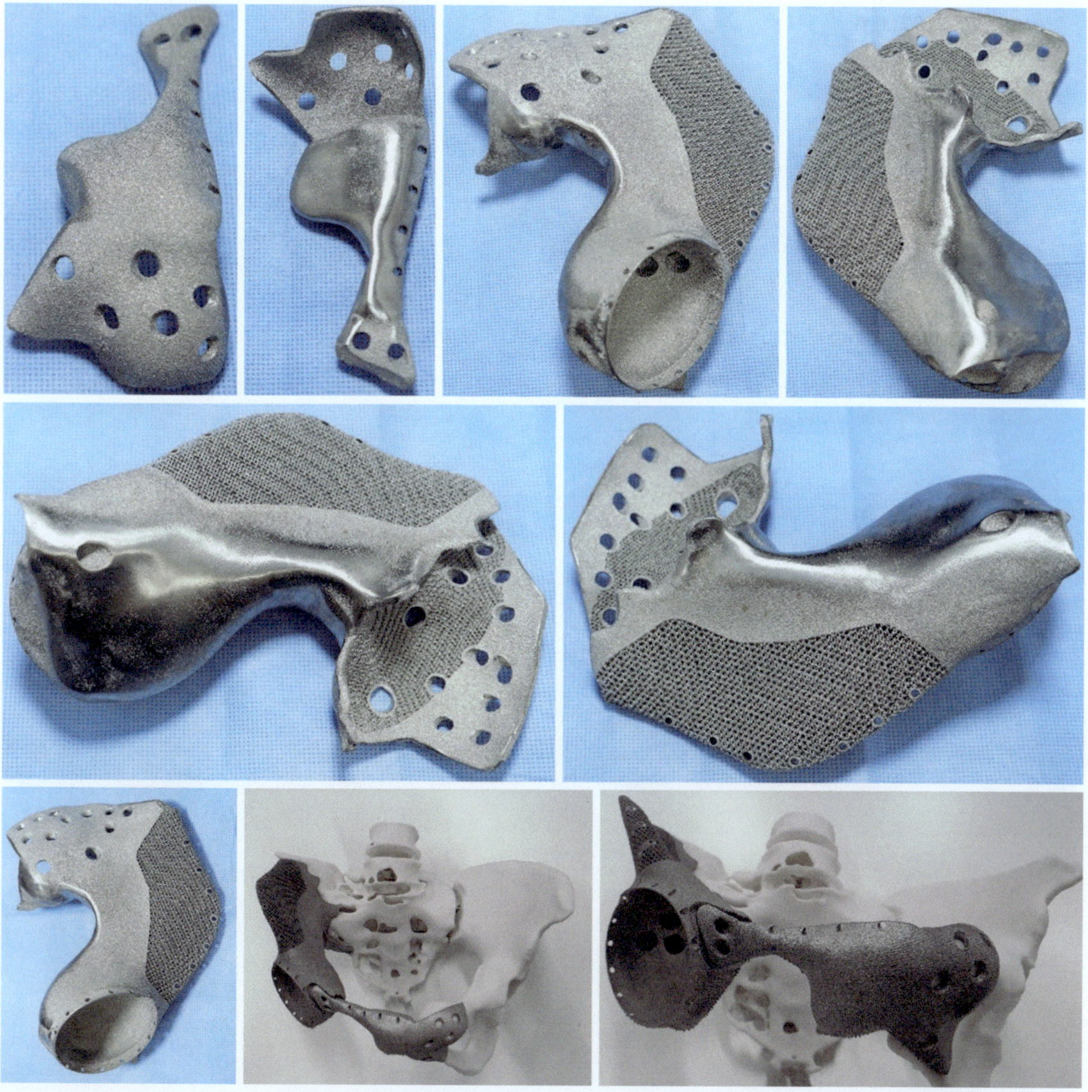

Fig. 13.6 Printed implant: designed supporting plate under the sacroiliac joint for stable fixation through a small ilium

13.5 Operation

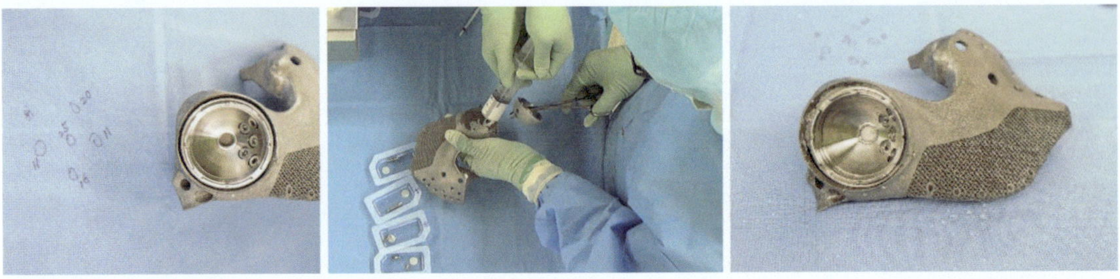

Fig. 13.7 Intraoperative photographs: during the surgical approach, attach the acetabular cup outside the surgical field using PMMA cement and trimmed screws

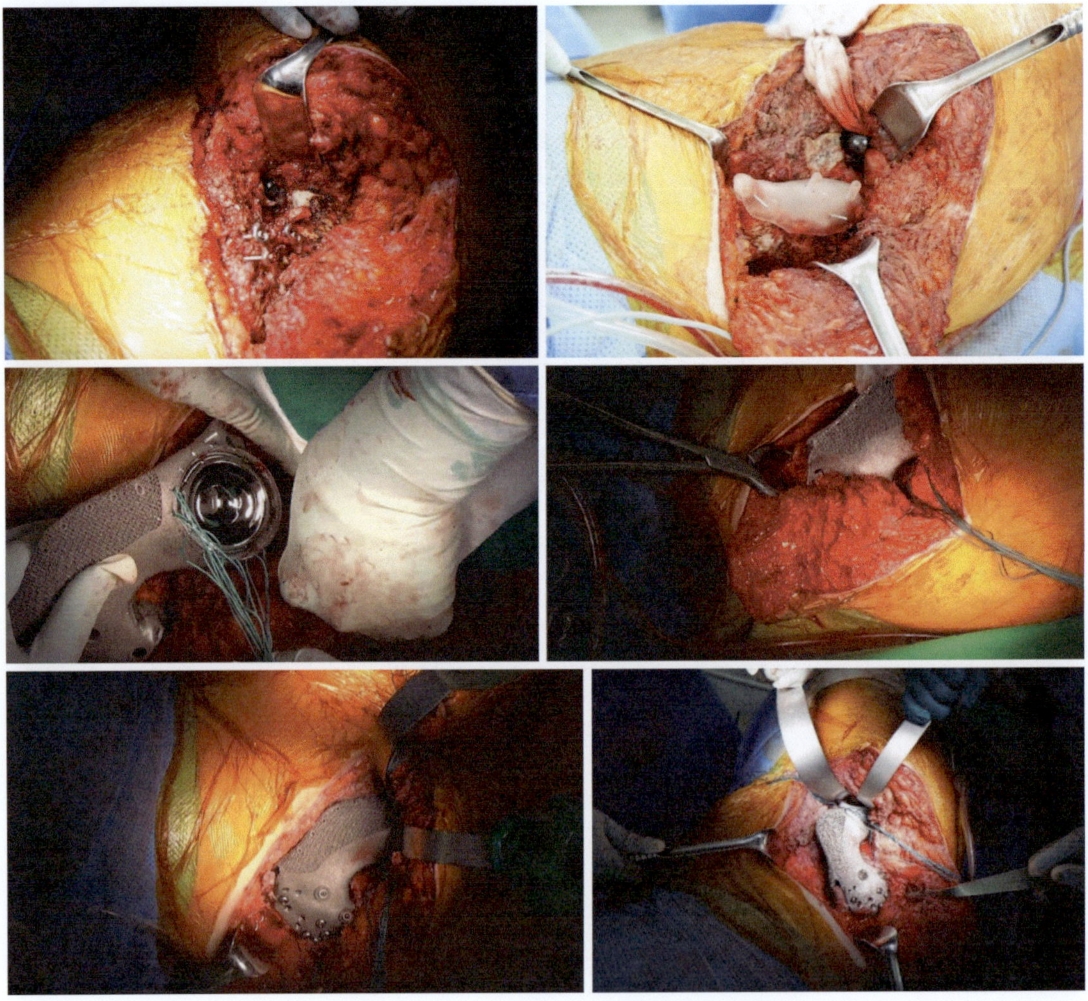

Fig. 13.8 Intraoperative photographs: the prepared pubic implant was not assembled

13.6 Postoperative Images

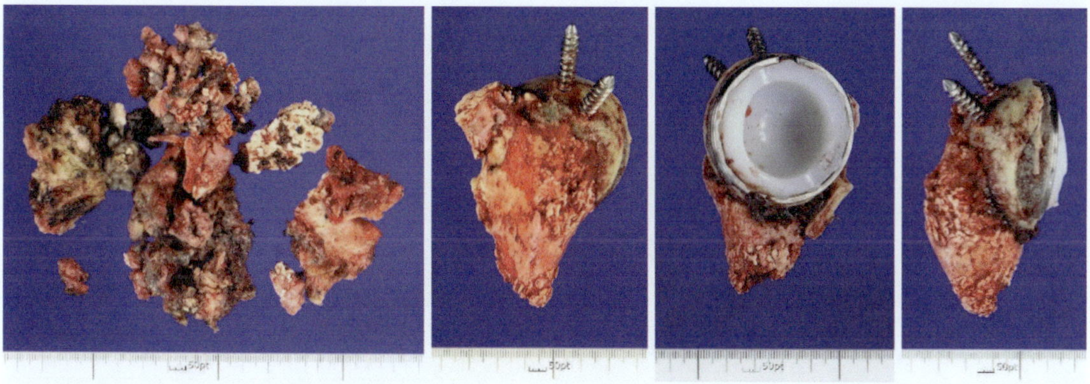

Fig. 13.9 Removed allograft and acetabular cup

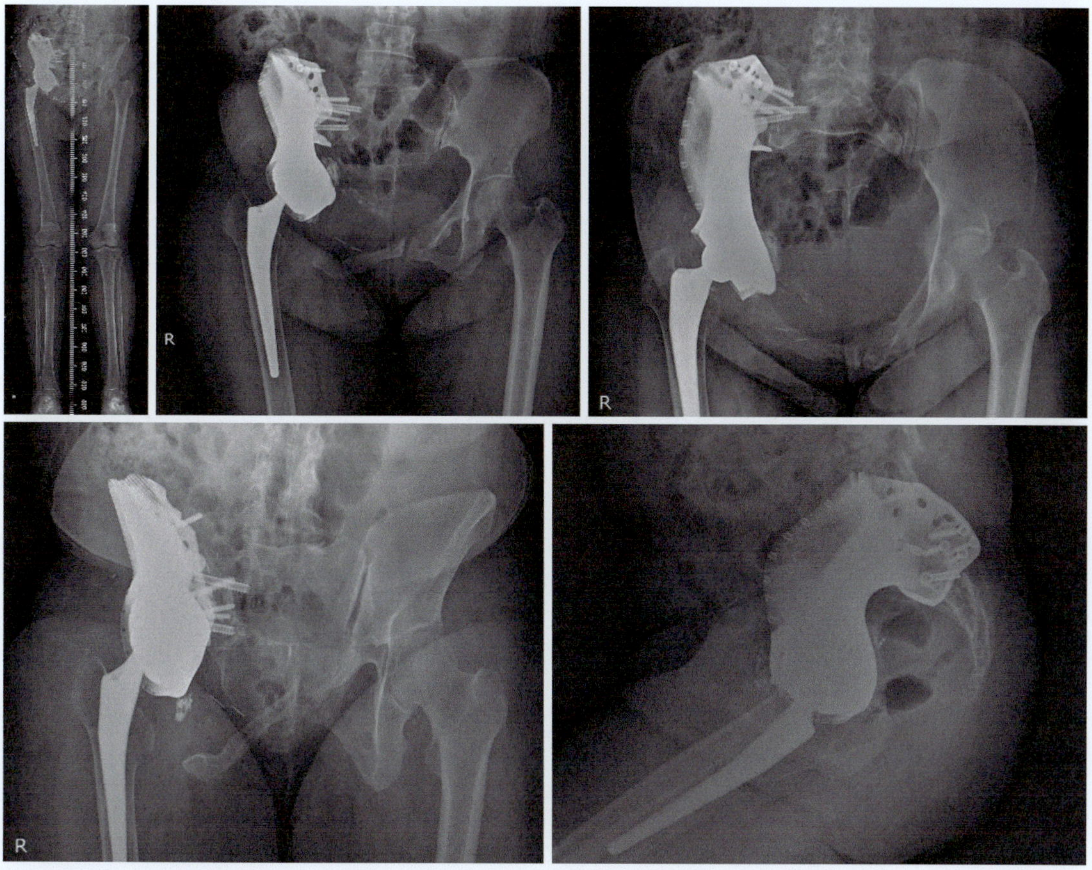

Fig. 13.10 Postoperative X-ray images

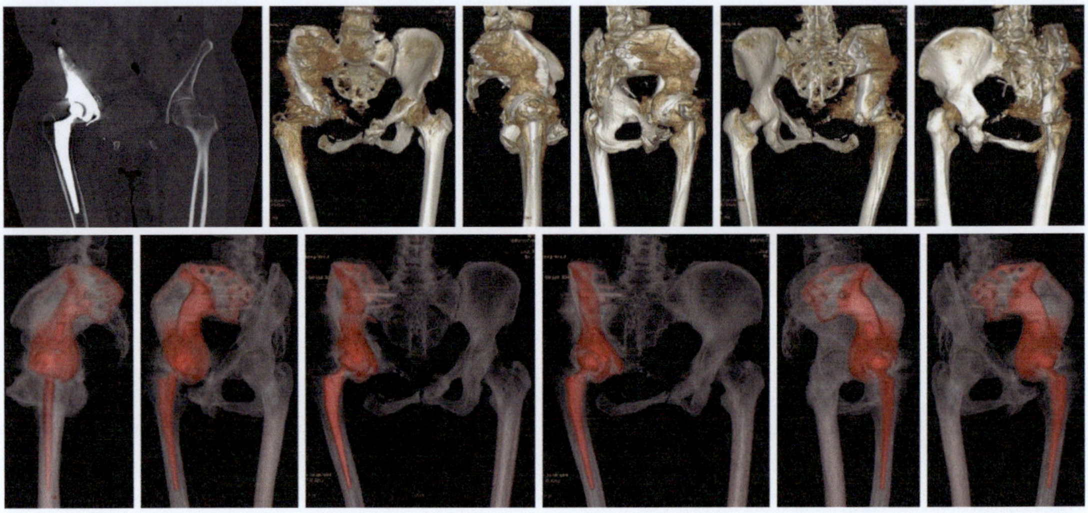

Fig. 13.11 Postoperative CT images: greater sciatic notch widening design restores common peroneal nerve paralysis

Patient Case 14: Revision: Failed Total Hip Arthroplasty

14

14.1 Patient Case 14

Age/sex	42/female
Location/site	Pelvis/left
Diagnosis	Loosening of pelvic artificial joint
Preoperative symptom	Wheelchair ambulation
Preoperative pain score	Resting 2/activity 5
Past history	Driver traffic accident 2 years ago Hospitalized 20 times and had 11 surgeries Left hip joint surgery 5 times
BMI (height/weight)	21.83 (163/58)
Present illness	Visited for 3D printing customized pelvic reconstruction

H.-G. Kang, *Clinical Atlas of 3D Printing Bone Reconstruction*,
https://doi.org/10.1007/978-981-16-2043-0_14

14.2 Preoperative Images

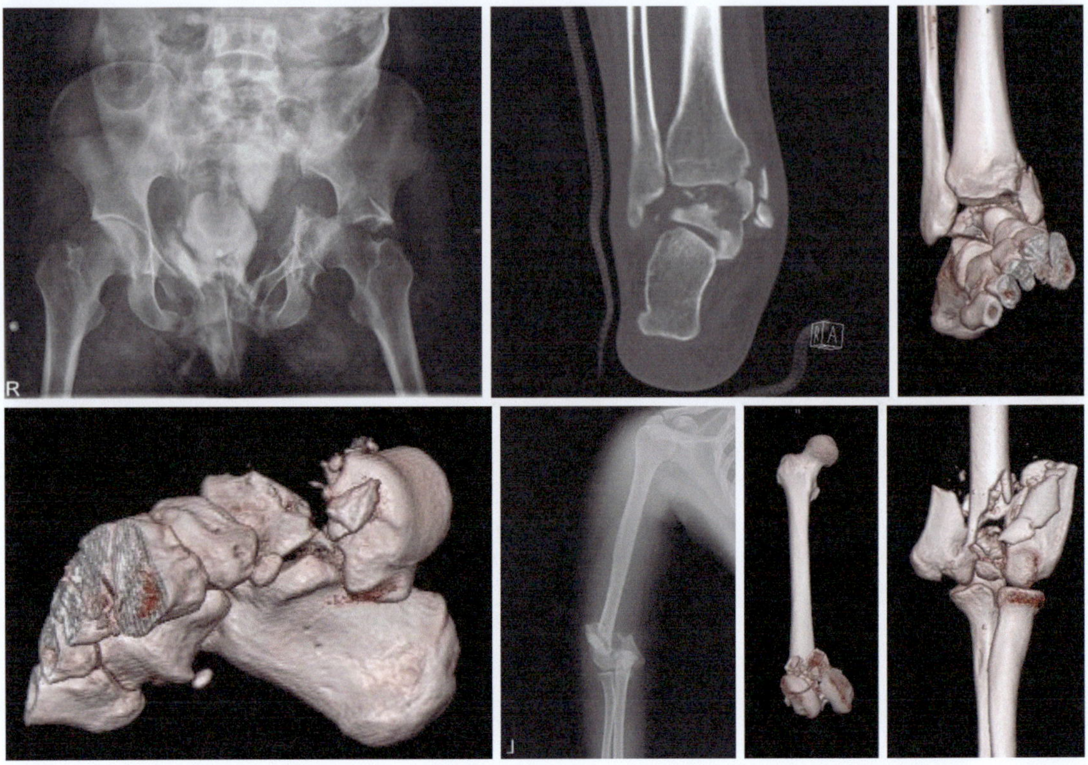

Fig. 14.1 Radiologic images of past traffic accident

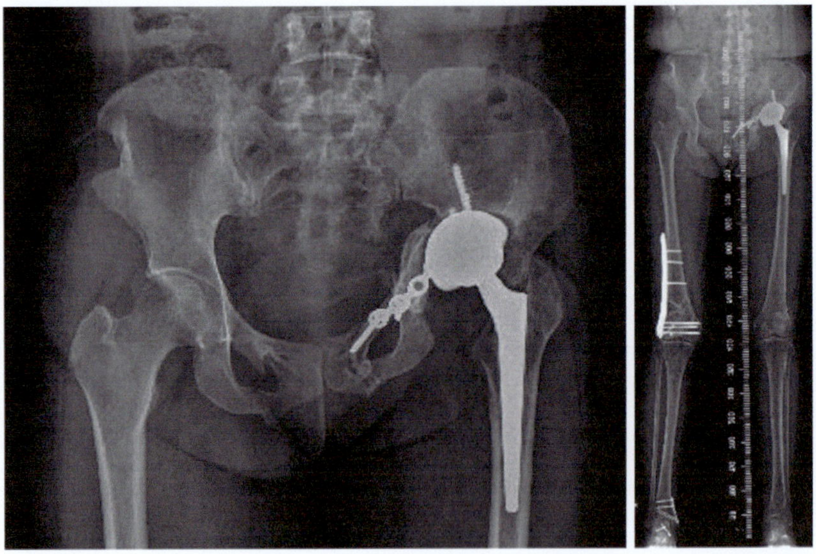

Fig. 14.2 Preoperative X-ray images

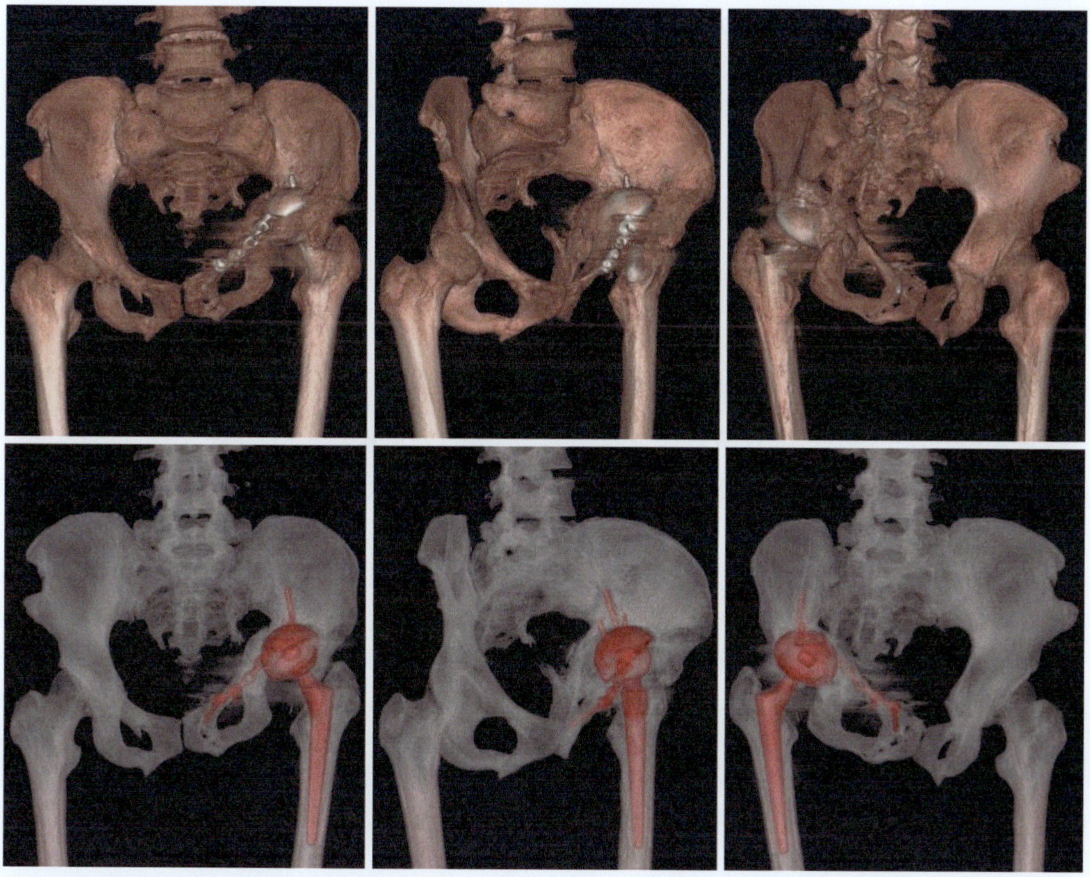

Fig. 14.3 Preoperative CT images

14.3 Planning of Surgery

Preserves the bones around the acetabular cup as much as possible

Thick solid iliac plate
The body is mesh style
Omit pubis and ischium
Maintained femoral stem

14.4 Design and Fabrication

- Implant measurement
- Implant weight (g): 198
- Size (mm): 131

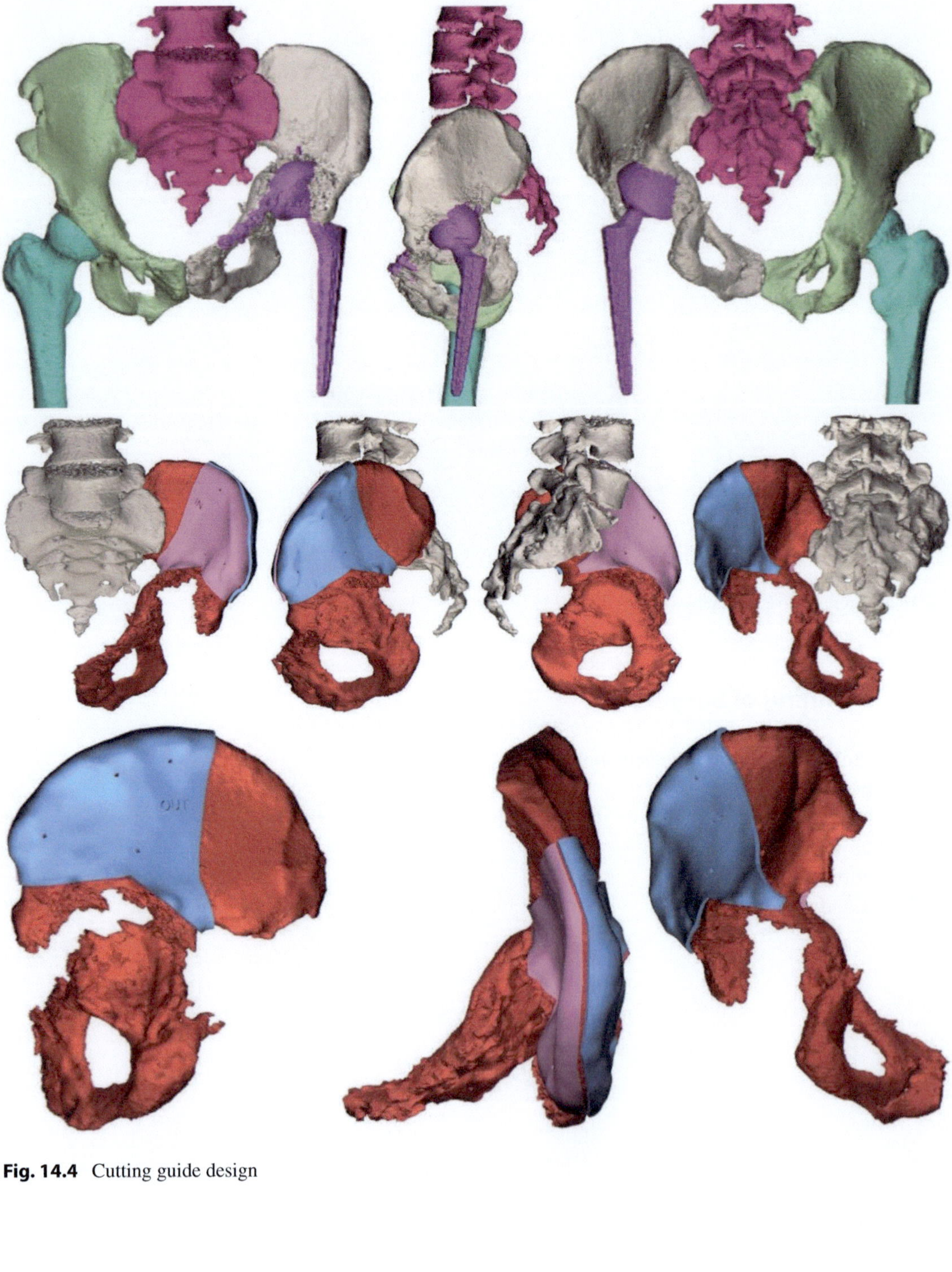

Fig. 14.4 Cutting guide design

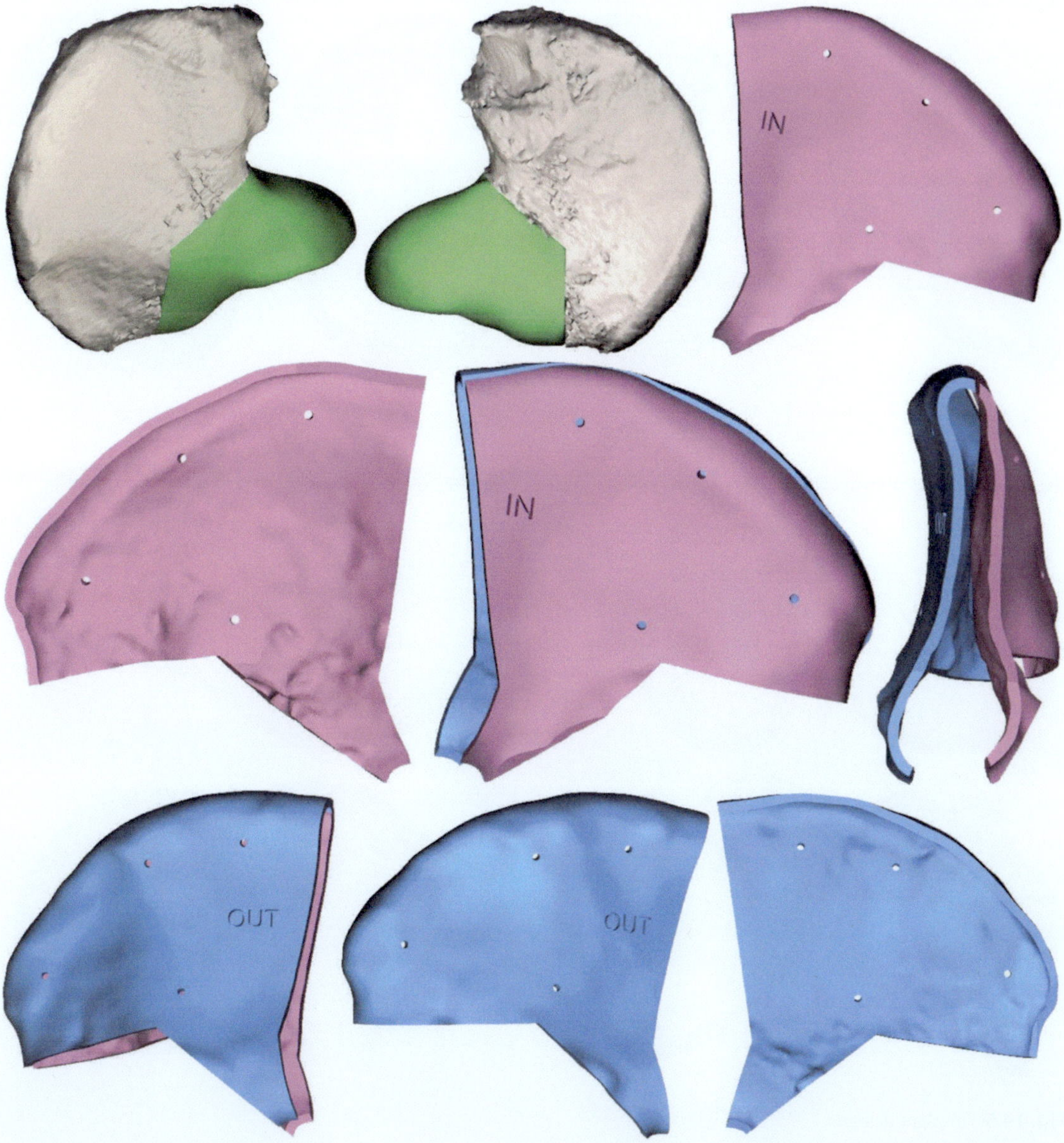

Fig. 14.4 (continued)

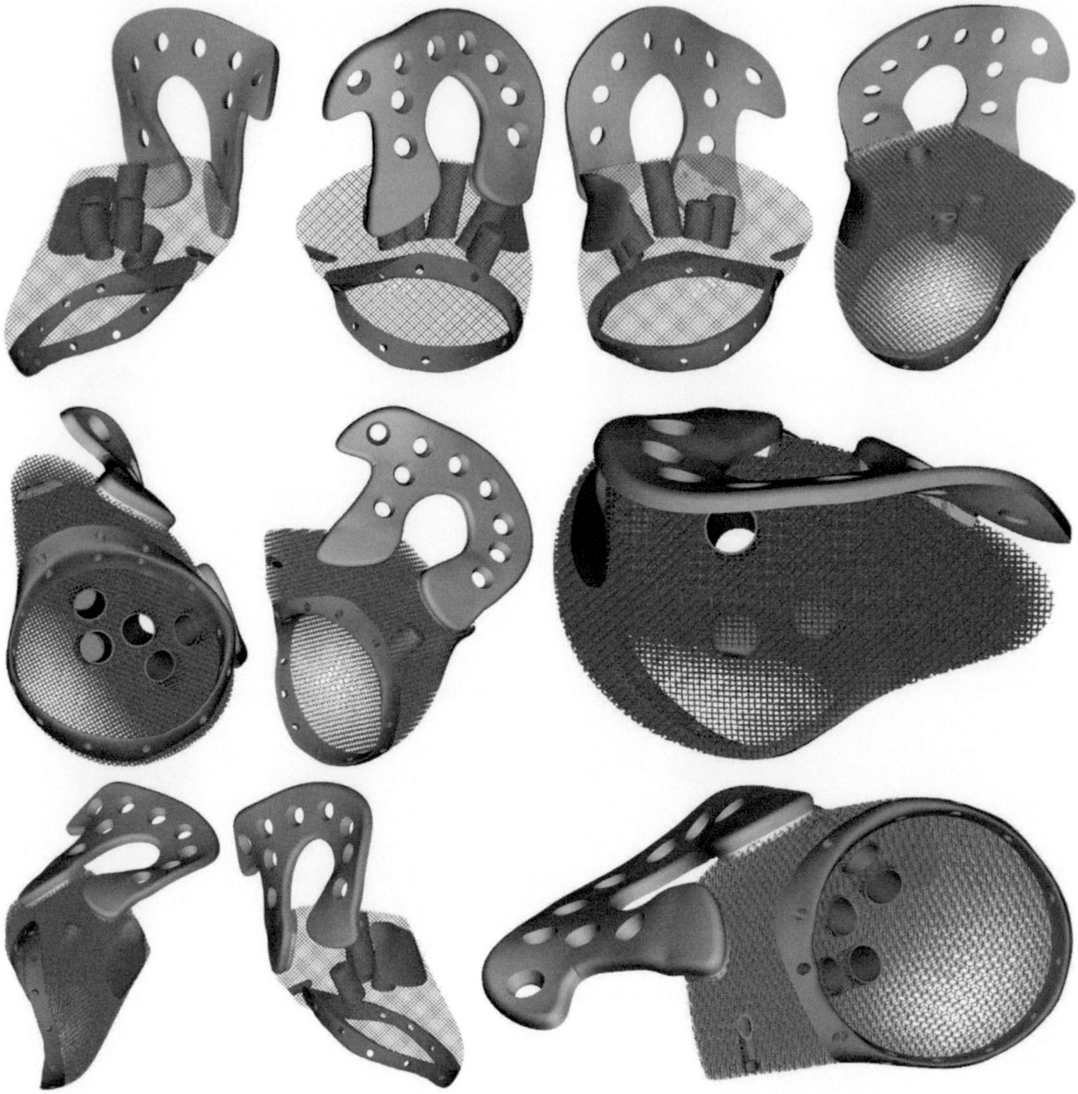

Fig. 14.5 Implant design

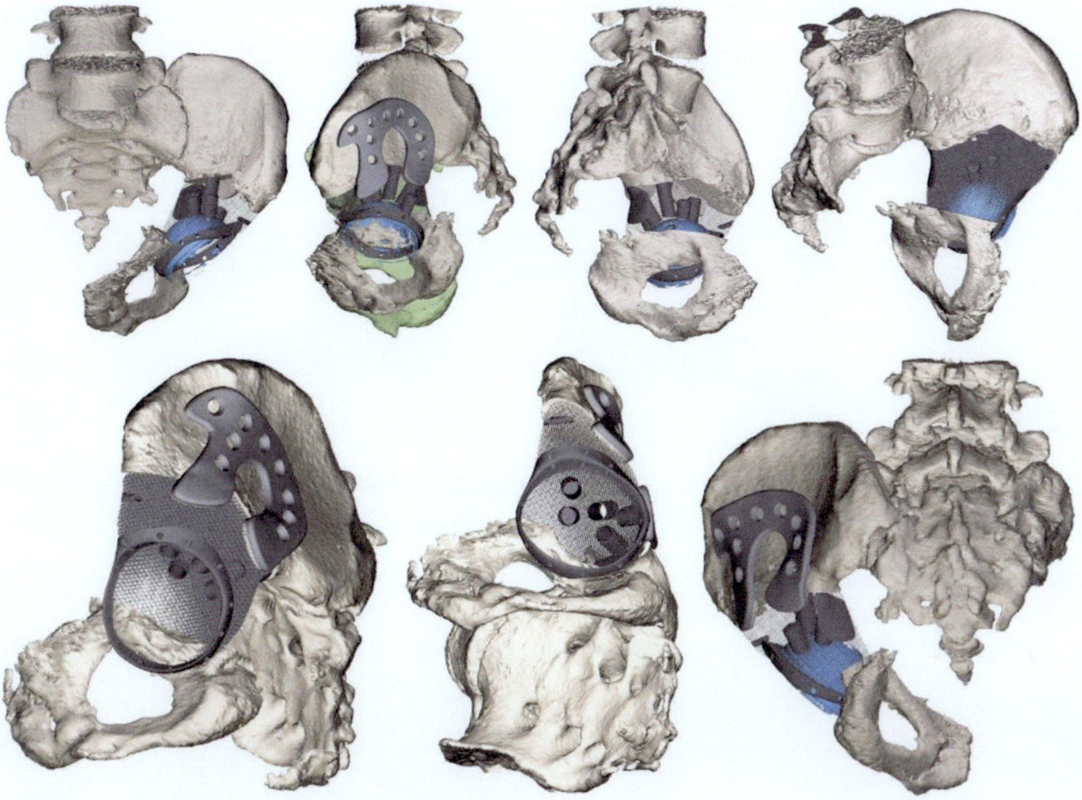

Fig. 14.5 (continued)

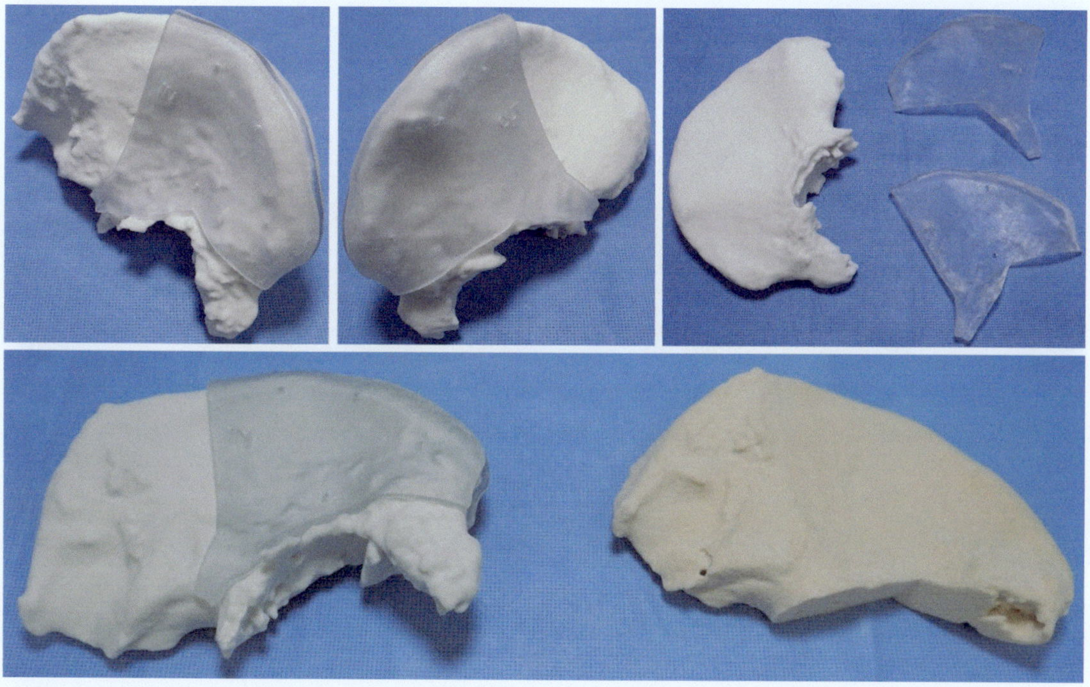

Fig. 14.6 Printed cutting guide

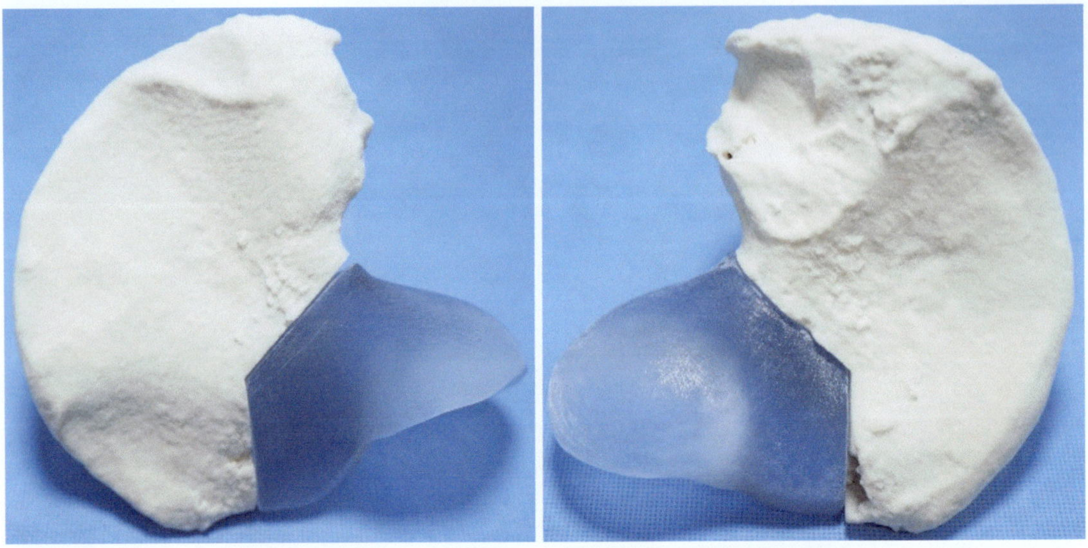

Fig. 14.7 Printed trial block

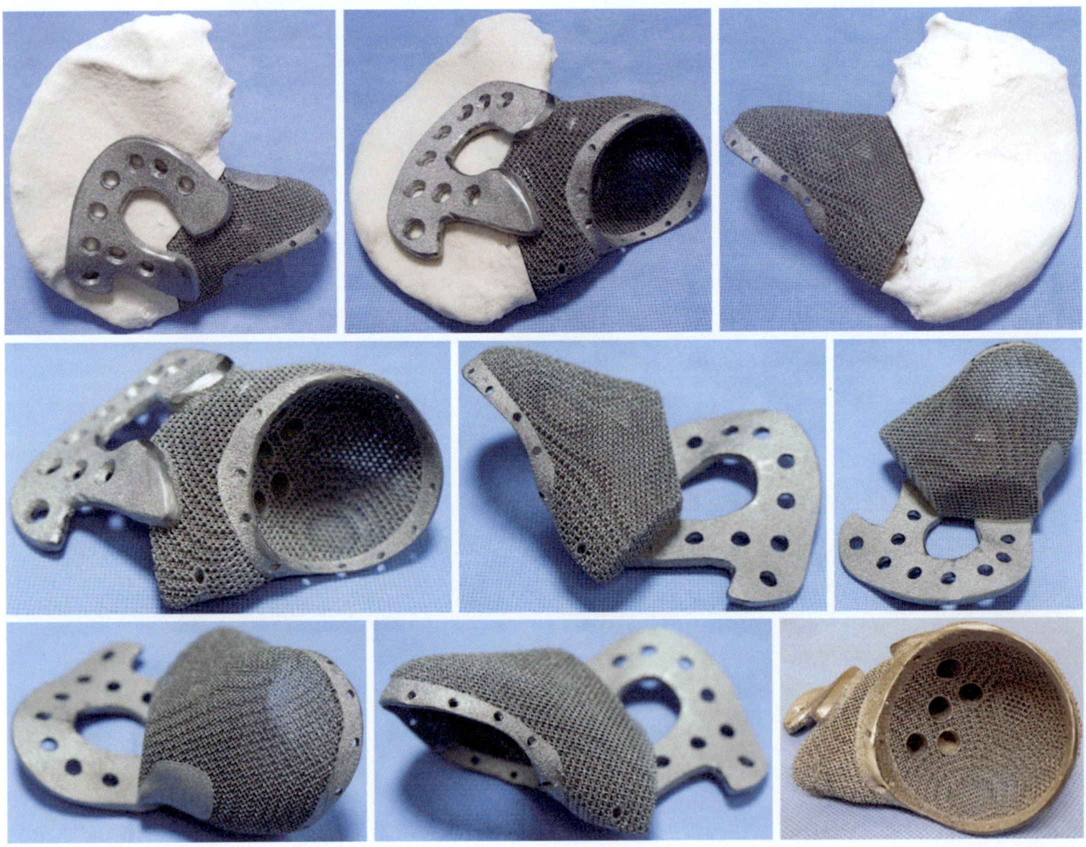

Fig. 14.8 Printed Implant

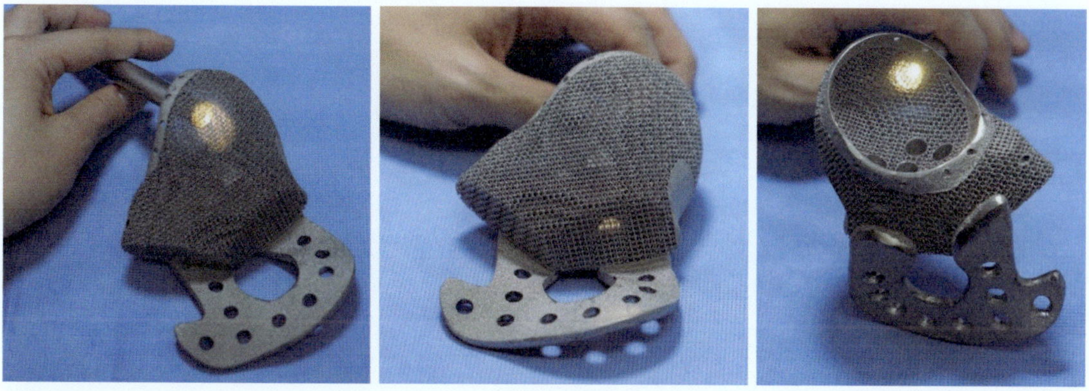

Fig. 14.9 Printed Implant: Mesh style enough to transmit light

14.5 Operation

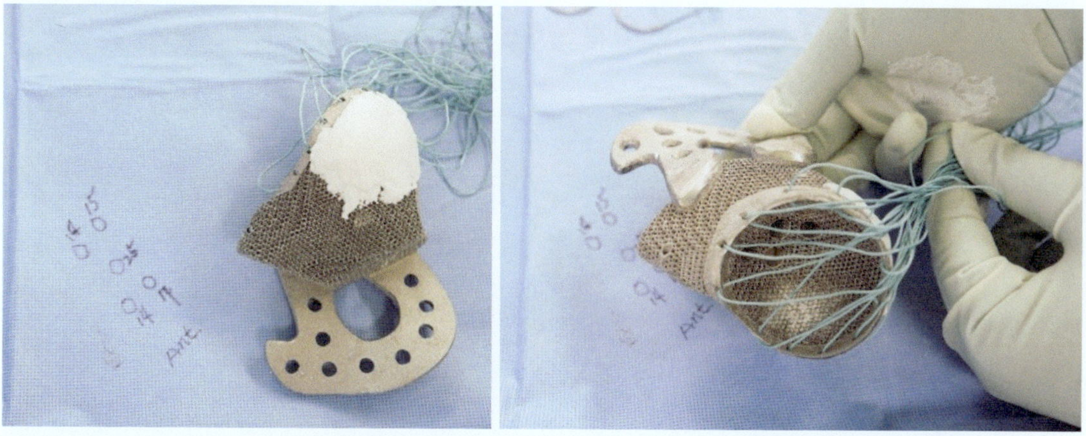

Fig. 14.10 Intraoperative photographs: attach a calcium-based bone substitute to the medial wall

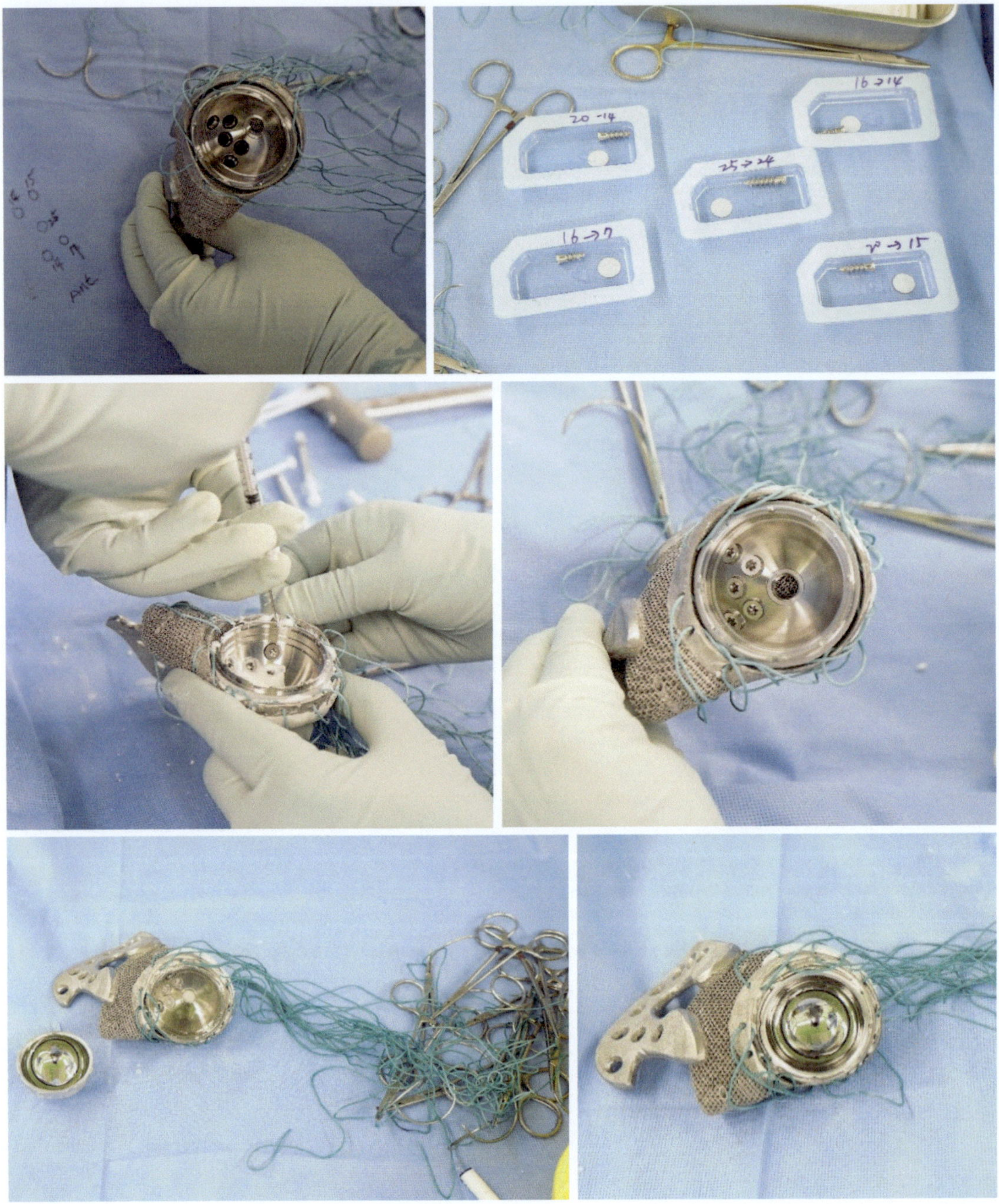

Fig. 14.11 Intraoperative photographs: after fixing the metal shell with PMMA cement and cup screws, connect the metal liner

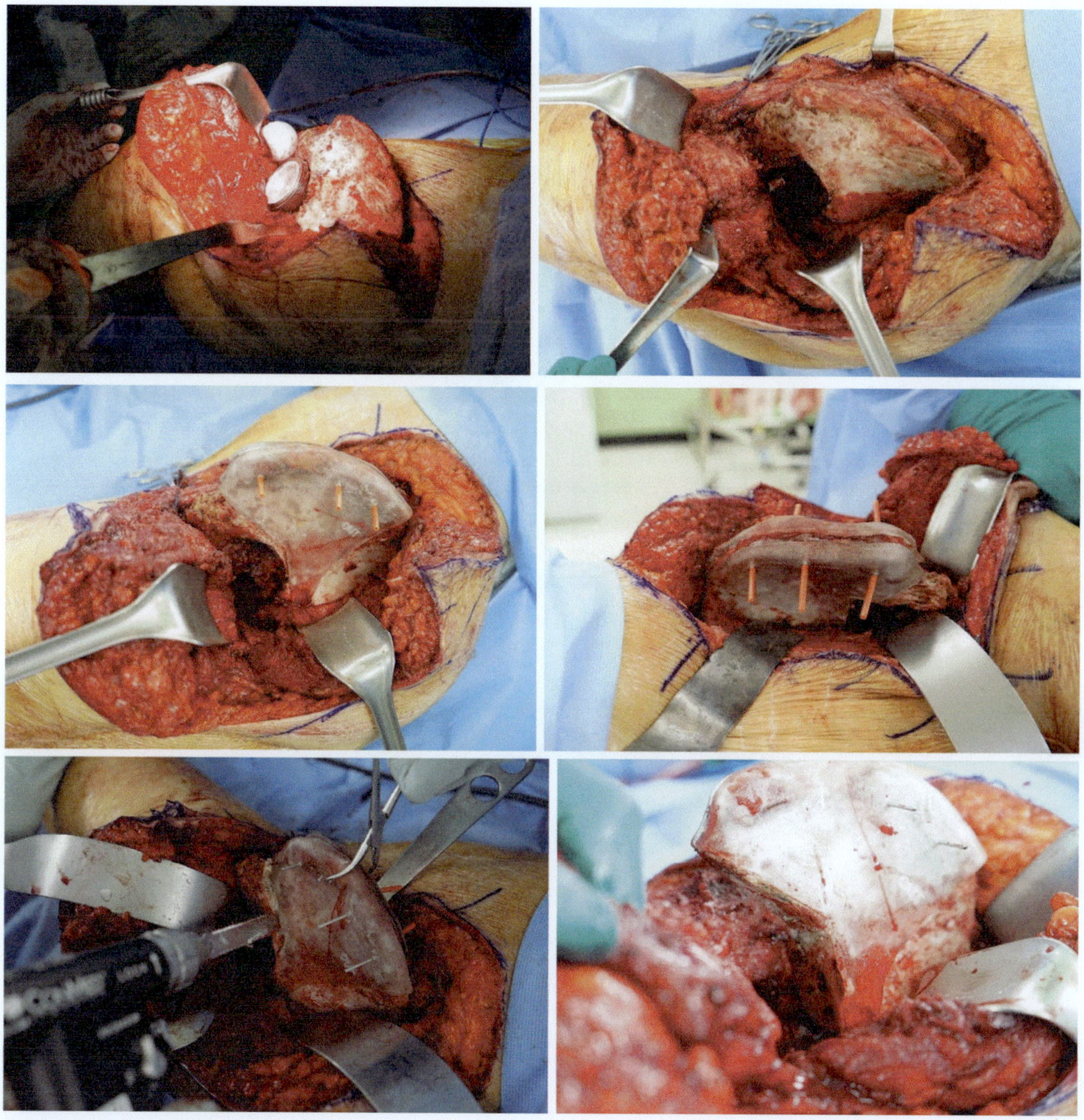

Fig. 14.12 Intraoperative photographs

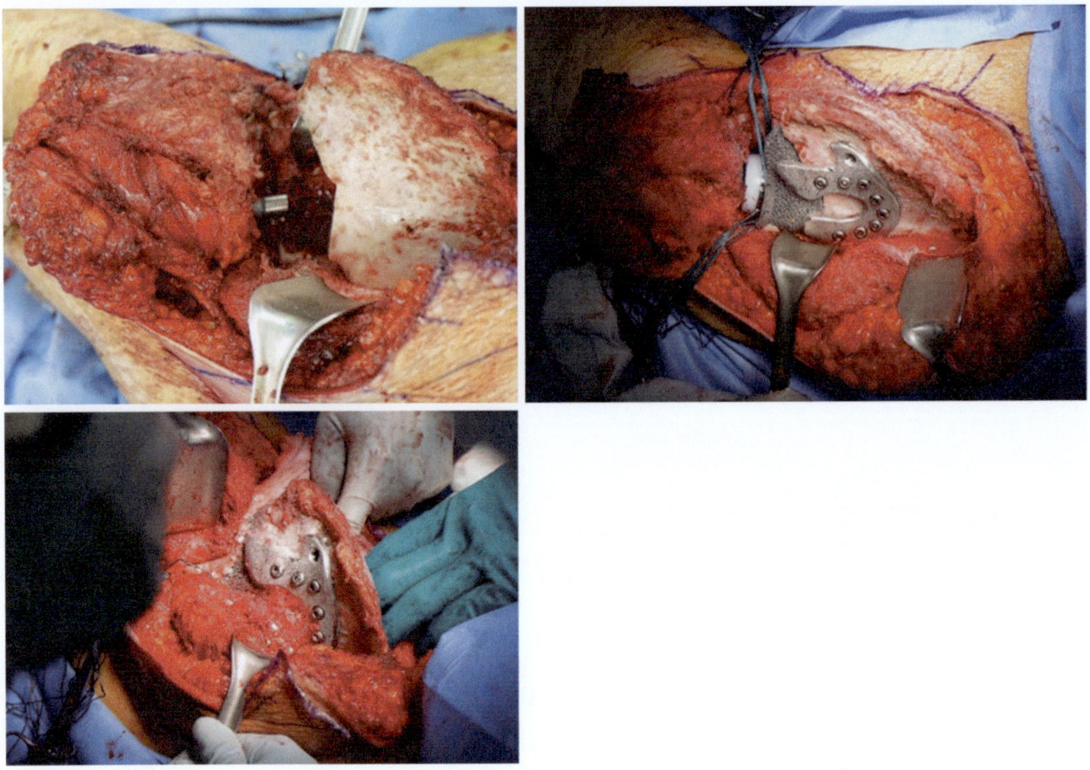

Fig. 14.12 (continued)

14.6 Postoperative Images

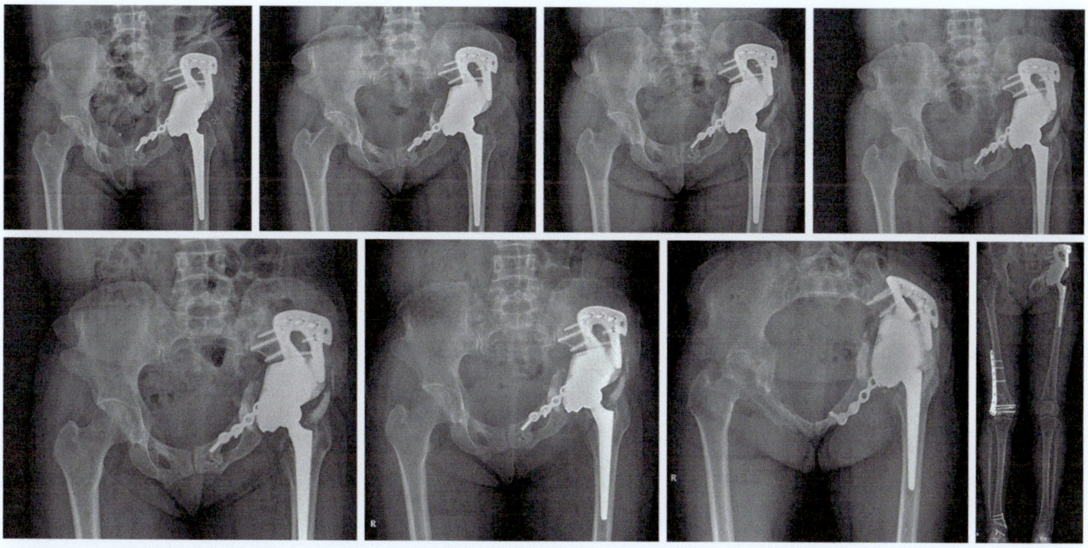

Fig. 14.13 Postoperative X-ray images

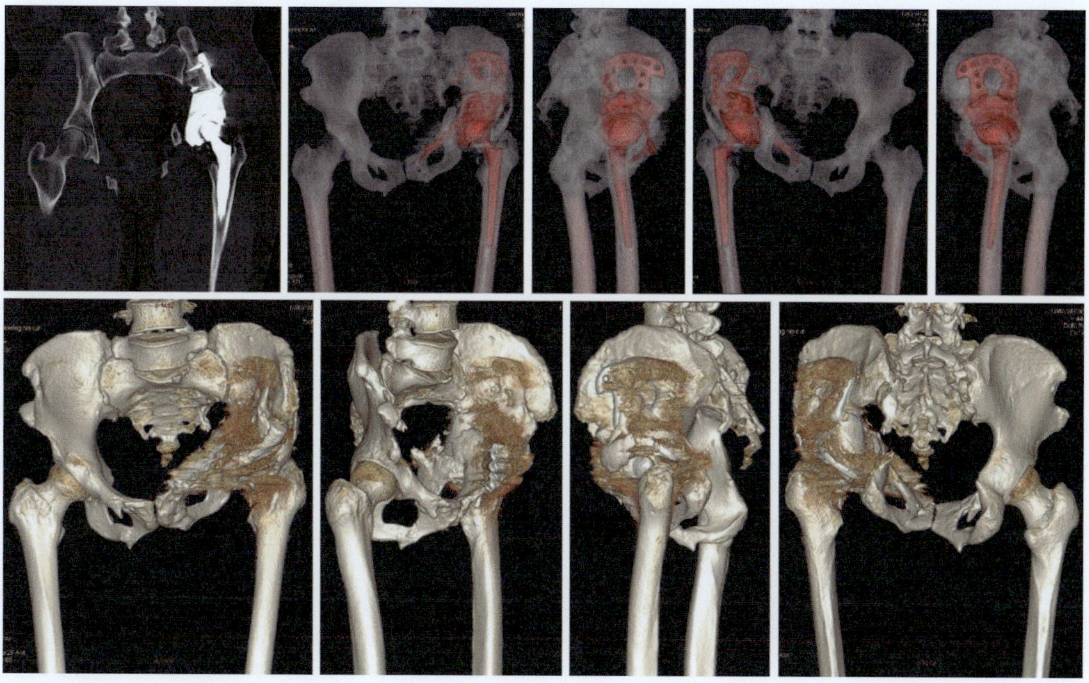

Fig. 14.14 Postoperative CT images

Patient Case 15: Revision: Complicated Saddle Prosthesis

15

15.1 Patient Case 15

Age/sex	56/male
Location/site	Pelvis/right
Diagnosis	Periprosthetic bone destruction
Preoperative symptom	Limping gate
BMI (height/weight)	24.22 (160/62)
Past history	Osteosarcoma pelvis at 20 years ago Saddle prosthesis bone reconstruction
Present illness	Increasing limping gait and difficult sitting posture

15.2 Preoperative Images

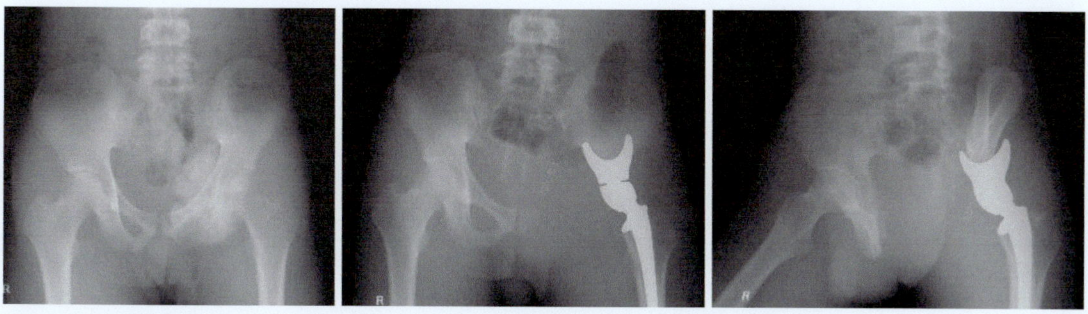

Fig. 15.1 Saddle prosthesis reconstruction of pelvic osteosarcoma at 20 years ago

H.-G. Kang, *Clinical Atlas of 3D Printing Bone Reconstruction*,
https://doi.org/10.1007/978-981-16-2043-0_15

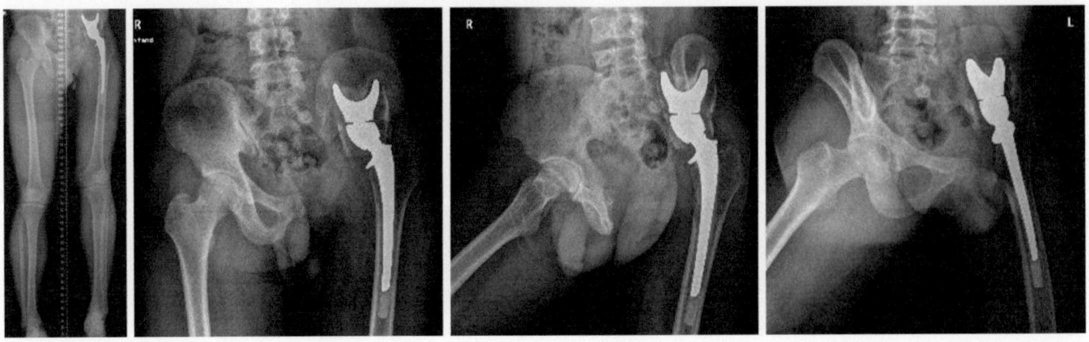

Fig. 15.2 Preoperative X-ray images

15.3 Planning of Surgery

Preserve bone around the acetabular cup as much as possible

Iliac fixation plate is a thick solid
The body is mesh style
Omit pubis and ischium
Femoral stem is maintained
Saddle stem femoral neck cone taper 14/16

- 3D printed pelvis
- Acetabular metal shell, metal liner, poly cup (Stryker, MDM® system) +
- 28 mm Femoral head, neck cone taper 14/16 (DePuy Synthes, BIOLOX® delta)

  Prepare screwdriver of Saddle prosthesis

15.4 Design and Fabrication

- Implant measurement
- Implant weight (g): 245
- Size (mm): 121

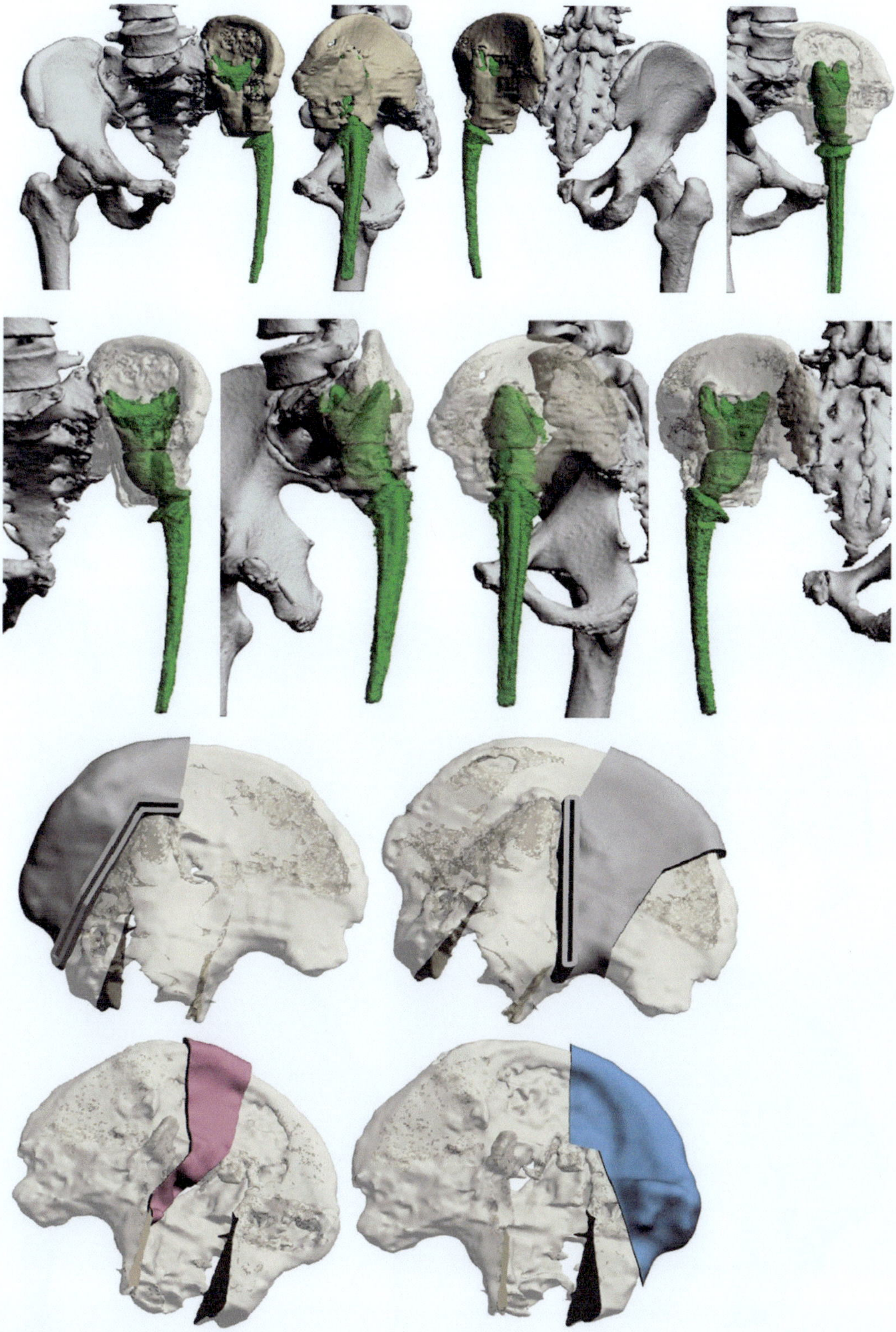

Fig. 15.3 Cutting guide design

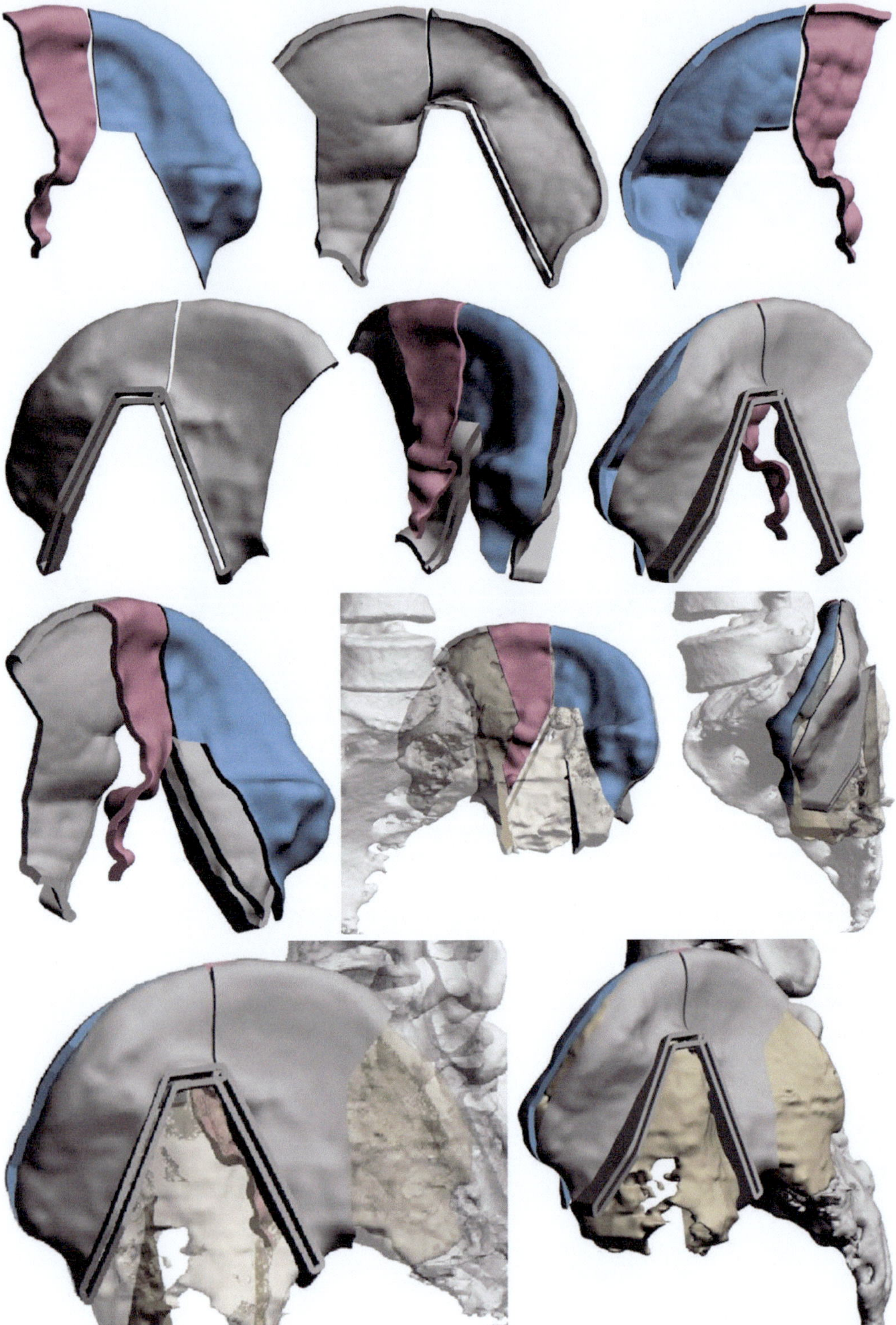

Fig. 15.3 (continued)

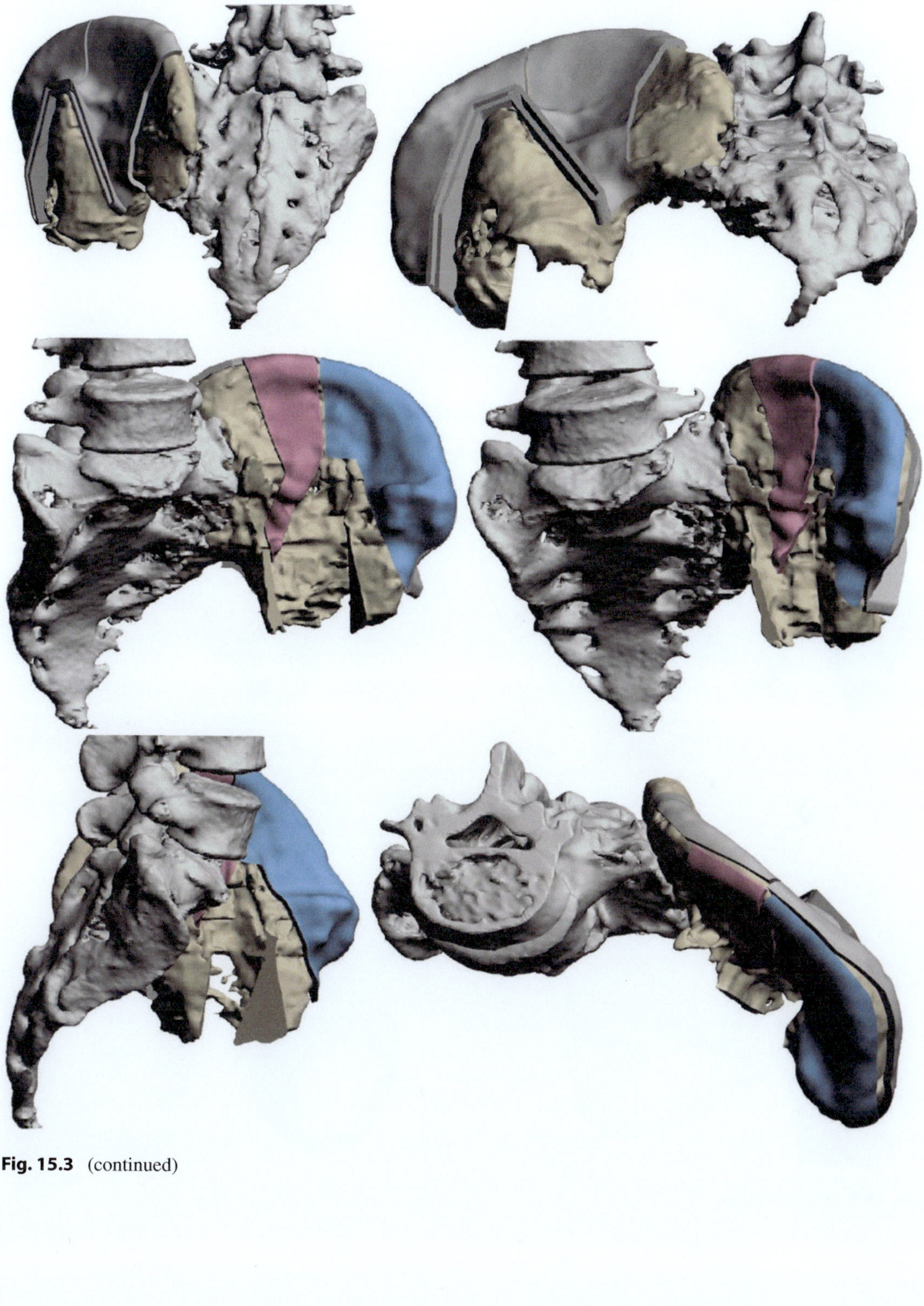

Fig. 15.3 (continued)

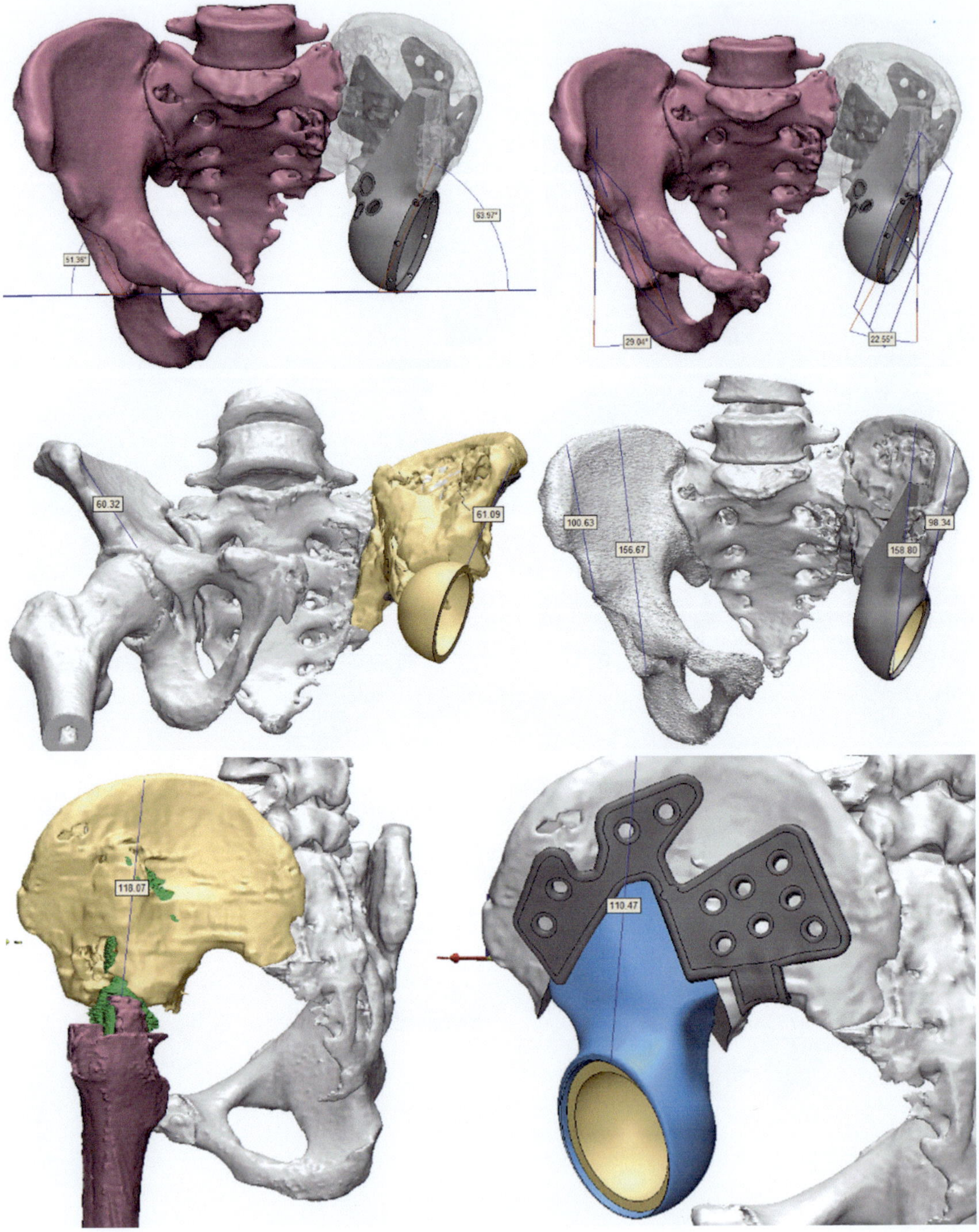

Fig. 15.4 Implant design

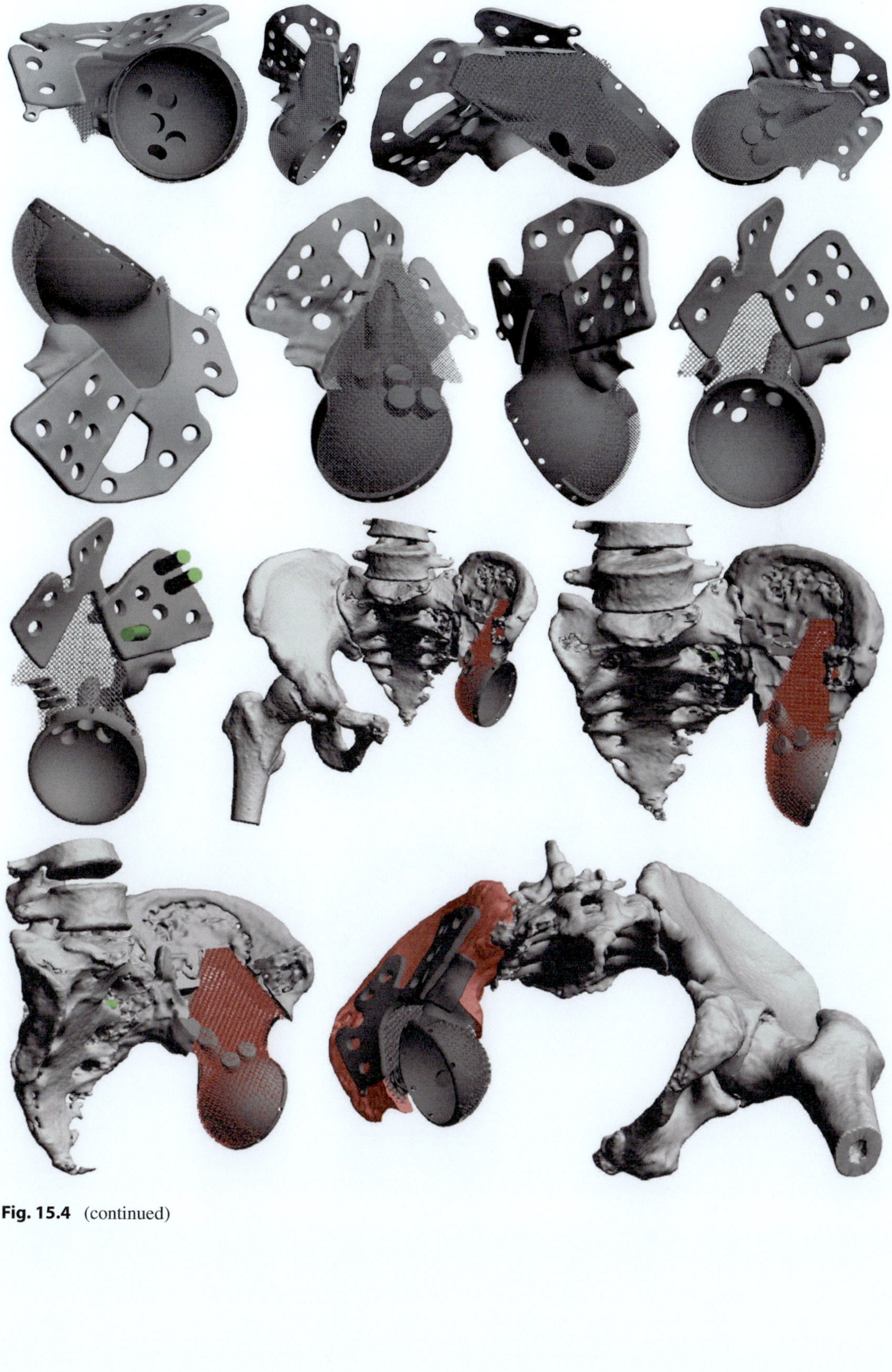

Fig. 15.4 (continued)

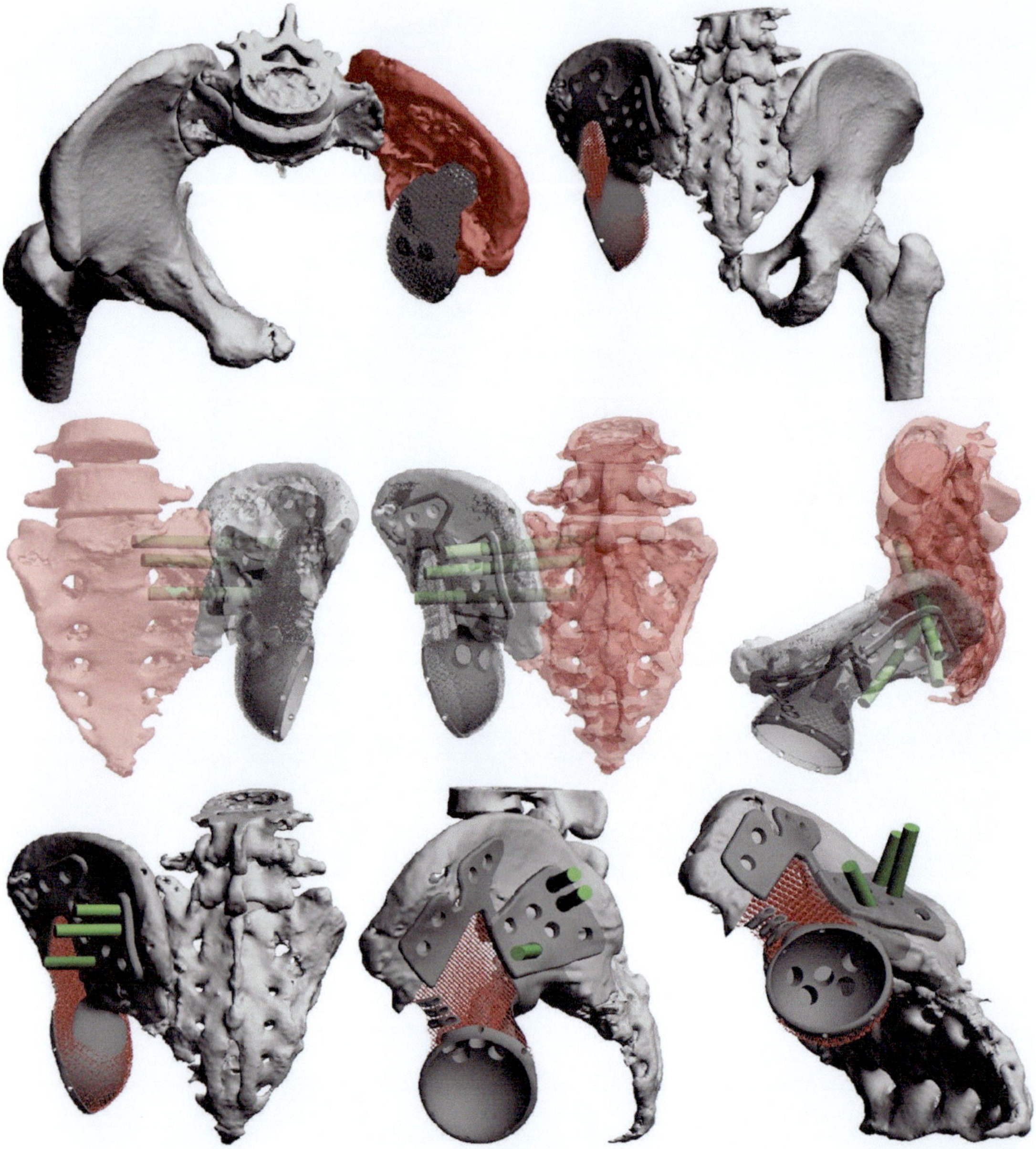

Fig. 15.4 (continued)

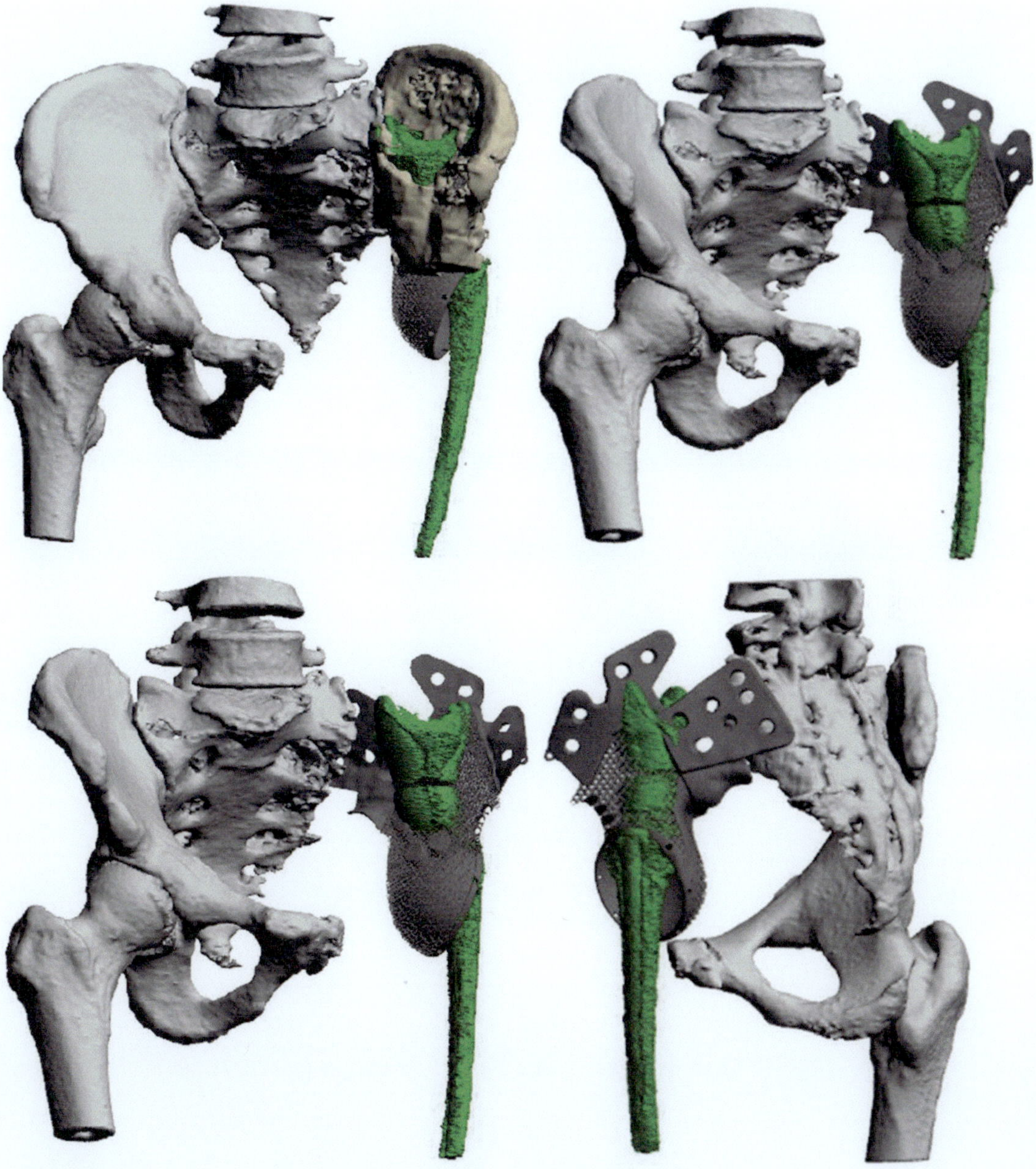

Fig. 15.5 Implant design: overlapping simulation before and after surgery

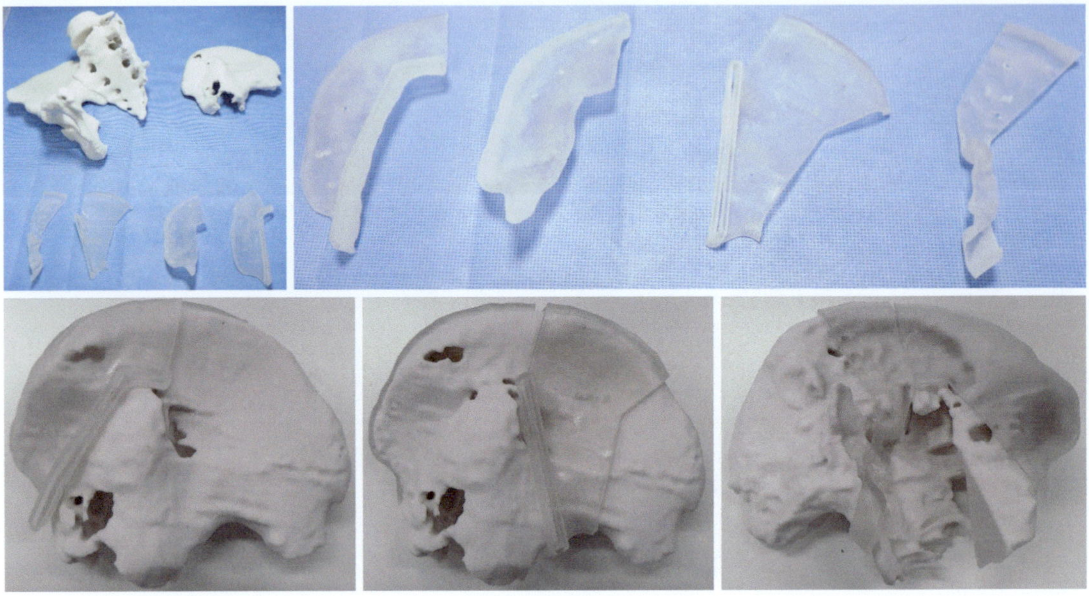

Fig. 15.6 Printed cutting guide

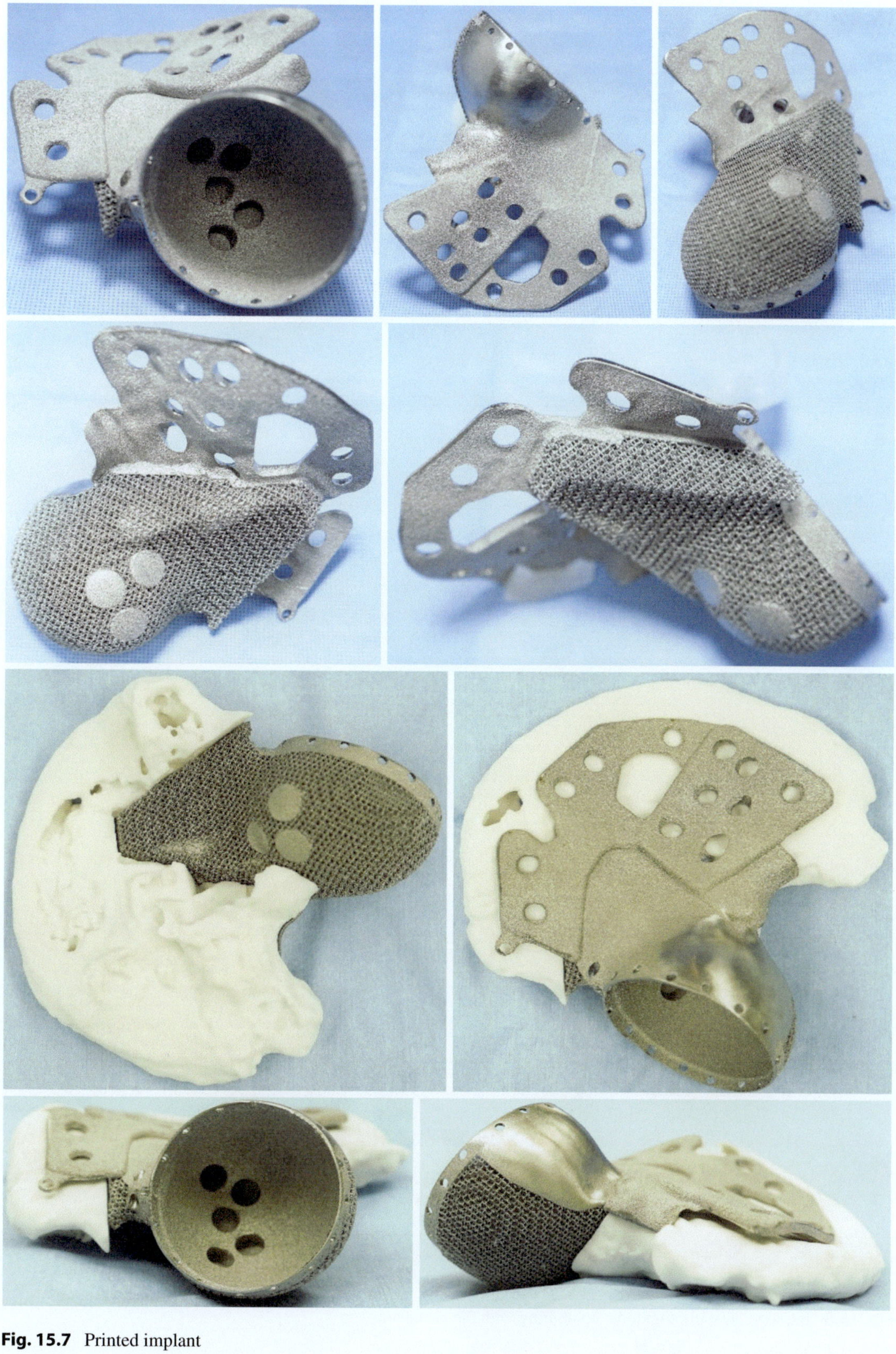

Fig. 15.7 Printed implant

15.5 Operation

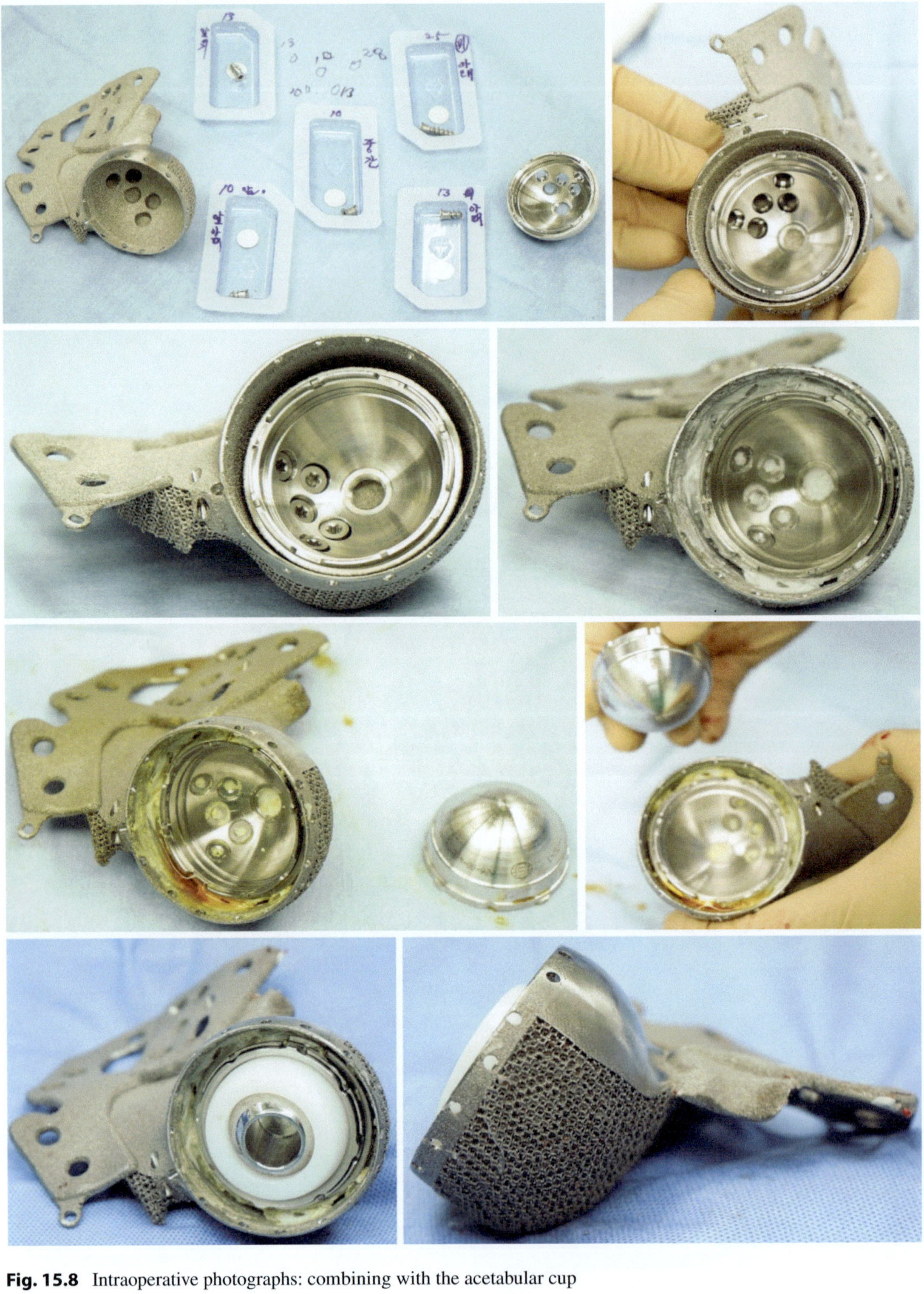

Fig. 15.8 Intraoperative photographs: combining with the acetabular cup

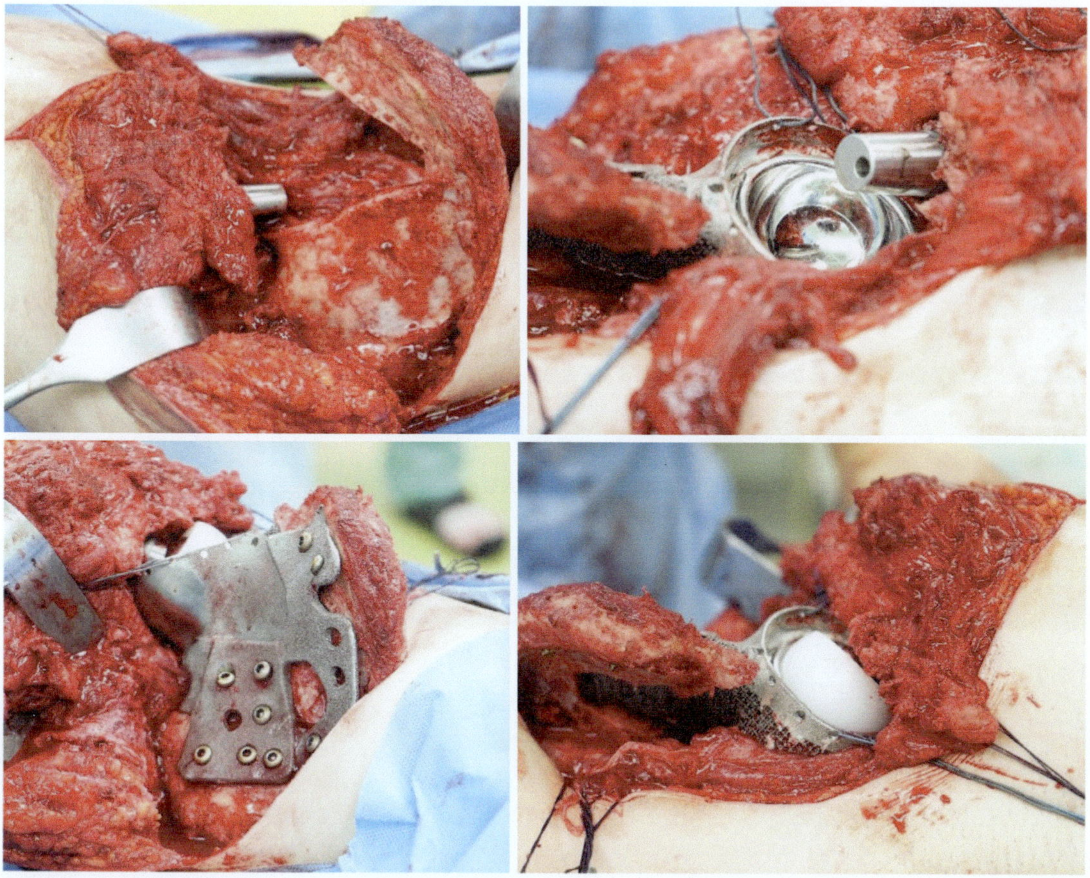

Fig. 15.9 Intraoperative photographs

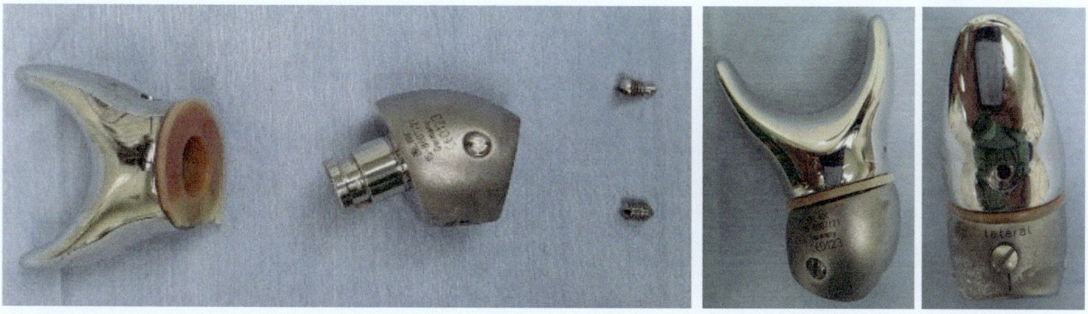

Fig. 15.10 Removed Saddle prosthesis

15.6 Postoperative Images

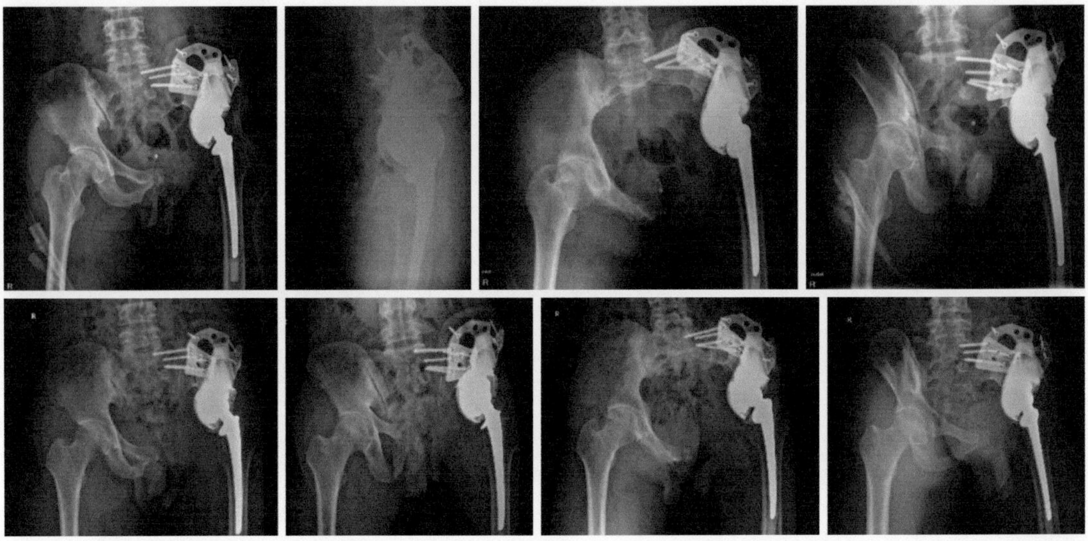

Fig. 15.11 Postoperative X-ray images

Part II

Femur

16 Patient Case 16: Allograft Bone Shaping Guide in the Cortical Resection

16.1 Patient 16

Age/sex	24/female
Location/site	Femur/left
Diagnosis	Parosteal osteosarcoma
Preoperative symptom	Pain on full flexion of the knee
Preoperative pain score	Resting 2/activity 2
BMI (height/weight)	24.23 (172.5/72.1)
Past history	Posterior knee pain aggravation
Present illness	Visits for save the joint

H.-G. Kang, *Clinical Atlas of 3D Printing Bone Reconstruction*,
https://doi.org/10.1007/978-981-16-2043-0_16

16.2 Preoperative Images

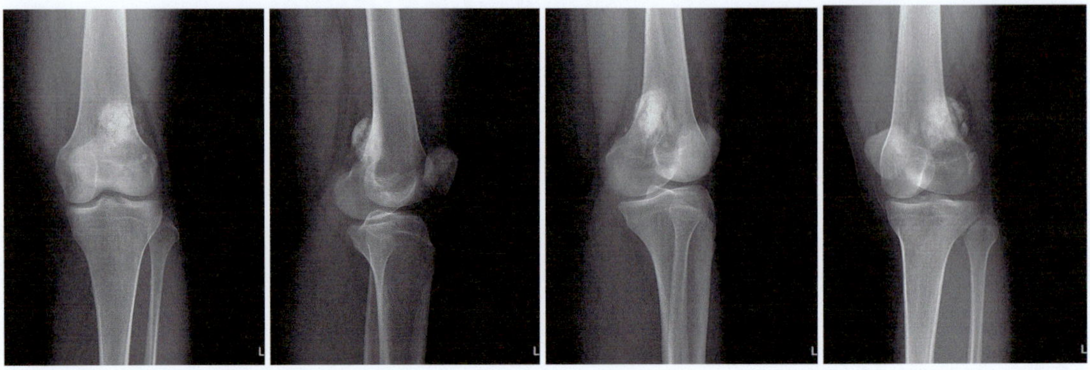

Fig. 16.1 Preoperative X-ray images: Tumor on the left distal femur

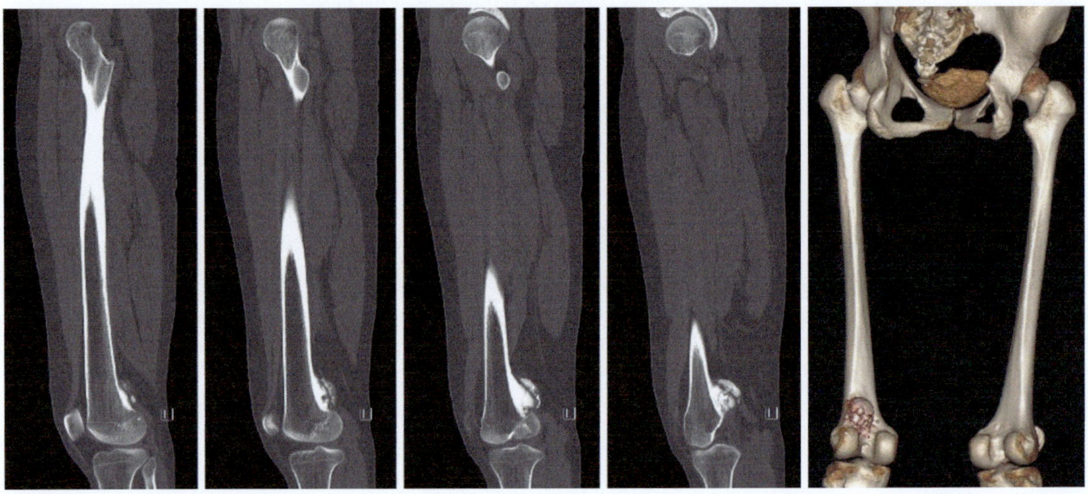

Fig. 16.2 Preoperative CT images

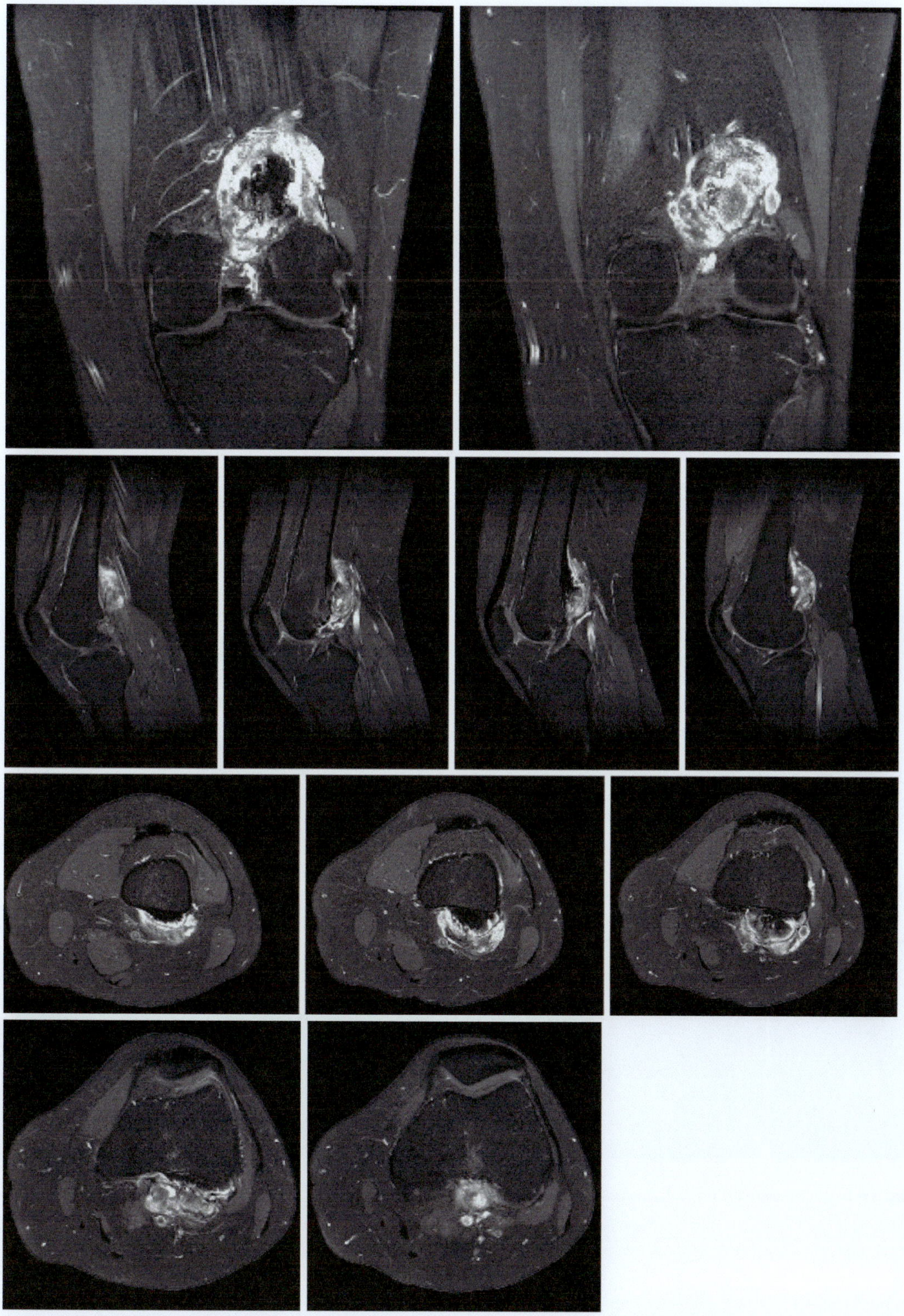

Fig. 16.3 Preoperative MRI images

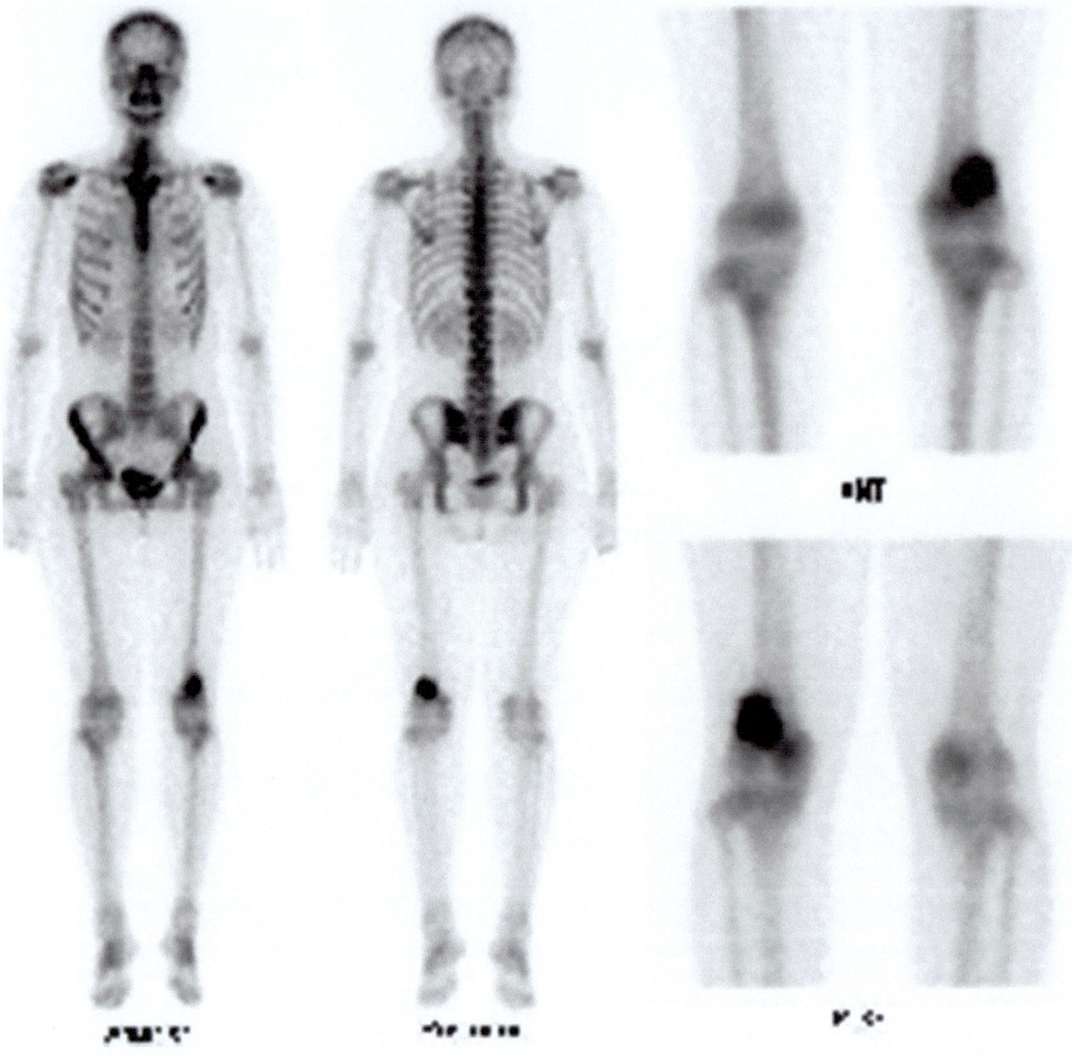

Fig. 16.4 Preoperative bone scan images

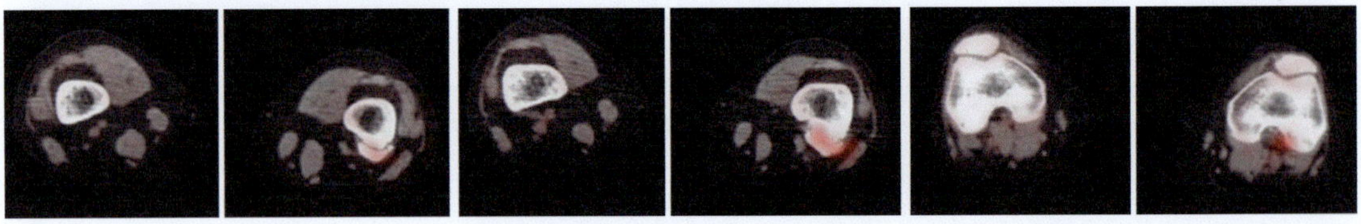

Fig. 16.5 Preoperative PET-CT images

16.3 Planning of Surgery

3D printed bone tumor resection guide
3D Printed allograft bone shaping guide

16.4 Design and Fabrication

A closed-type cutting guide is advantageous when there is no cortical breakage, no soft tissue tumor extension, no cartilaginous tumor, and there is limited soft tissue dissection.

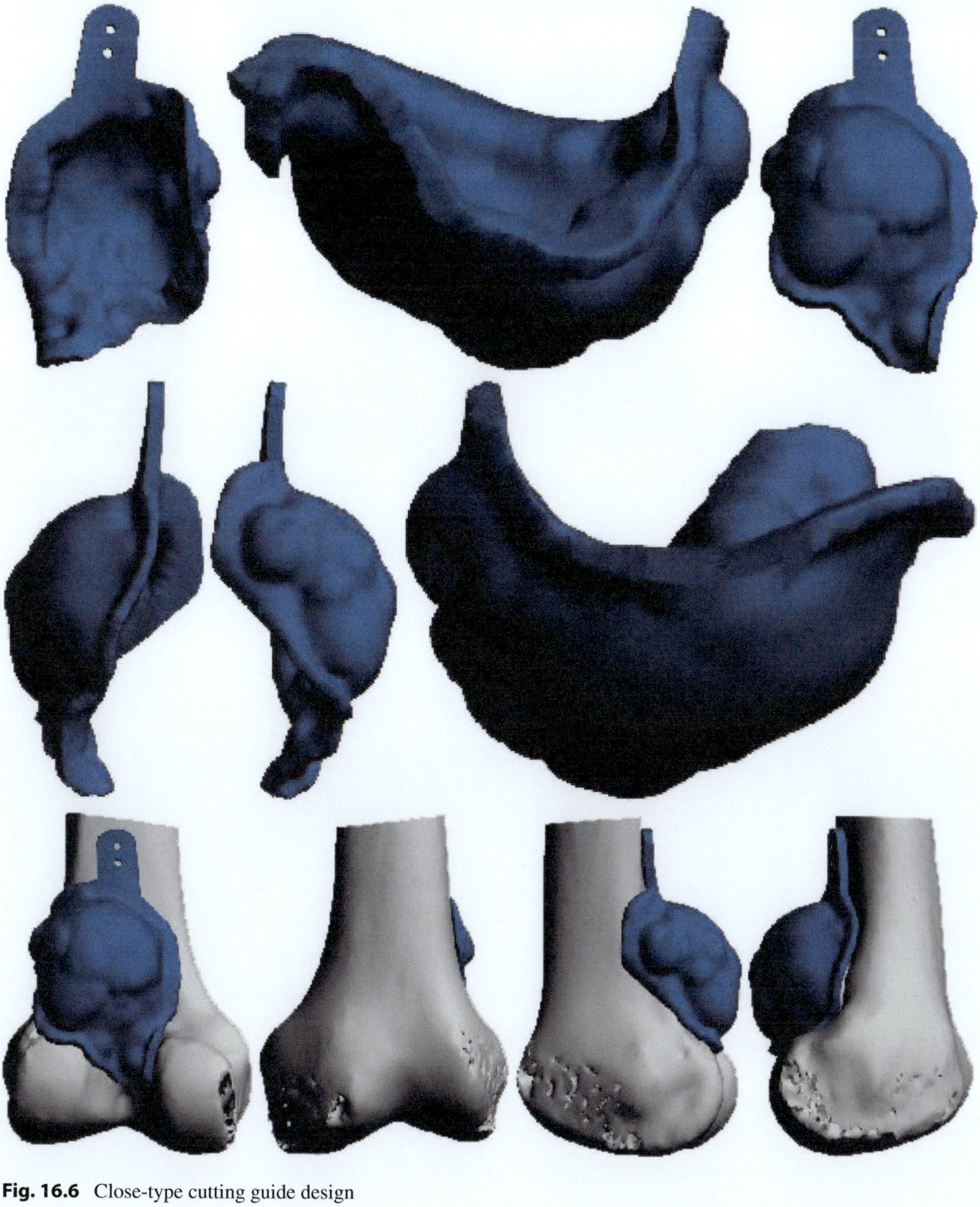

Fig. 16.6 Close-type cutting guide design

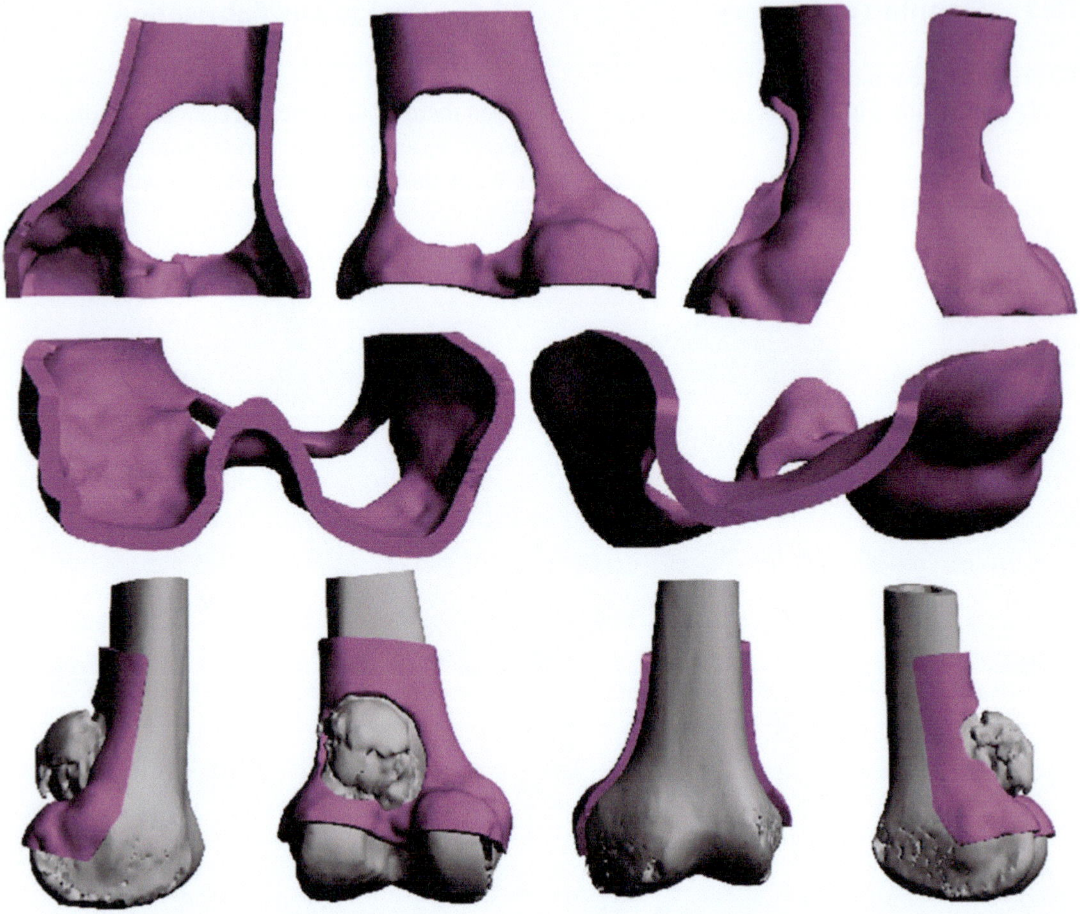

Fig. 16.7 Open-type cutting guide design

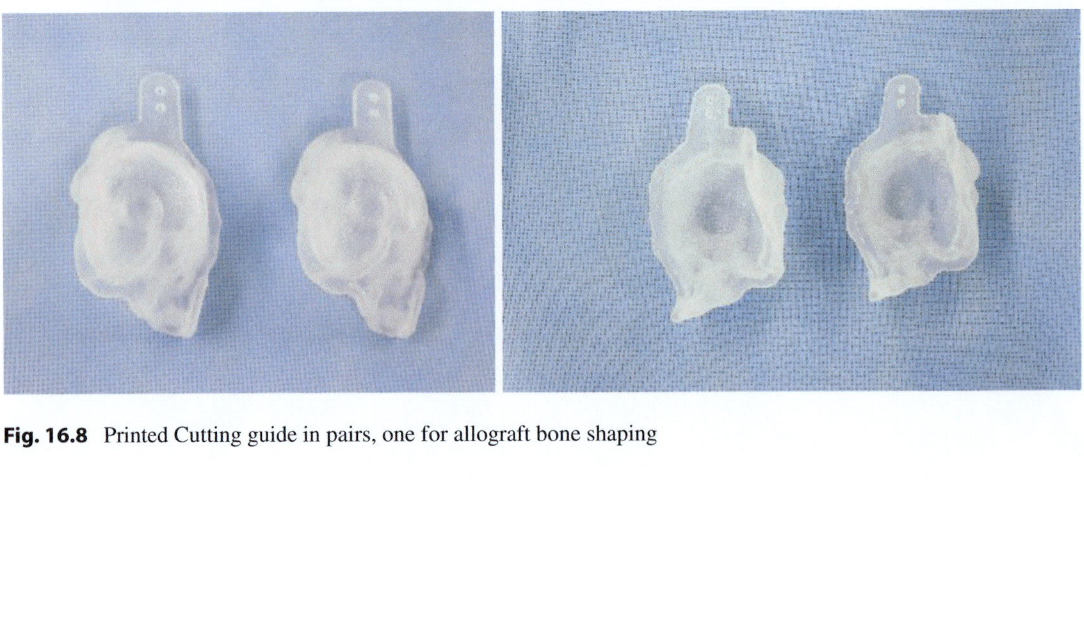

Fig. 16.8 Printed Cutting guide in pairs, one for allograft bone shaping

16.5 Operation

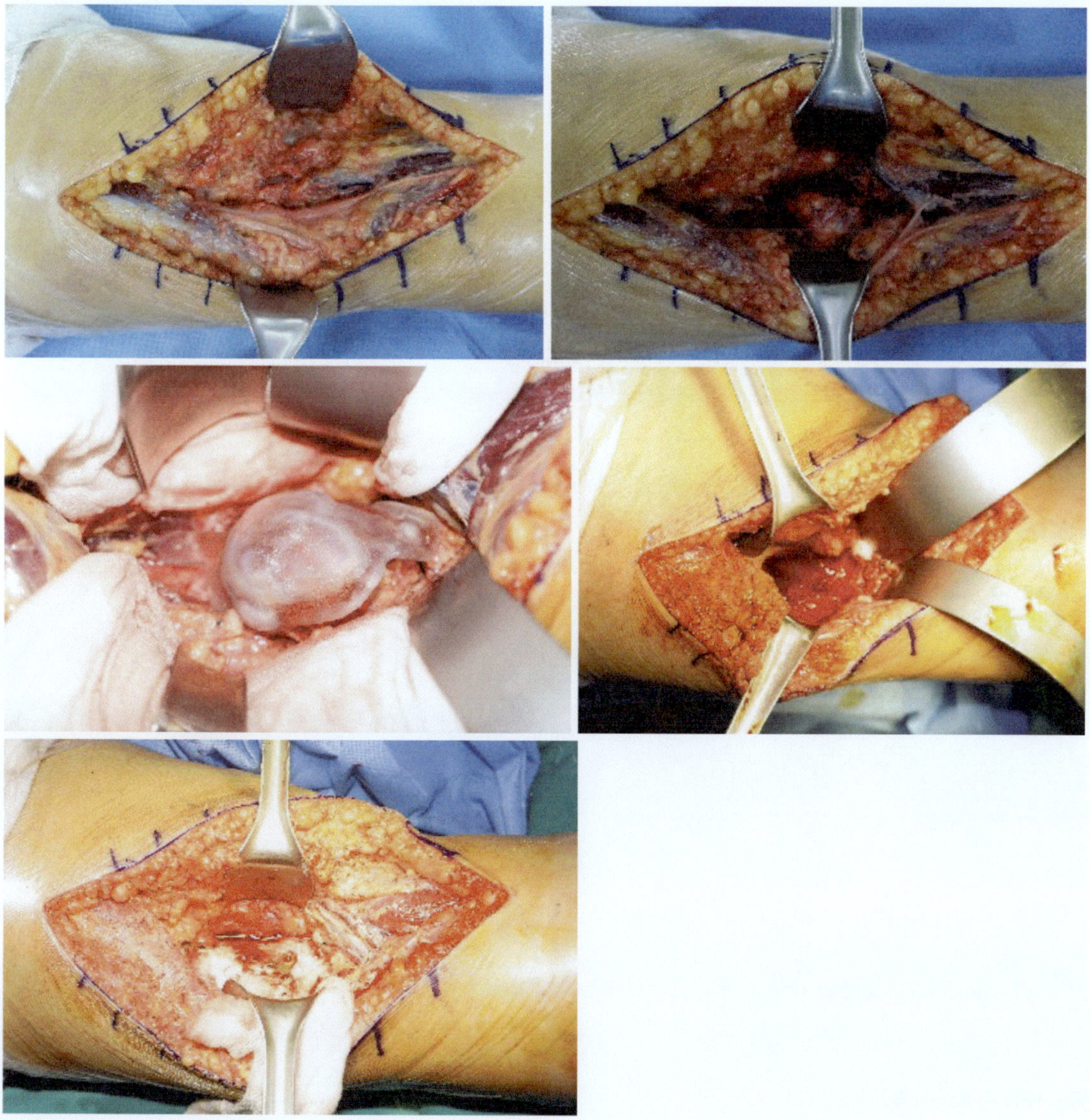

Fig. 16.9 Intraoperative photographs

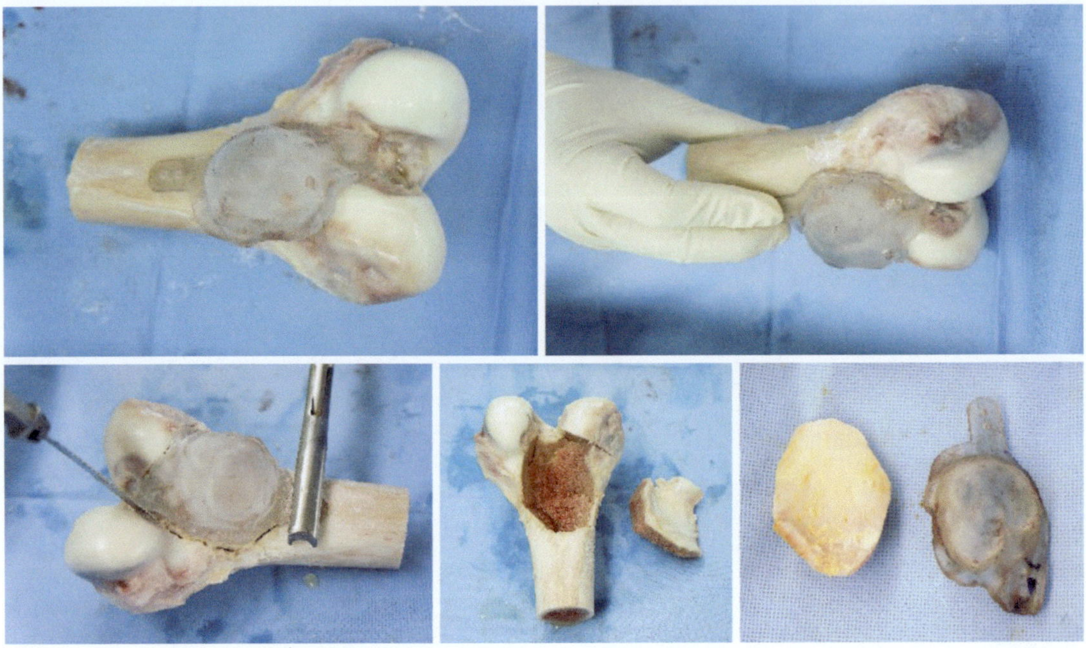

Fig. 16.10 Allograft bone shaping guide

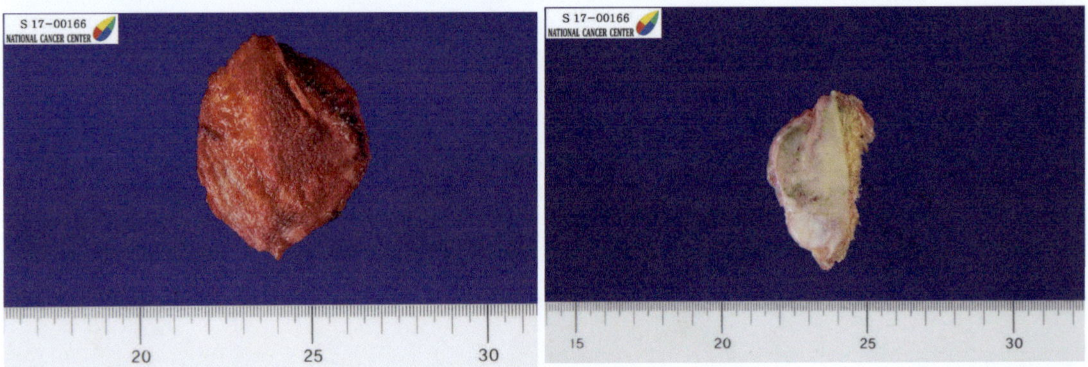

Fig. 16.11 Resected tumor

16.6 Postoperative Images

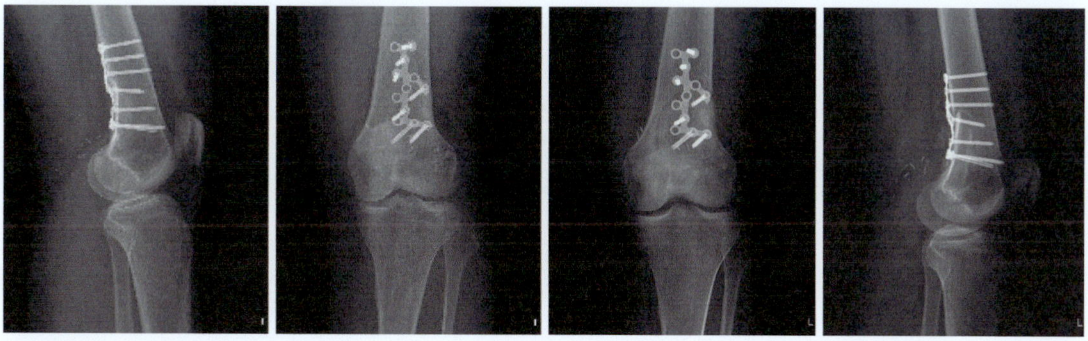

Fig. 16.12 Postoperative X-ray images

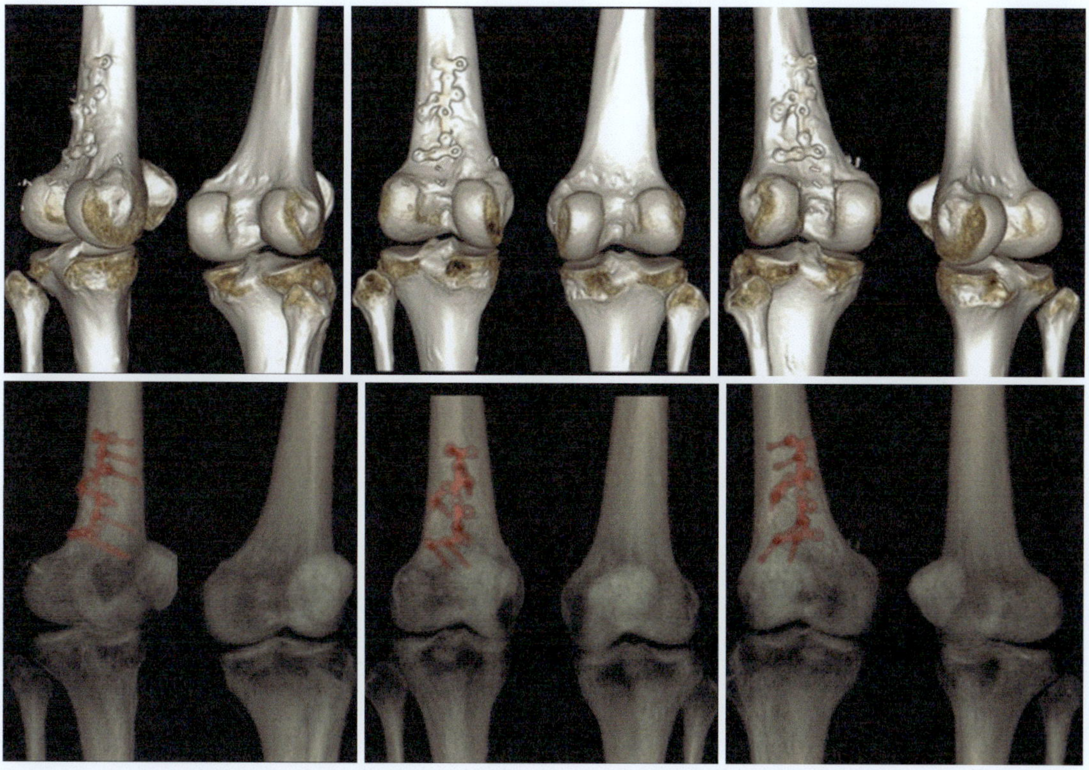

Fig. 16.13 Postoperative CT images

Patient Case 17: Plate with Reinforcement Ridge

17

17.1 Patient 17

Age/sex	68/male
Location/site	Femur/right
Diagnosis	Melorheostosis
Preoperative symptom	Restricted knee flexion
Preoperative pain score	Resting 1/activity 1
BMI (height/weight)	22.56 (165.9/62.1)
Past history	Discomfort for over 10 years
Present illness	Palpable mass with progressive nerve compression symptom Surgery planning under the possibility of malignant bone tumor such as parosteal osteosarcoma

H.-G. Kang, *Clinical Atlas of 3D Printing Bone Reconstruction*,
https://doi.org/10.1007/978-981-16-2043-0_17

17.2 Preoperative Images

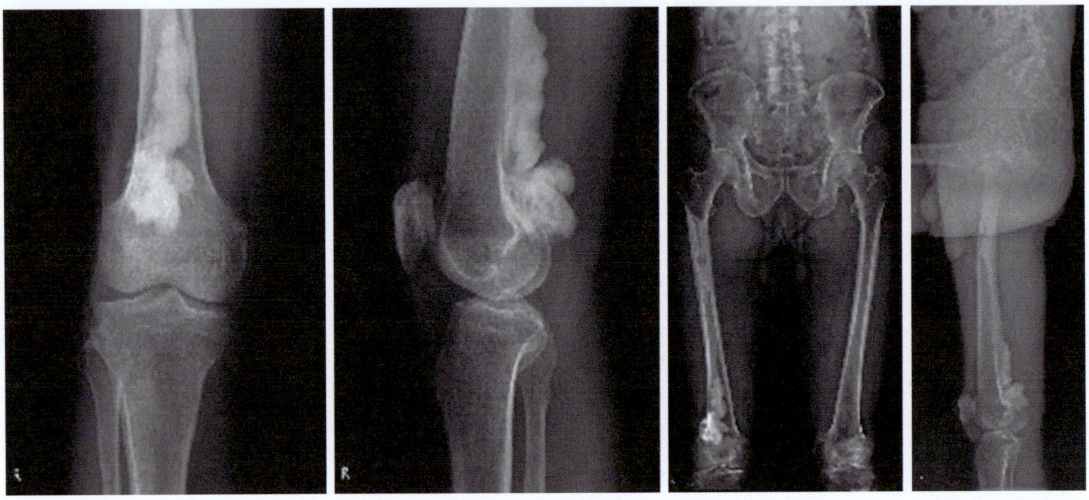

Fig. 17.1 Preoperative X-ray images: tumor elongated to the diaphysis

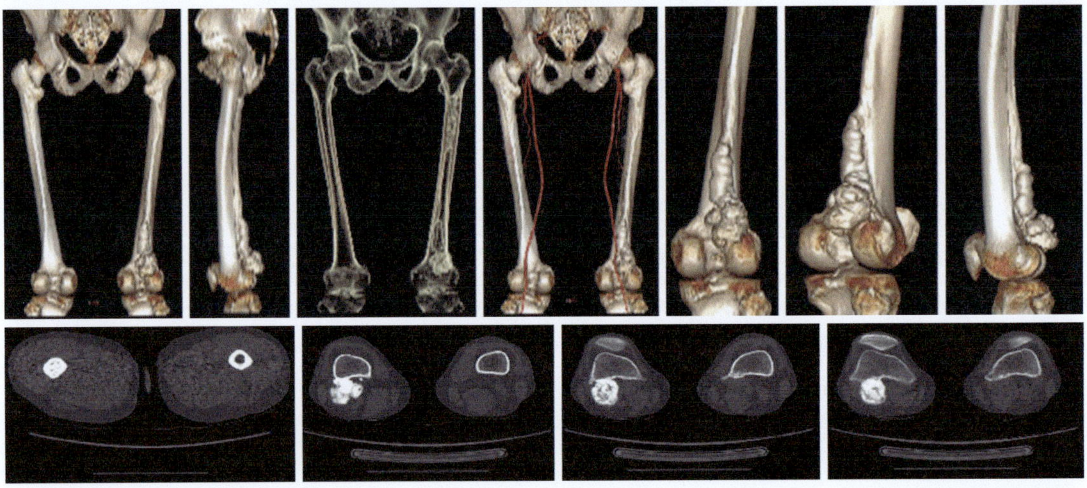

Fig. 17.2 Preoperative CT images

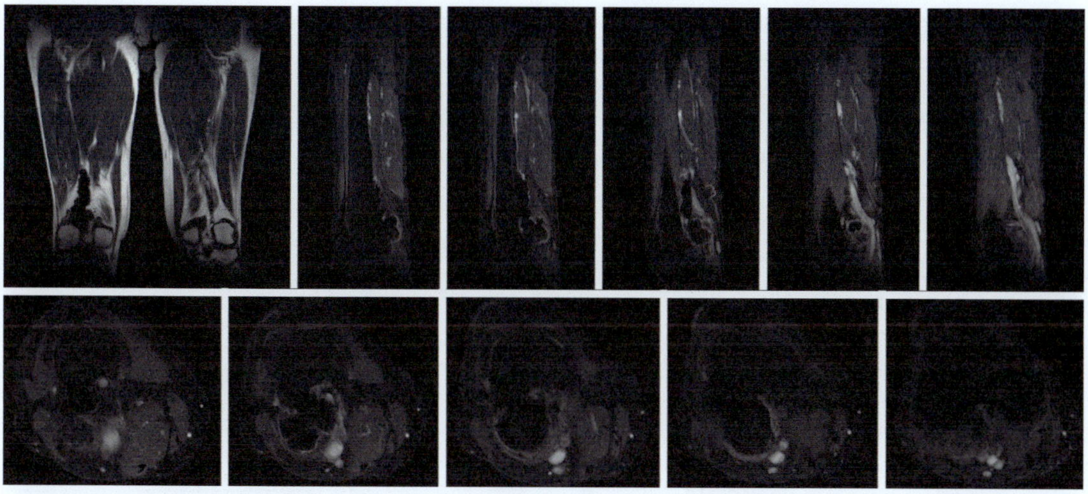

Fig. 17.3 Preoperative MRI images: partial enhancement area of contrast on the metaphysis

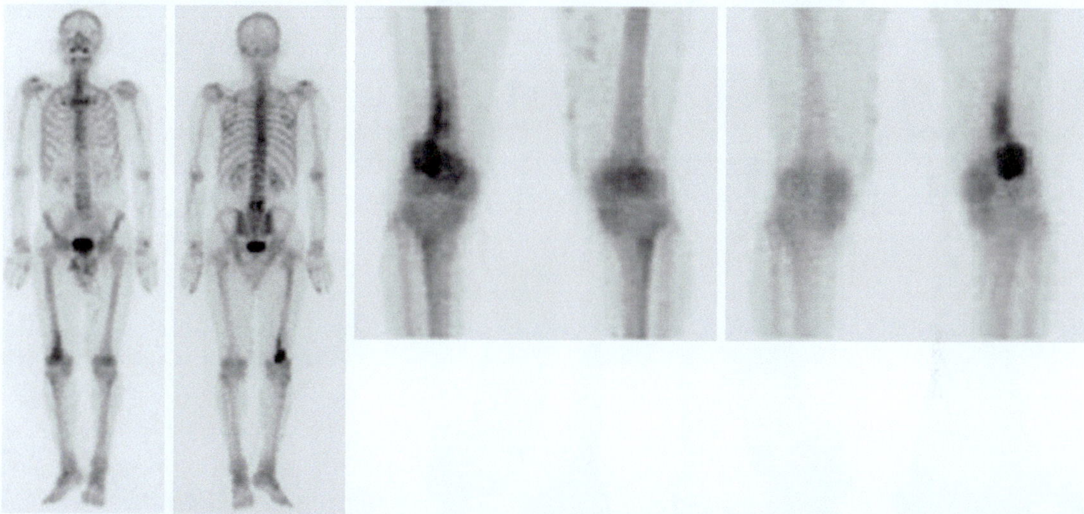

Fig. 17.4 Preoperative bone scan images

17.3 Planning of Surgery

Surgery only for tumors in the popliteal region due to the symptomatic.

Possibility of parosteal osteosarcoma on the findings of MRI and bone scan.

3D printed condylar plate of distal femur.

17.4 Design and Fabrication

- Implant measurement
- Implant weight (g): 82
- Size (mm): 110

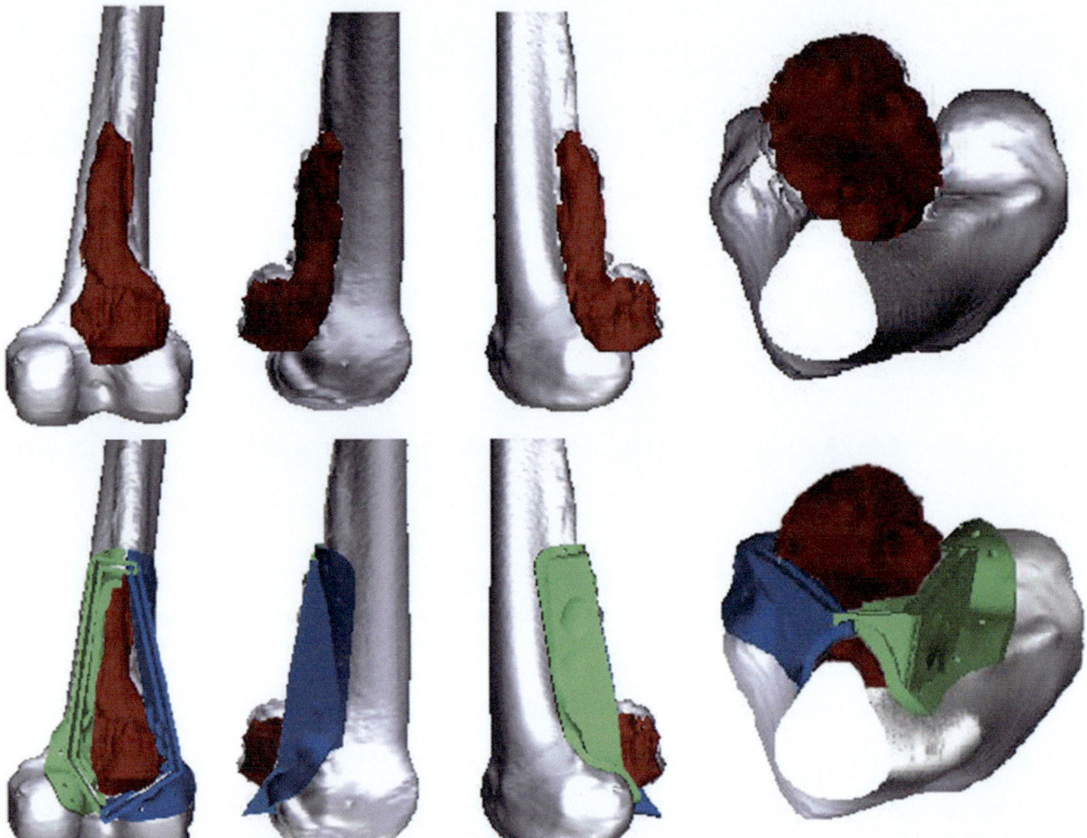

Fig. 17.5 Cutting guide design

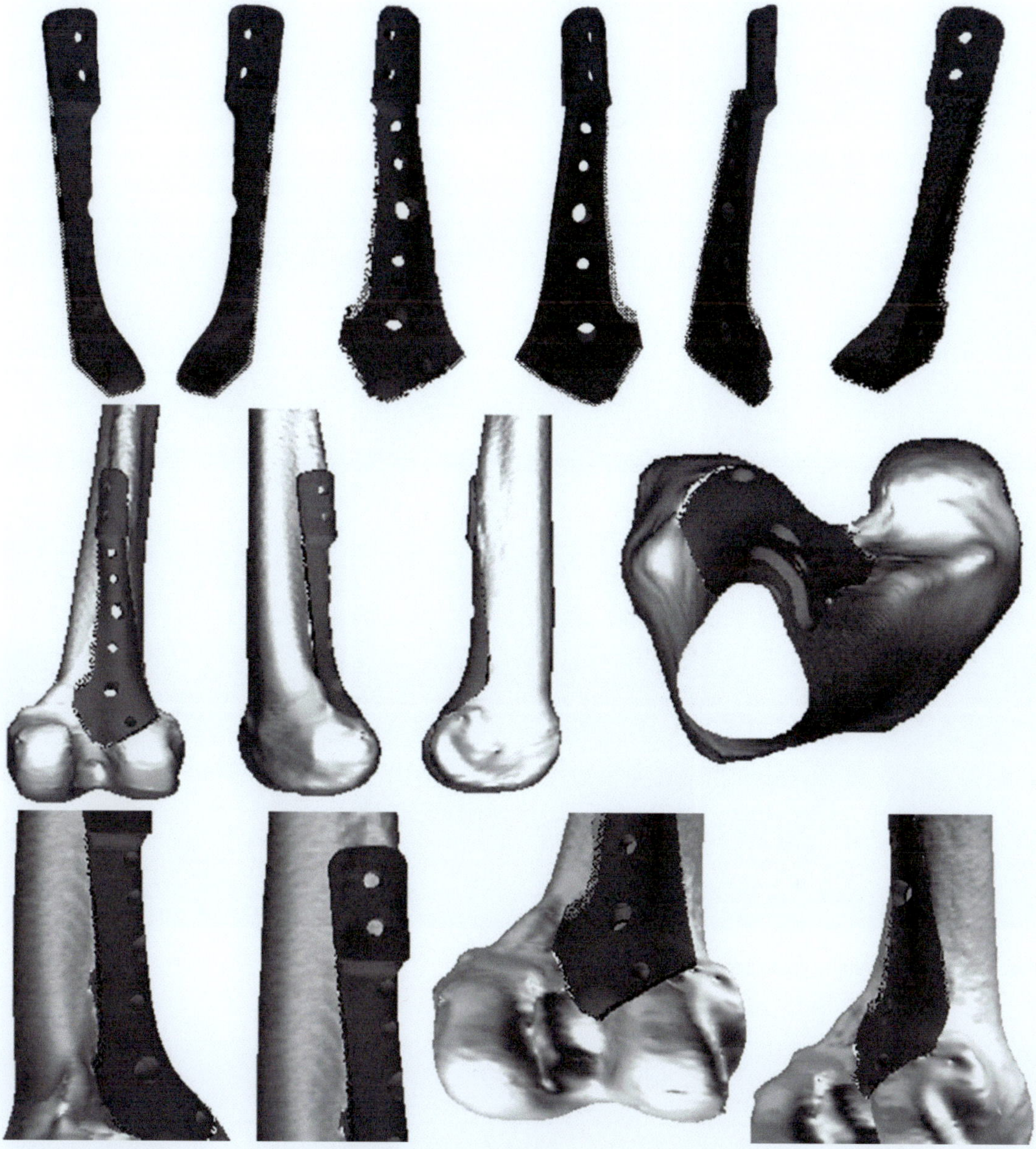

Fig. 17.6 Implant design

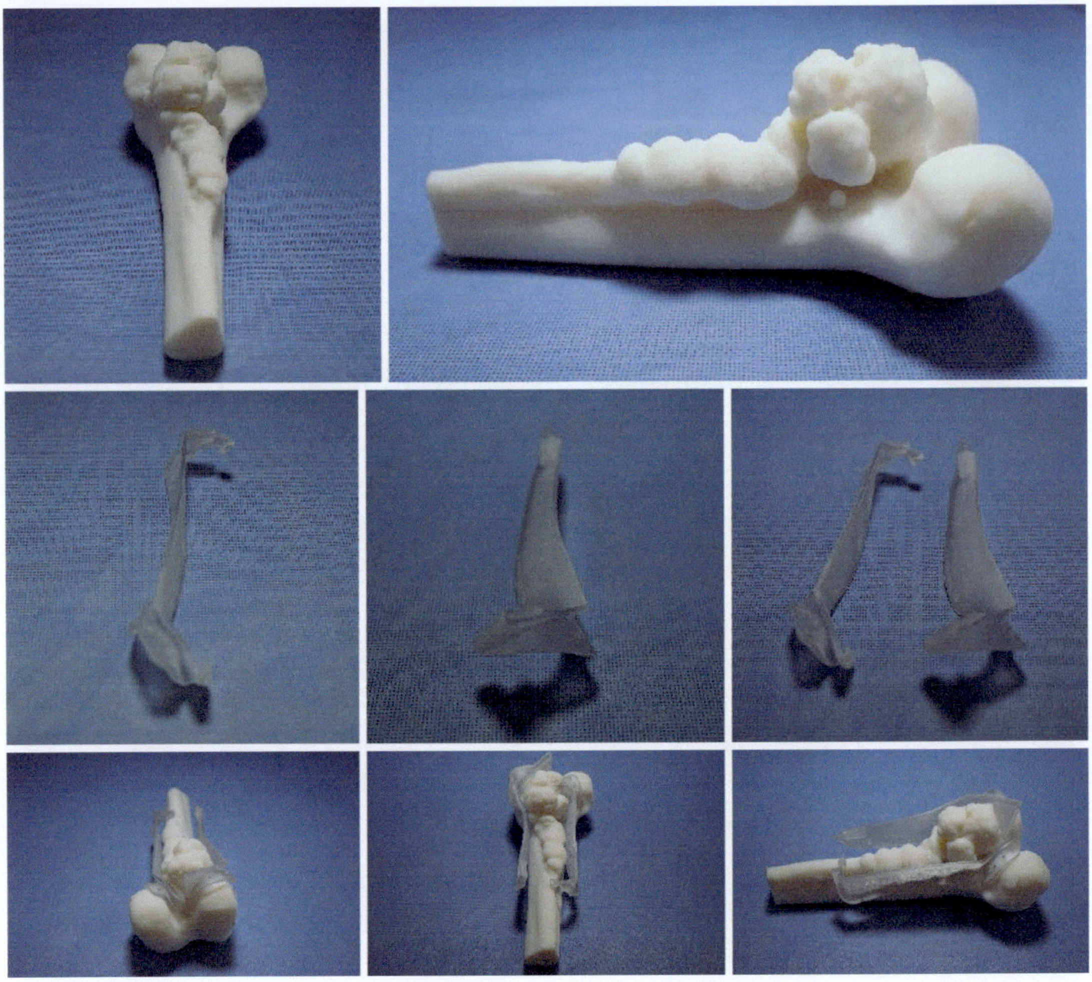

Fig. 17.7 Printed cutting guide and bone tumor model

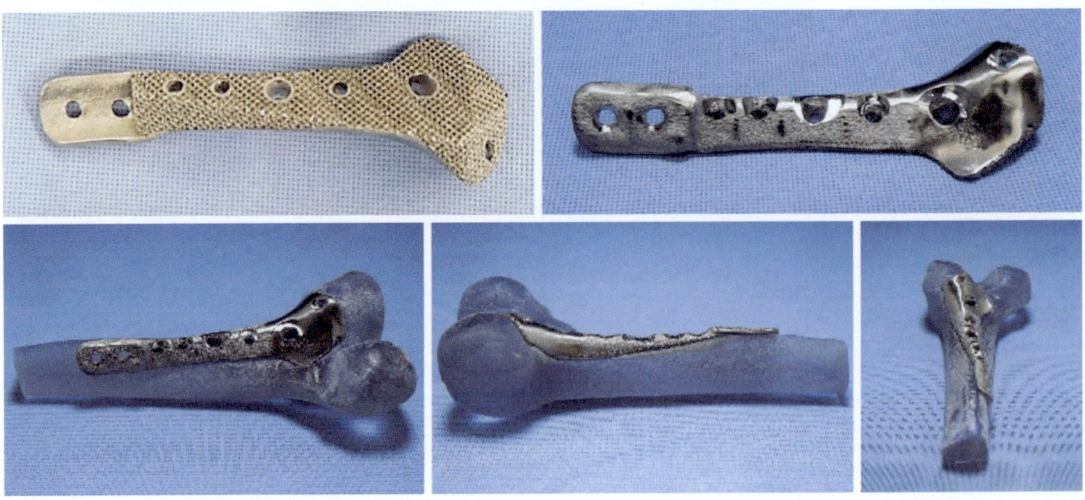

Fig. 17.8 3D printed condyle plate of distal femur

17.5 Operation

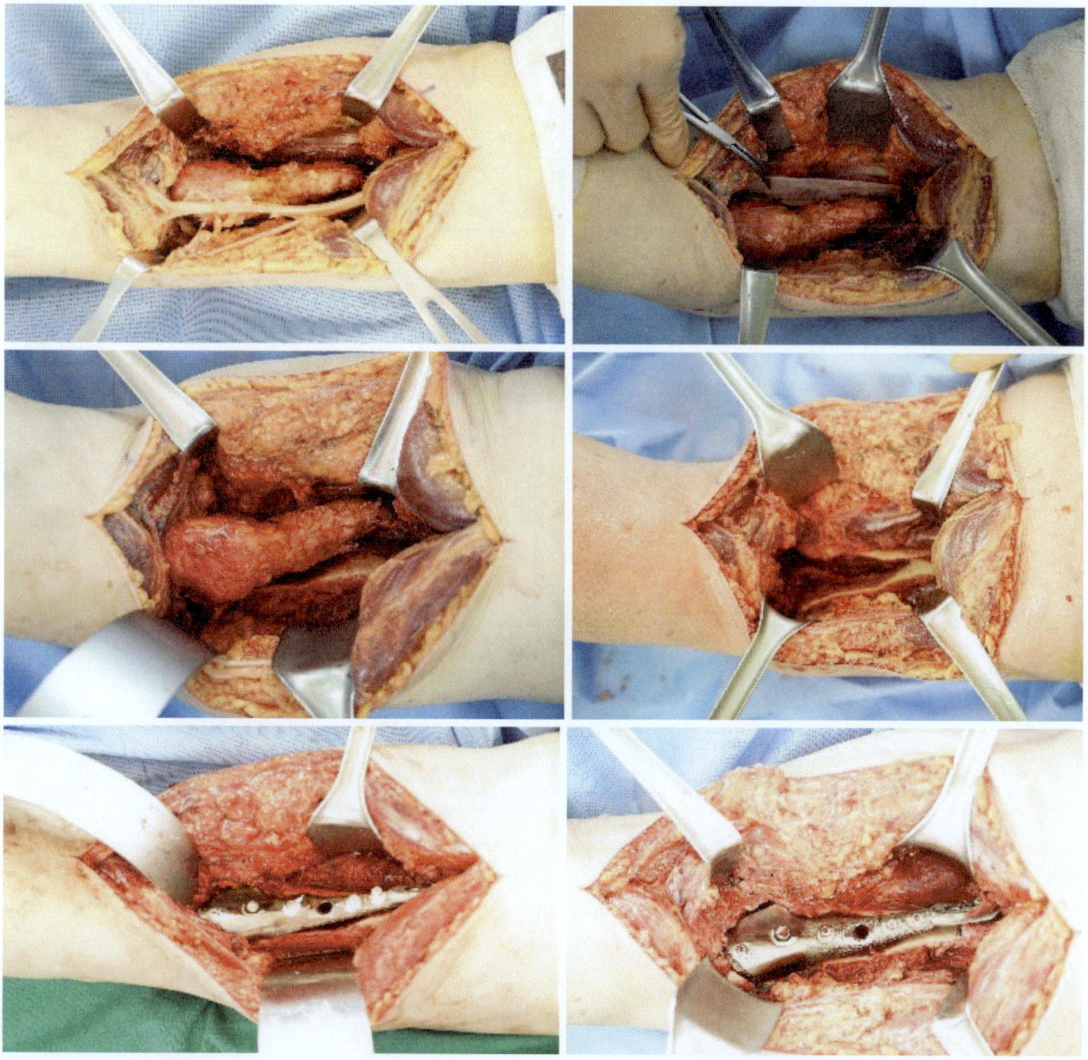

Fig. 17.9 Intraoperative photographs: using artificial bone graft between bone and implant

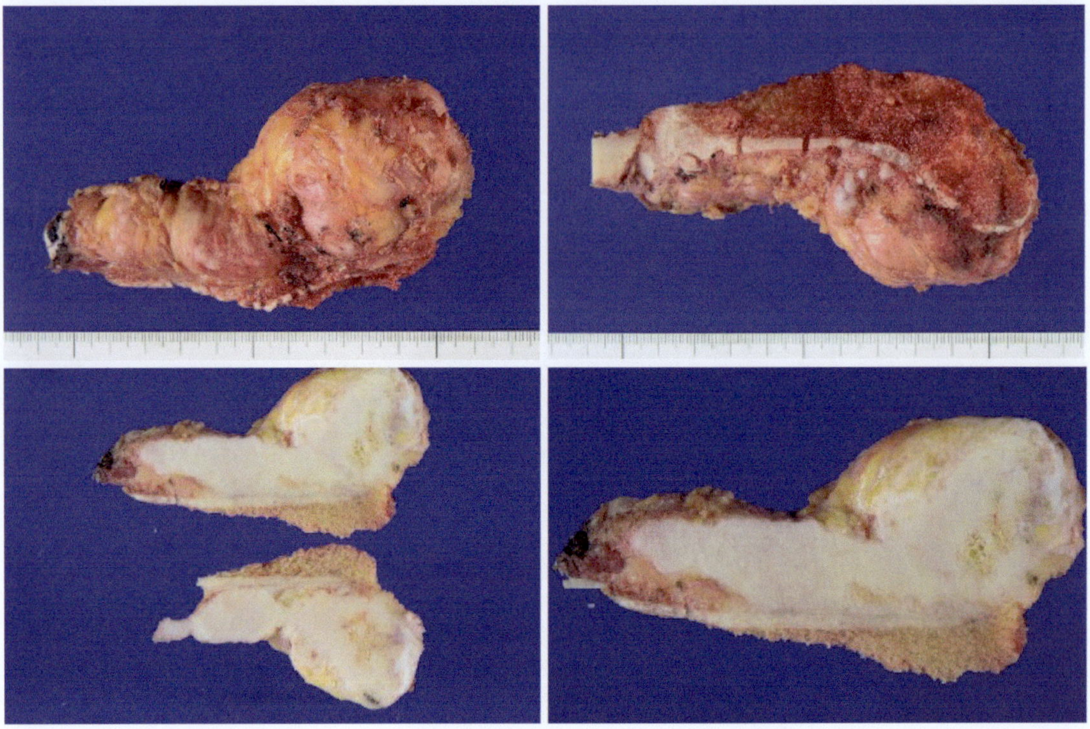

Fig. 17.10 Resected tumor

17.6 Postoperative Images

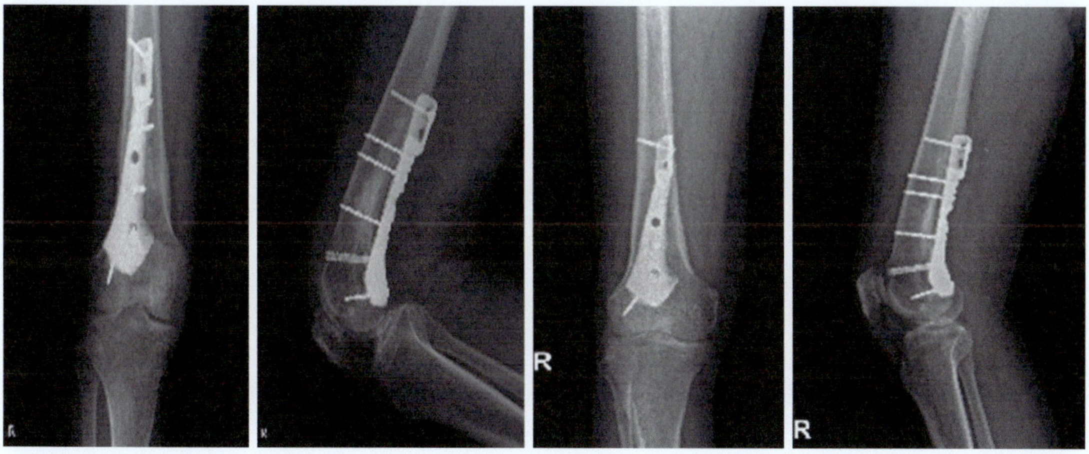

Fig. 17.11 Postoperative X-ray images

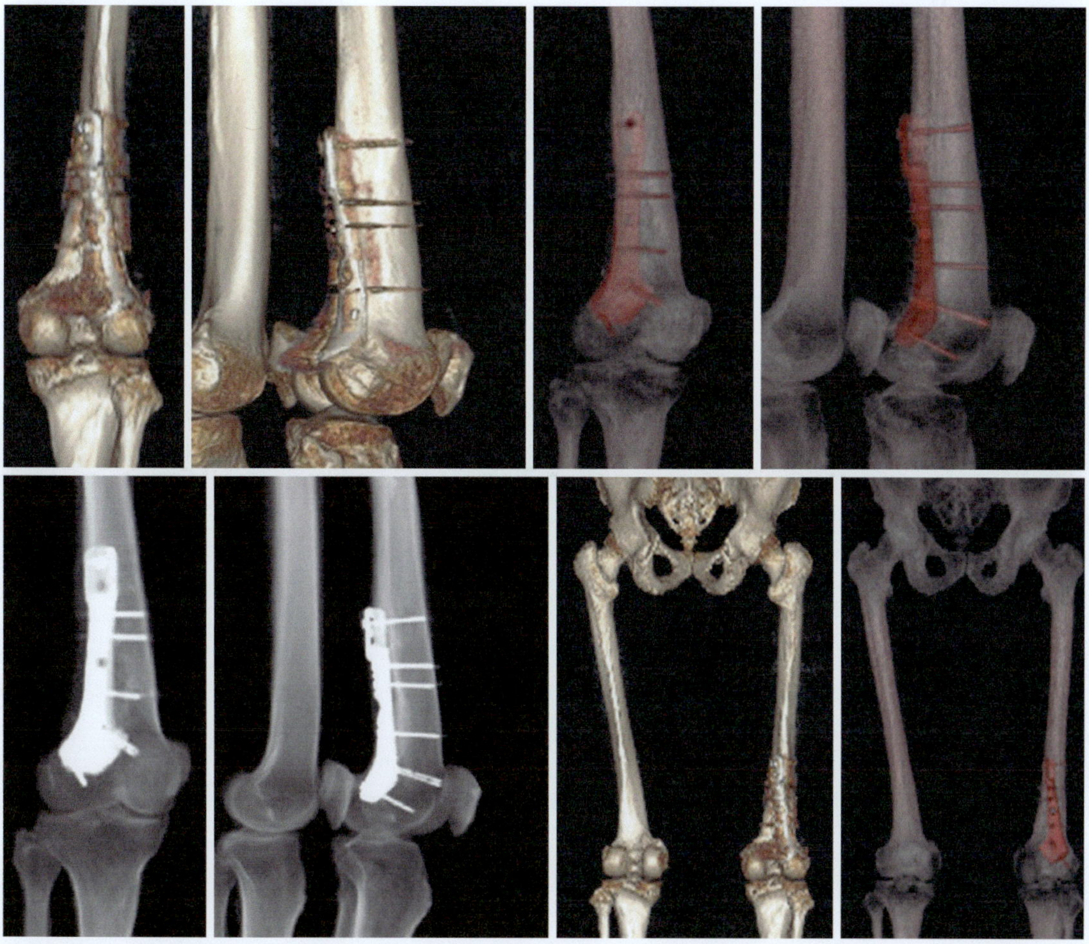

Fig. 17.12 Postoperative CT images

Patient Case 18: Posterior Intercondylar Y Plate

18

18.1 Patient Case 18

Age/sex	27/male
Location/site	Femur distal/right
Diagnosis	Recurred giant cell tumor of the bone
Preoperative symptom	Antalgic gait
Preoperative pain score	Resting 0/activity 5
BMI (height/weight)	26.01 (172.6/77.5)
Past history	Operated at another hospital 1 year ago
Present illness	Visit due to persistent knee pain after surgery

H.-G. Kang, *Clinical Atlas of 3D Printing Bone Reconstruction*,
https://doi.org/10.1007/978-981-16-2043-0_18

18.2 Preoperative Images

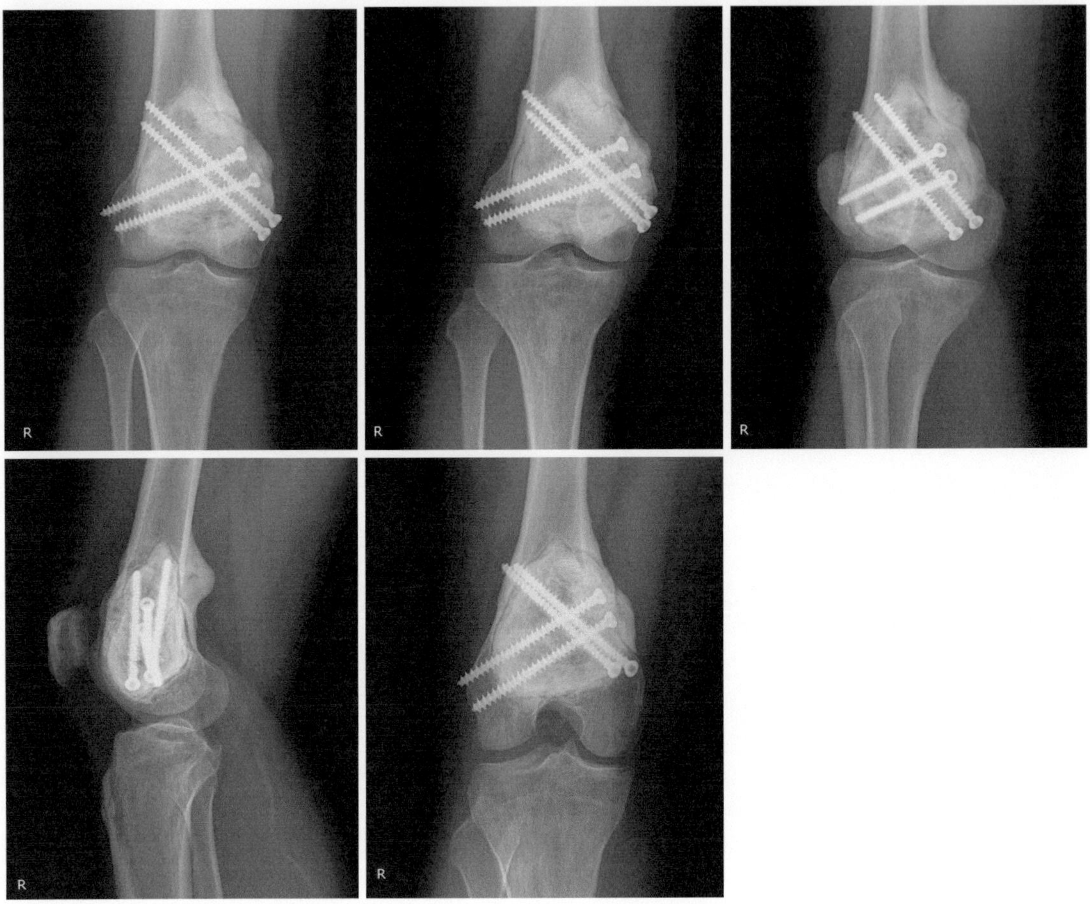

Fig. 18.1 Preoperative X-ray images

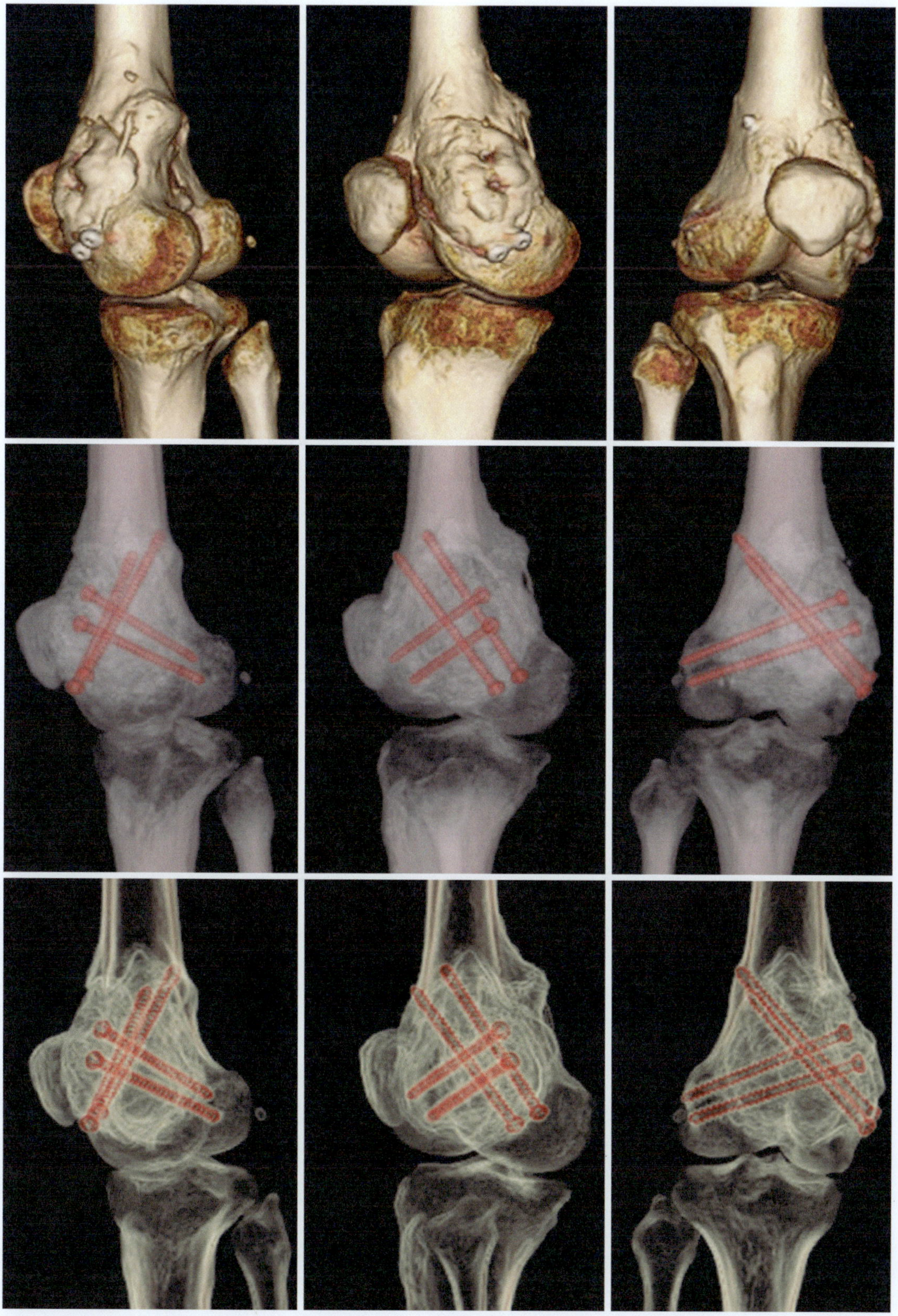

Fig. 18.2 Preoperative CT images

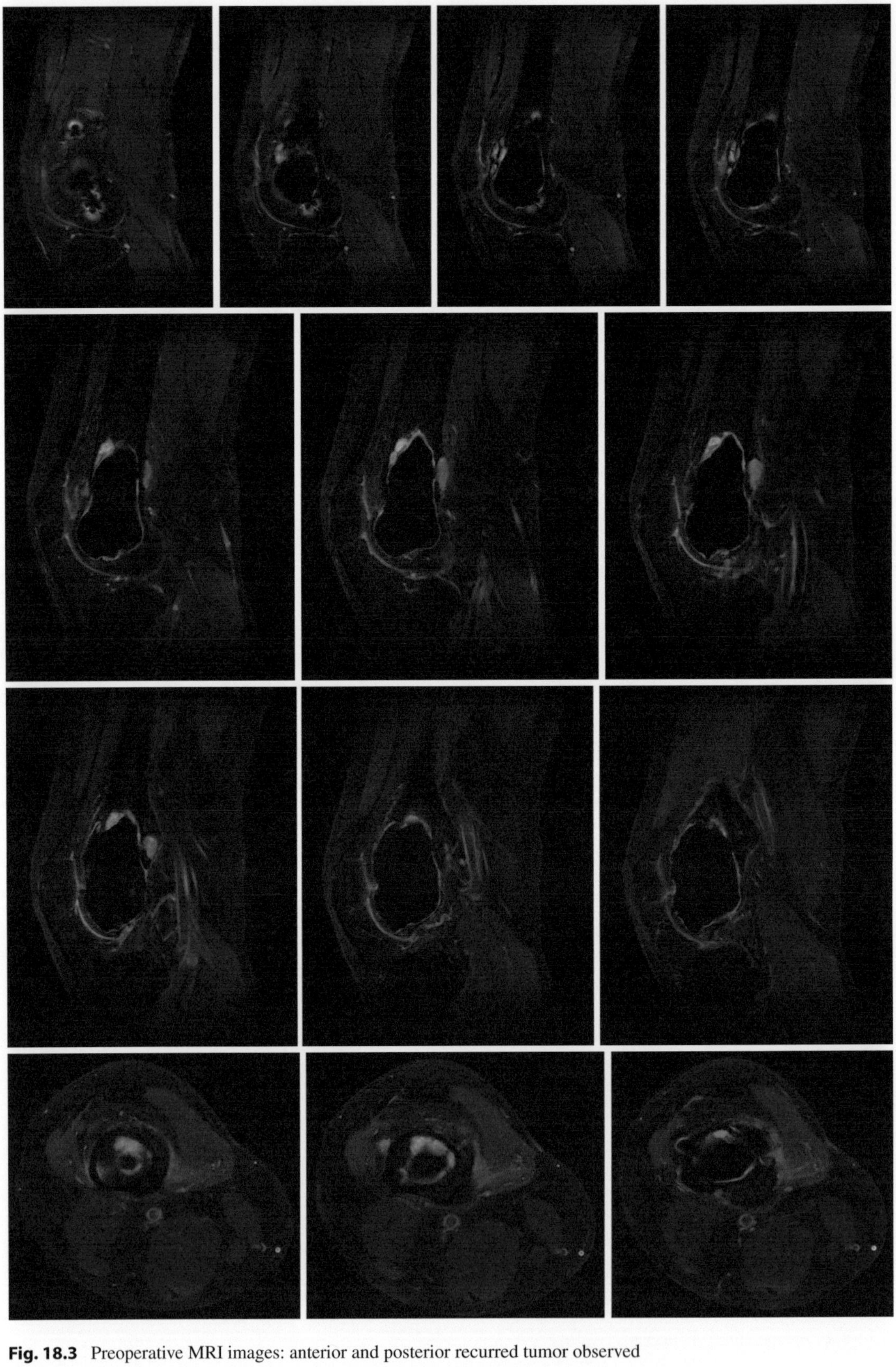

Fig. 18.3 Preoperative MRI images: anterior and posterior recurred tumor observed

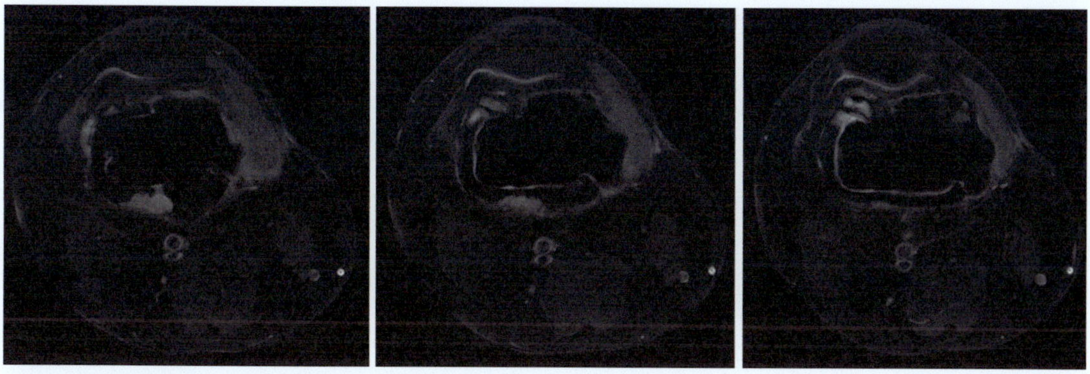

Fig. 18.3 (continued)

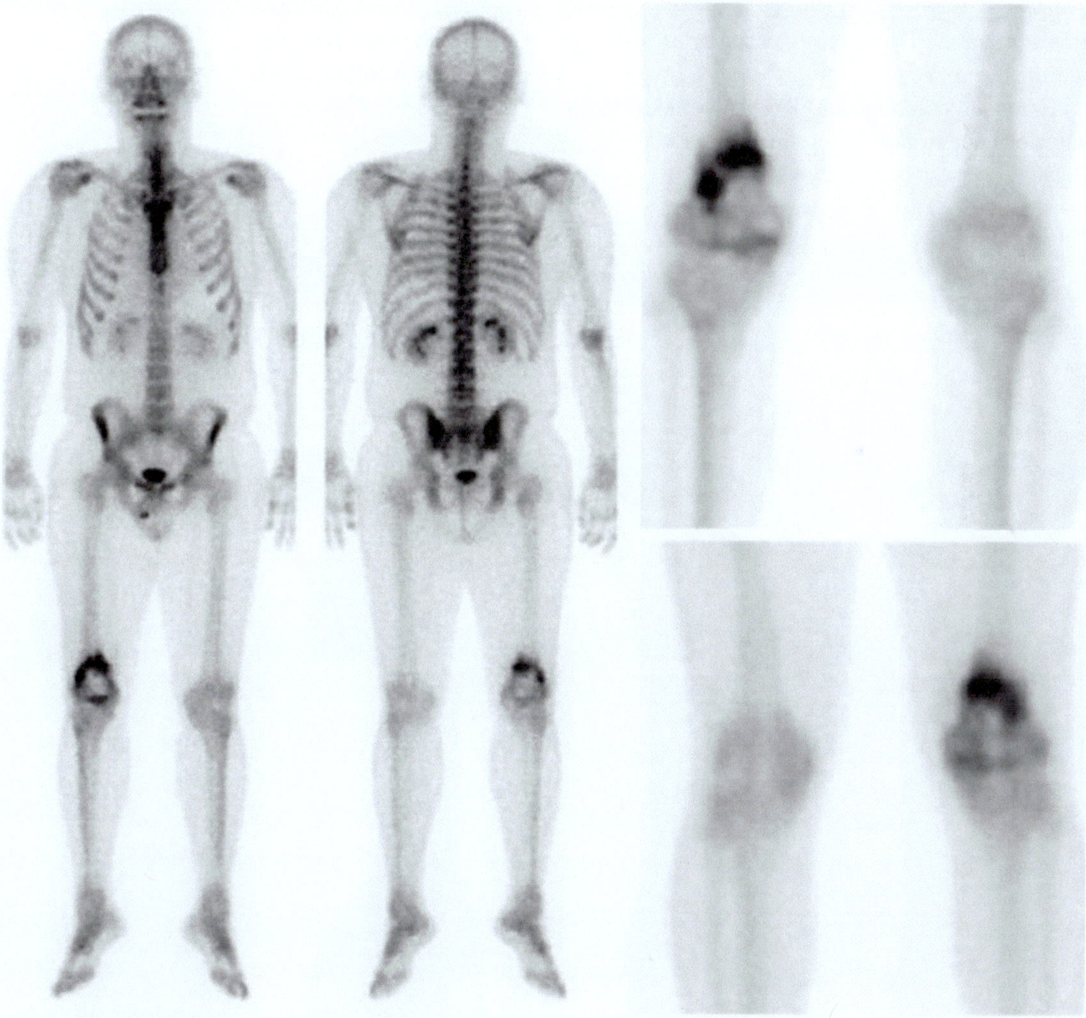

Fig. 18.4 Preoperative bone scan images

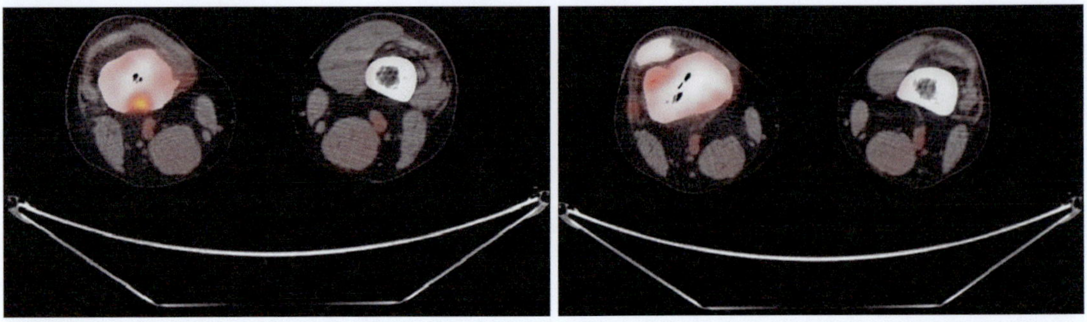

Fig. 18.5 Preoperative PET-CT images

18.3 Planning of Surgery

Resection and 3D-printed intercondylar plate for popliteal tumor

Extended curettage and PMMA cementing for anterior knee tumor

18.4 Design and Fabrication

- Implant measurement
- Implant weight (g): 82
- Size (mm): 129

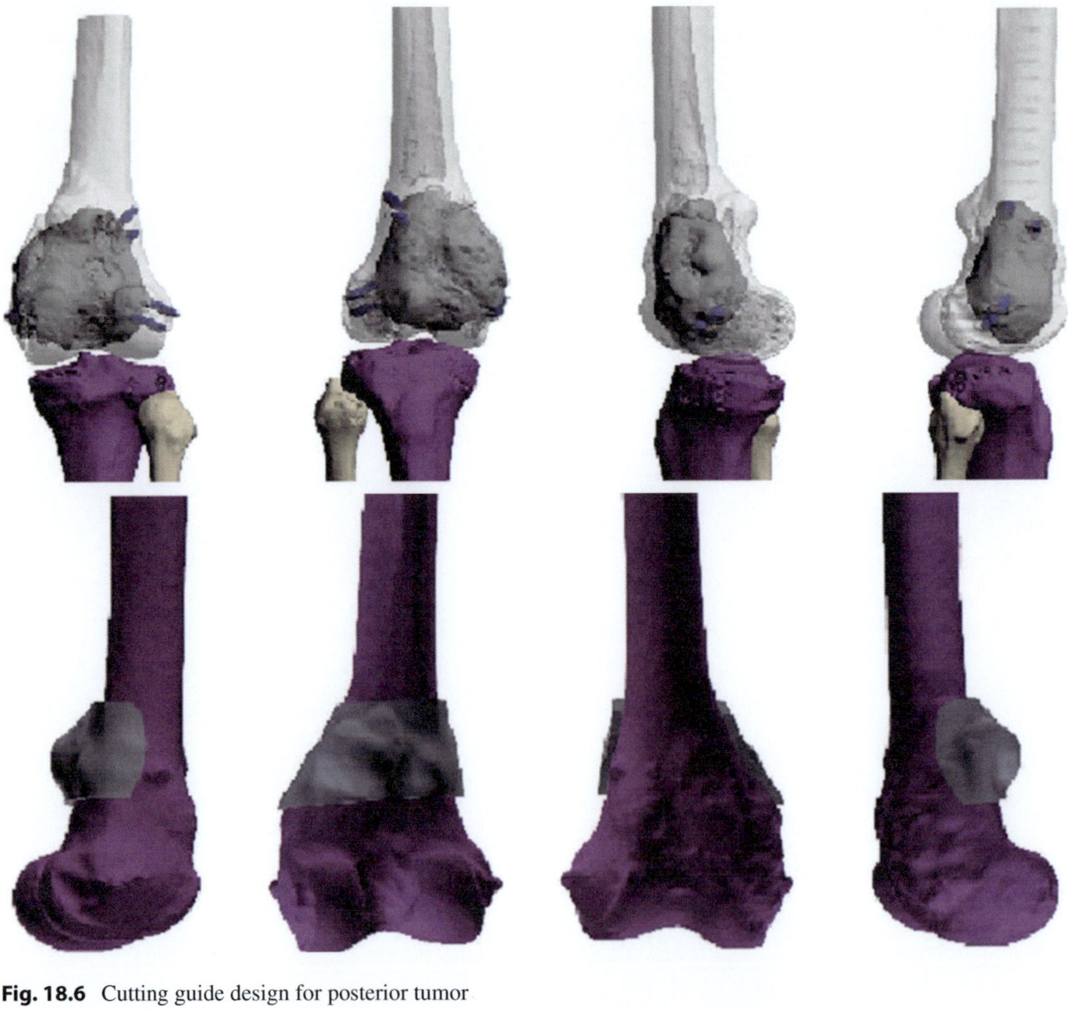

Fig. 18.6 Cutting guide design for posterior tumor

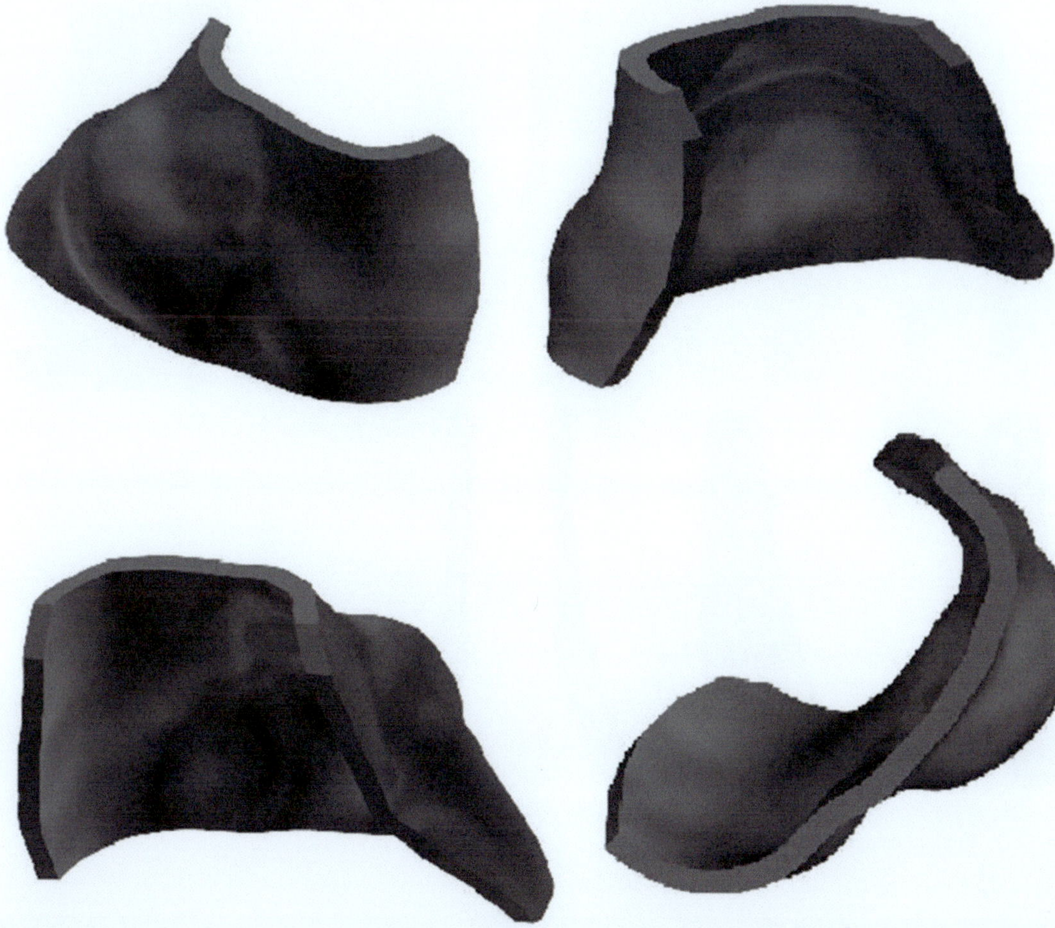

Fig. 18.6 (continued)

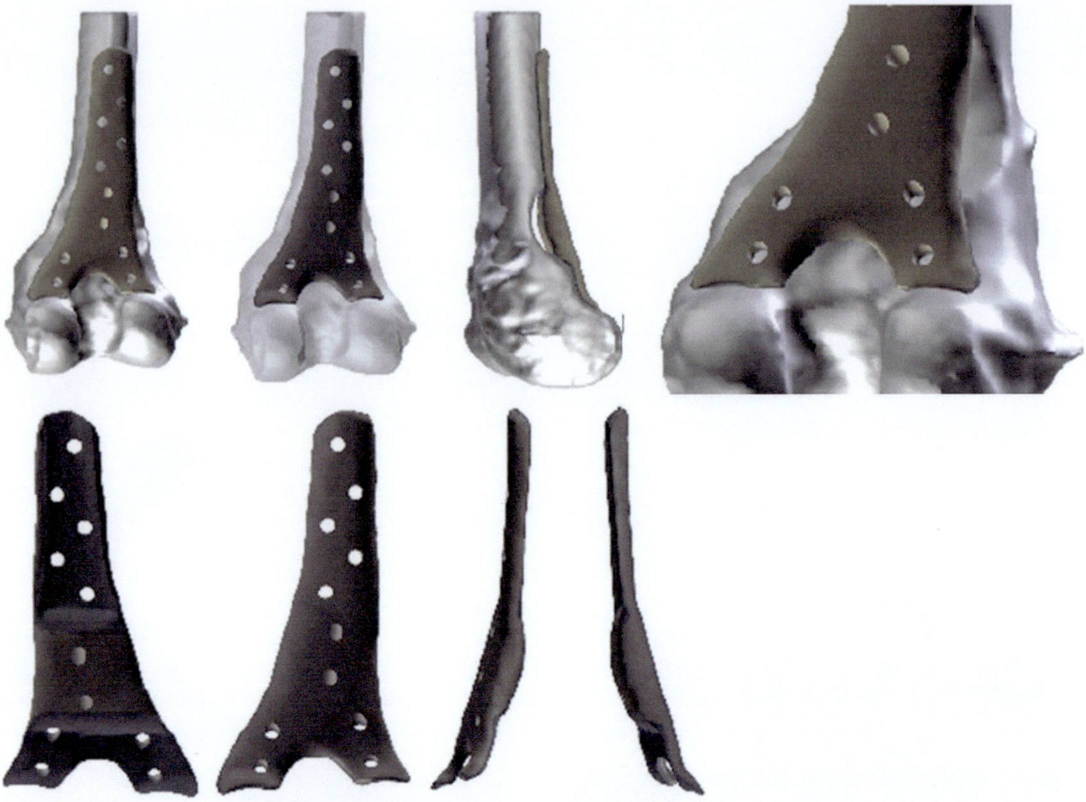

Fig. 18.7 Implant design

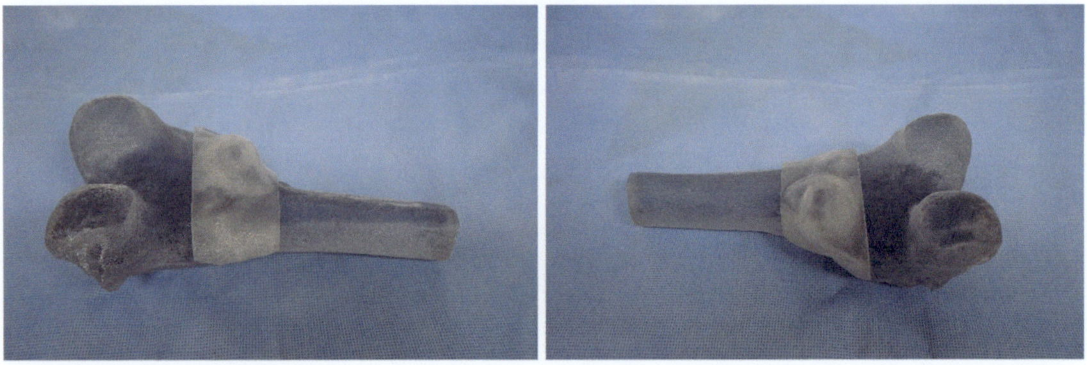

Fig. 18.8 Printed cutting guide

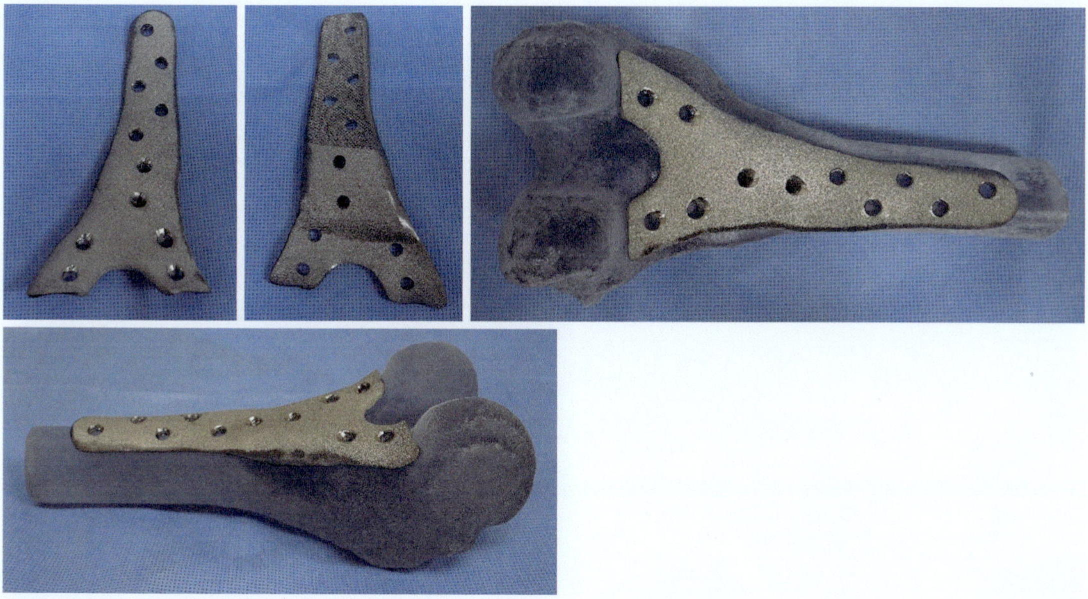

Fig. 18.9 3D-printed intercondylar plate of distal femur

18.5 Operation

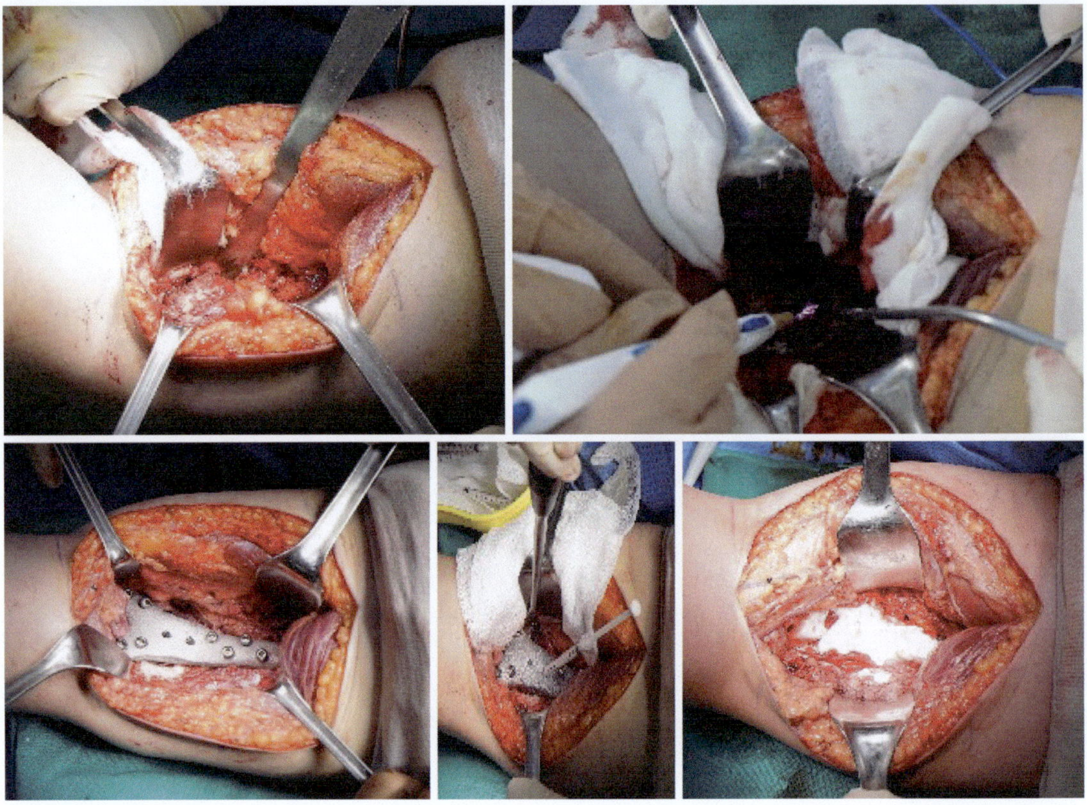

Fig. 18.10 Intraoperative photographs of popliteal tumor: resection and argon laser ablation, PMMA bone cement augmentation

18.6 Postoperative Images

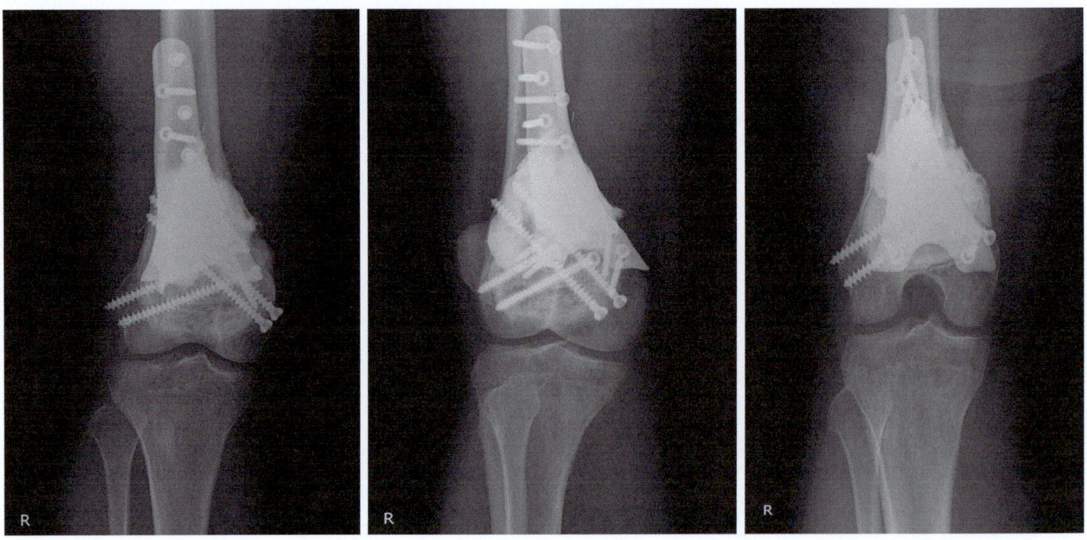

Fig. 18.11 Postoperative X-ray images

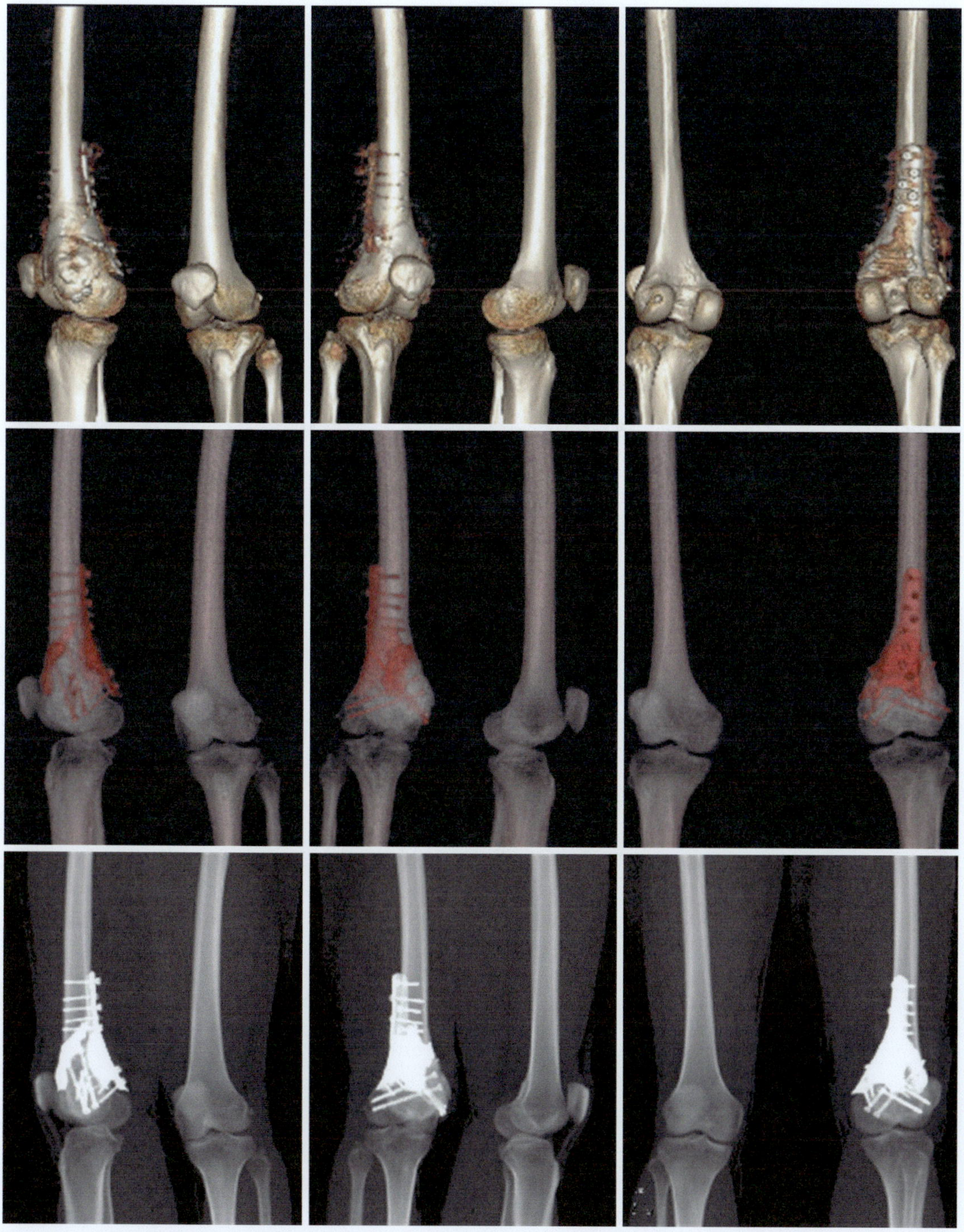

Fig. 18.12 Postoperative CT images

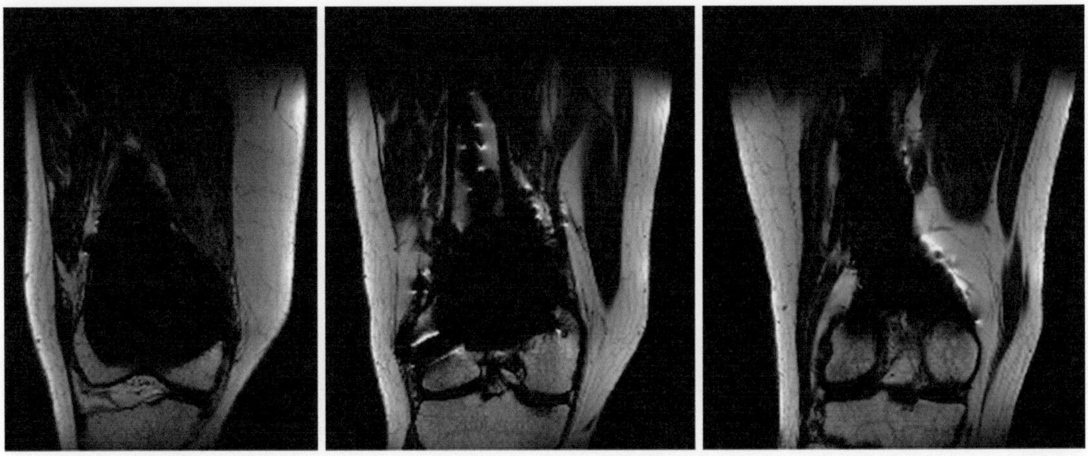

Fig. 18.13 Postoperative MRI images

Patient Case 19: Segmental Distal Femur Combined with IM Nail

19

19.1 Patient Case 19

Age/sex	54/female
Location/site	Femur distal/right
Diagnosis	High-grade undifferentiated spindle cell sarcoma of bone
Preoperative symptom	Limping gate with cane
Preoperative pain score	Resting 2/activity 7
BMI (height/weight)	18.29 (161/47.4)
Present illness	Visited after hearing surgical methods at several hospitals

H.-G. Kang, *Clinical Atlas of 3D Printing Bone Reconstruction*,
https://doi.org/10.1007/978-981-16-2043-0_19

19.2 Preoperative Images

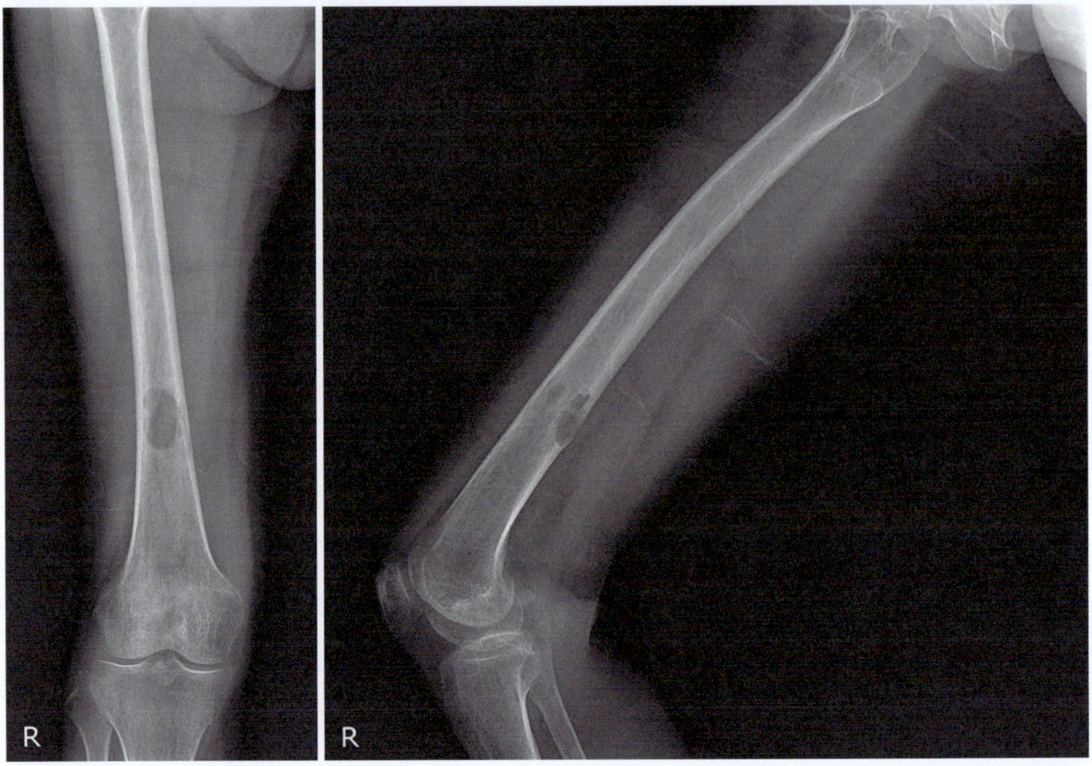

Fig. 19.1 Preoperative X-ray images

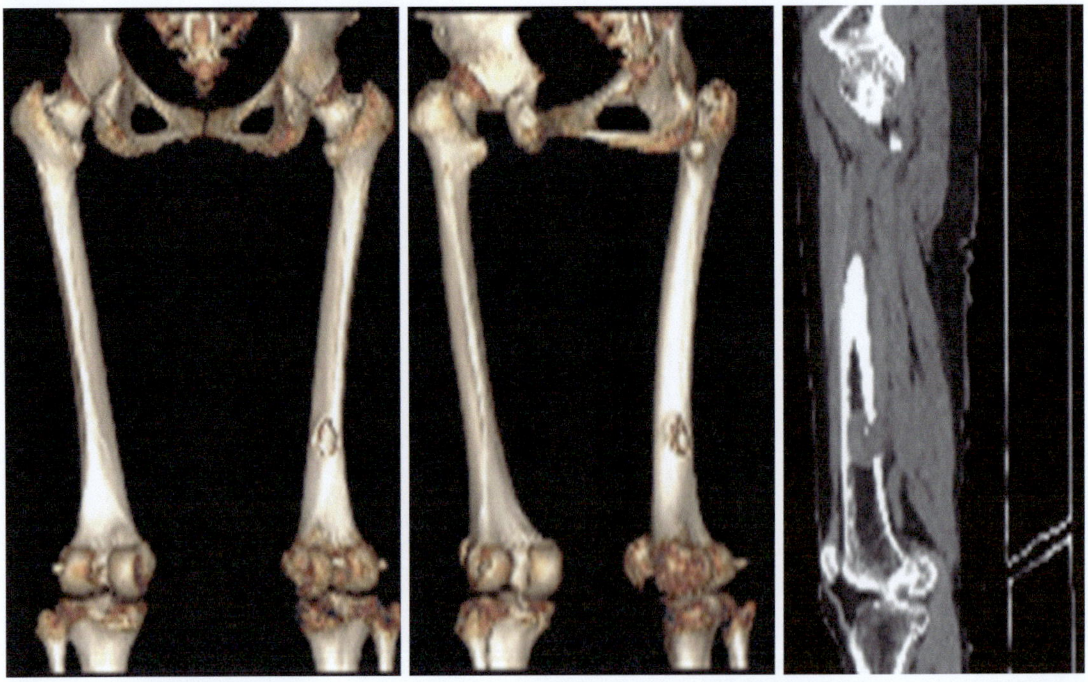

Fig. 19.2 Preoperative CT images

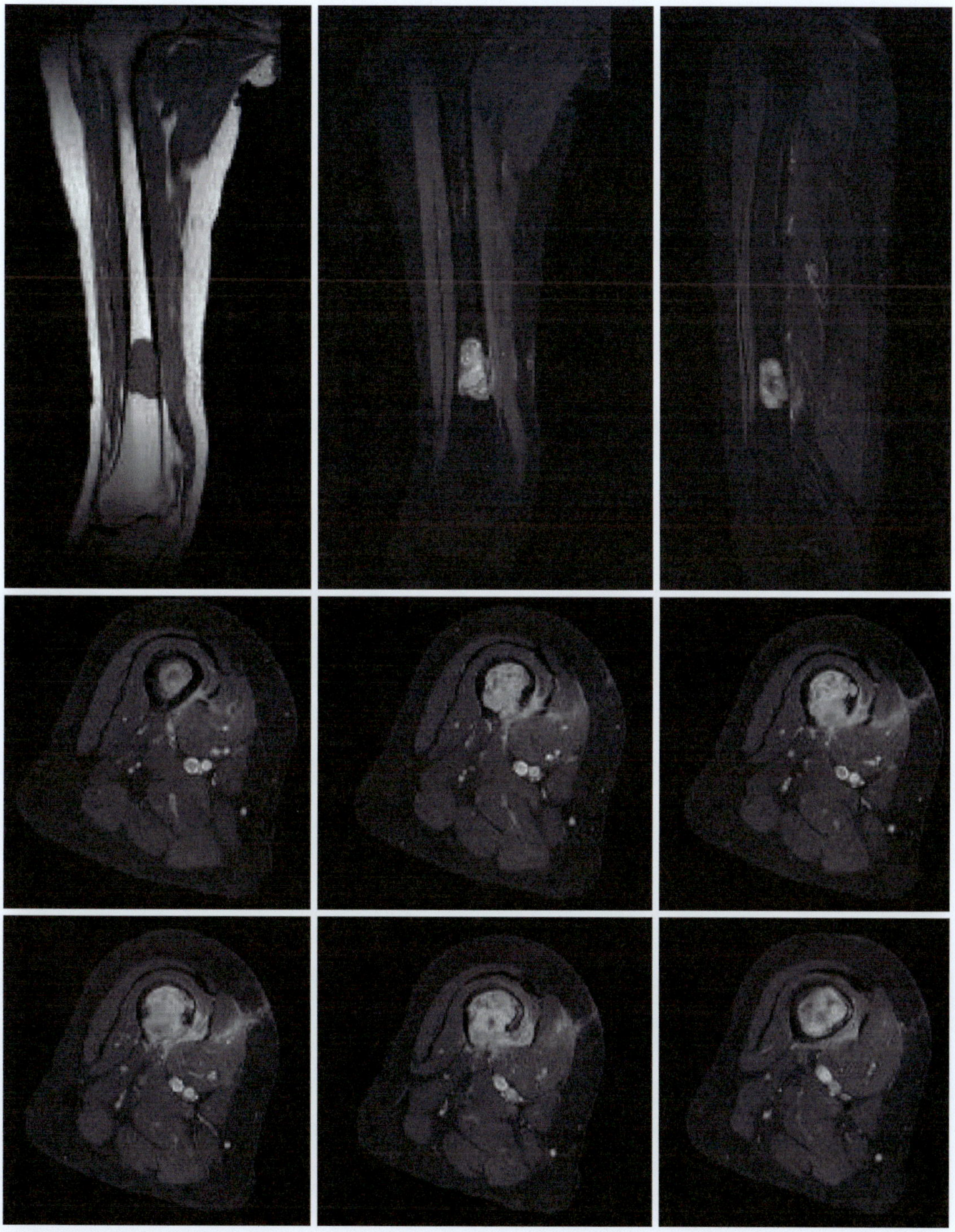

Fig. 19.3 Preoperative MRI images

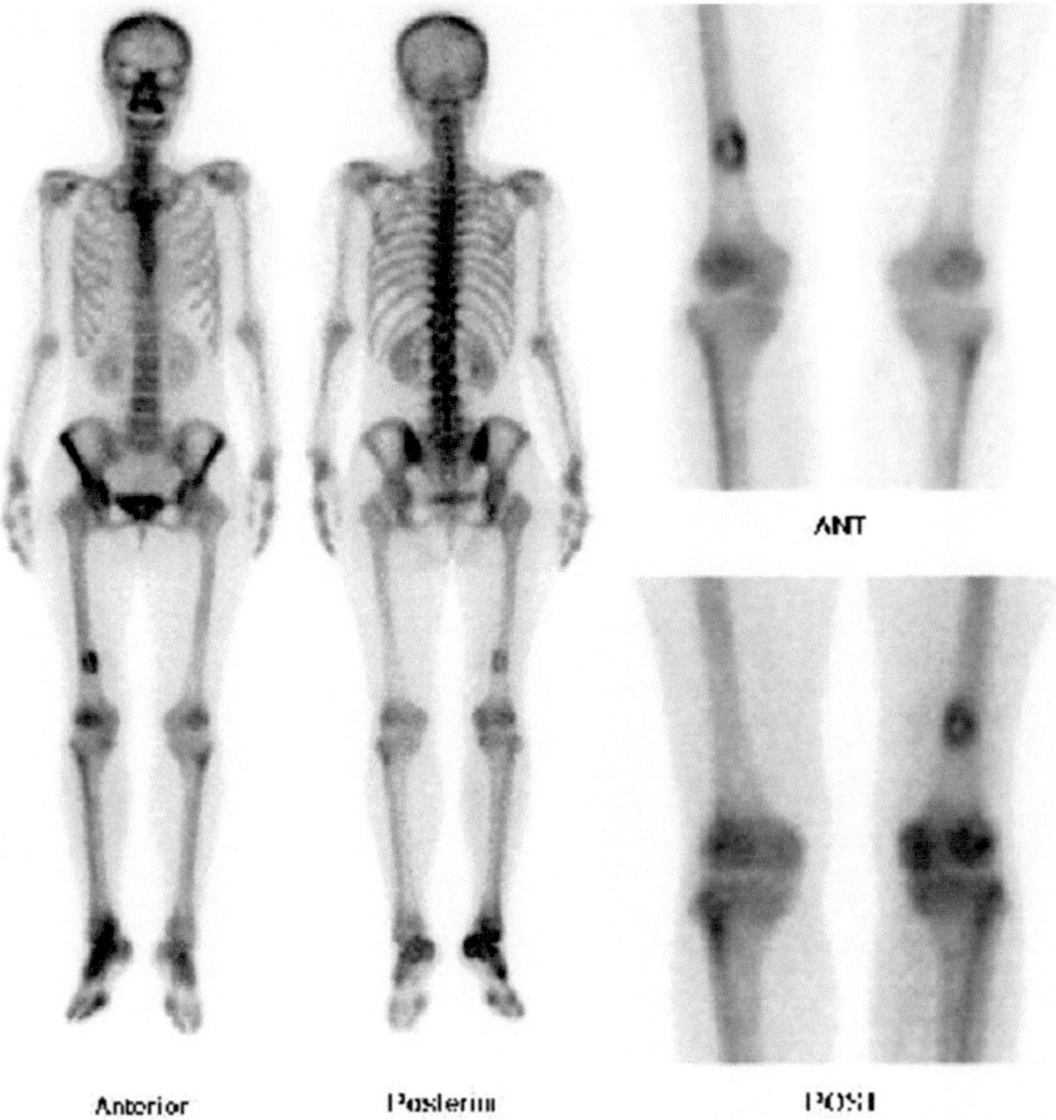

Fig. 19.4 Preoperative bone scan images

19.3 Planning of Surgery

Segmental resection (9.5 cm) and intercalary reconstruction

3D-printed segmental femur prosthesis

Retrograde IM nailing

19.4 Design and Fabrication

Circular wrapped for each side bone end

Polishing posteromedial neuro-vascular contact area

The central canal is straight of a 3D-printed implant.

- Implant measurement
- Implant weight (g): 350
- Size (mm): 157

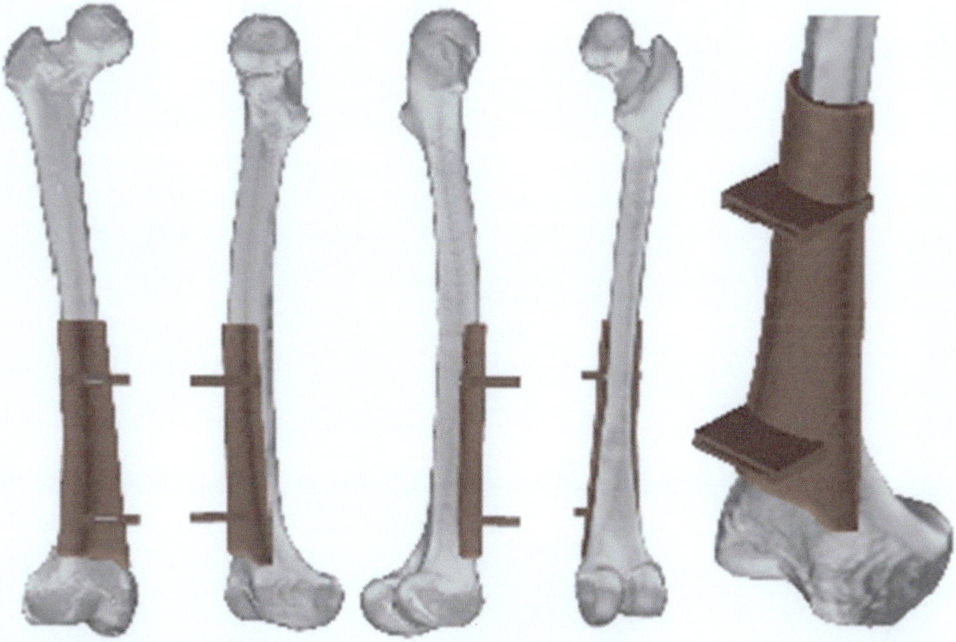

Fig. 19.5 Cutting guide for segmental bone cut

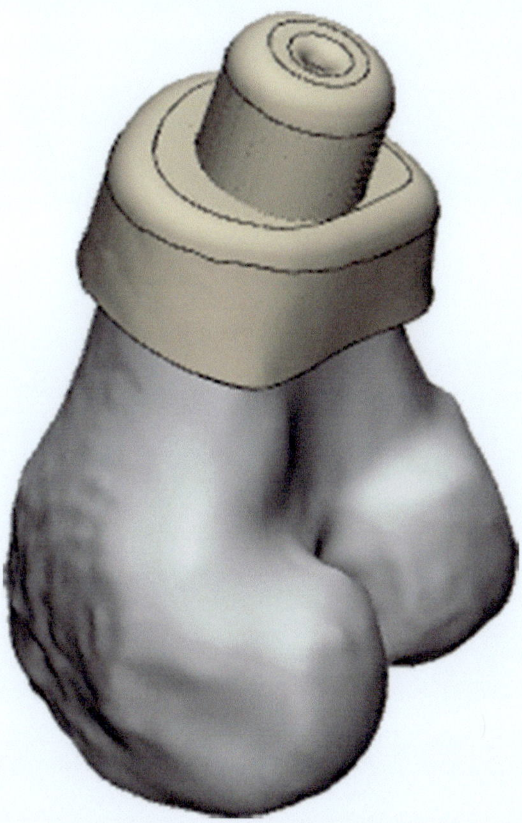

Fig. 19.6 Center pin guide for retrograde IM nailing

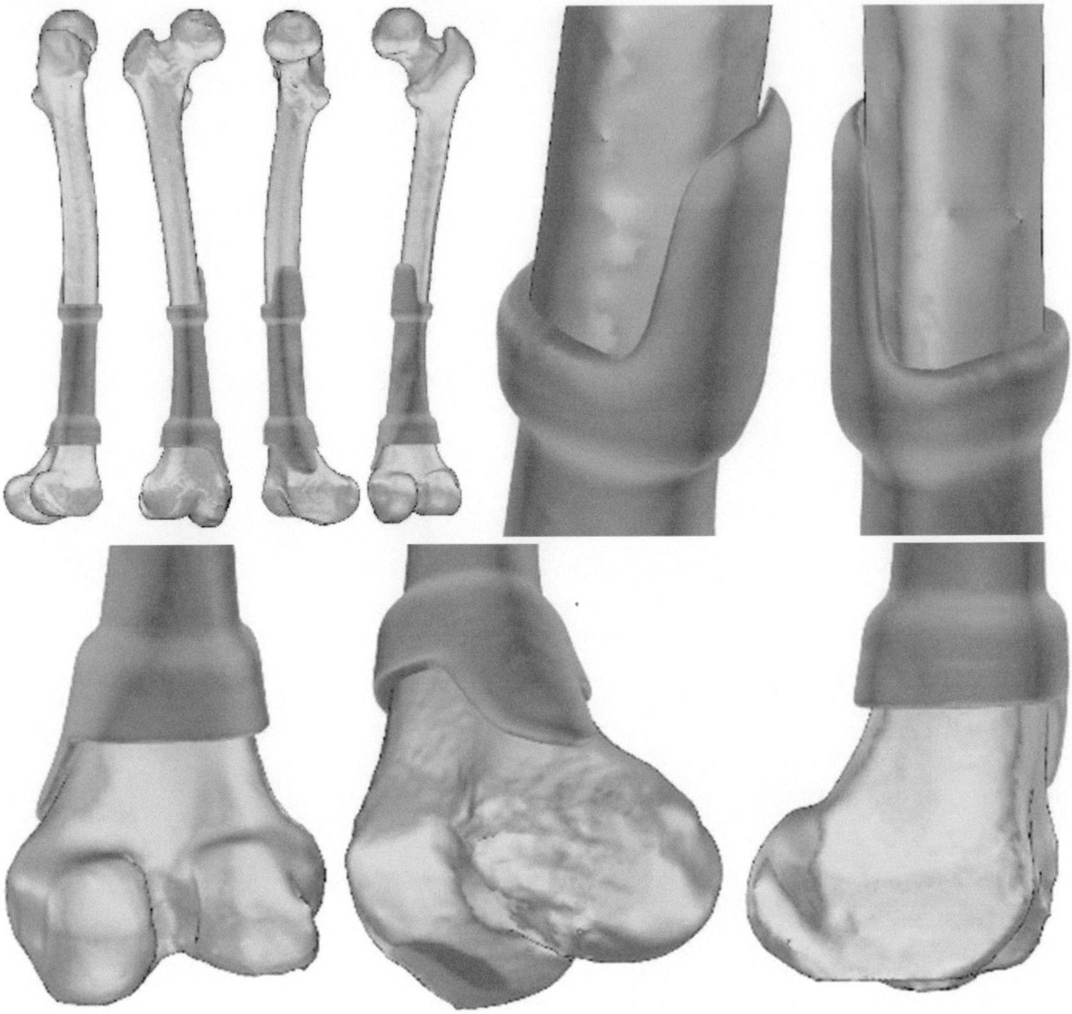

Fig. 19.7 Implant design

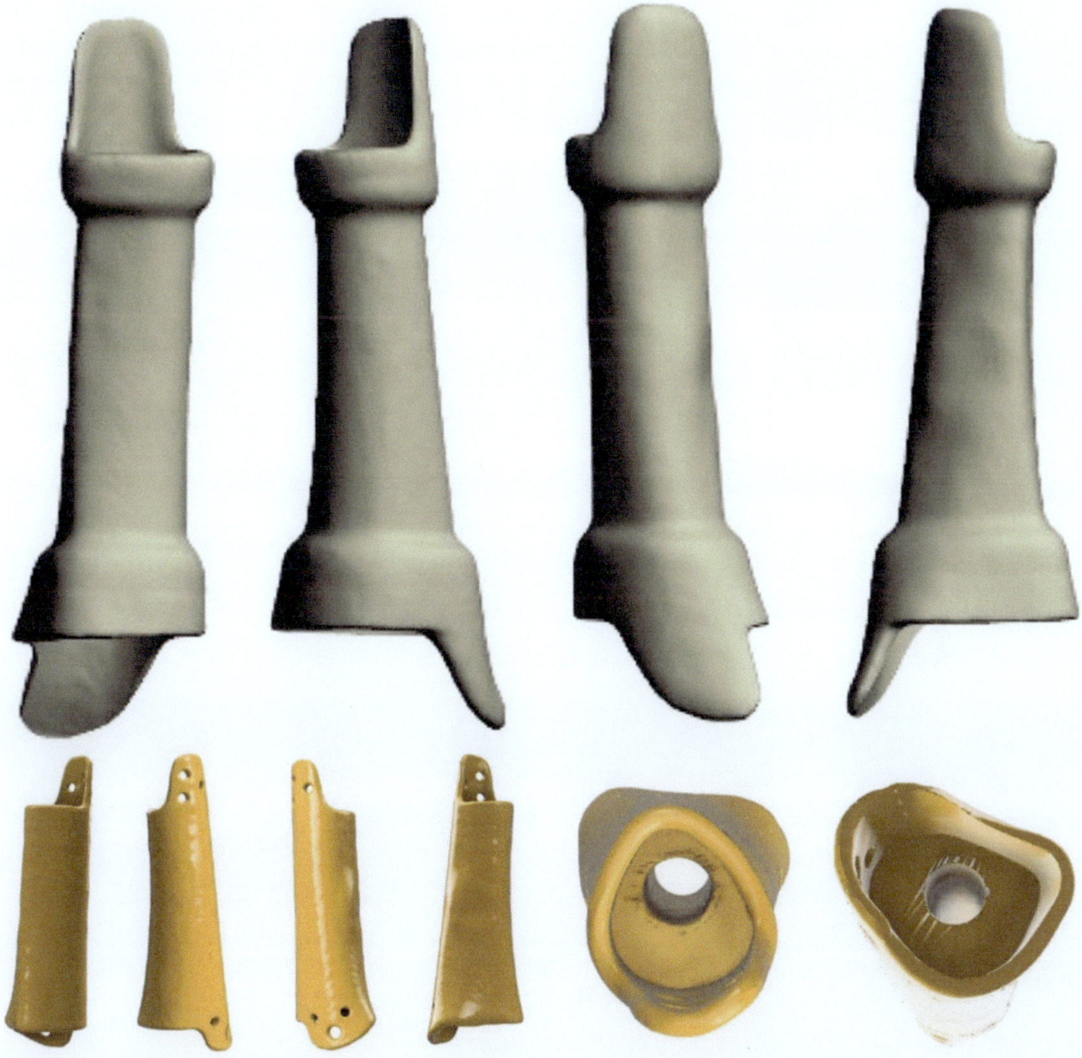

Fig. 19.7 (continued)

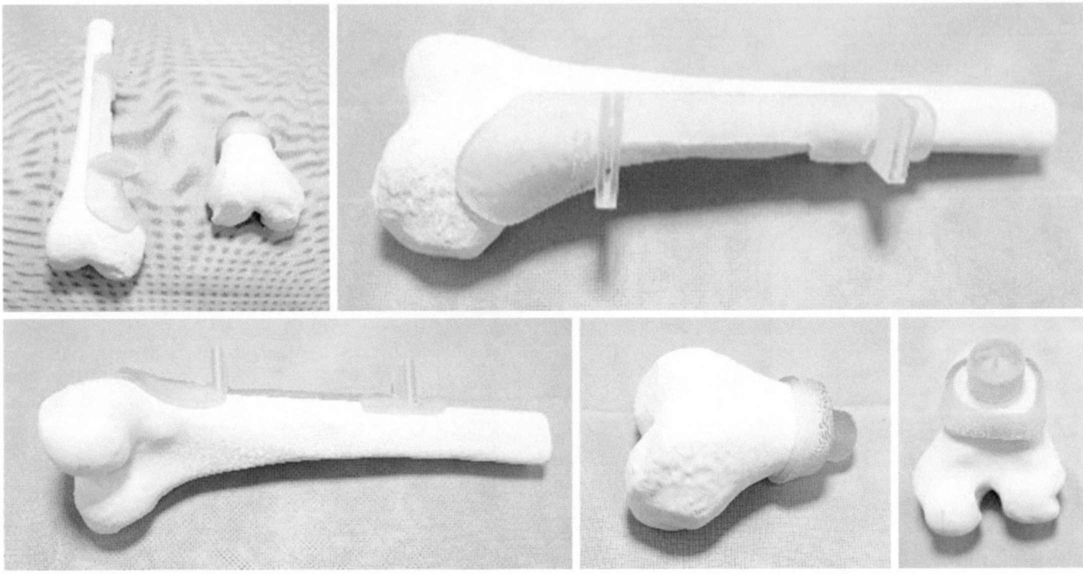

Fig. 19.8 Printed cutting guide and center pin guide

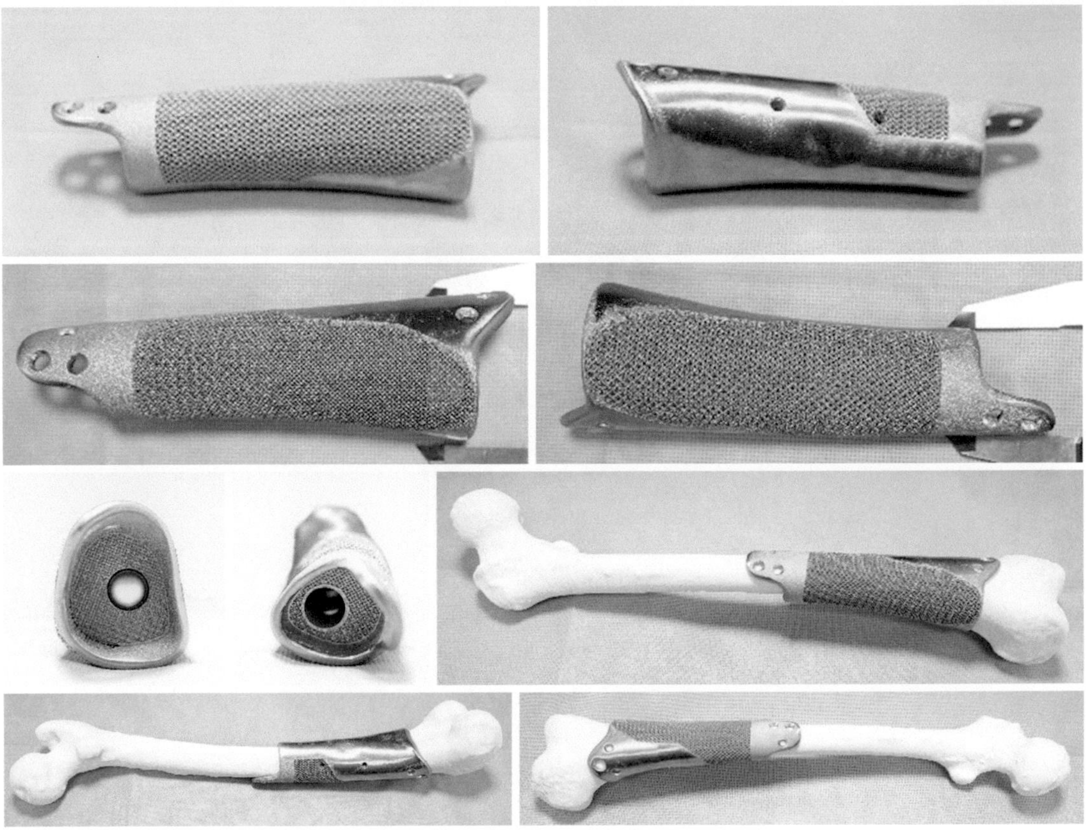

Fig. 19.9 3D-printed segmental femur prosthesis: lateral two perforated holes connected central canal for cement injection to the peri-IM nail

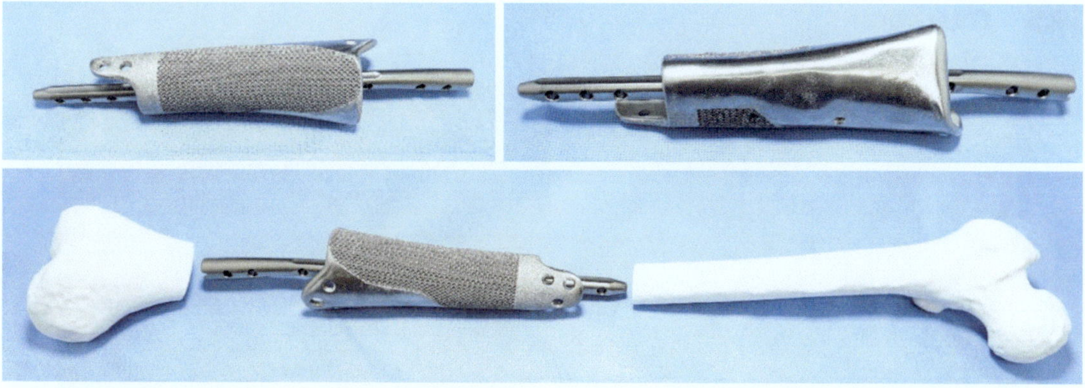

Fig. 19.10 The length and direction of the retrograde

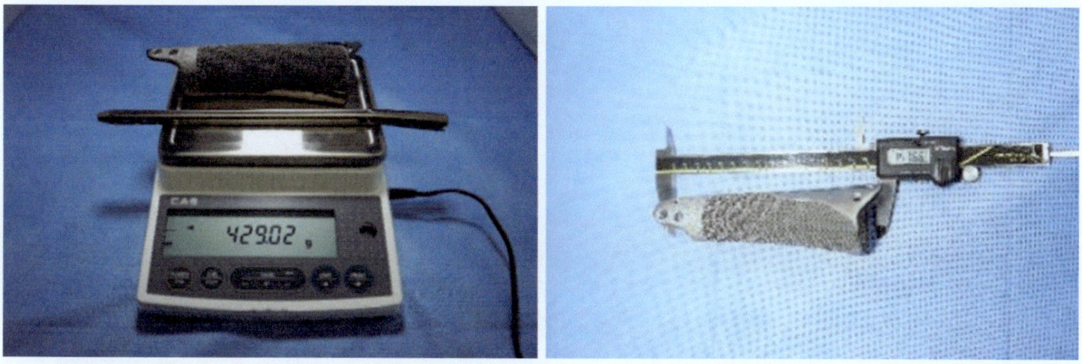

Fig. 19.11 Measurement of 3D-printed implant

19.5 Operation

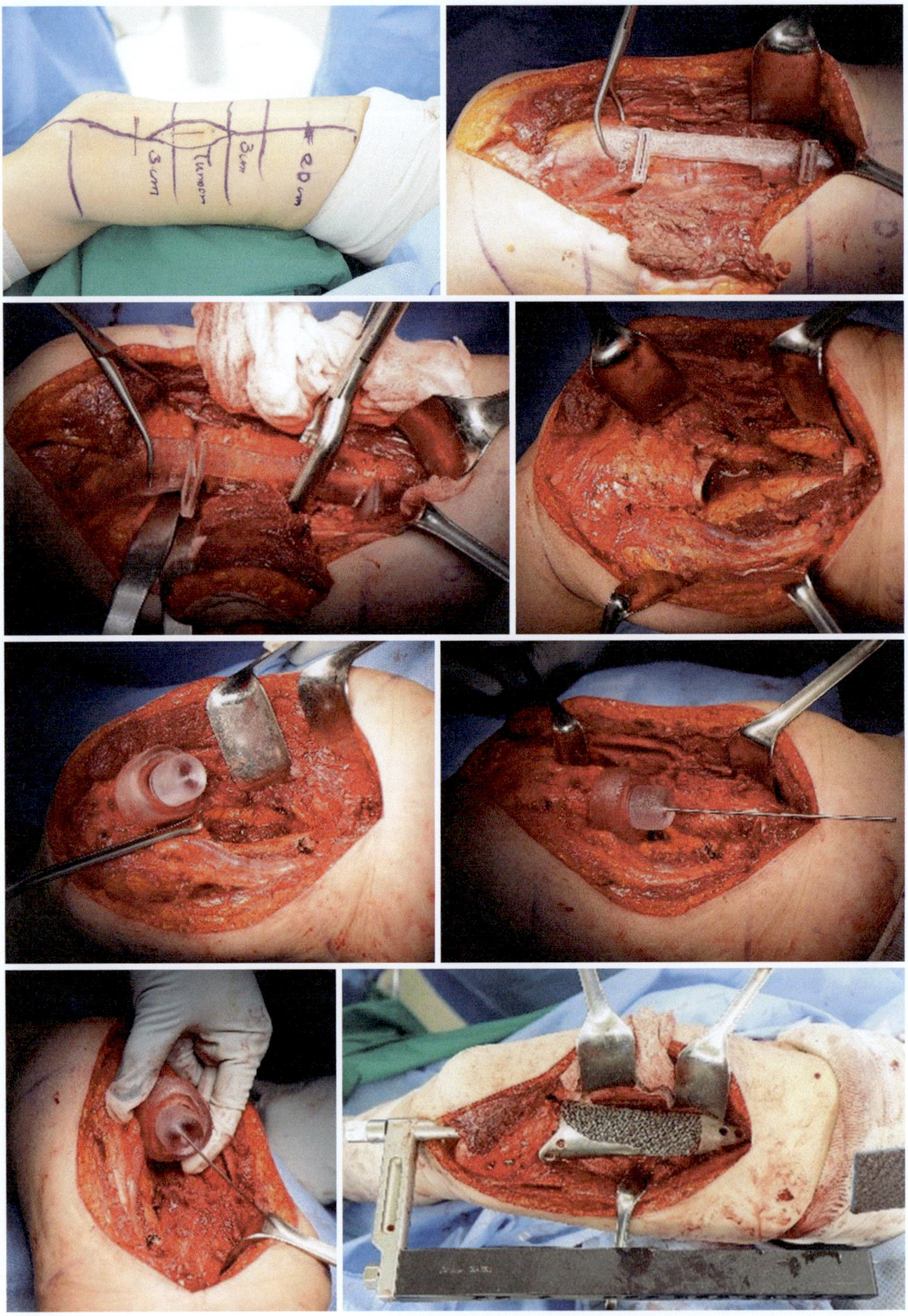

Fig. 19.12 Intraoperative photographs: low viscosity PMMA bone cement injection into the peri-nail canal of 3D printed implant

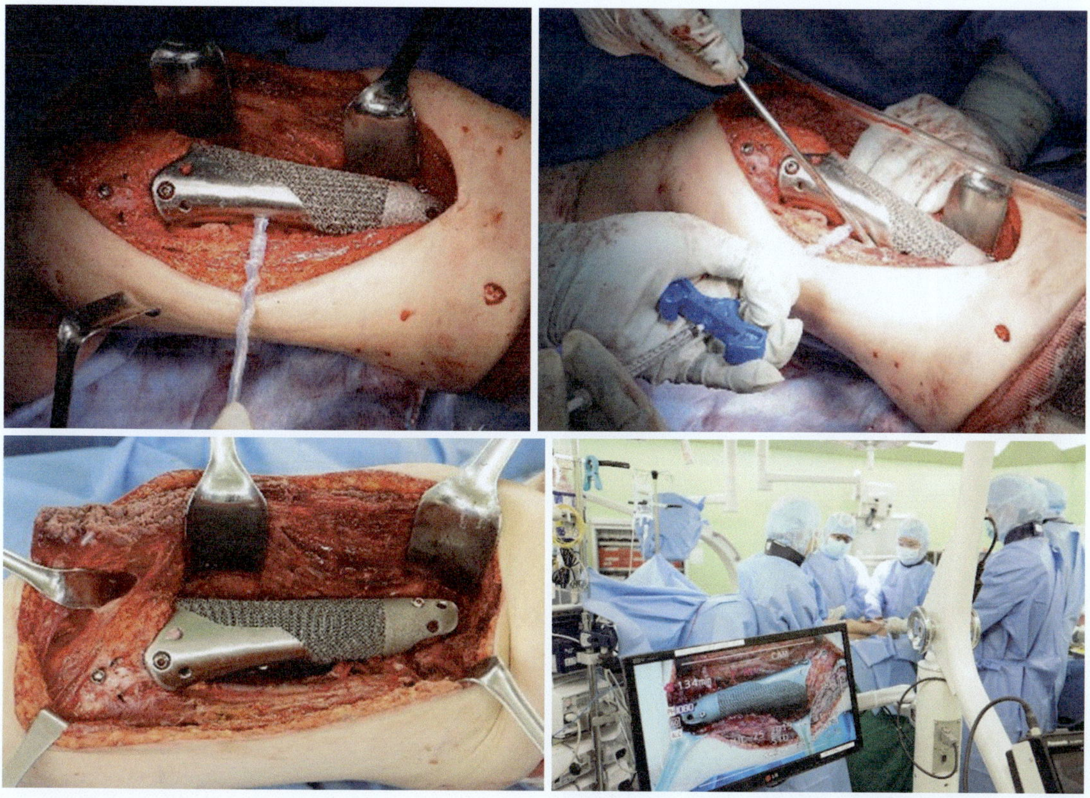

Fig. 19.12 (continued)

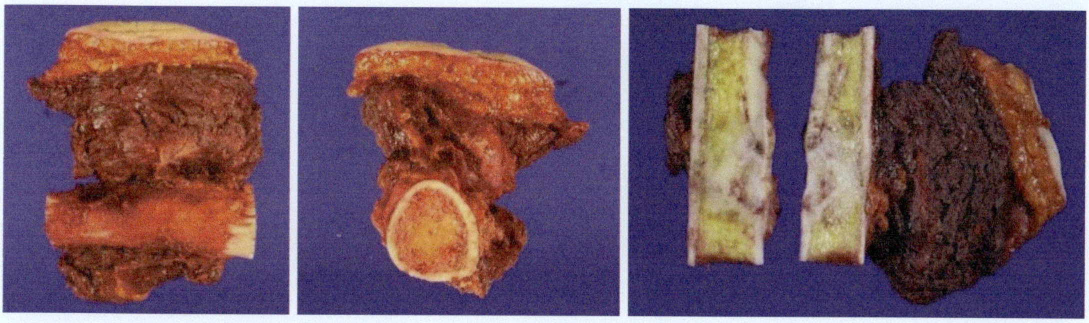

Fig. 19.13 Resected bone tumor

19.6 Postoperative Images

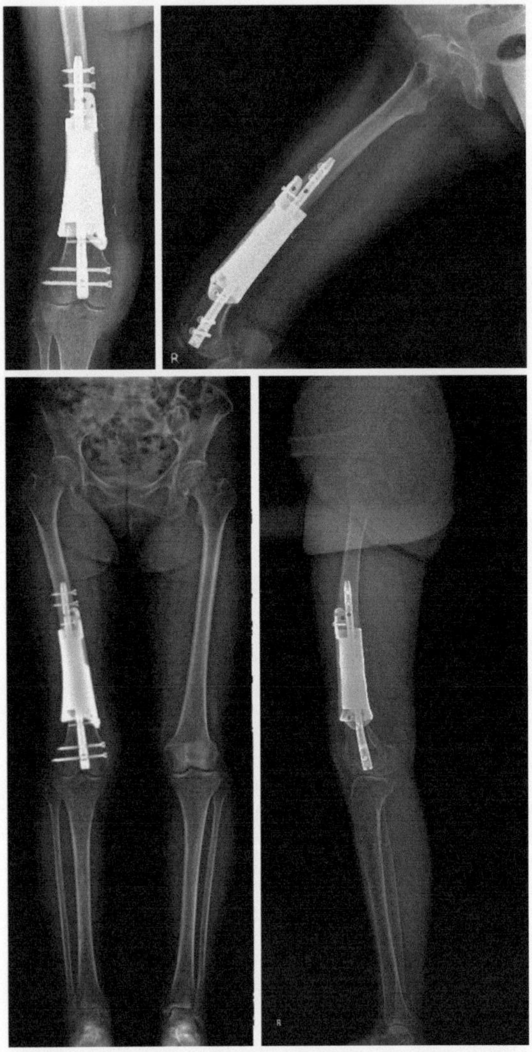

Fig. 19.14 Postoperative X-ray images

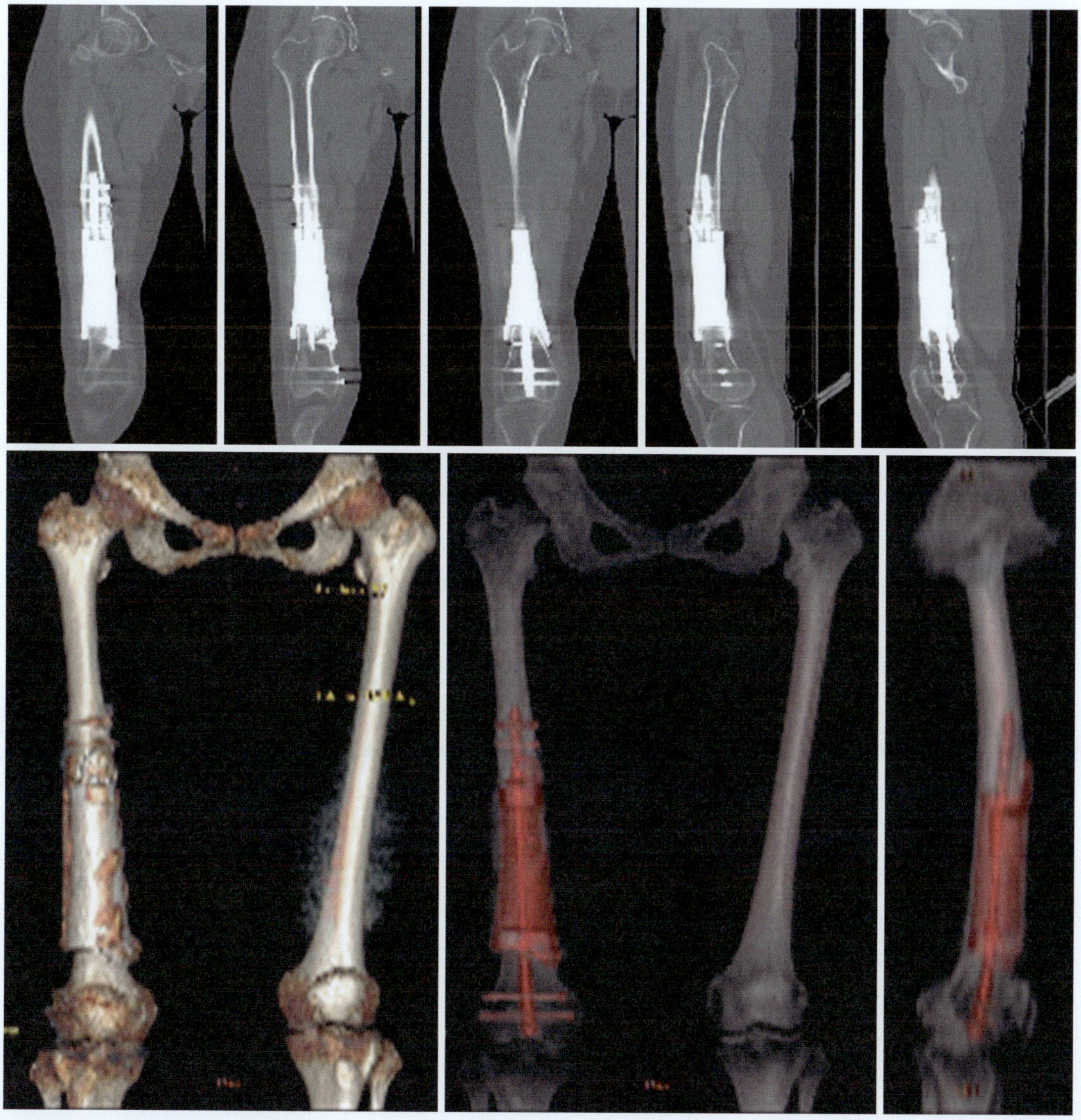

Fig. 19.15 Postoperative CT images

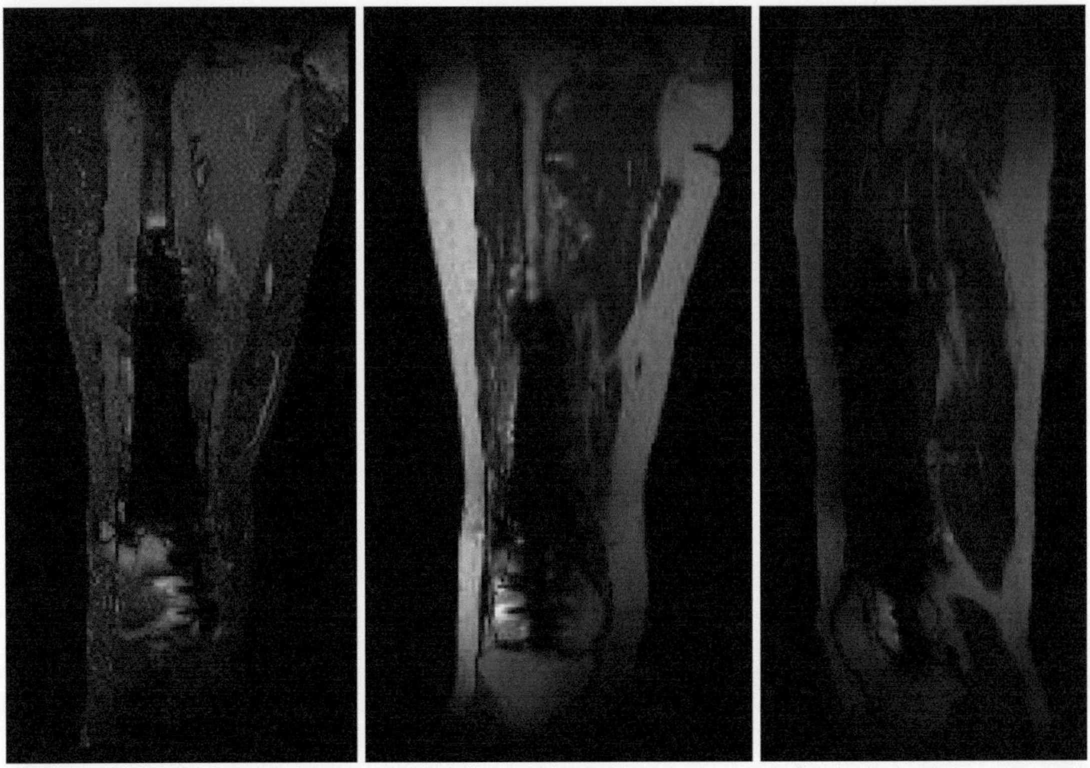

Fig. 19.16 Postoperative MRI images

Patient Case 20: Cortical Mesh Covering IM Nail and Cement

20

20.1 Patient Case 20

Age/sex	68/female
Location	Femur diaphysis/left
Diagnosis	Metastatic bone cancer (solitary) Renal cell carcinoma (RCC) left
Preoperative symptom	Wheelchair ambulation
Preoperative pain score	Resting 4/activity 8
BMI (height/weight)	20.17 (154.6/48.2)
Past history	RCC clear cell type, left Total nephrectomy at 3 years ago
Present illness	Requested complete resection from the urology department

H.-G. Kang, *Clinical Atlas of 3D Printing Bone Reconstruction*,
https://doi.org/10.1007/978-981-16-2043-0_20

20.2 Preoperative Images

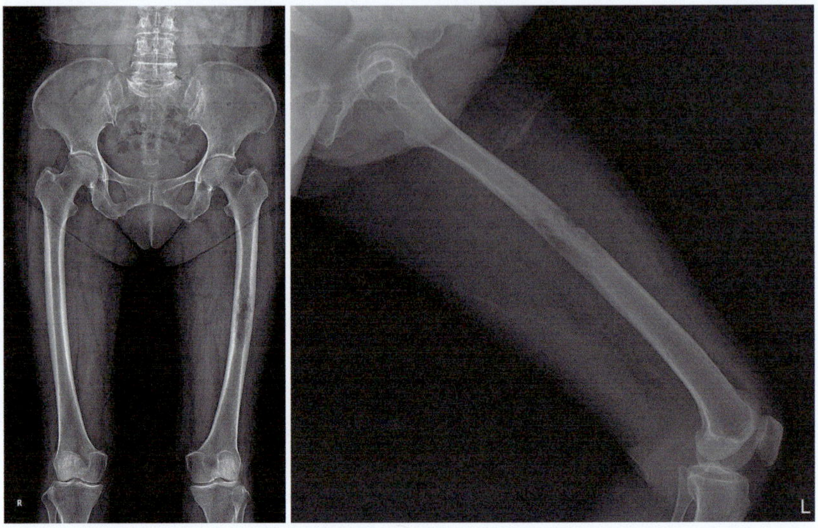

Fig. 20.1 Preoperative X-ray images

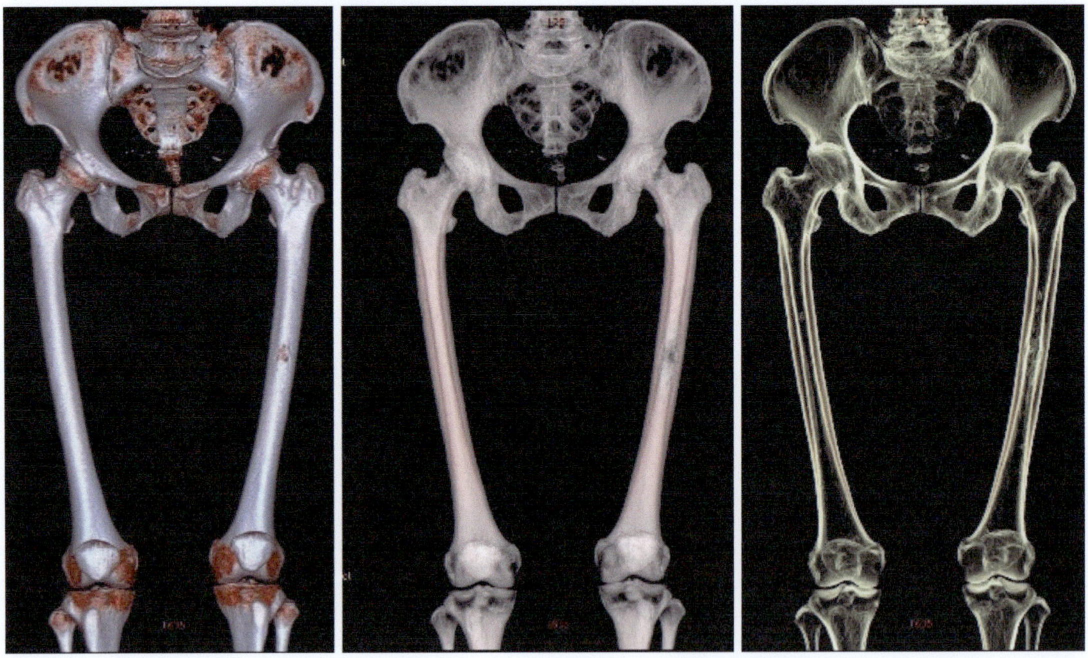

Fig. 20.2 Preoperative CT images

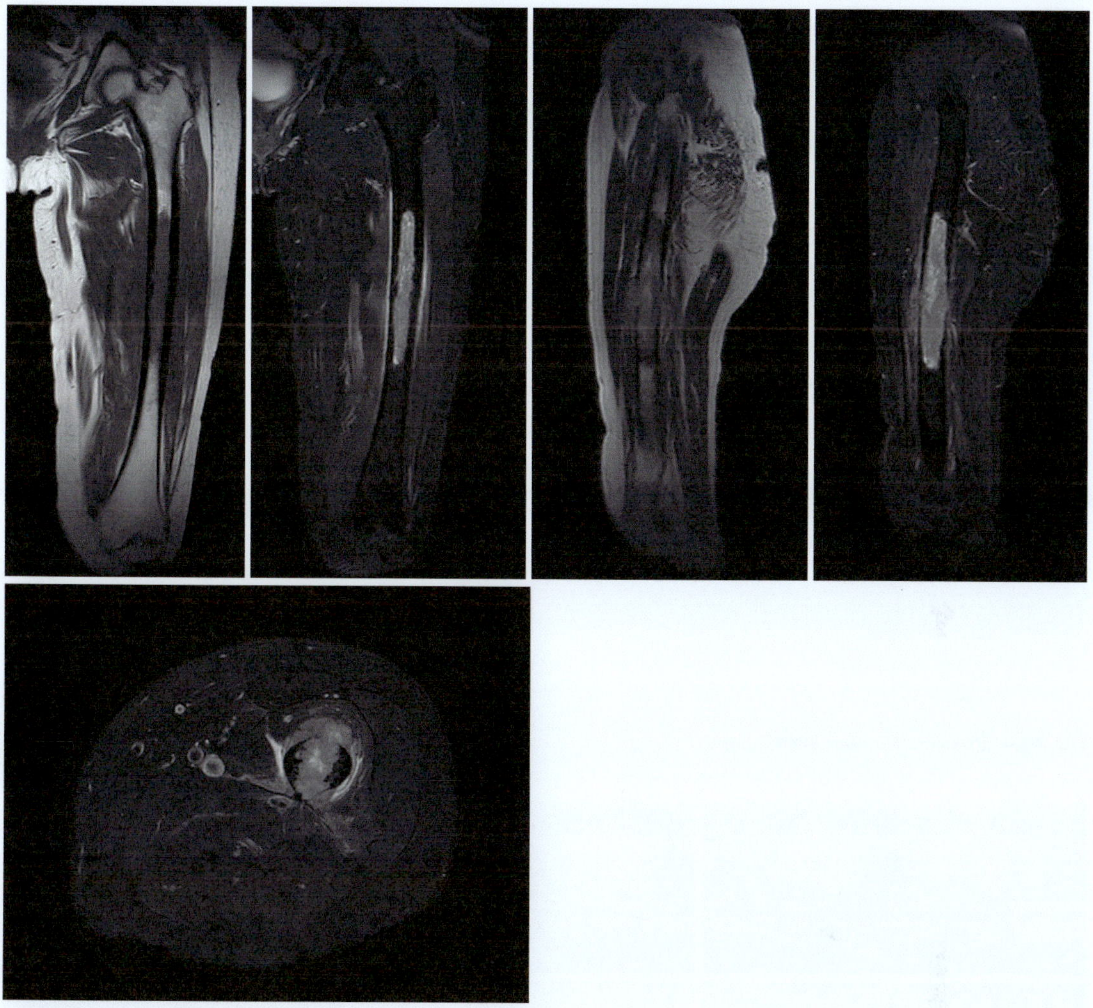

Fig. 20.3 Preoperative MRI images

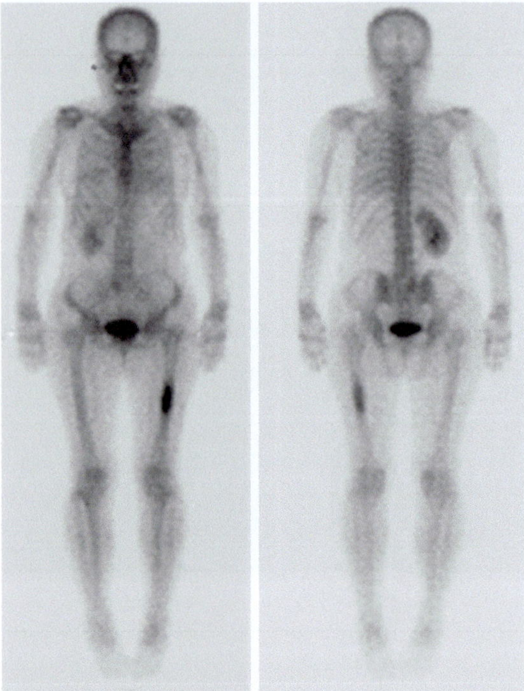

Fig. 20.4 Preoperative bone scan images

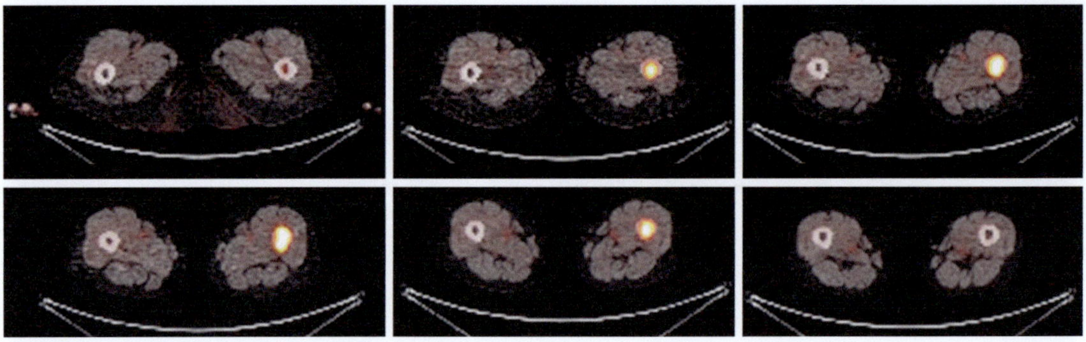

Fig. 20.5 Preoperative PET-CT images

20.3 Planning of Surgery

Segmental resection left femur diaphysis
  Long gamma nail fixation
  Bone cement augmentation around nail
  3D printed cortical mesh implant

- Divided into anterior and posterior blocks for easy attachment
- 3D-printed segmental prosthesis may be difficult to adjust the length if there is an intraoperative change
- There is also a difficulty in matching the antebowing of the nail if it is used with an intramedullary nail
- Sometimes, there are patients who need to easily and simply prepare 3D-printed implants
- Stability can be obtained by mixing various methods

20.4 Design and Fabrication

Whole mesh style

Longer than Segmental defect to cover the upper and lower normal bones sufficiently

Cutting guide

Insufficient reference point to attach guide to femur diaphysis

- Implant measurement
- Implant weight (g): 56
- Size (mm): 164

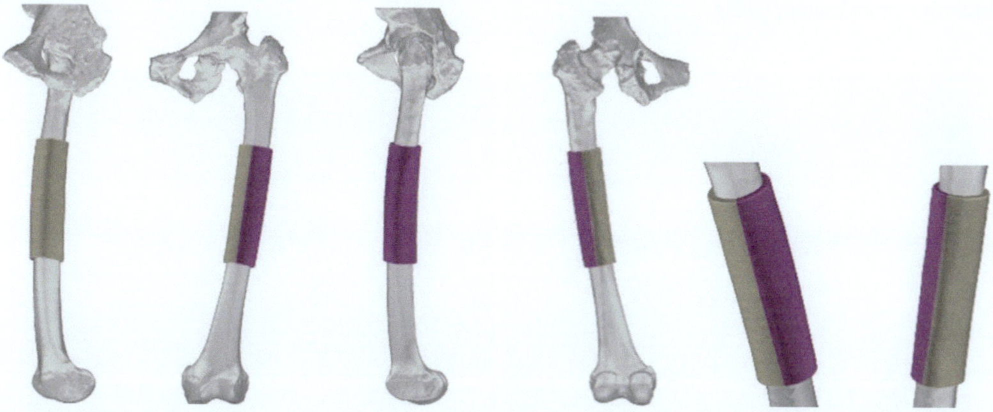

Fig. 20.6 Cutting guide: segmental bone resection using a combination of intraoperative fluoroscopy and length measurement

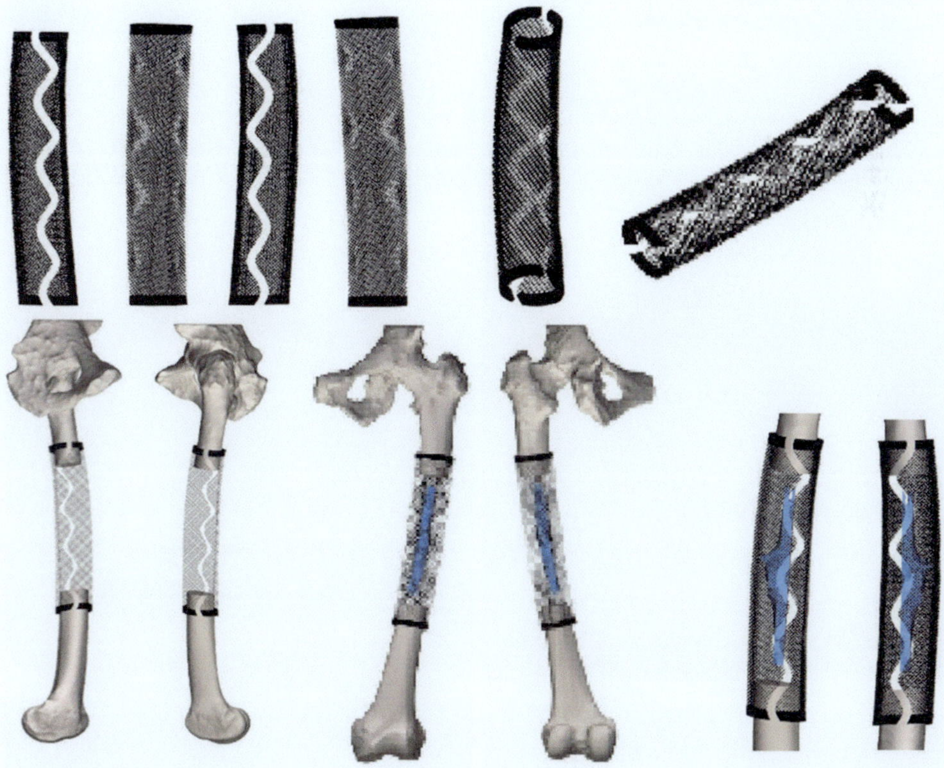

Fig. 20.7 Implant design: longer than bone defect space

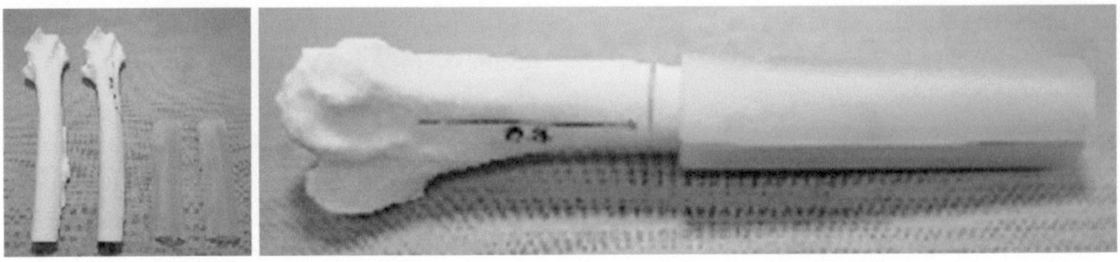

Fig. 20.8 3D-printed cutting guide

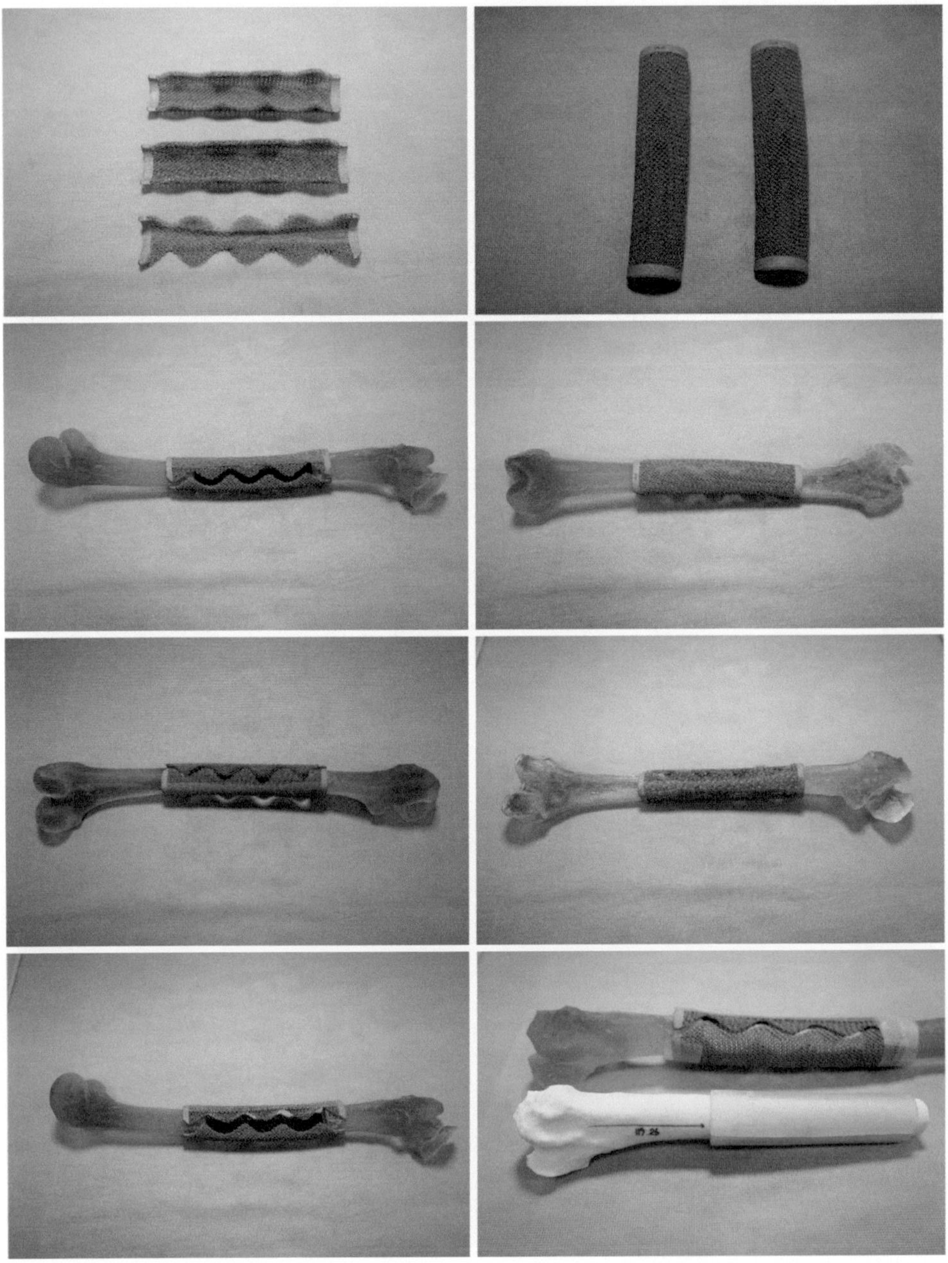

Fig. 20.9 Printed implant

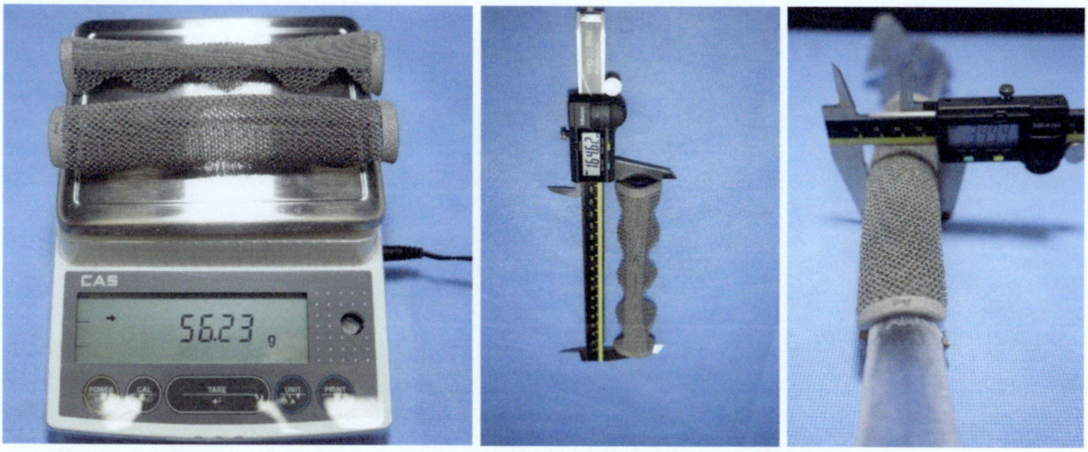

Fig. 20.9 (continued)

20.5 Operation

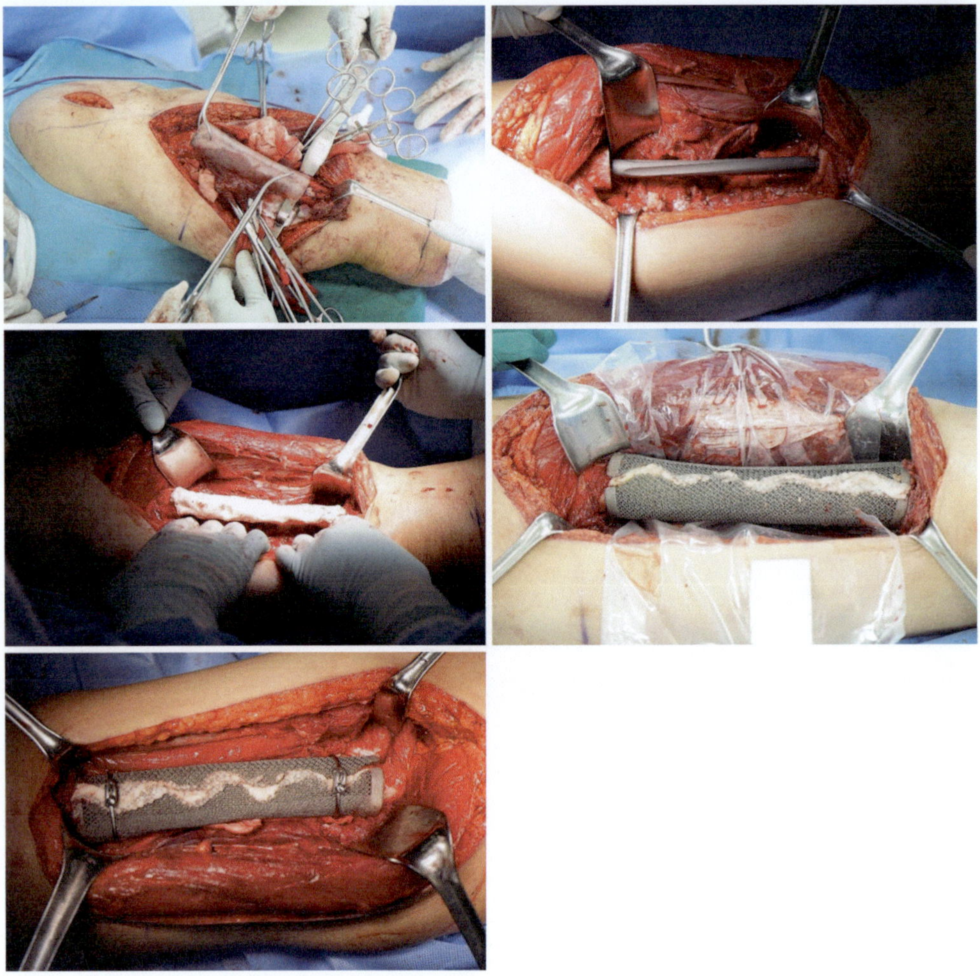

Fig. 20.10 Intraoperative photographs: cortical mesh implant attached before the PMMA bone cement hardening

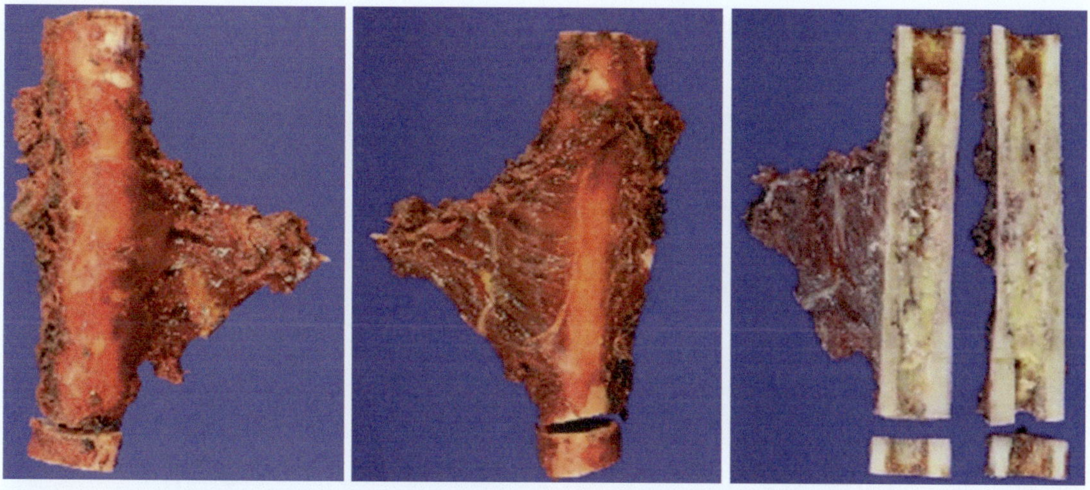

Fig. 20.11 Resected bone tumor: additional distal resection due to margin tumor positive

20.6 Postoperative Images

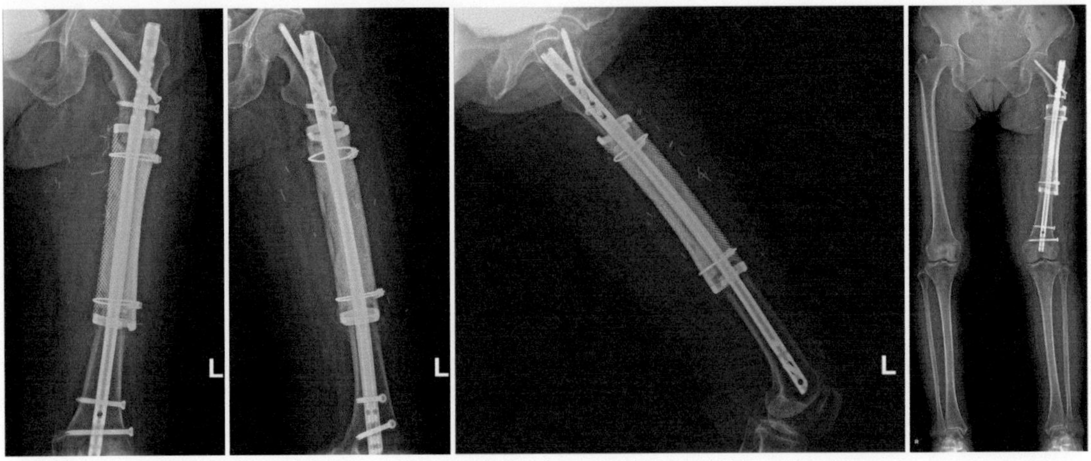

Fig. 20.12 Postoperative X-ray images: cortical bony bridging showing between the implant and bone

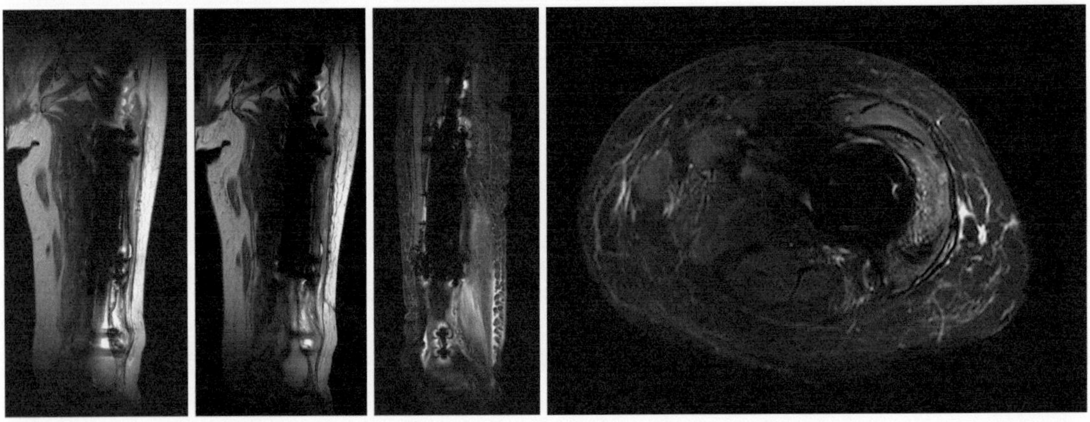

Fig. 20.13 Postoperative MRI images: much reduced metal artifact by mesh style implant

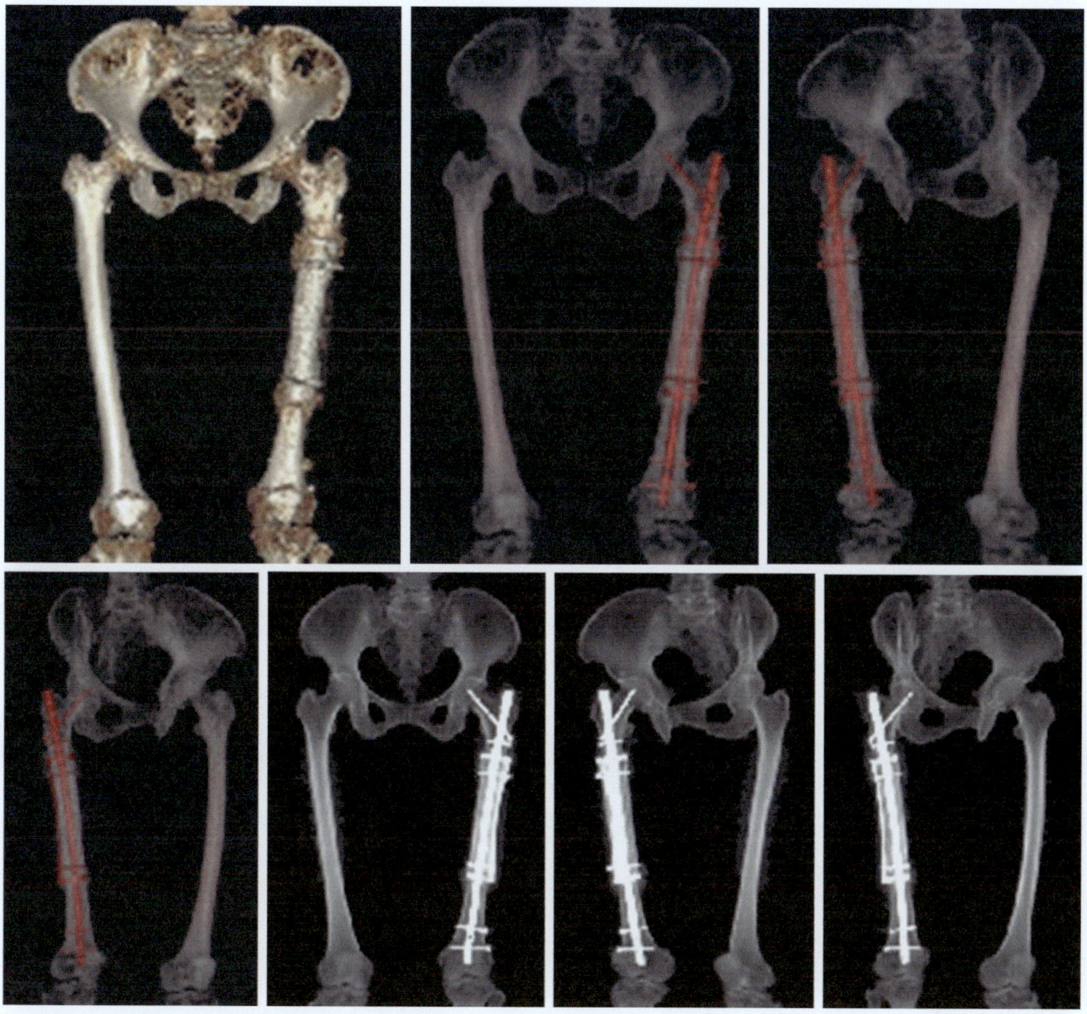

Fig. 20.14 Postoperative CT images

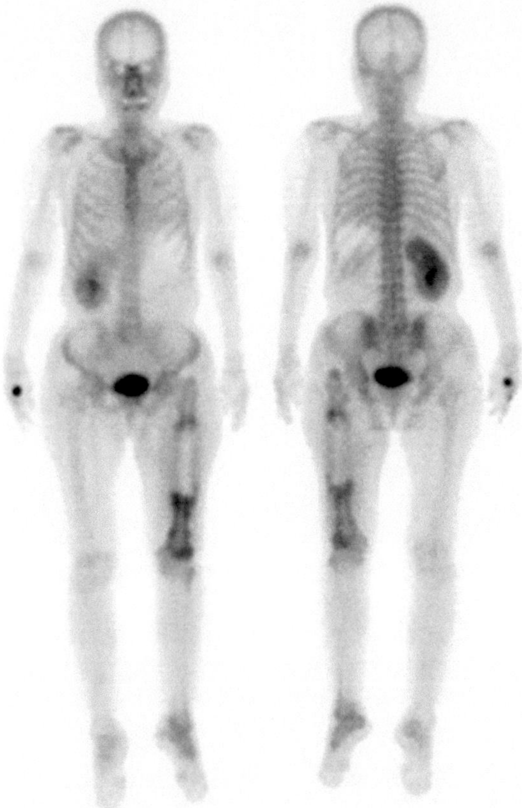

Fig. 20.15 Postoperative bone scan images

Patient Case 21: Deformity Correction: Open Wedge Spacer and Supporting Plate

21

21.1 Patient Case 21

Age/sex	42/female
Location/site	Femur/left
Diagnosis	Fibrous dysplasia Linear pathologic fracture
Preoperative symptom	Limping gait
Preoperative pain score	Resting pain 0/activity 5
BMI (height/weight)	26.68 (155.6/64.6)
Past history	Femoral tumor accidentally discovered as a pathological fracture
Present illness	No fracture healing of subtrochanteric until 6 months' observation

H.-G. Kang, *Clinical Atlas of 3D Printing Bone Reconstruction*,
https://doi.org/10.1007/978-981-16-2043-0_21

21.2 Preoperative Images

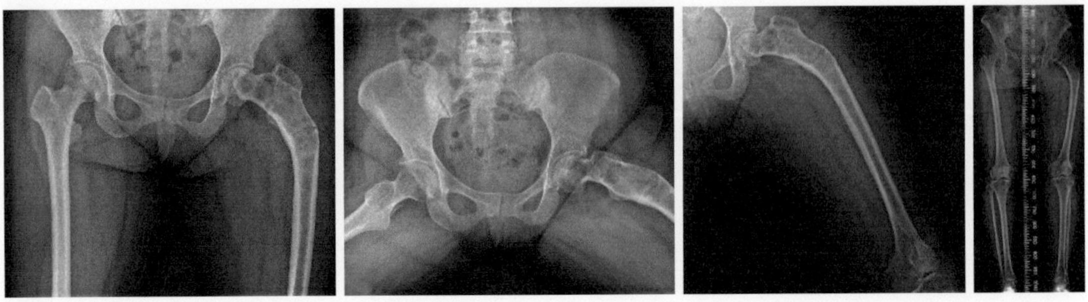

Fig. 21.1 Preoperative X-ray images: linear pathologic fracture with Varus angulation, leg shortening 2.5 cm

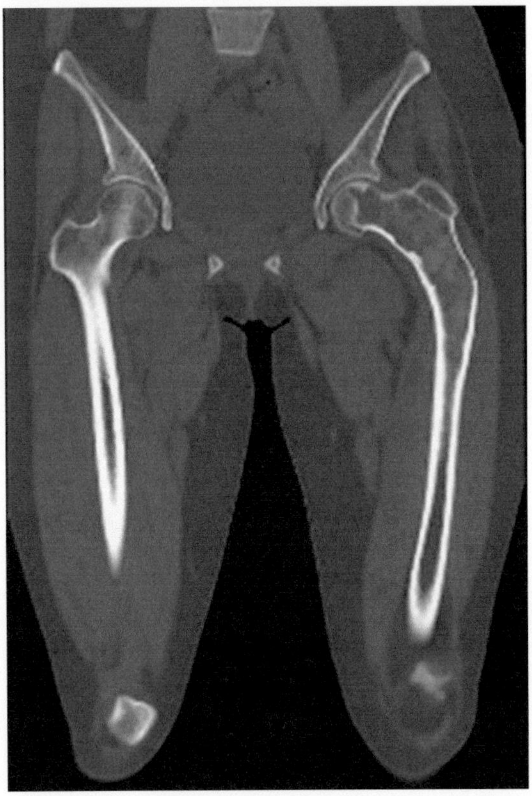

Fig. 21.2 Preoperative CT images

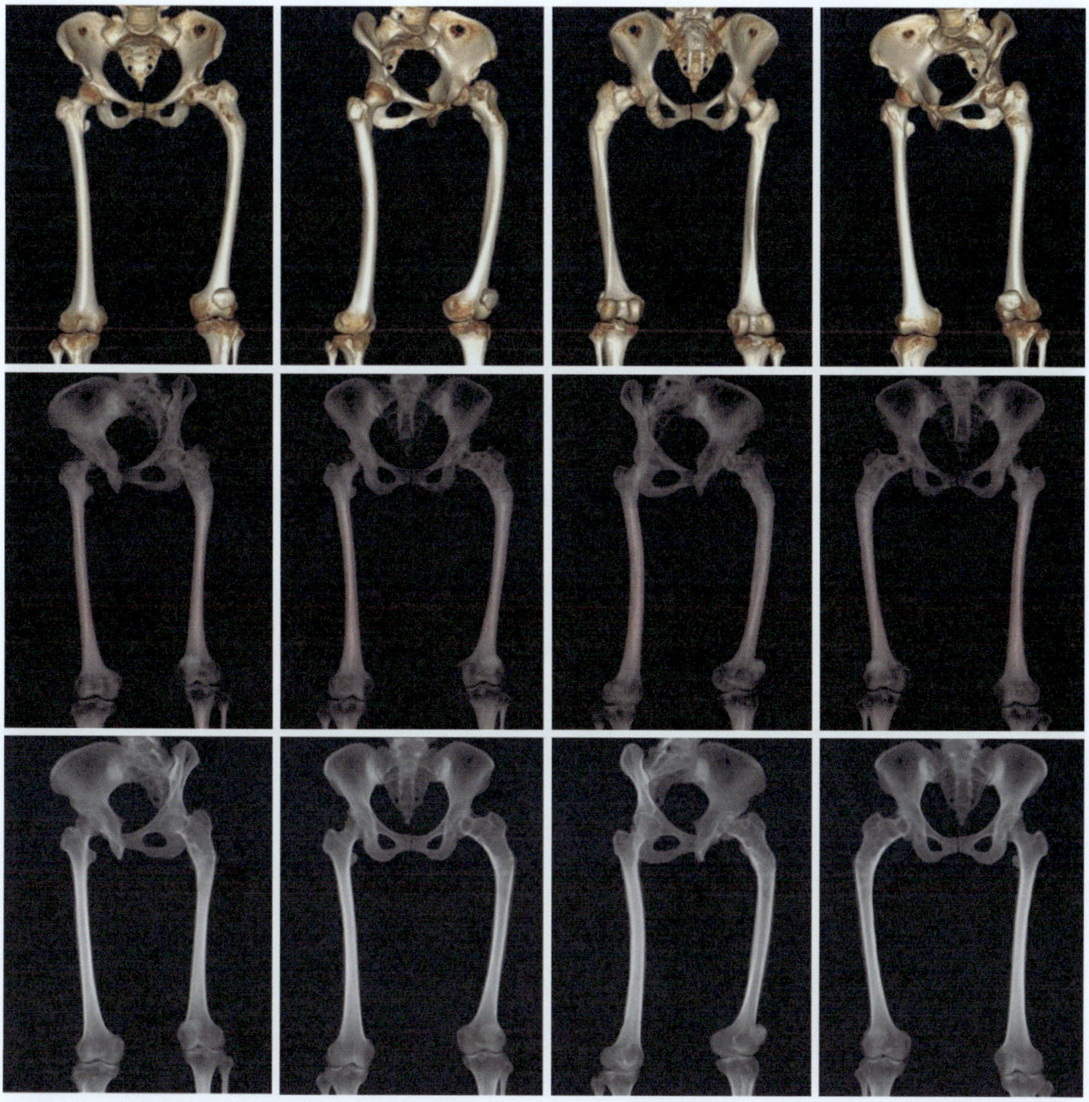

Fig. 21.2 (continued)

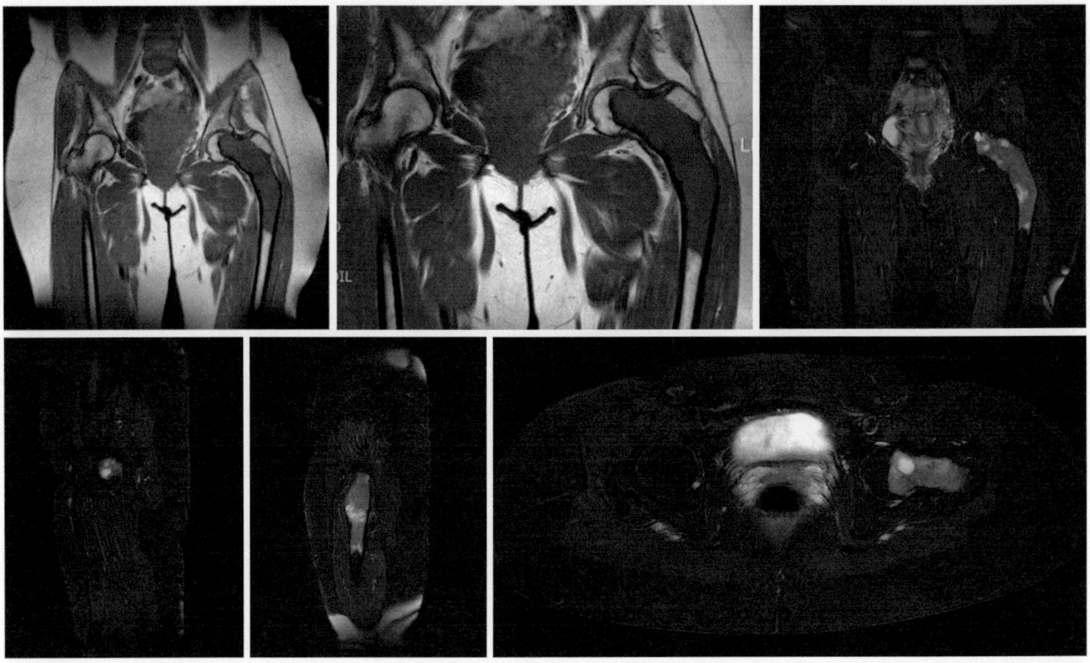

Fig. 21.3 Preoperative MRI images: tumor extended to the femoral head and neck

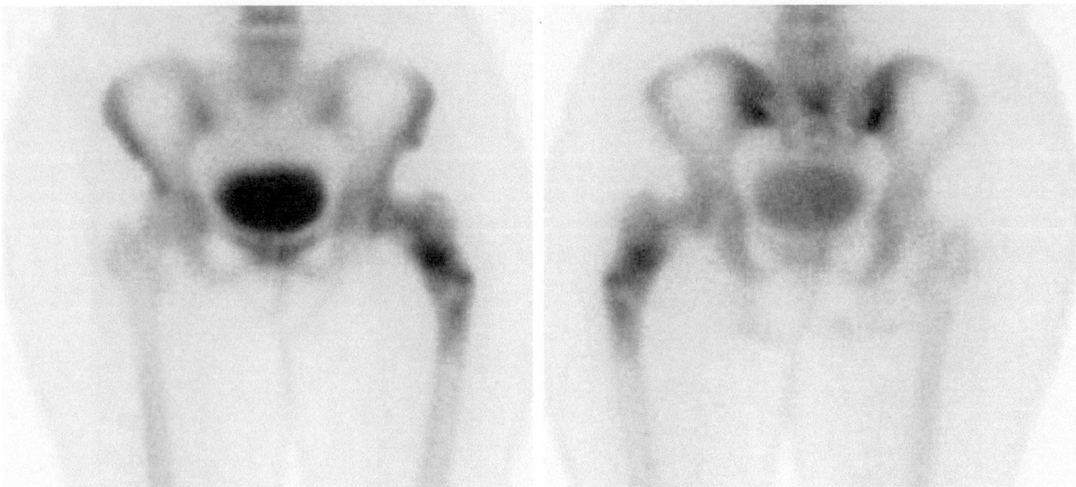

Fig. 21.4 Preoperative bone scan images

21.3 Planning of Surgery

Open wedge osteotomy

3D-printed plate +3D-printed open wedge spacer implant

Femoral head and neck preservation

Tumor removal

Deformity correction at the subtrochanteric area

- Bone cutting and curettage of tumor
- Varus deformity correction with open wedge
- Femur neck retroversion and rotational deformity correction
- Two pieces 3D-printed implant—open wedge spacer (medial side) and plate (lateral side)
- PMMA bone cement augmentation femoral head and neck
- Allograft bone chip for medullary cavity
- Muscle reattachment of vastus lateralis and gluteus maximus

21.4 Design and Fabrication

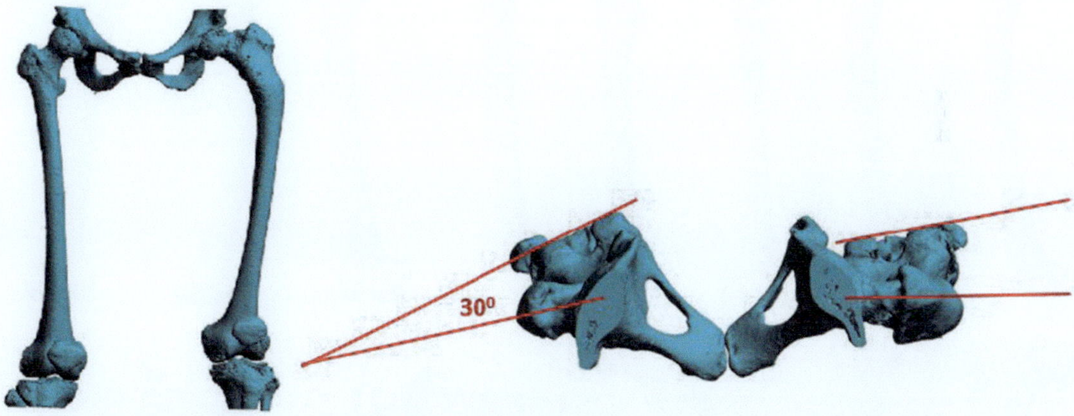

Fig. 21.5 Preoperative 3D modeling: varus angulation and retroversion deformity, leg shortening

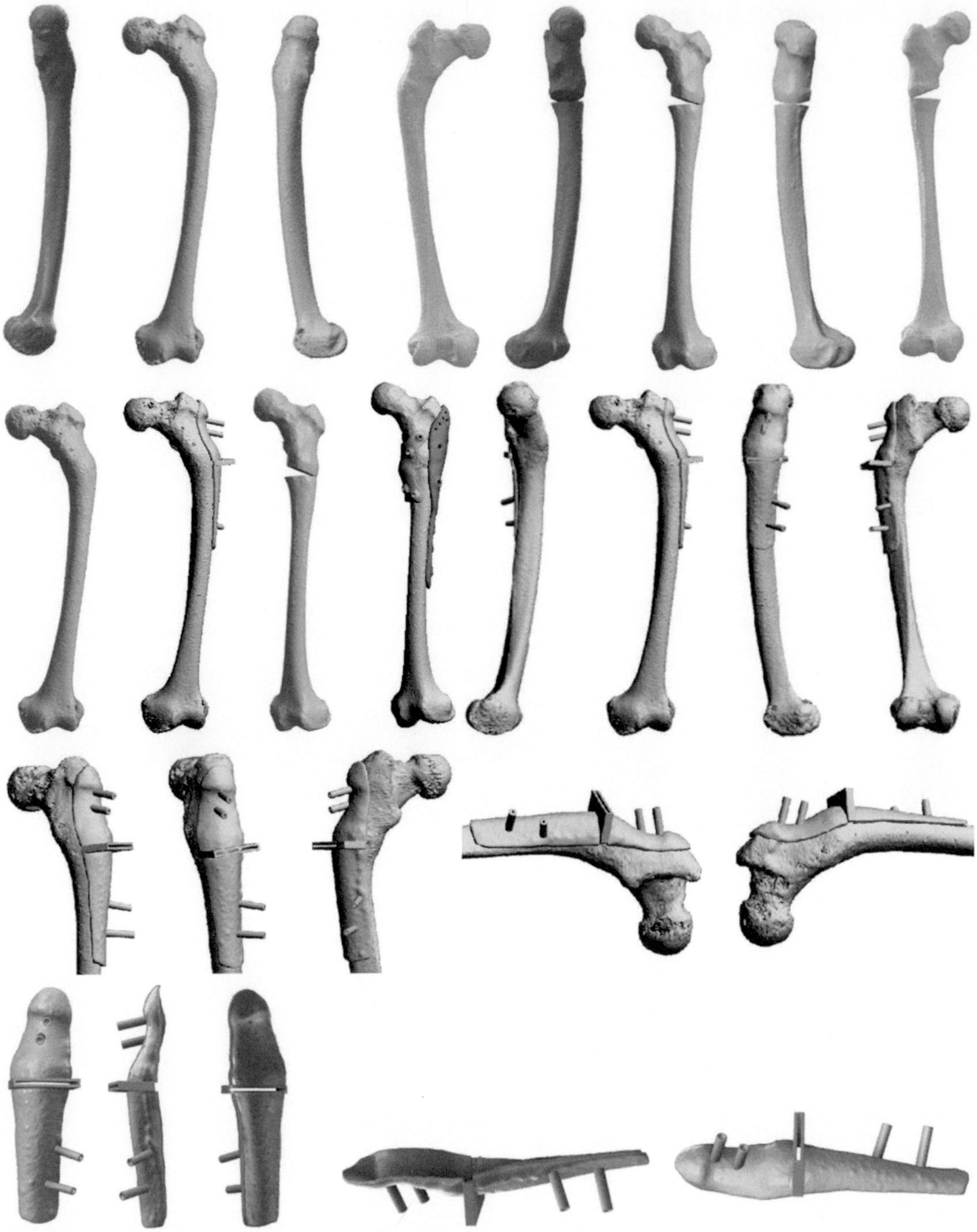

Fig. 21.6 Cutting guide for open wedge osteotomy

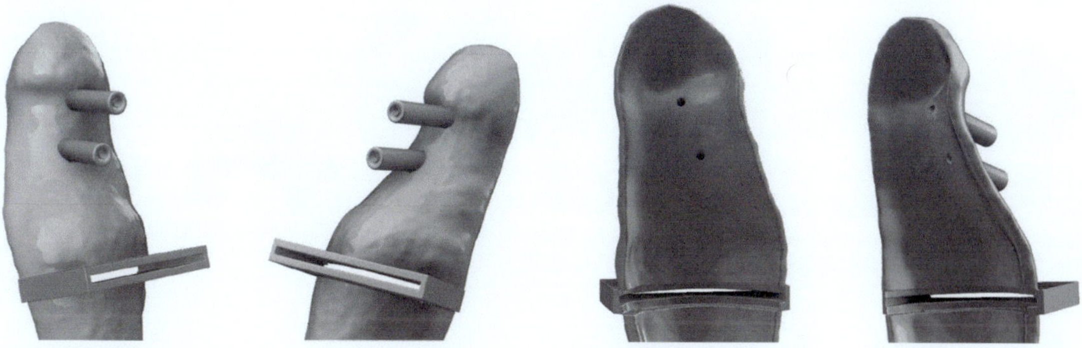

Fig. 21.7 Proximal pin guides for screw direction to the femur head and neck

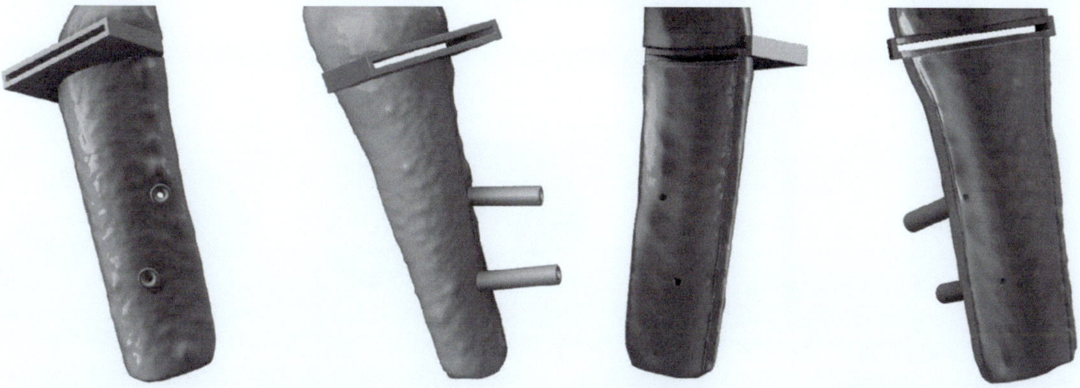

Fig. 21.8 Distal pin guides for correction of rotational deformity. Distal femur should be lateral rotation for the insertion of the screws on the guide pin holes

21.5 Implant design

Two 3D implant designs—buttress plate and open wedge spacer

- Open wedge osteotomy for 2.5 cm shorten leg length correction
- Cortical bone expansion and thinning by tumor
- No metal filling of medullary cavity for revision stem insertion of hip arthroplasty in the future

1. Open wedge spacer block (medial)
    - Cortical bone contact only and empty of medullary cavity
    - Short plate wing for screw fixation
    - Screw holes—Like a volcanic uplift: increase screw and plate contact, screw head deepening
    - PMMA bone cementing in the screw fixation—like locking plate
    - Whole meshed wedge implant—cortical bone contact area
2. Buttress plate (lateral)
    - Multiple suture holes on the trochanteric end
    - Reinforcement of subtrochanteric area
    - Meshed inner surface for limited periosteal contact

- Implant measurement
- Implant weight (g): 159/64
- Size (mm): 172/84

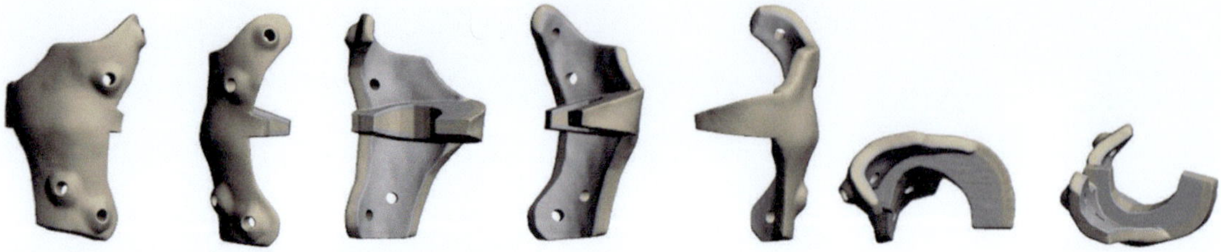

Fig. 21.9 Implant design: open wedge spacer block (medial)

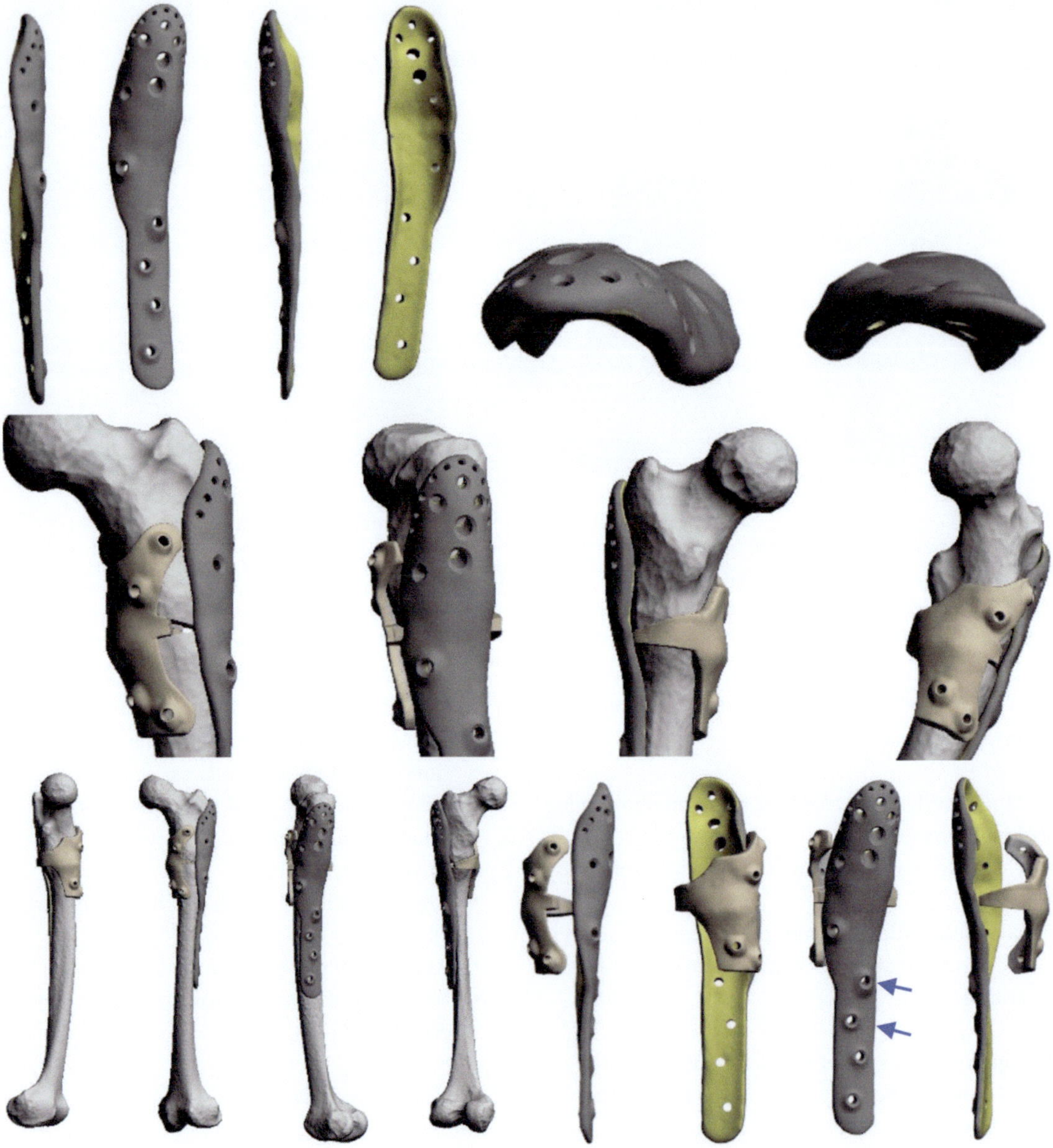

Fig. 21.10 Buttress plate (lateral): the distal femur should be lateral rotation to fit with screw's guide pin holes(arrows)

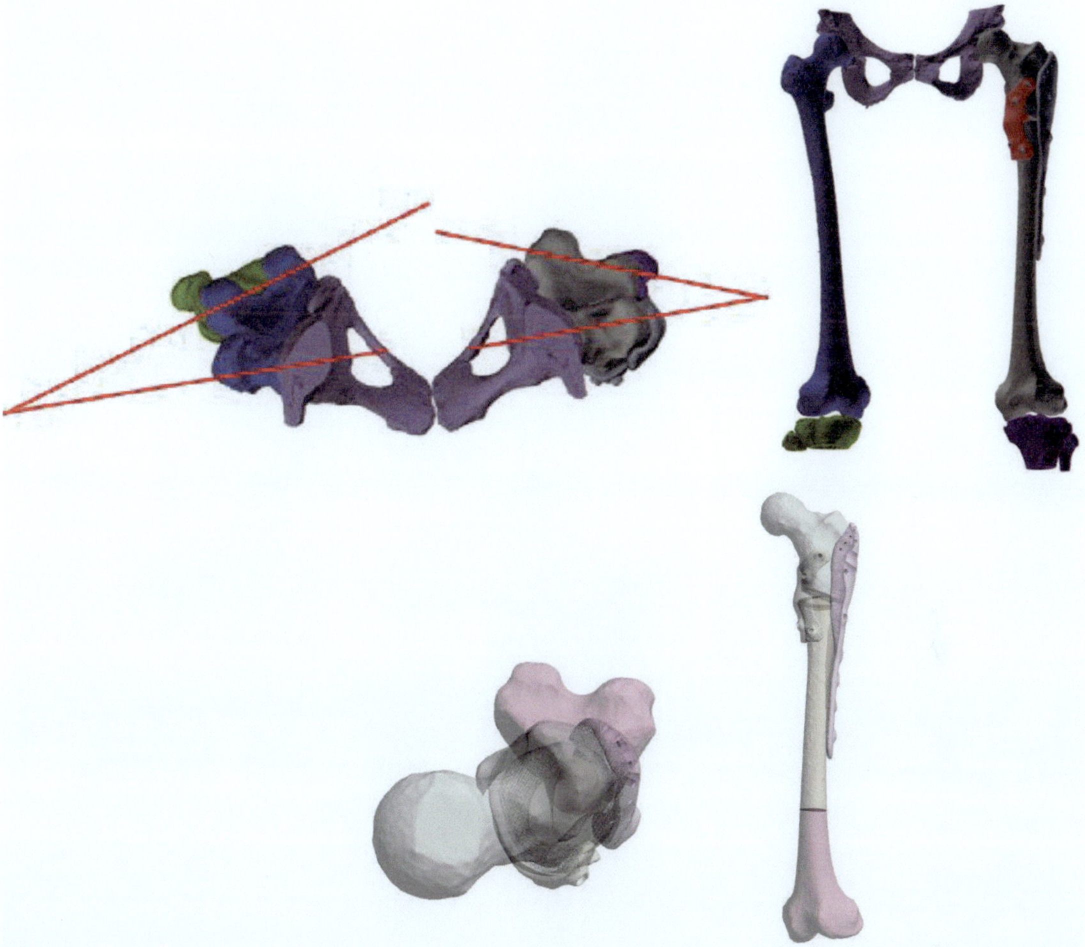

Fig. 21.11 Simulation of postoperative 3D modeling: correction of all the deformity including shortening, varus, and rotation

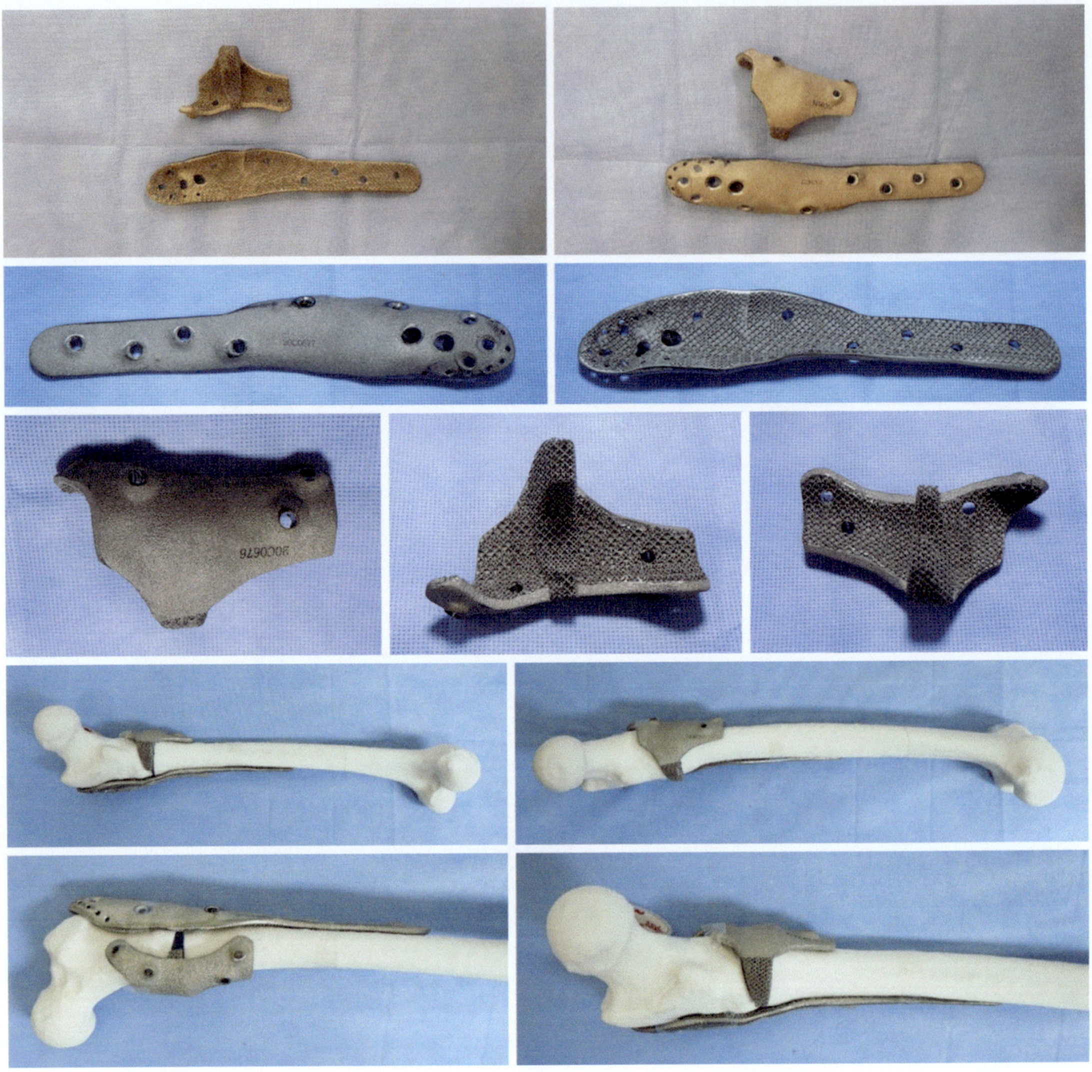

Fig. 21.12 Printed implant

21.6 Operation

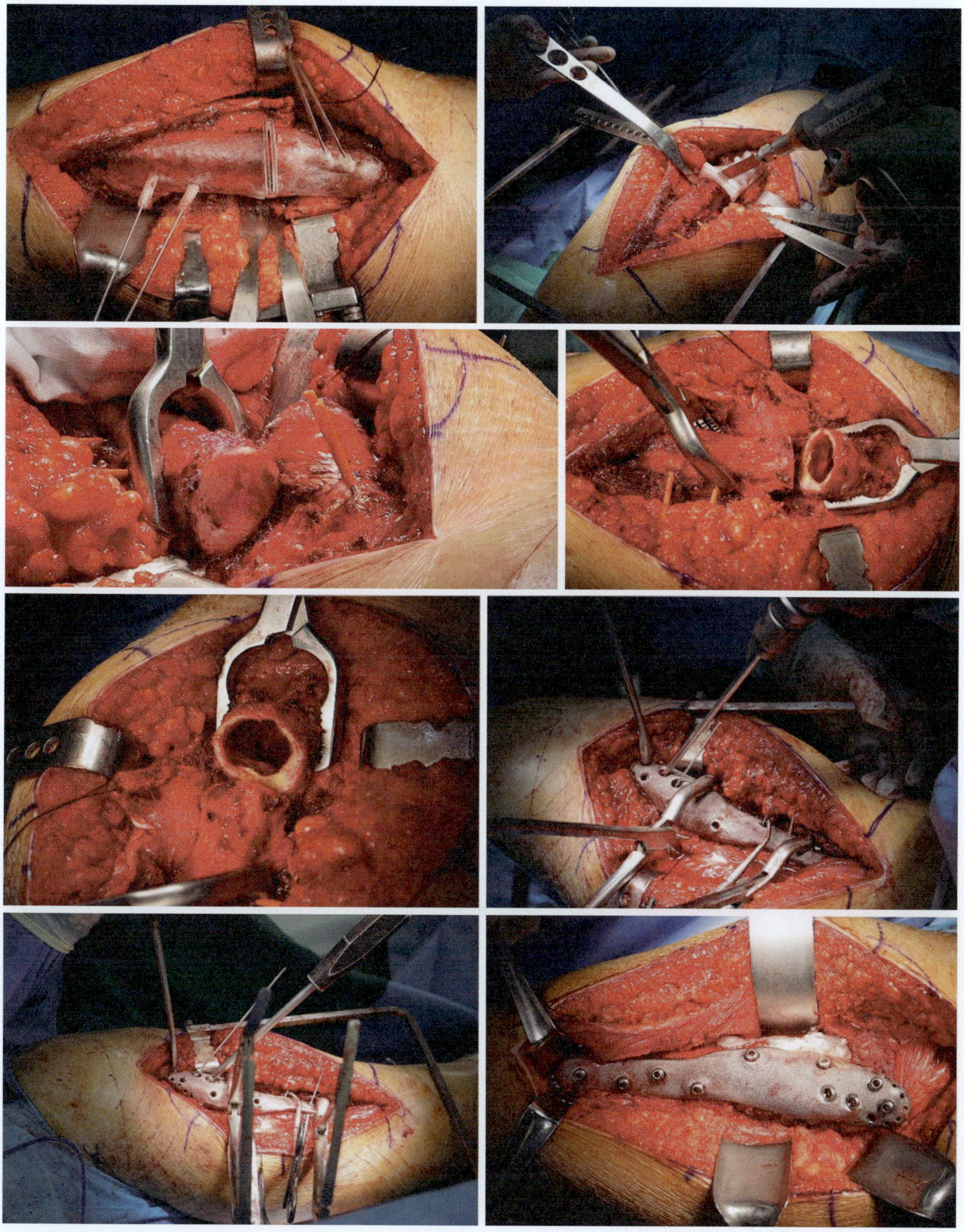

Fig. 21.13 Intraoperative photographs

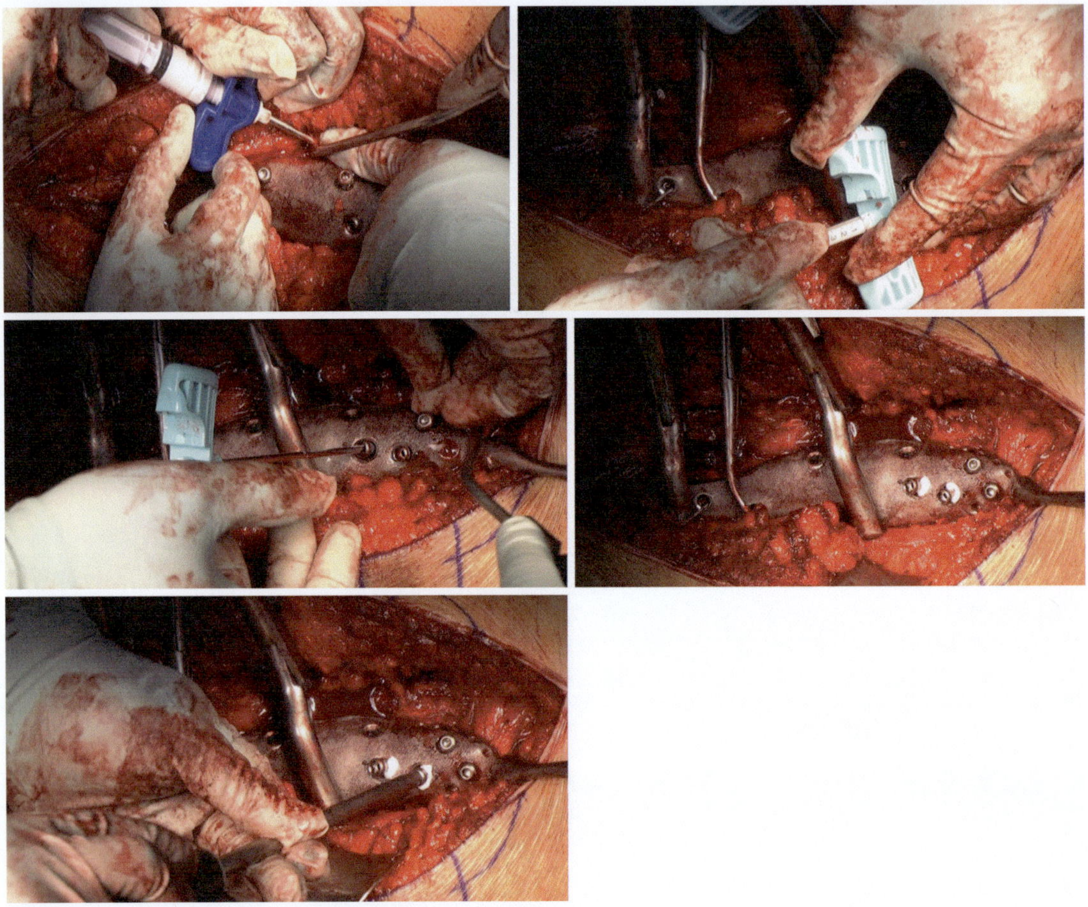

Fig. 21.13 (continued)

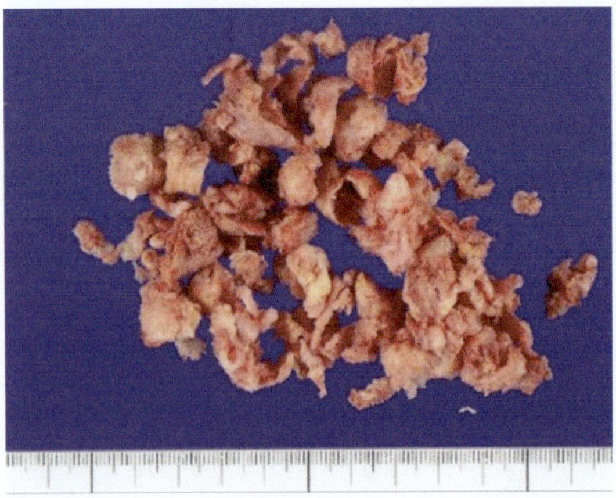

Fig. 21.14 Fibrous dysplasia curettage

21.7 Postoperative Images

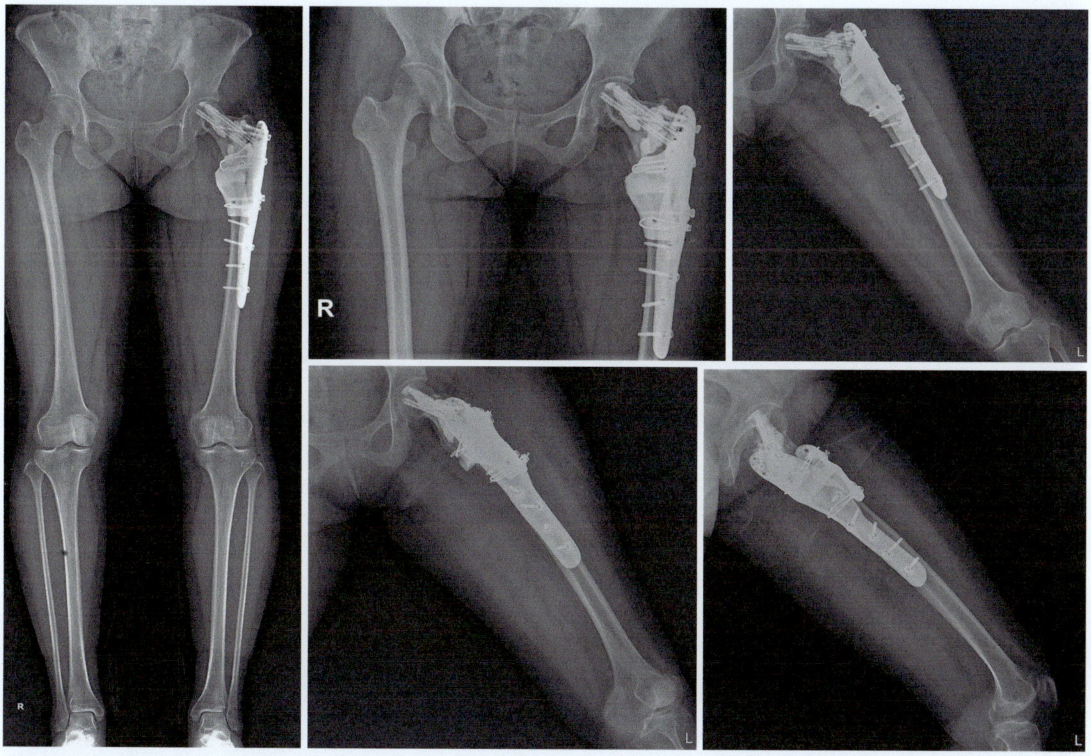

Fig. 21.15 Postoperative X-ray images

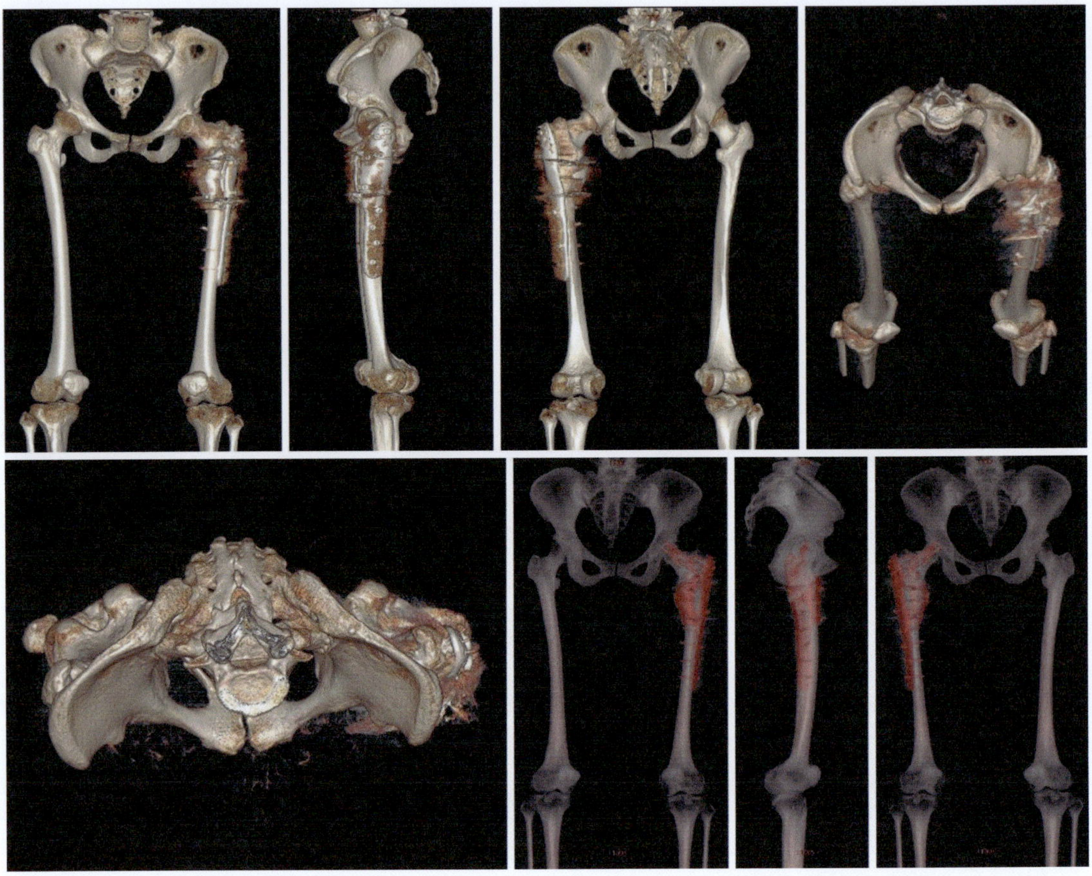

Fig. 21.16 Postoperative CT images

22 Patient Case 22: Segmental Femur and Implant-Bone Connector

22.1 Patient Case 22

Age/sex	67/female
Location/site	Femur/right
Diagnosis	Chondrosarcoma, grade 2
Preoperative symptom	Limping gate
Preoperative pain score	Resting 2/Activity 5
BMI (weight/height)	26.17(144.7/54.8)
Past history	Left leg growth disorder after injury at her middle school period Left heel does not touch the ground
Present illness	Wants to save the patient's own knee joint

Leg length discrepancy: 10 cm longer right leg (femur 7 cm longer + tibia 3 cm longer) due to adolescence trauma left leg

H.-G. Kang, *Clinical Atlas of 3D Printing Bone Reconstruction*,
https://doi.org/10.1007/978-981-16-2043-0_22

22.2 Preoperative Images

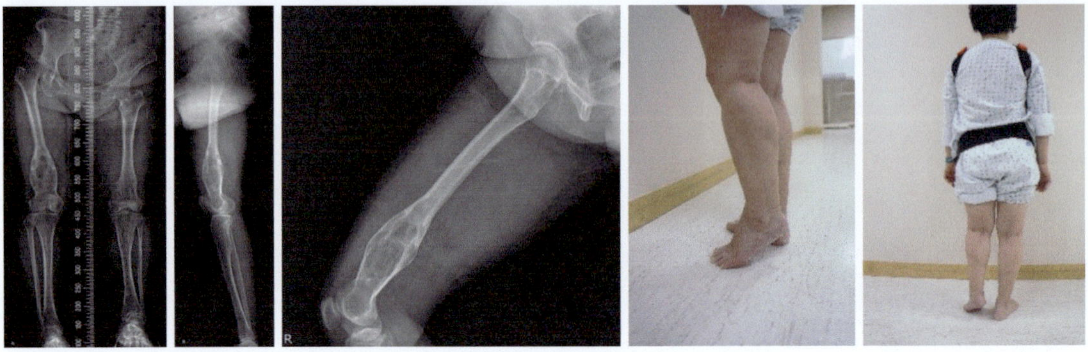

Fig. 22.1 Preoperative X-ray images and photographs

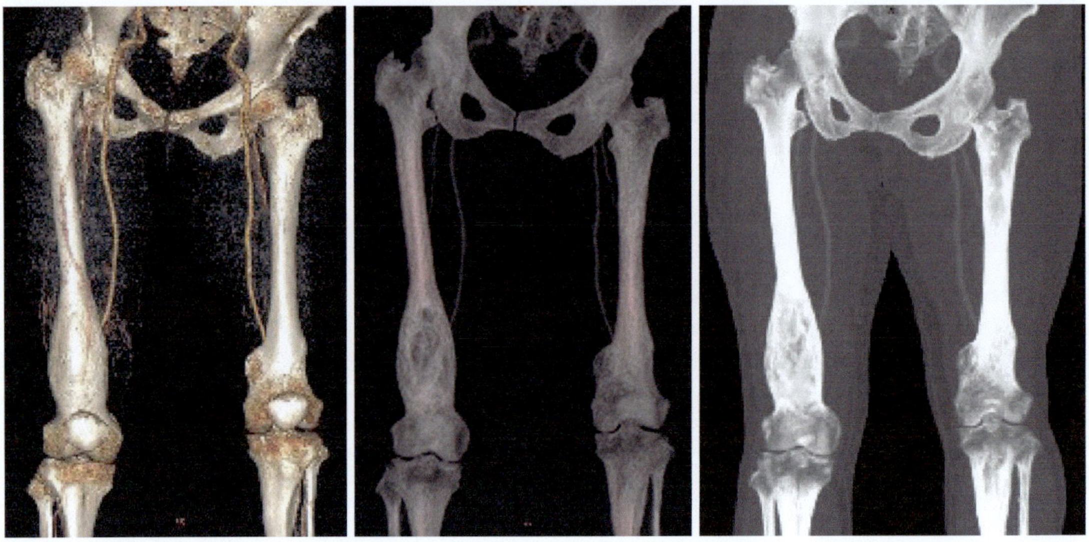

Fig. 22.2 Preoperative CT images

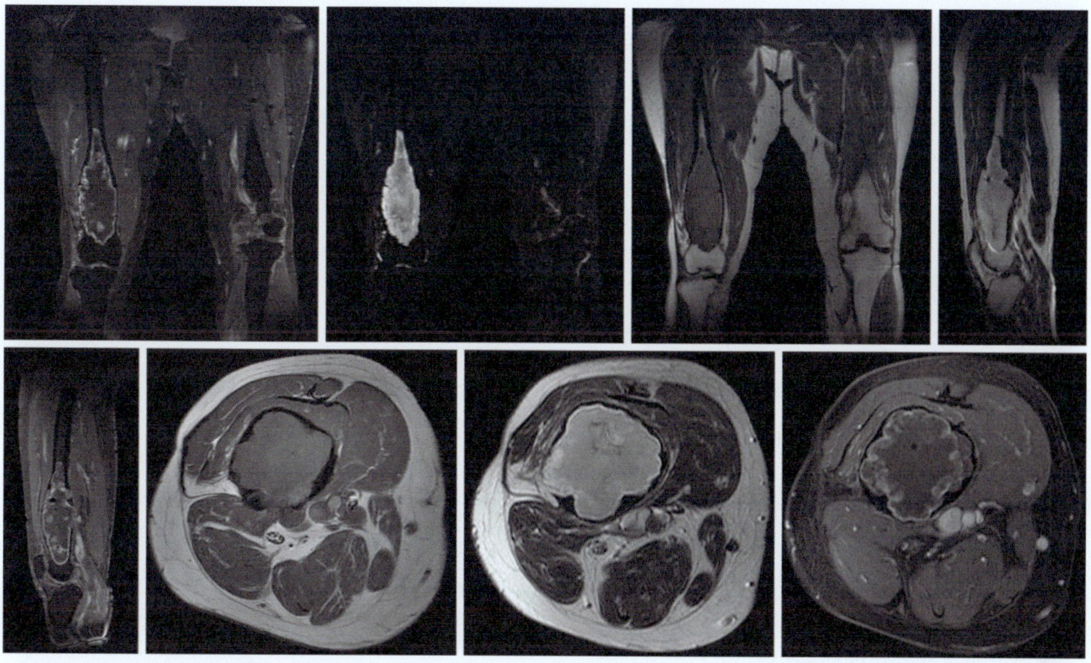

Fig. 22.3 Preoperative MRI images

22.3 Planning of Surgery

- 3D-printed segmental femur implant
- Approved 3D metal printing machine has a limitation of its product length less than 20 cm length
- Too much one-stage shortening of the femur makes the knee extension power weak
- Painful symptomatic knee arthritis in the future: designed to enable total knee arthroplasty combination

22.4 Design and Fabrication

- Segmental femur cut: 23 cm
- Femur segmental reconstruction 15 cm: 8 cm shortening of femur length
- Only 5 cm left for the proximal fixation portion of implant due to the 20 cm printing limitation
- Distal bone cutting guide
  - Joint open and intra-articular V-shaped bone cut
  - Bone cut through four directions—anterior and poster, medial and lateral saw cutting
  - Wing of each saw direction

Knee condylar area

- Mesh style of square pyramid
- Thin metal plate wrapping the joint condyle
- Multiple screw holes and suture holes
- Polishing the Patella-femoral surface area

Femur prosthesis body

- Solid core and mesh surface
- Three transverse screw holes in case of additional plate

Proximal osteosynthesis

- Circular bone wrapping 1 cm
- C-shaped plate to wrap half-diameter the femur
- Multiple screw holes
- Intramedullary inserted small peg at bone cut area
- Mesh style bone cut contact surface

- Implant measurement
- Implant weight (g): 346
- Size (mm): 198

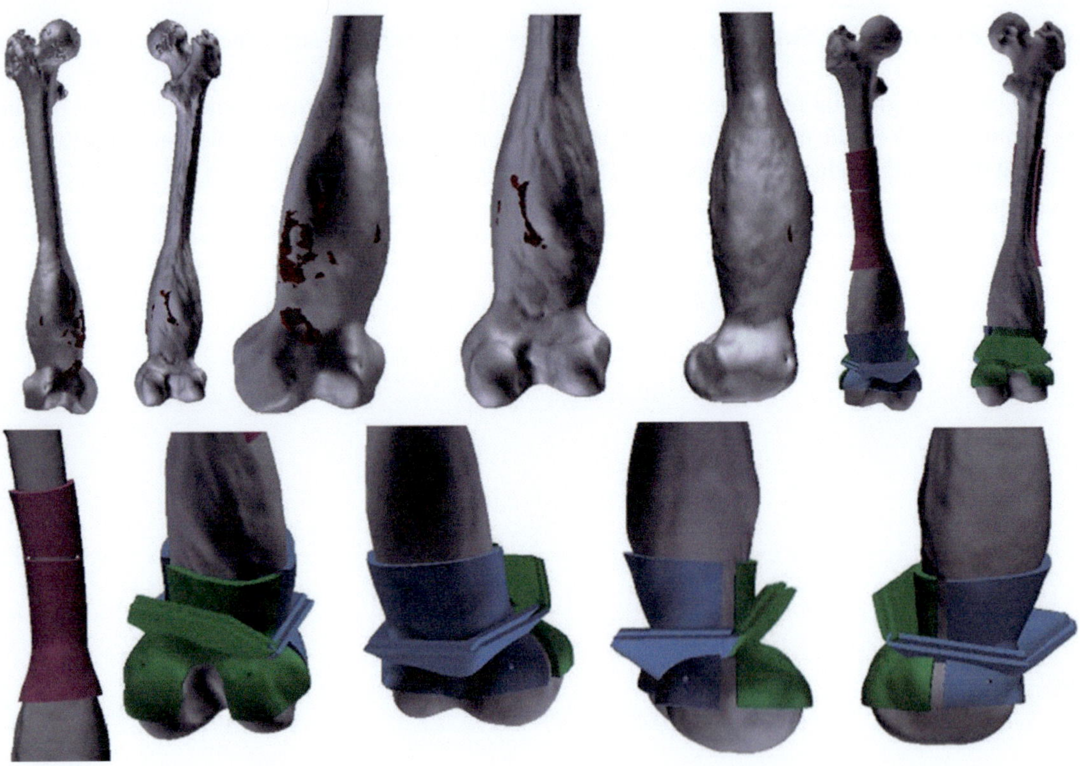

Fig. 22.4 Cutting guide design

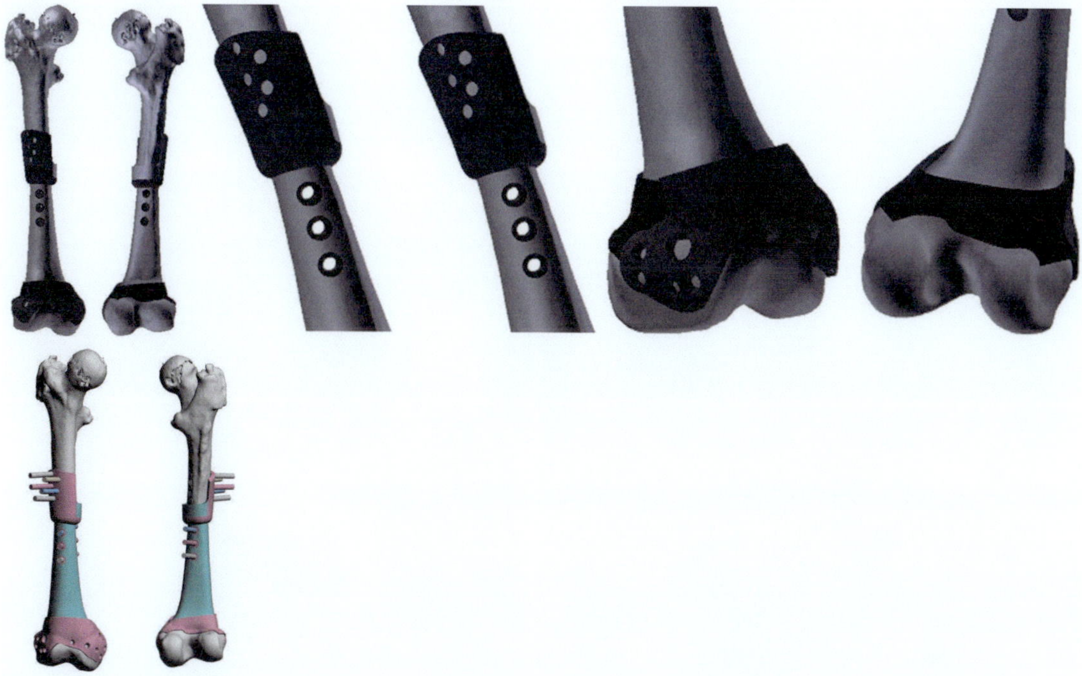

Fig. 22.5 Implant design

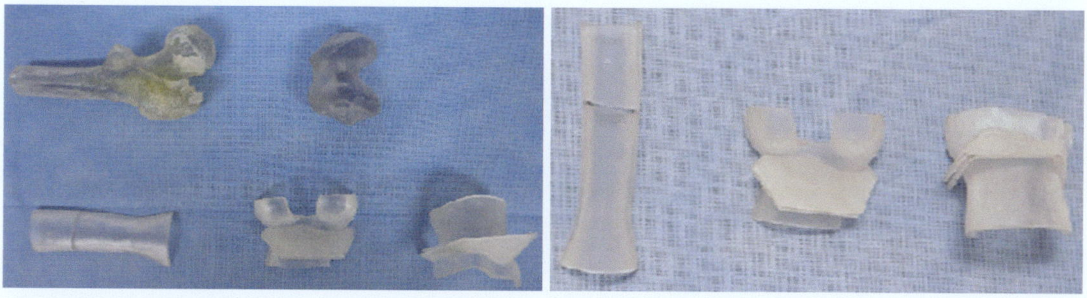

Fig. 22.6 Printed cutting guide

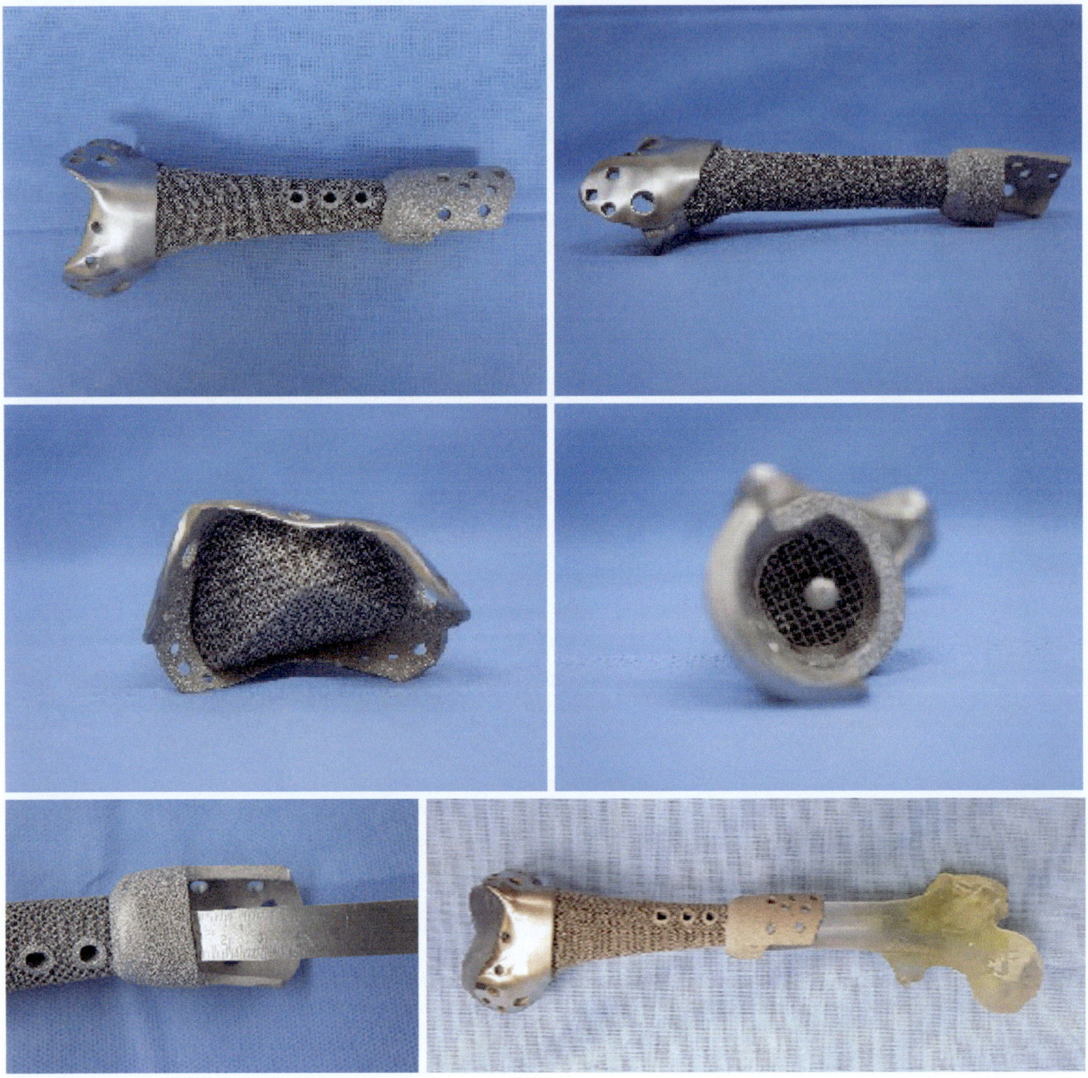

Fig. 22.7 Printed implant

22.5 Operation

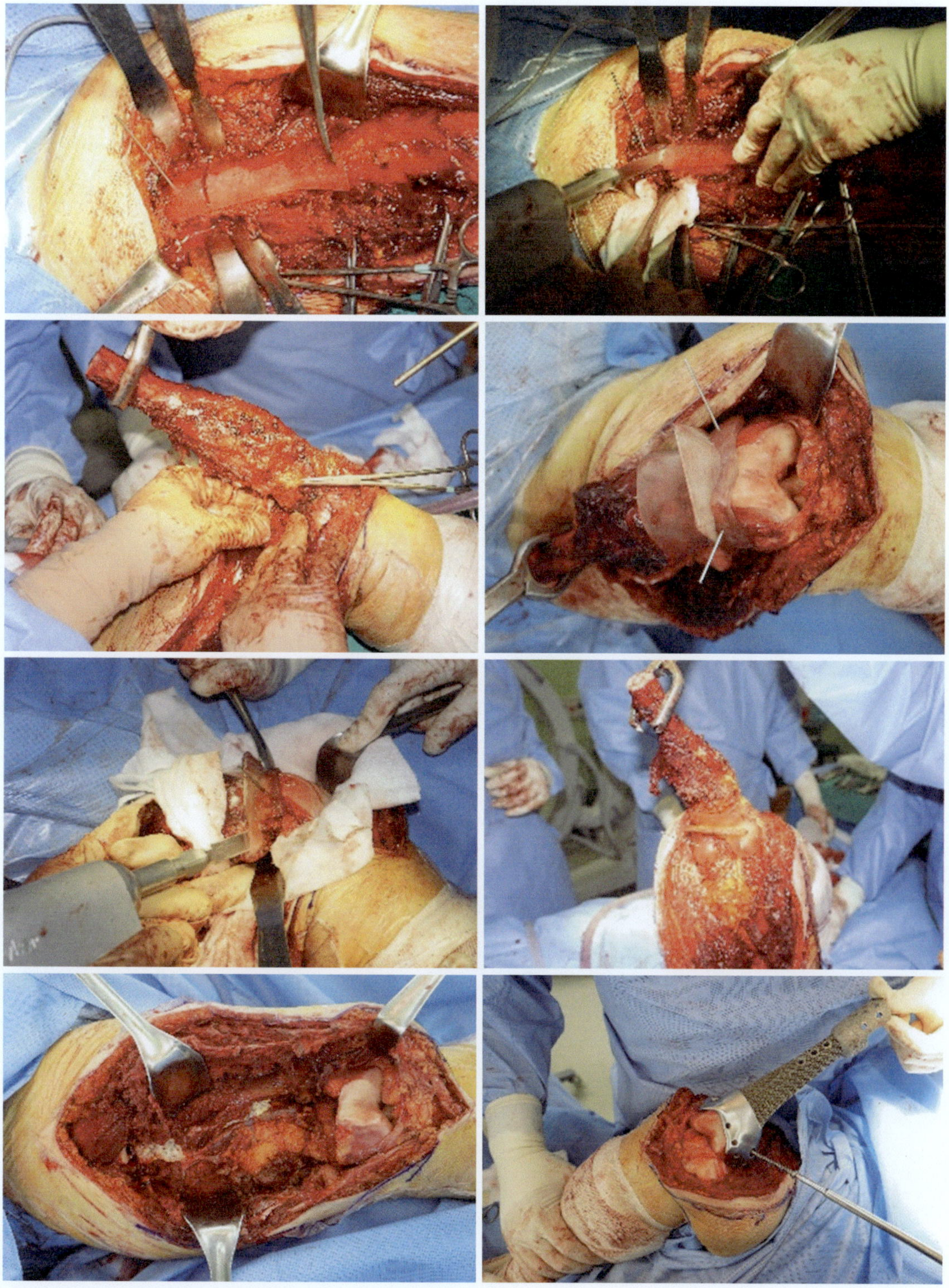

Fig. 22.8 Intraoperative photograph

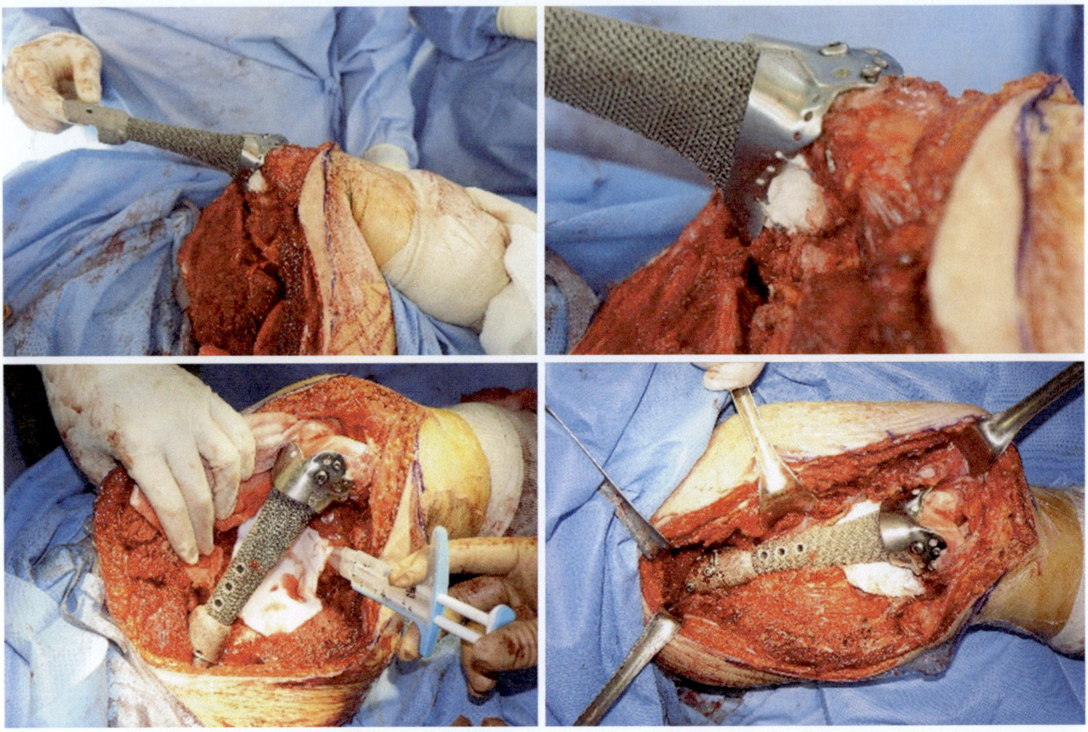

Fig. 22.8 (continued)

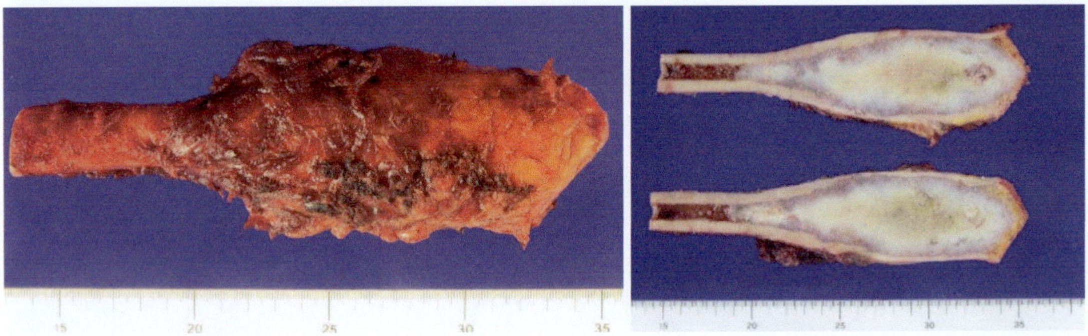

Fig. 22.9 Resected tumor

22.6 Postoperative Images

- 3D-printed femur implant breakage at the junction of body to plate transition zone
- Emergency operation
  - Removal of 3D-printed implant (plate part)
  - Fixation with two plates and five cable wires

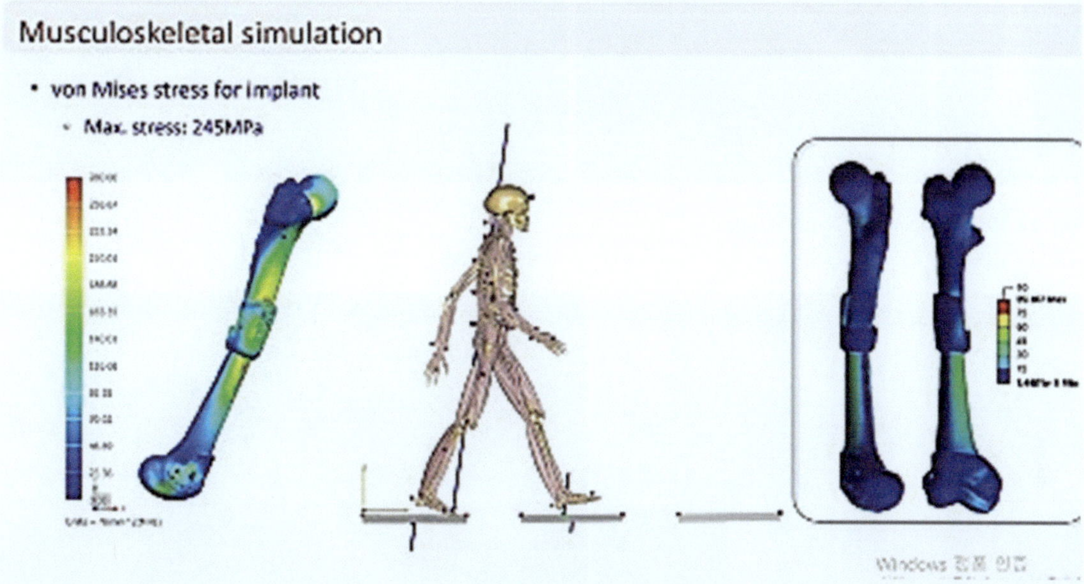

The transition site is the biggest stressful area in the simulation research

Titanium melting is not uniform at the transition site between the solid body and plate

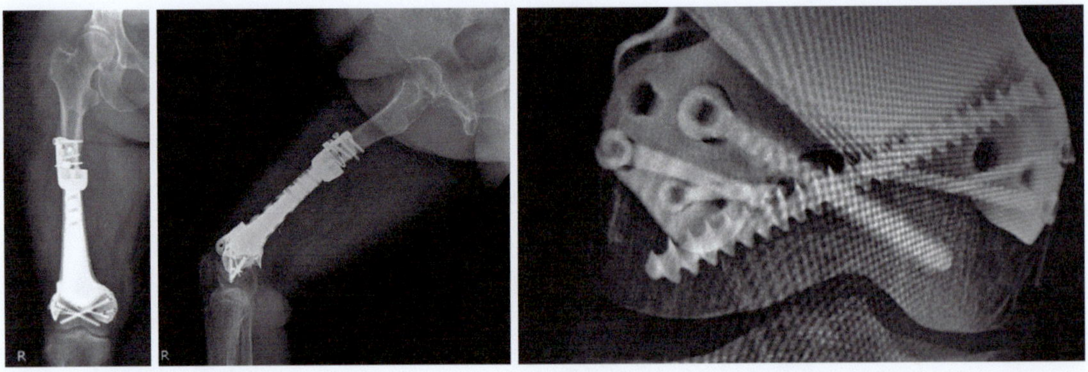

Fig. 22.10 Postoperative X-ray images

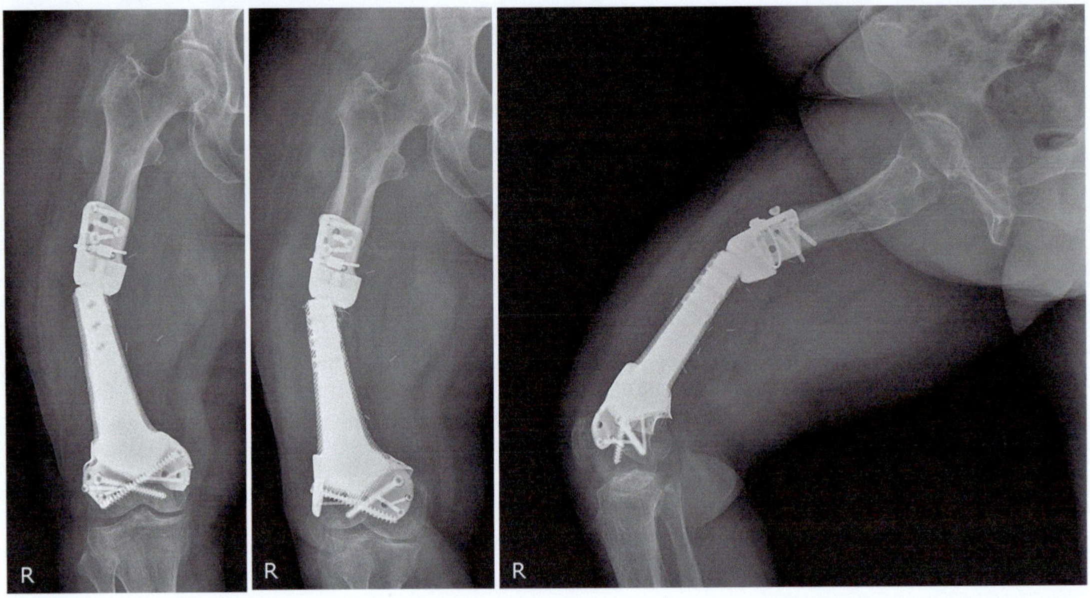

Fig. 22.11 Metal breakage occurs 7 months after surgery due to slip down

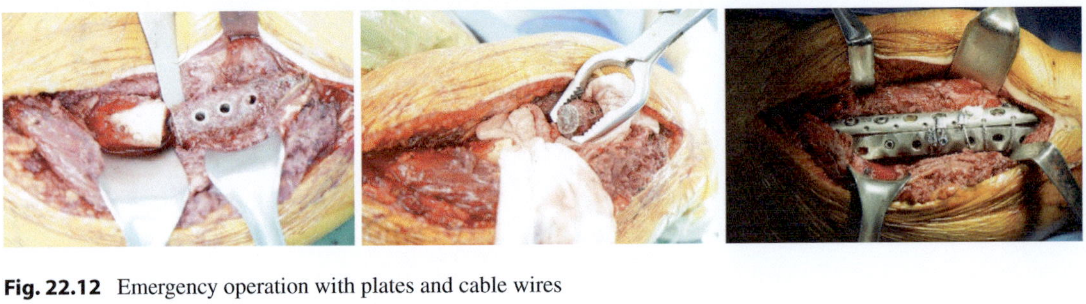

Fig. 22.12 Emergency operation with plates and cable wires

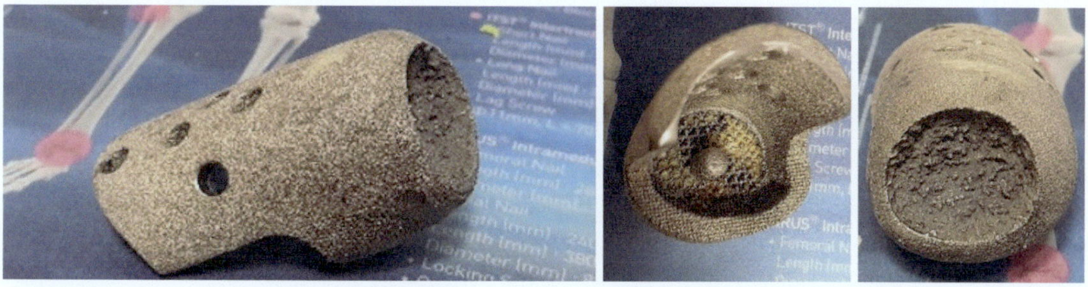

Fig. 22.13 Removed broken piece of 3D implant

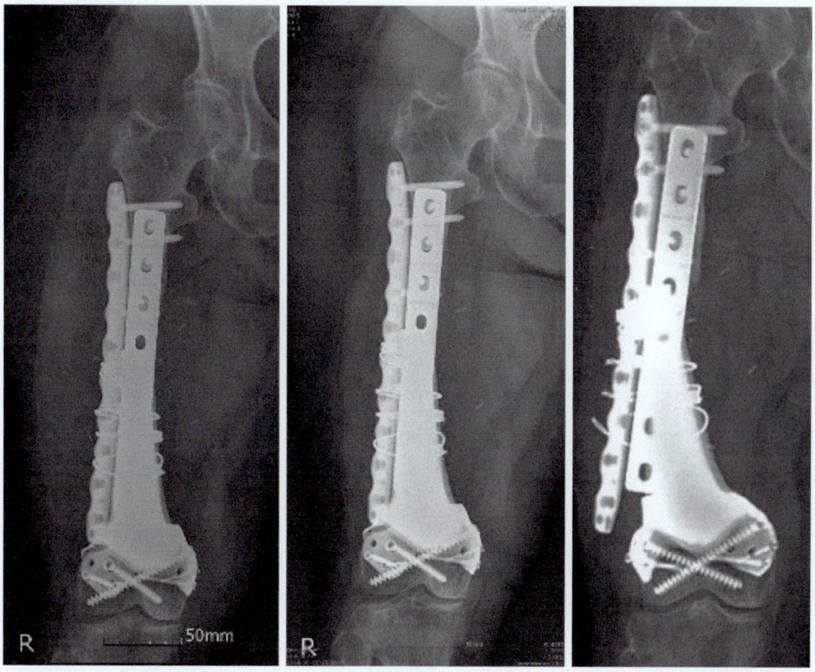

Fig. 22.14 Follow-up X-ray images of second operation: Cable wires breakage and progressive varus angular deformity

22.7 Planning of Third Operation

- Knee joint preservation
- 3D-printed connector between the bone and previous 3D-printed implant
- Valgus angulation implant to prevent knee medial arthritis

22.8 Design and Fabrication for Revision Surgery

3D-printed connector

- Hollow cylinder to insert broken 3D implant
- Valgus angulation at the junction of bone and implant
- The valgus angulation area is reinforced thicker
- Bone end wrapped 1 cm height and wider plate
- 6.5 cancellous screw holes toward femur neck: prepared screw direction
- Mesh style periosteal contact surface of plate

- Implant measurement
- Implant weight (g): 164
- Size (mm): 171

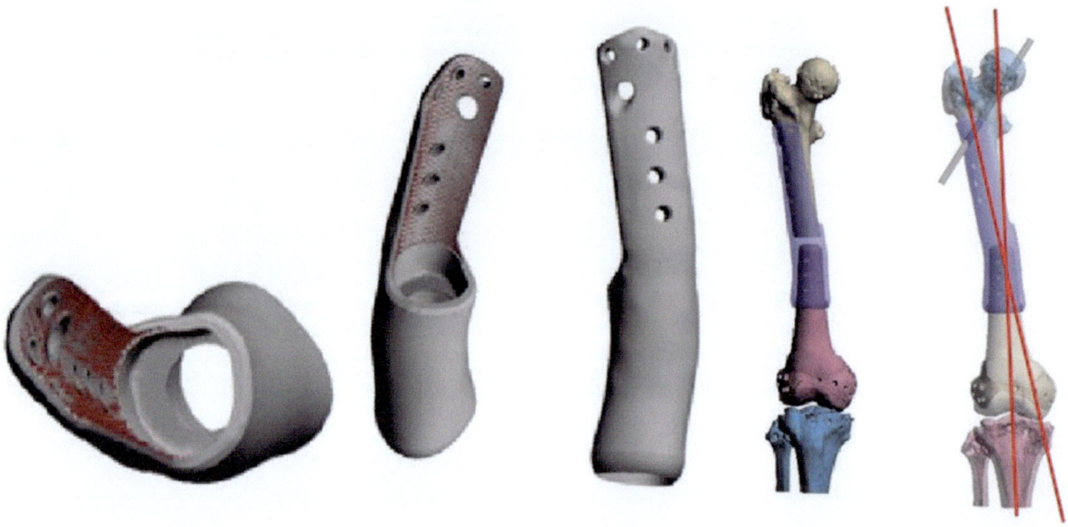

Fig. 22.15 Implant design

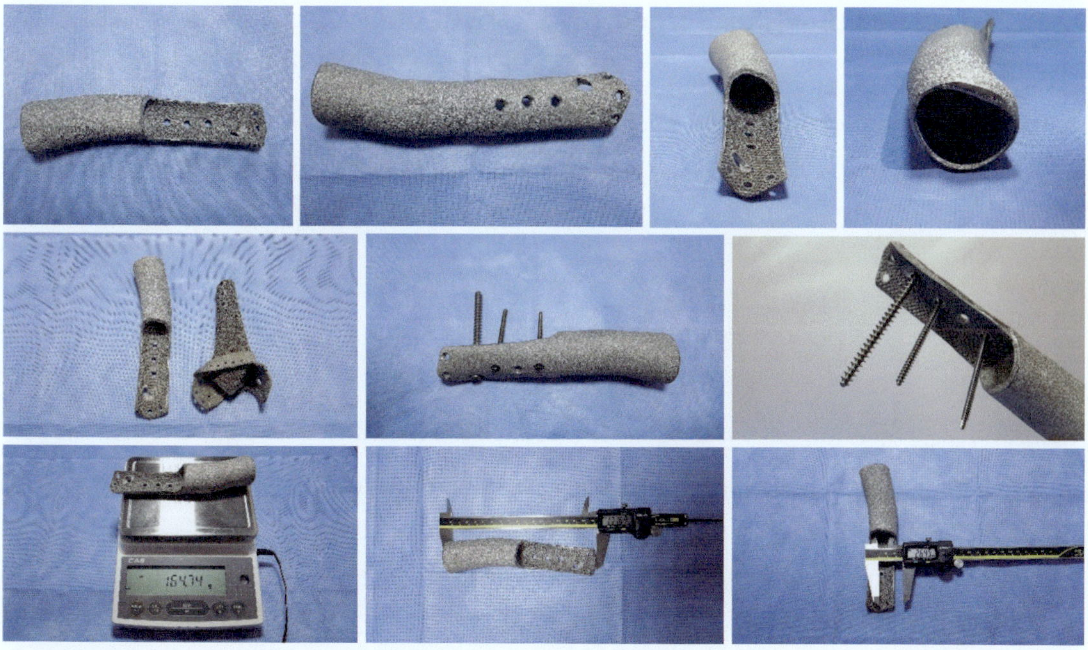

Fig. 22.16 Printed implant

22.9 Operation (Revision Surgery)

Low viscosity PMMA cement is used to connect the broken implant into the 3D printed connector.

Femur shortening 1.5 cm: leg length almost equalized (10 cm longer initially → 0.5 cm longer now)

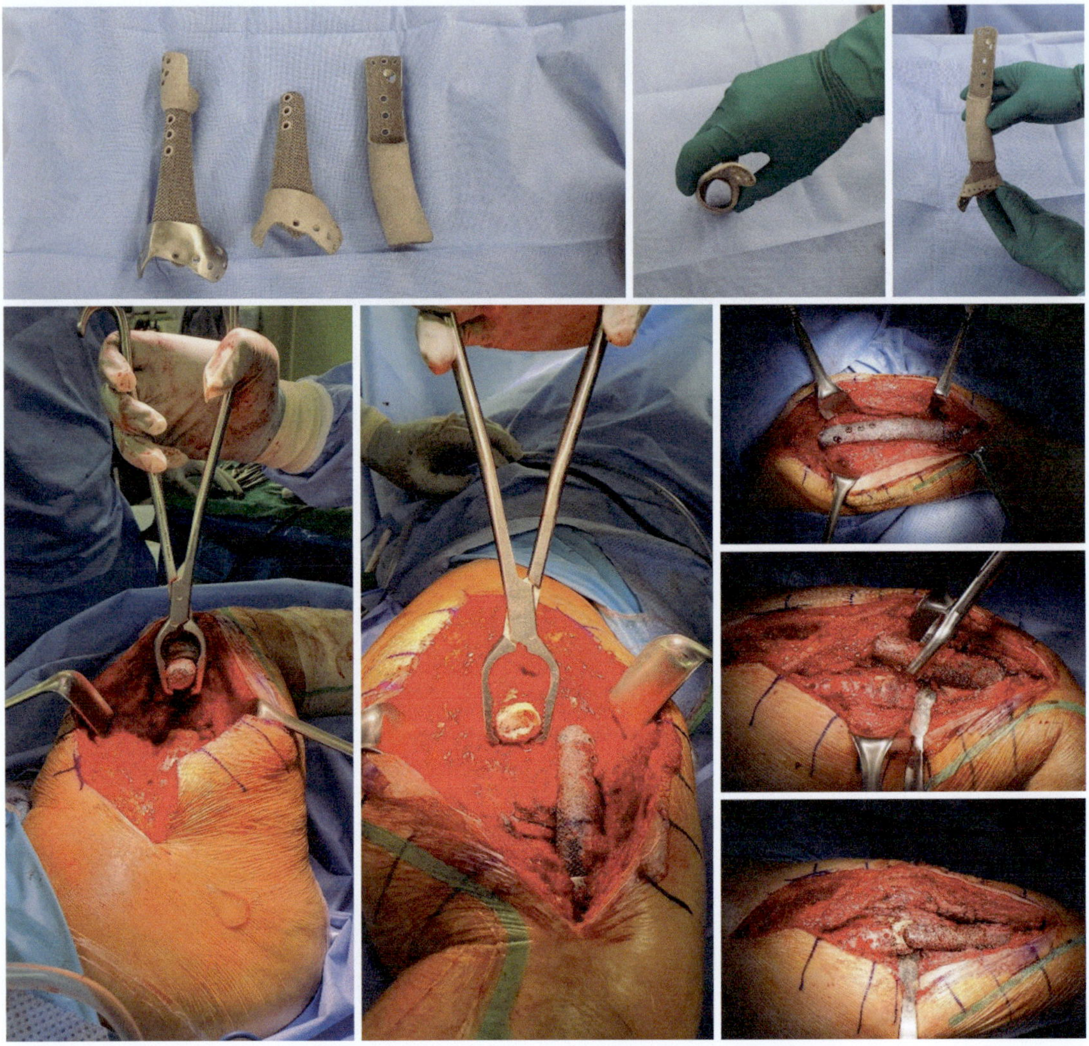

Fig. 22.17 Intraoperative photographs

22.10 Postoperative Images

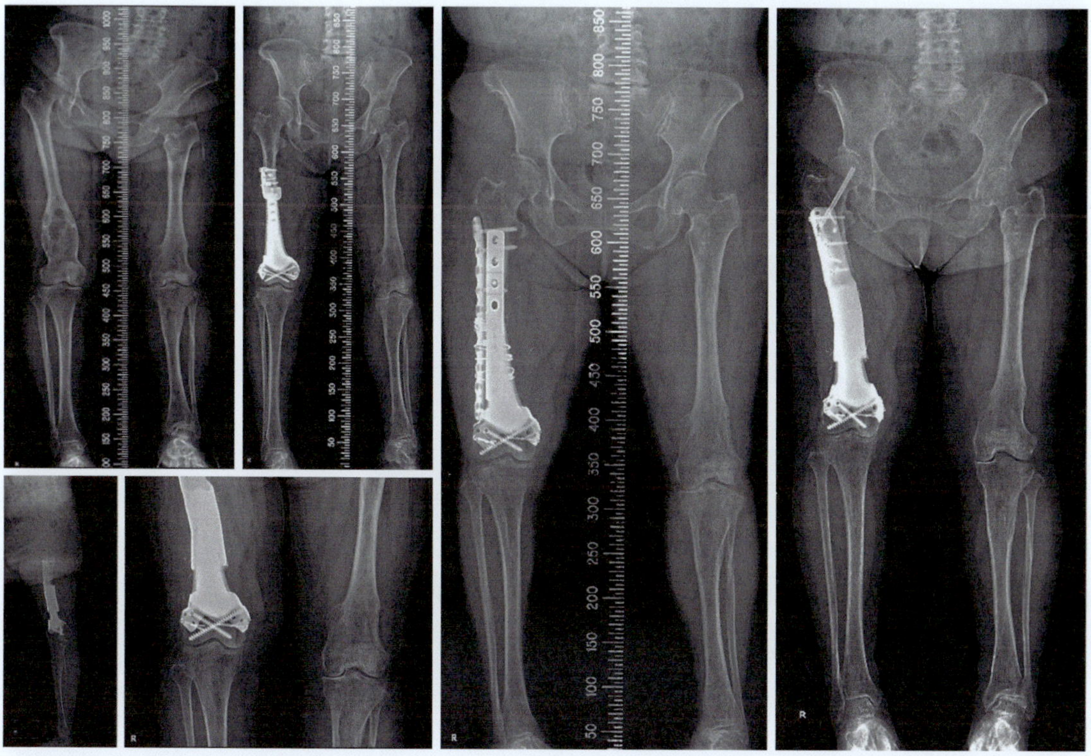

Fig. 22.18 Postoperative X-ray images

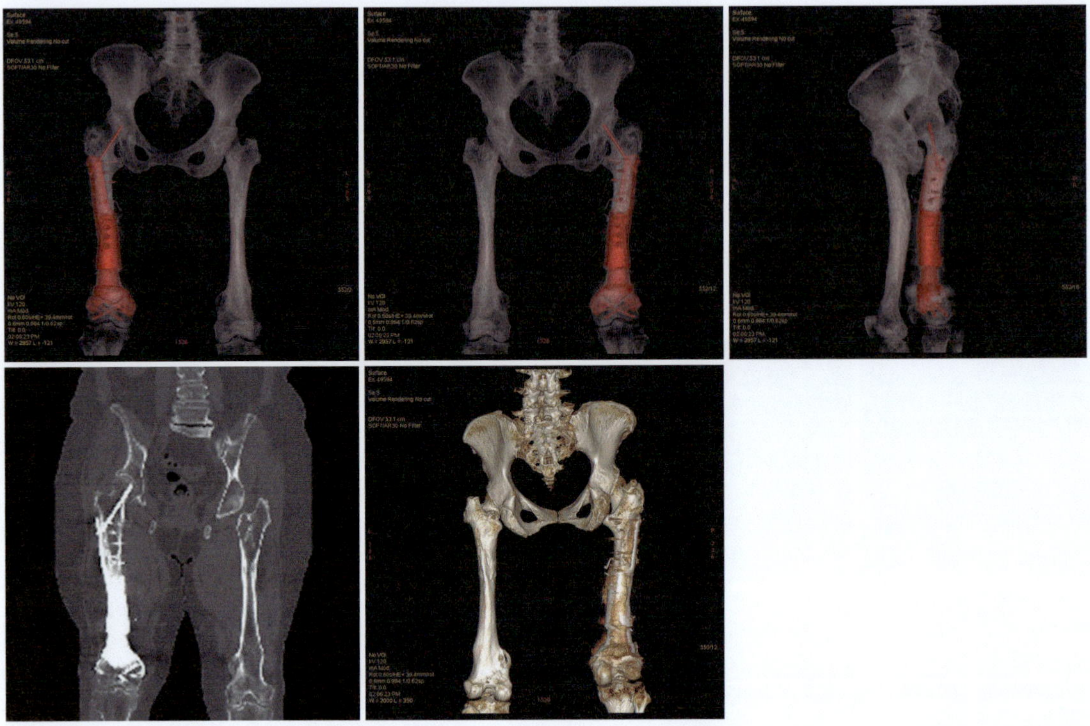

Fig. 22.19 Postoperative CT images

Part III

Tibia

23 Patient Case 23: Targeting Guide for Small Lesion

23.1 Patient Case 23

Age/sex	70/male
Location/site	Tibia/right
Diagnosis	Fibrosarcoma of bone/secondary sarcoma from fibrous dysplasia
Preoperative symptom	Normal gait
Preoperative pain score	Resting 0/activity 3
BMI (height/weight)	25.29 (156.7/62.1)
Past history	No X-ray checked tibia in his life
Present illness	Malignant bone tumor confirmed by incisional biopsy

H.-G. Kang, *Clinical Atlas of 3D Printing Bone Reconstruction*,
https://doi.org/10.1007/978-981-16-2043-0_23

23.2 Preoperative Images

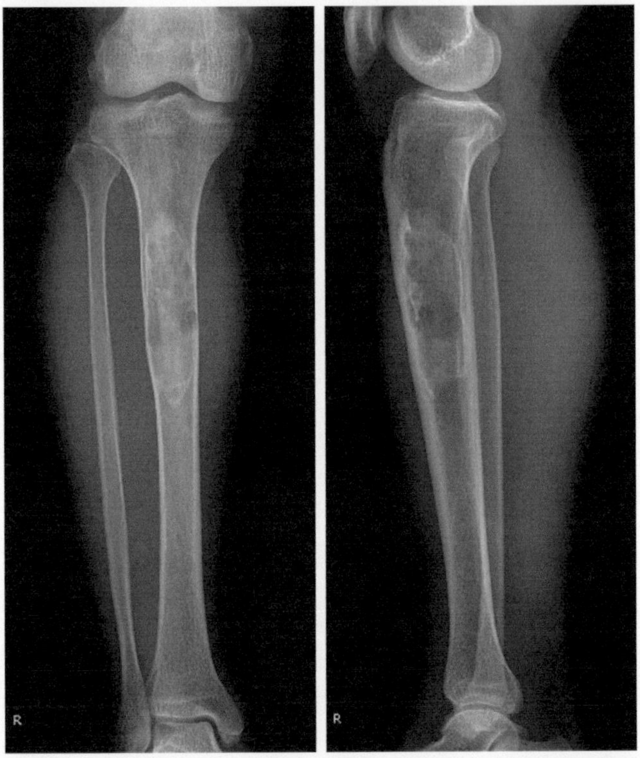

Fig. 23.1 Preoperative X-ray images

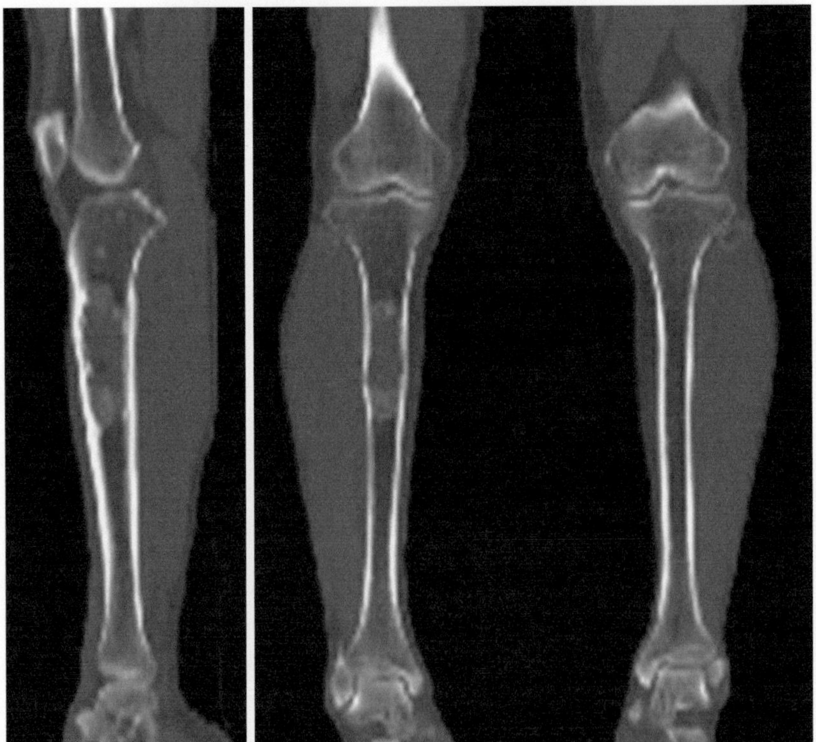

Fig. 23.2 Preoperative CT images

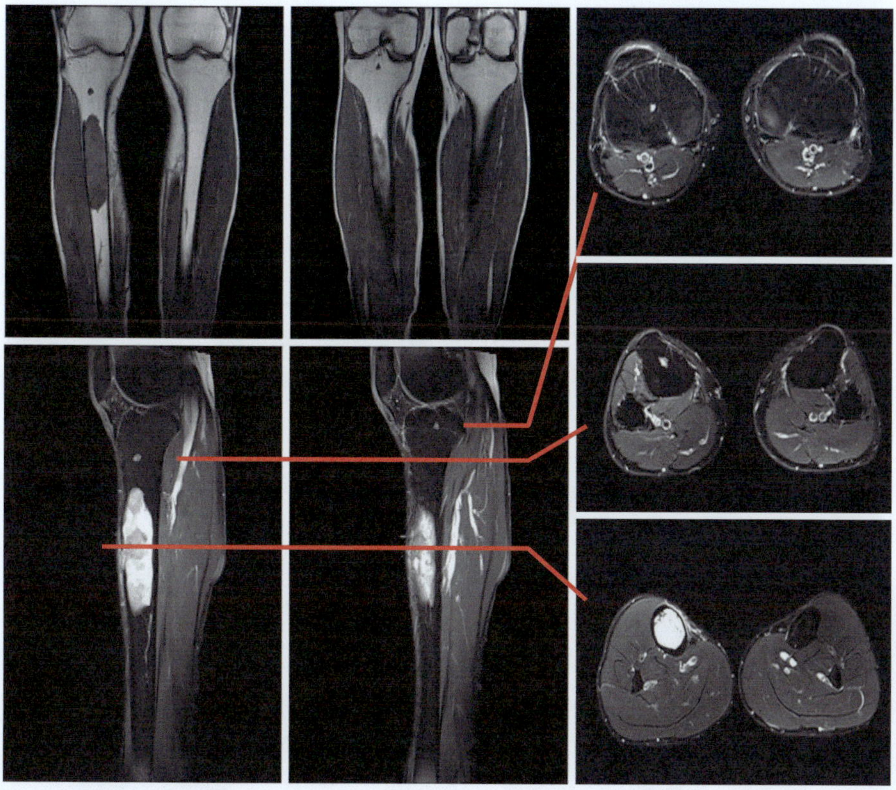

Fig. 23.3 Preoperative MRI images

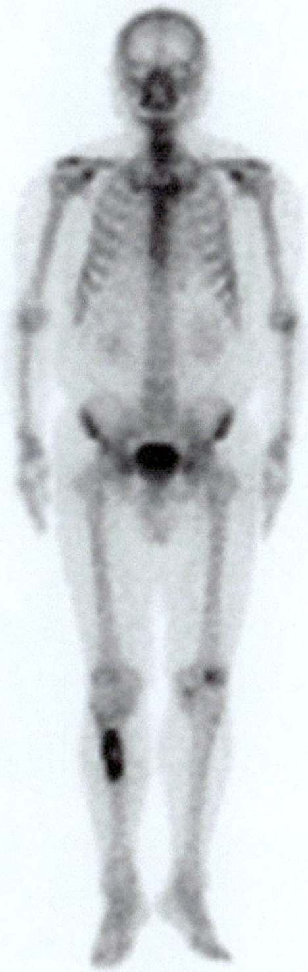

Fig. 23.4 Preoperative bone scan image

23.3 Planning of Surgery

Segmental resection of the main tumor
  Save patellar tendon attachment area
  Save the knee joint

  Extended curettage of subchondral skip lesion
  3D-printed targeting guide of tumor

23.4 Design and Fabrication

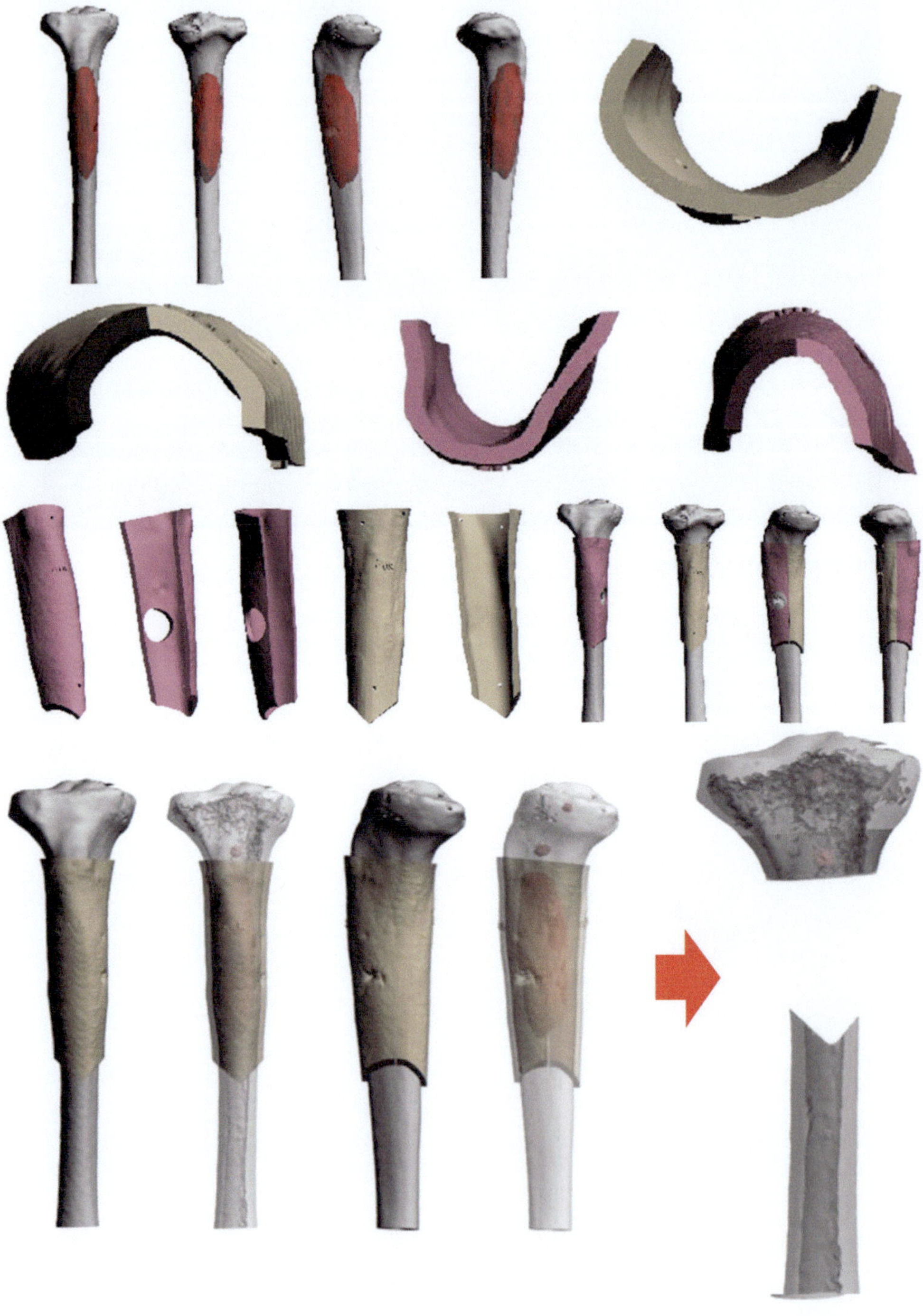

Fig. 23.5 Cutting guide design: segmental tumor resection guide

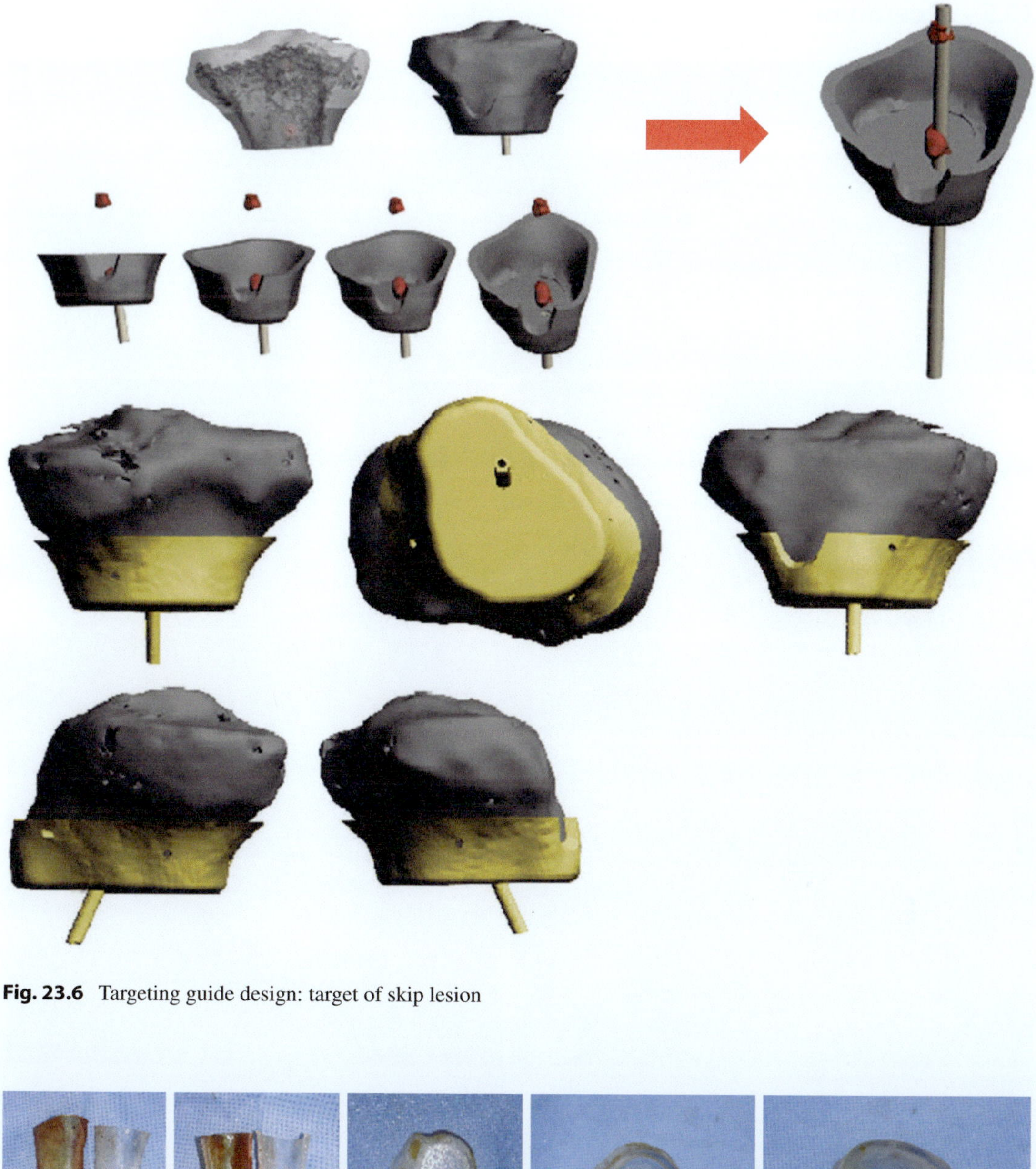

Fig. 23.6 Targeting guide design: target of skip lesion

Fig. 23.7 Printed cutting guide

23.5 Operation

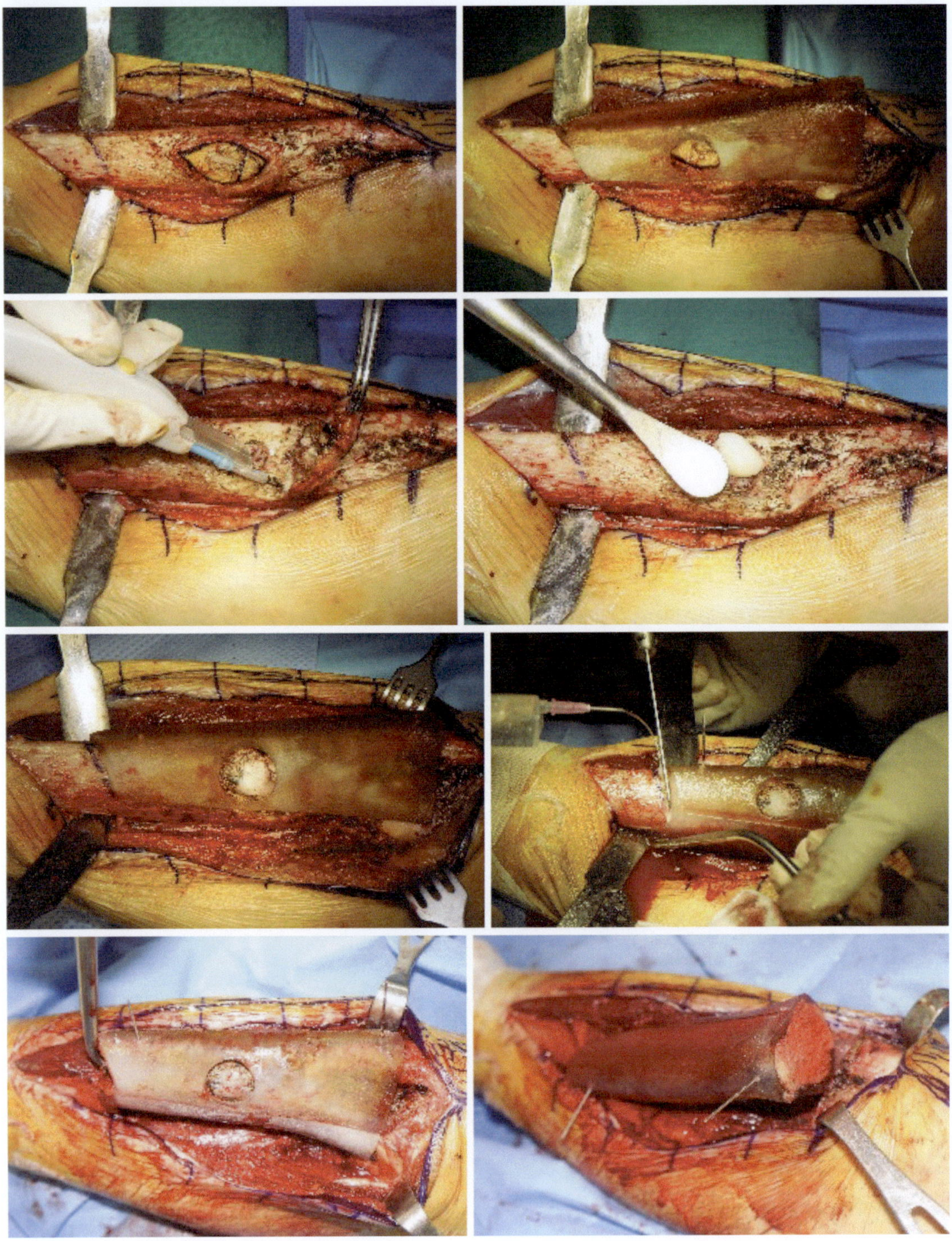

Fig. 23.8 Intraoperative photographs: segmental tibia resection guide

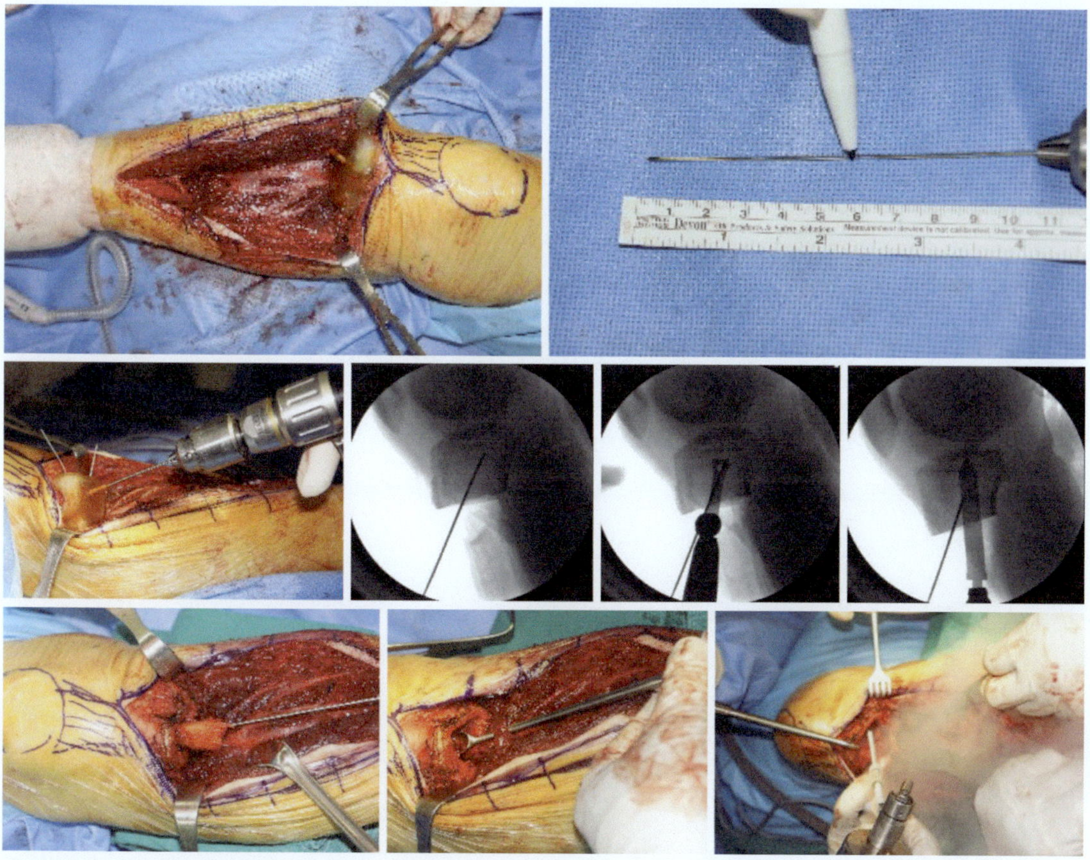

Fig. 23.9 Intraoperative photographs: target pinning guide

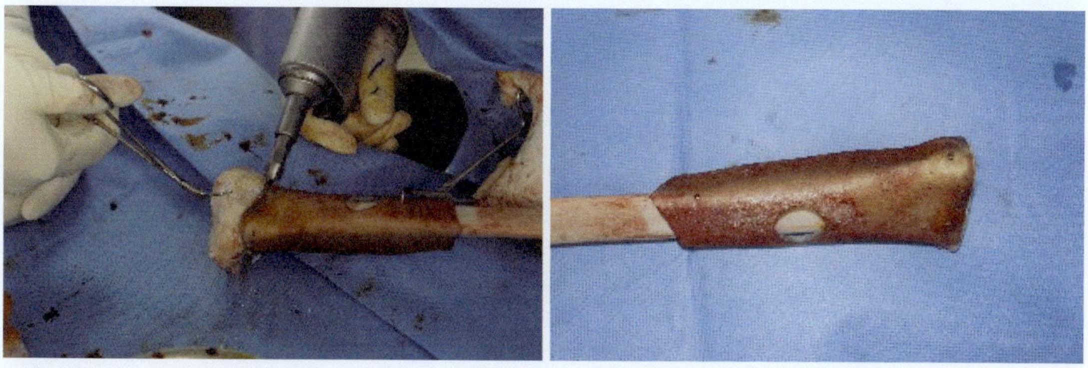

Fig. 23.10 Intraoperative photograph: reconstruction using an allograft bone

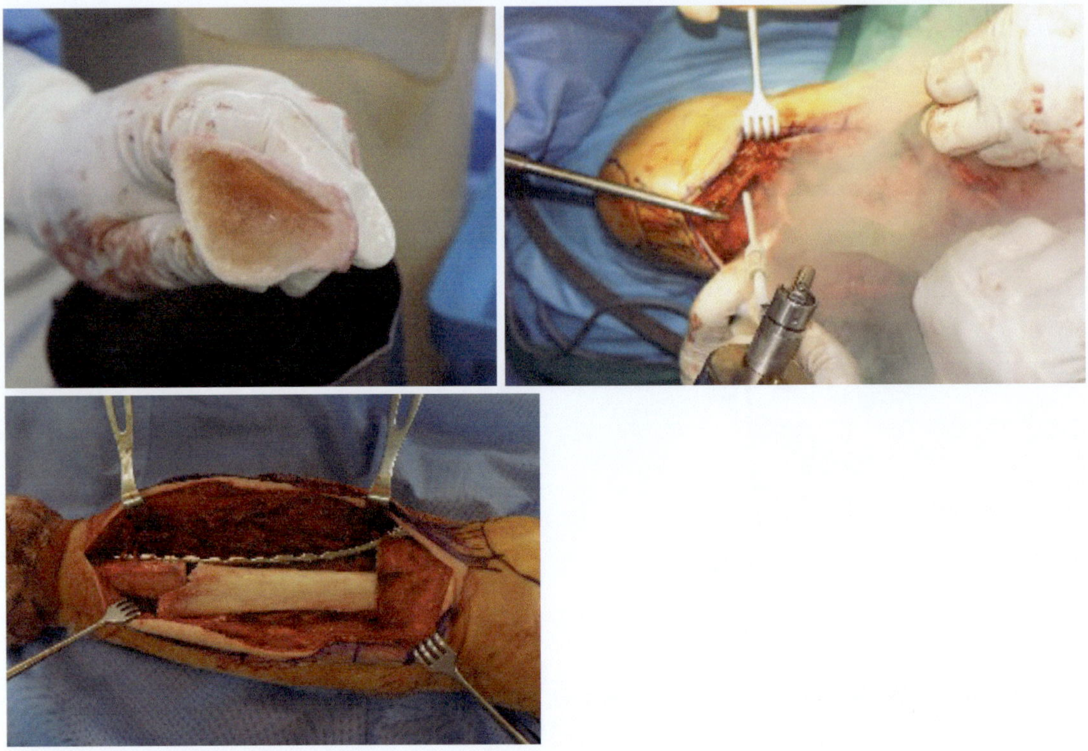

Fig. 23.10 (continued)

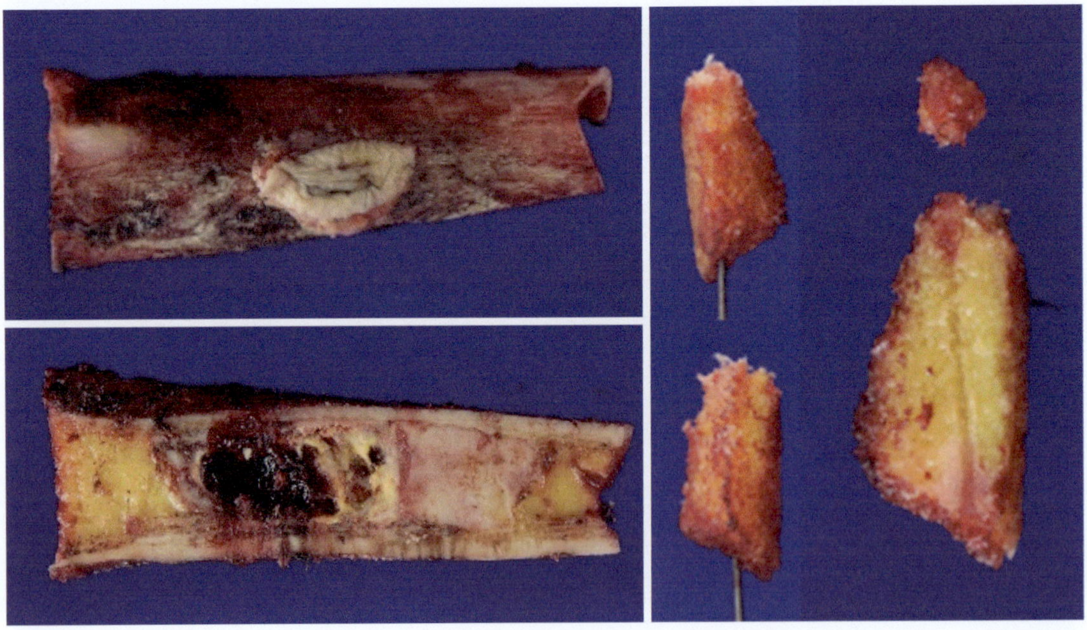

Fig. 23.11 Resected tumor pathology segmental resected tumor: Fibrosarcoma targeting two small lesion: Fibrous dysplasia

23.6 Postoperative Images

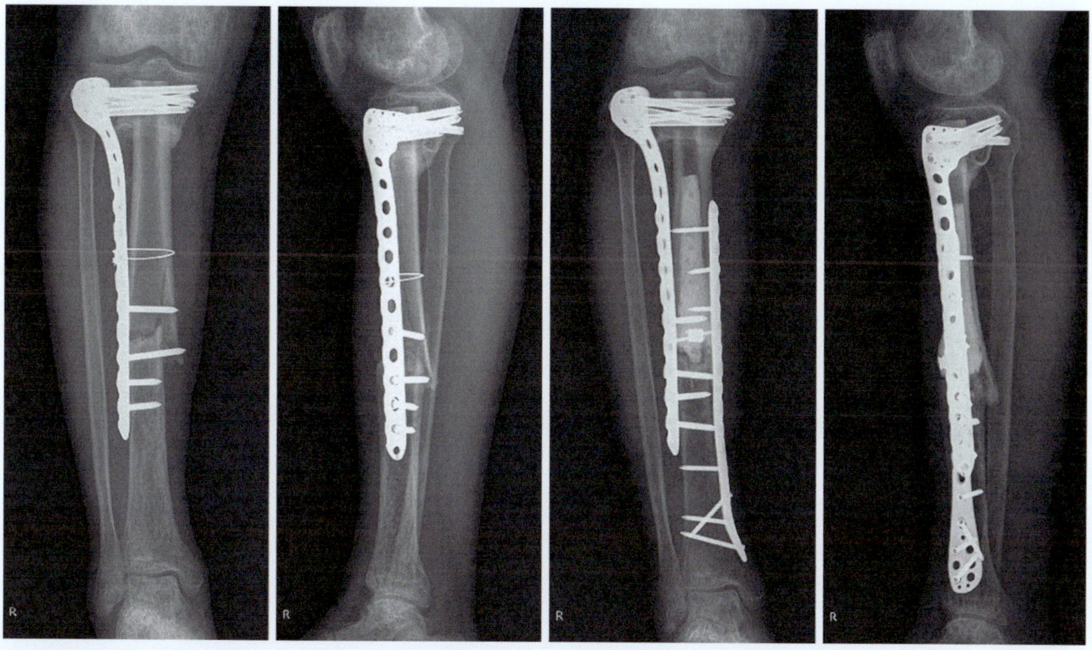

Fig. 23.12 Postoperative X-ray images: secondary operation for plate adding and PMMA cemmenting

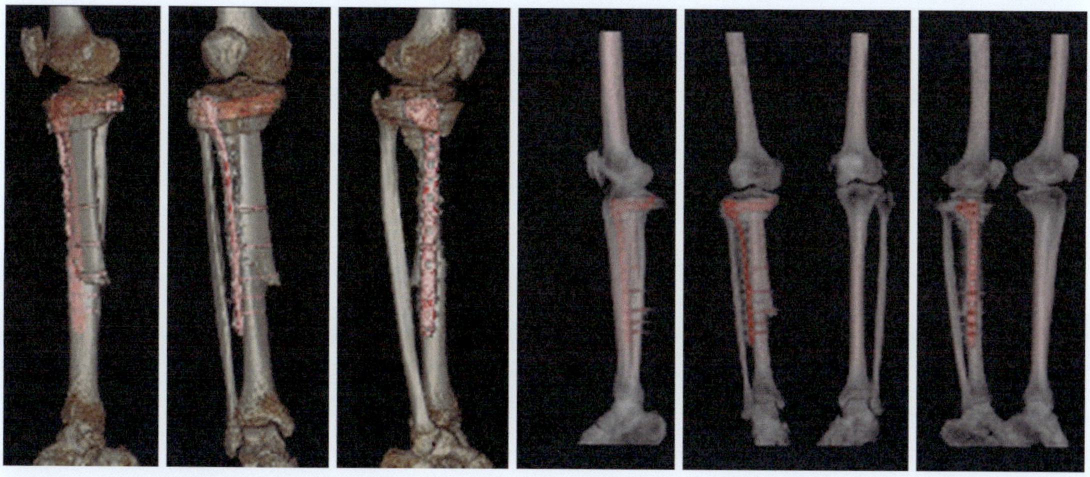

Fig. 23.13 Postoperative CT images

Patient Case 24: Segmental Tibia Diaphysis

24

24.1 Patient Case 24

Age/sex	13/male
Location/site	Tibia/left
Diagnosis	Adamantinoma Pathologic fracture
Preoperative symptom	Wheelchair ambulation
Preoperative pain score	Resting 2/Activity 8
BMI (height/weight)	15.43 (180/50)
Past history	Tibia diaphysis pathologic fractured 2 weeks ago
Present illness	Adamantinoma confirmed by incisional biopsy Patient's father wants 3D-printed customized bone reconstruction

H.-G. Kang, *Clinical Atlas of 3D Printing Bone Reconstruction*,
https://doi.org/10.1007/978-981-16-2043-0_24

24.2 Preoperative Images

- Cortical thinning at pathologic fracture area
- Distal tibia intramedullary sclerotic lesion: need to distinguish whether it is the same lesion
- Growth plate open

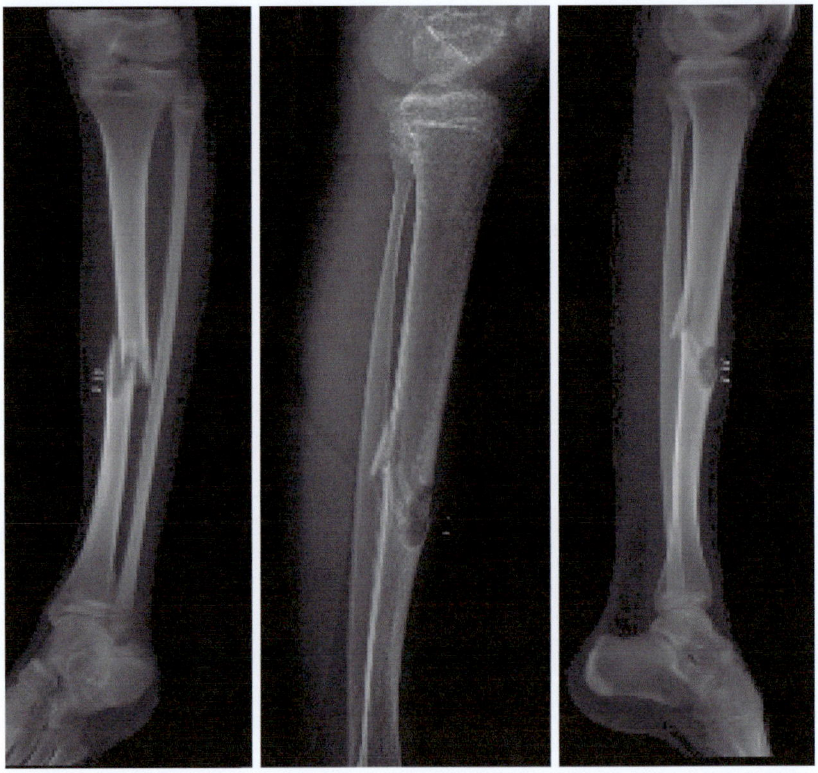

Fig. 24.1 Preoperative X-ray images

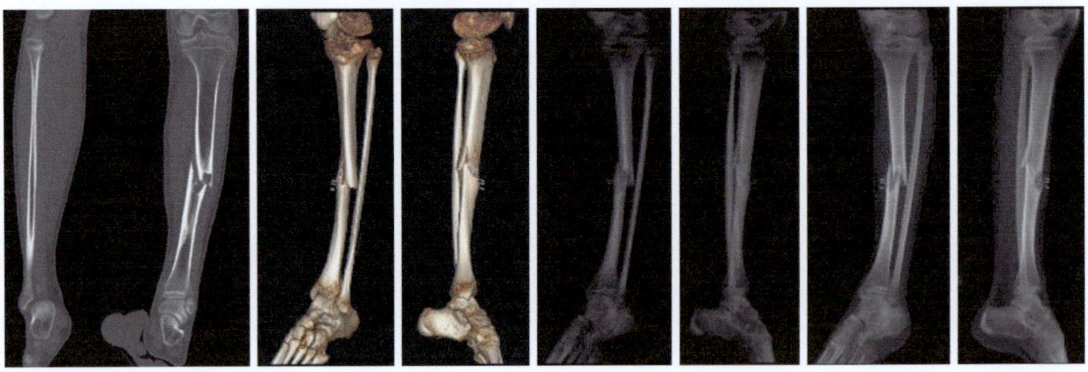

Fig. 24.2 Preoperative CT images

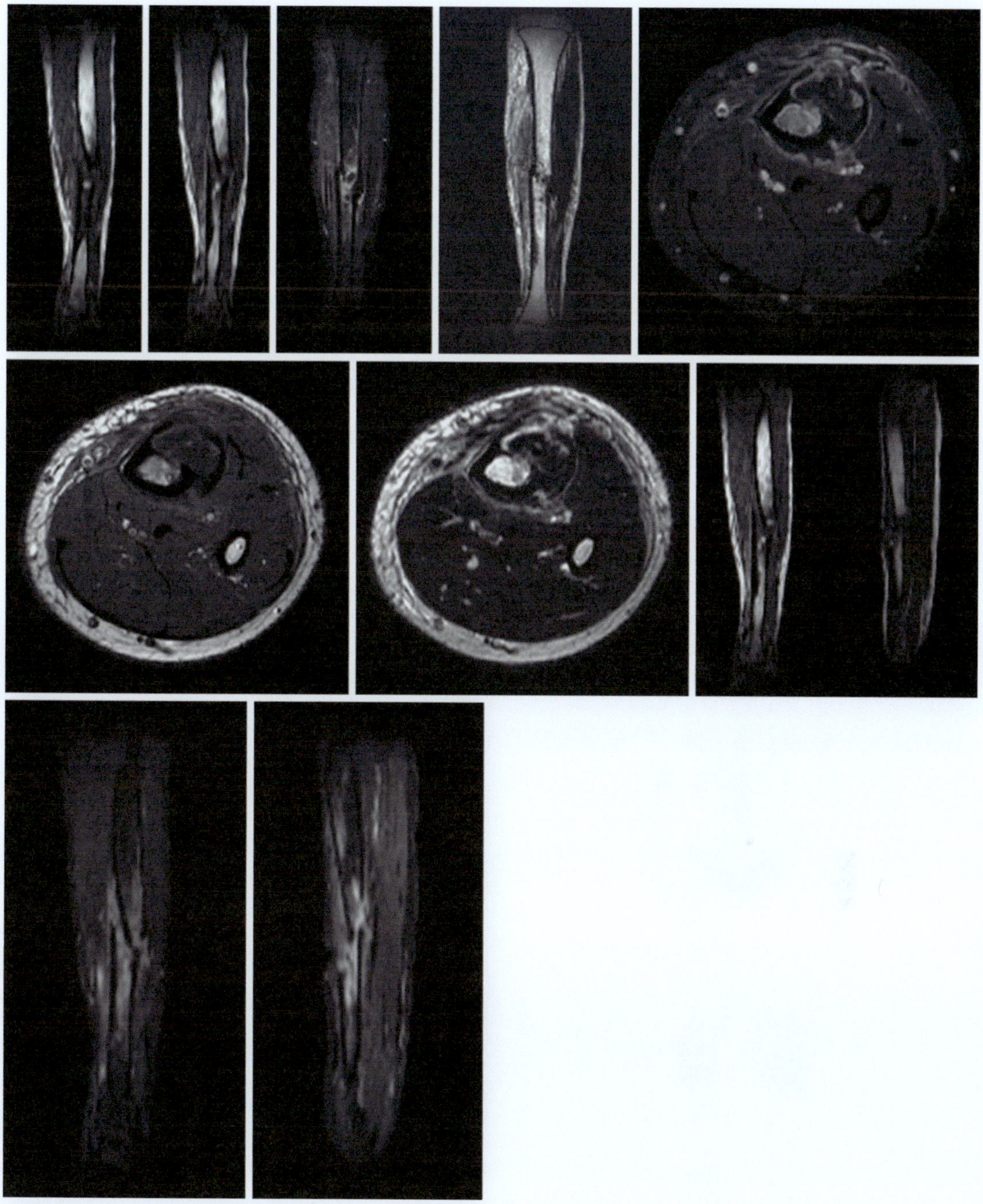

Fig. 24.3 Preoperative MRI images

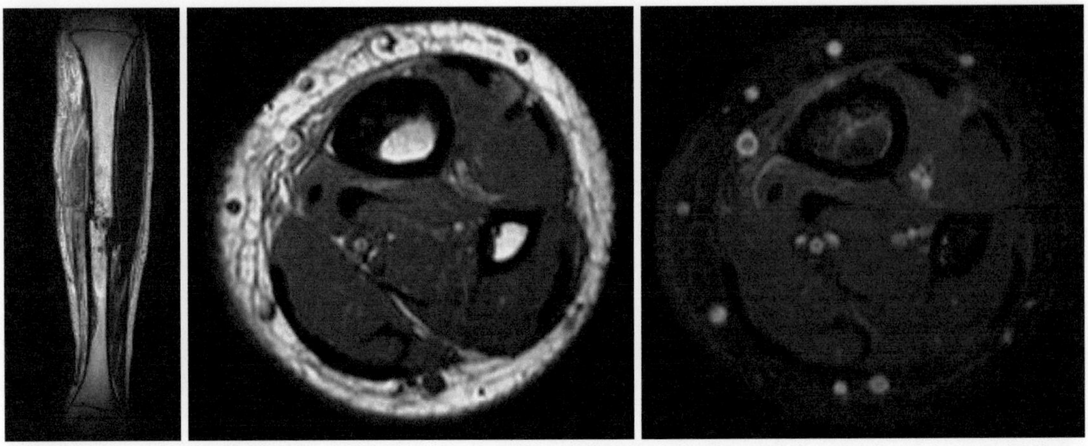

Fig. 24.4 Preoperative MRI images: distal intramedullary lesion also observed

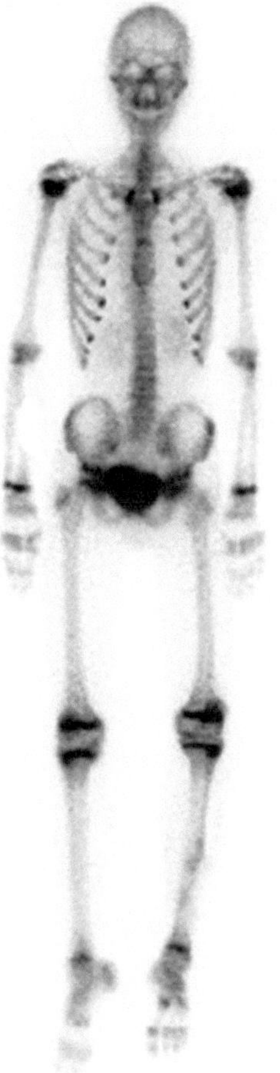

Fig. 24.5 Preoperative bone scan images

24.3 Planning of Surgery

- 10 cm segmental resection of pathologic fracture area
- Distal tibia intramedullary lesion
  - Intramedullary curettage for permanent biopsy
  - Intraoperative adjuvant with argon laser and liquid nitrogen gun
- 3D-printed tibia prosthesis
  - 10 cm implant body
  - 5-cm-long metal plate in each upper and lower parts

24.4 Design and Fabrication

Cutting guide

- There is no protruding part as a reference
  - Using C-arm fluoroscopy and measuring the distance from the knee joint line
- Proximal and distal two parts
  - Proximal: tibial tuberosity and tibial angled border fitting
  - Distal: tibial border fitting

Implant

- Mesh style bone contact end: 2 cm in length each proximal and distal end
- Tibial anterior crest-size reduction and slightly concave
- Tibia cross-section is a slightly rounded body rather than triangular
- Tibial posterior surface-thicker reinforcement
- For stable fixation with 5 cm plate each upper and lower
  - Almost half surrounding plate posterior and lateral located
  - Multiple 4.5 mm screw holes.
- Thicker plate and prominent screw area like volcano uplift for screw head seating.
- The inner screw hole wider to make the screw direction flexible.
- Screw insertion avoids the fibula in the antero-lateral area.

- Implant measurement.
- Implant weight (g): 359
- Size (mm): 195

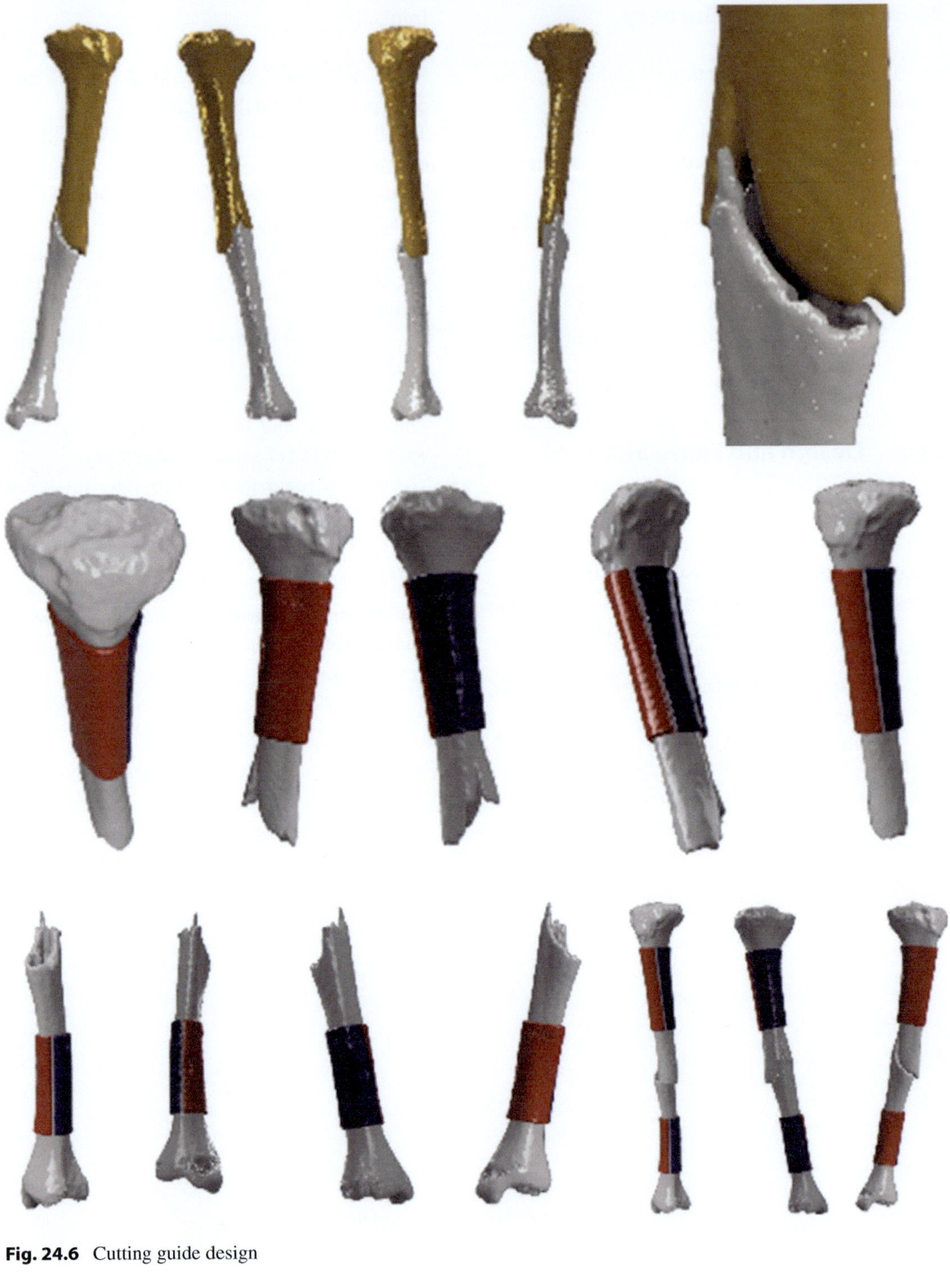

Fig. 24.6 Cutting guide design

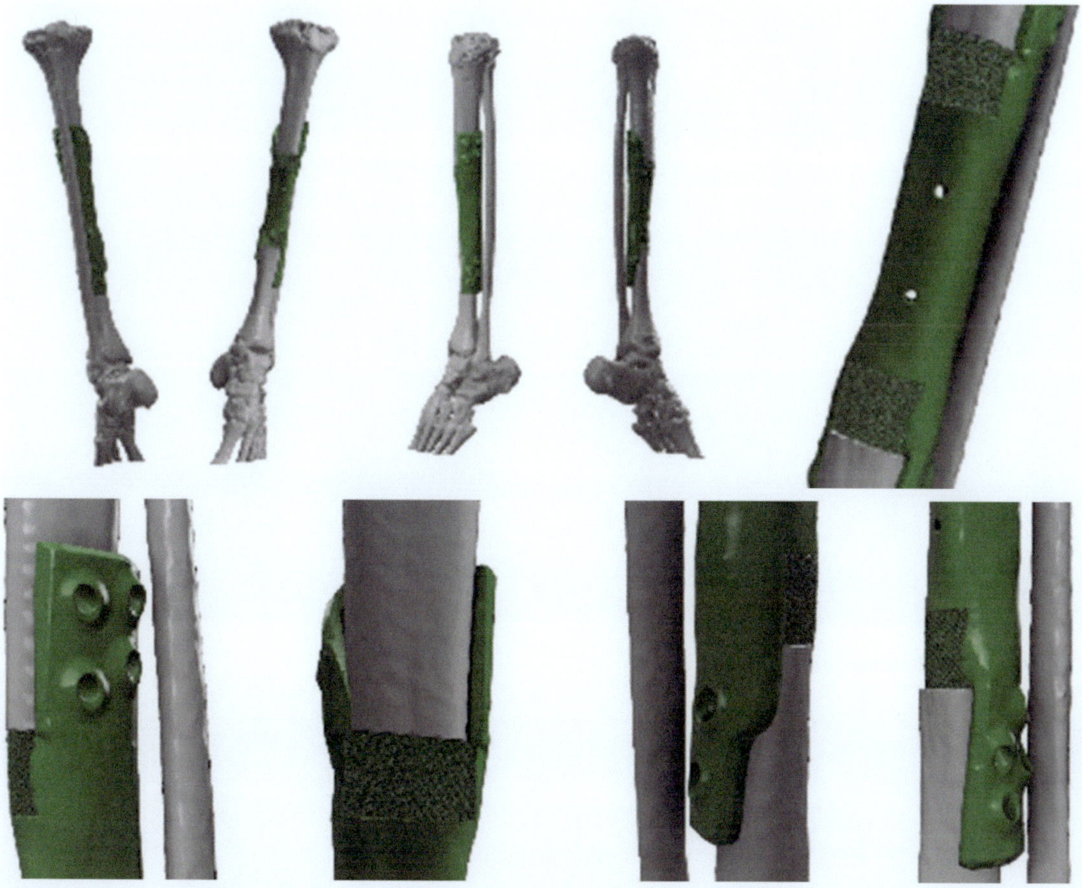

Fig. 24.7 Implant design

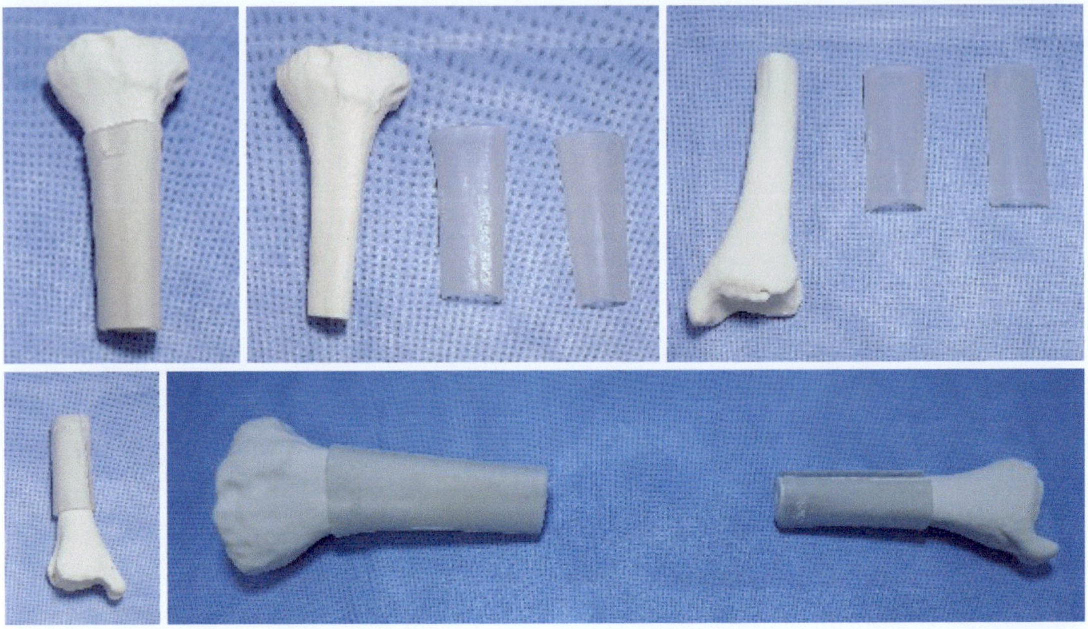

Fig. 24.8 Printed cutting guide

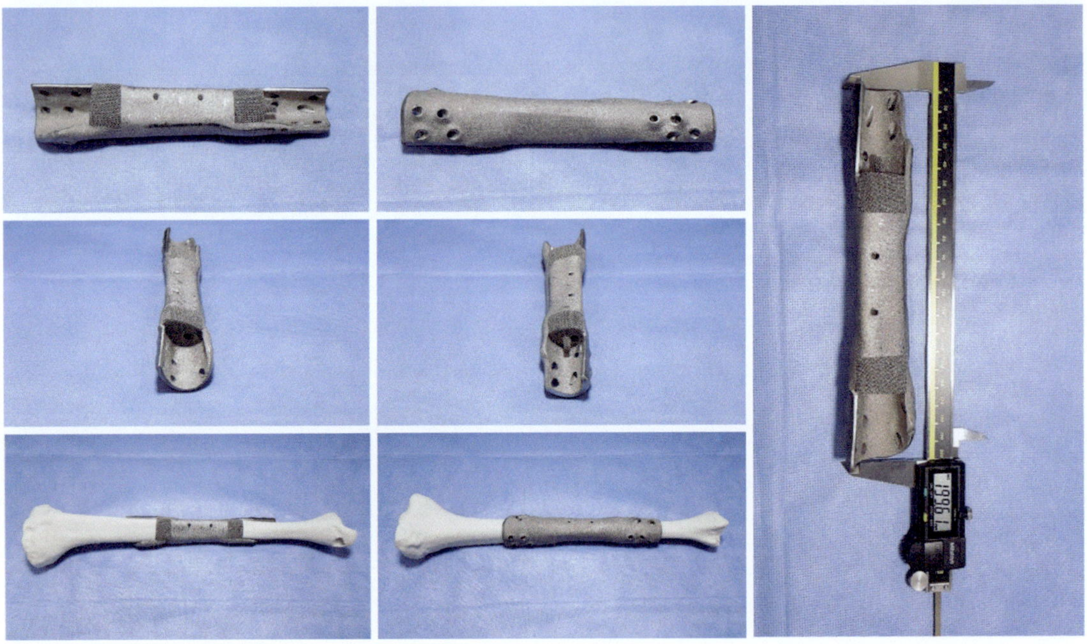

Fig. 24.9 Printed implant

24.5 Operation

Pathology: Segmental resected tumor: Adamantinoma.

Curettage of distal medullary cavity: No tumor

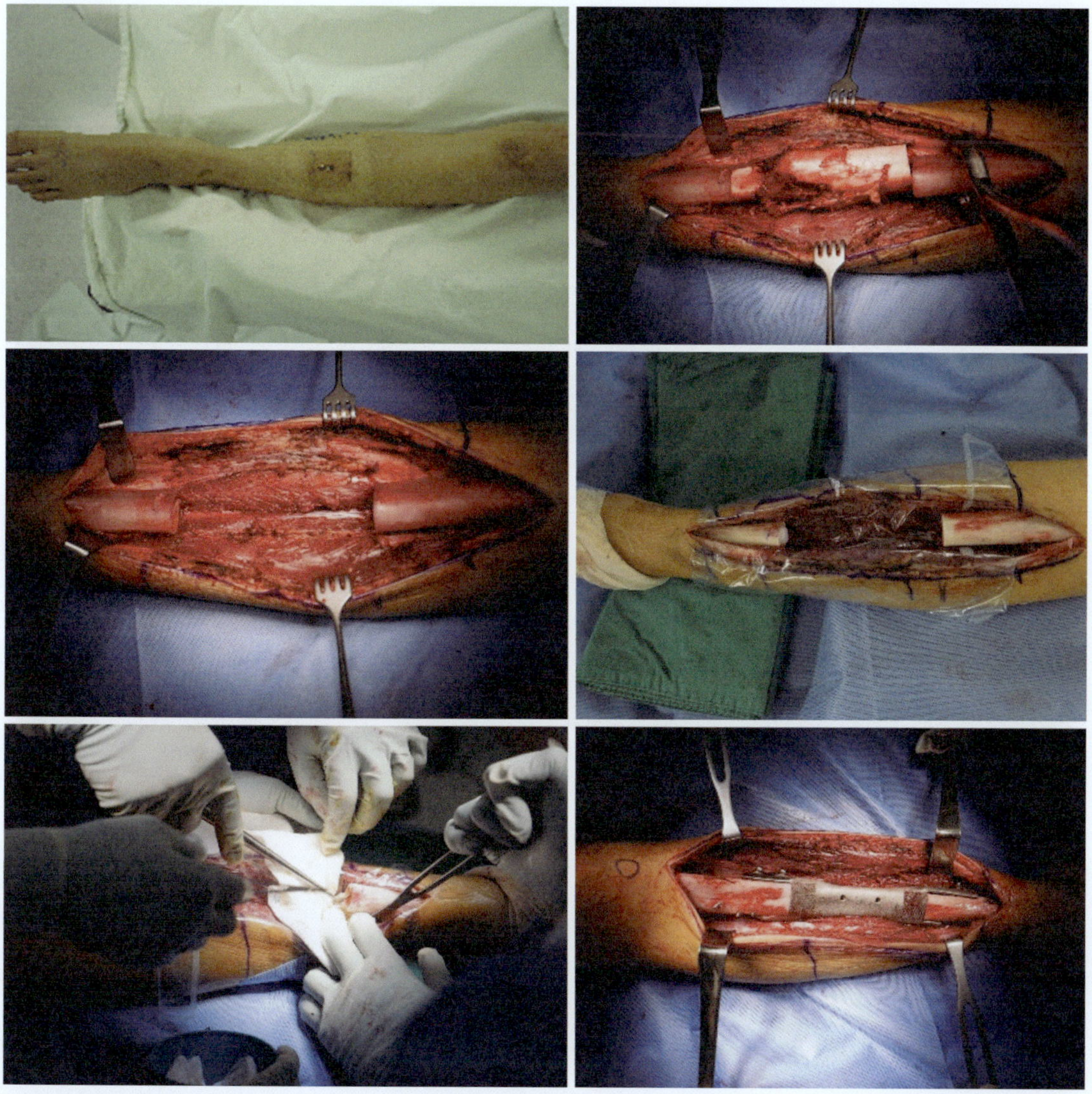

Fig. 24.10 Intraoperative photographs: 3D printing implant reconstruction within 1 week of patient visit

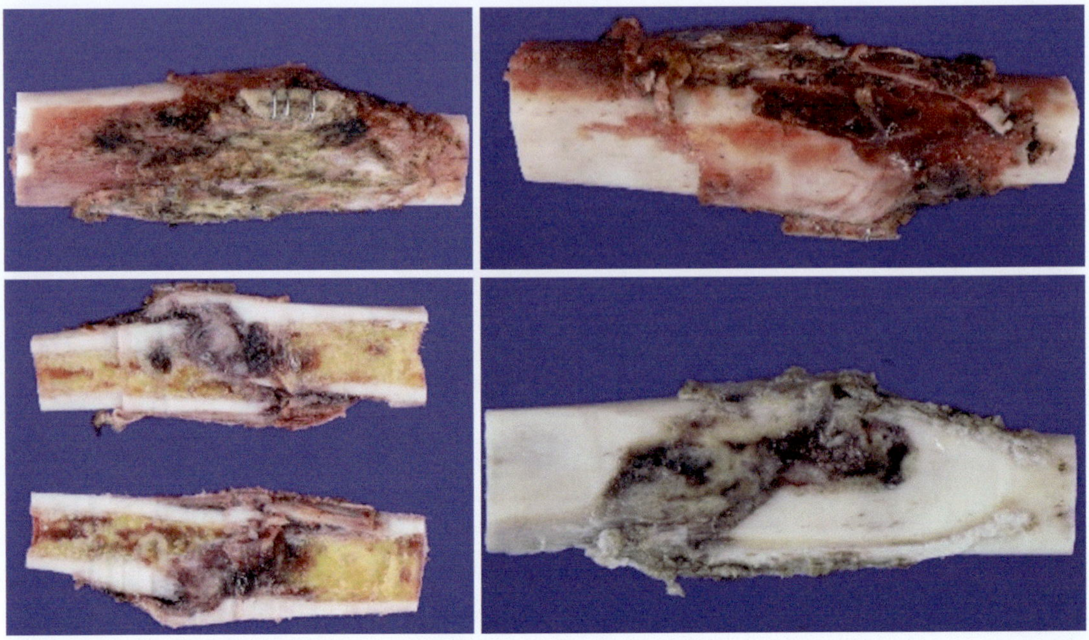

Fig. 24.11 Resected tumor

24.6 Postoperative Images

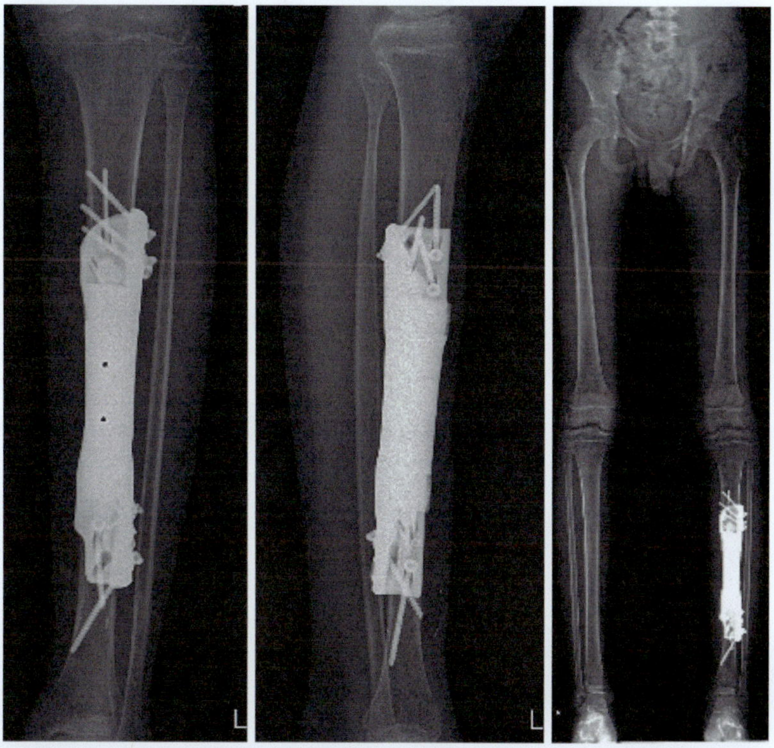

Fig. 24.12 Post-operative X-ray images

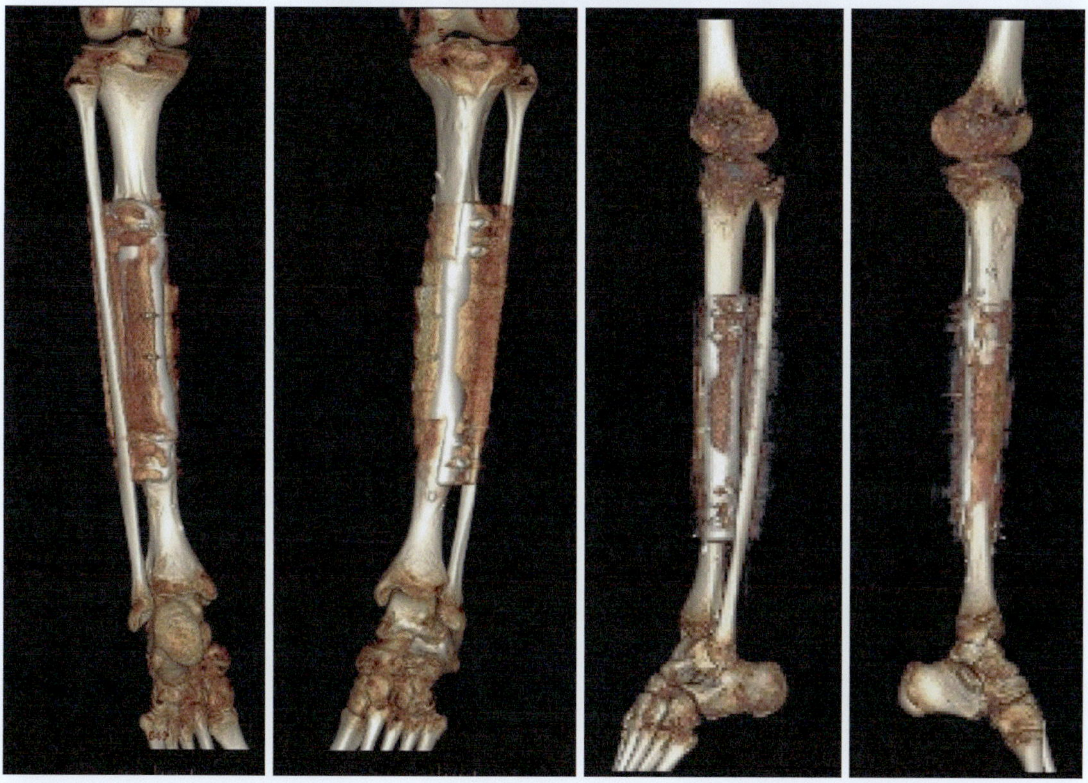

Fig. 24.13 Postoperative CT images

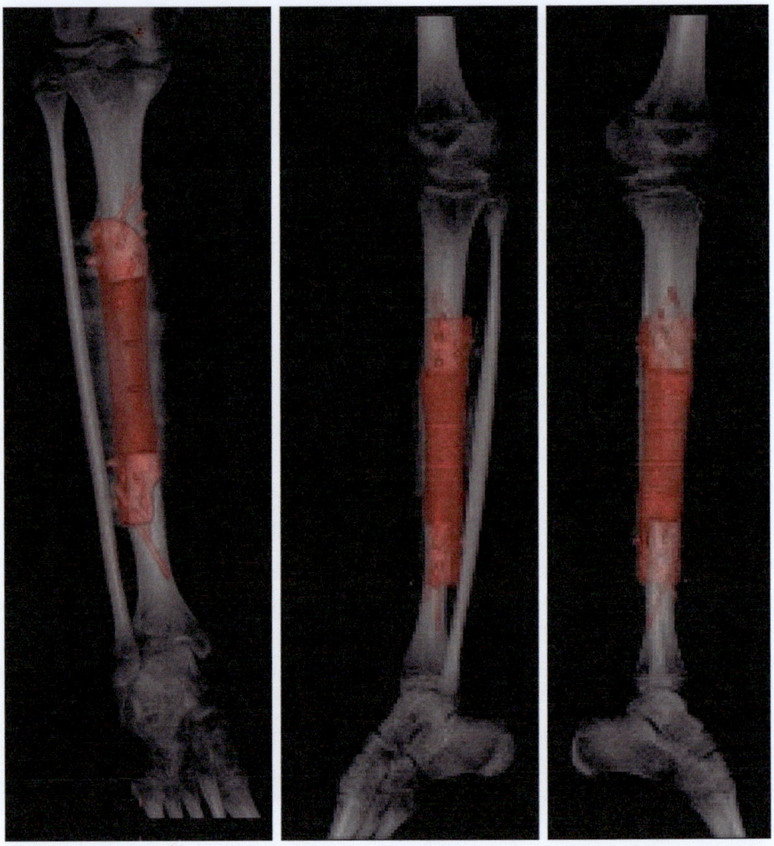

Fig. 24.13 (continued)

25 Patient Case 25: Proximal Tibia for Knee Joint Preserving

25.1 Patient Case 25

Age/sex	12/female
Location/site	Tibia proximal/left
Diagnosis	Osteosarcoma
Preoperative symptom	Antalgic gait
Preoperative pain score	Resting 0/Activity 4
BMI (height/weight)	18.53 (151.8/42.7)
Past history	Diagnosed by incisional biopsy
Present illness	Two times preoperative chemotherapy Reluctance to artificial joint and osteoarticular allograft

25.2 Preoperative Images

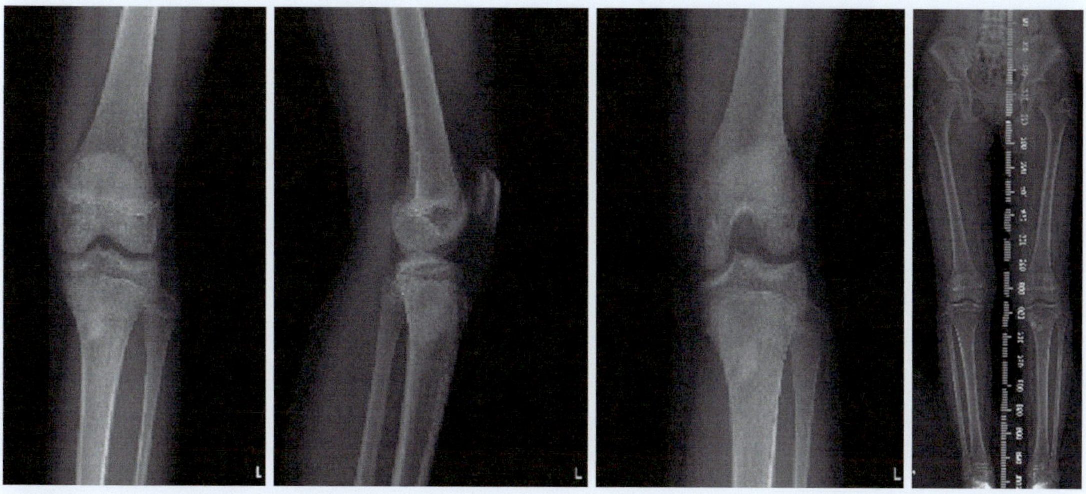

Fig. 25.1 Preoperative X-ray images

H.-G. Kang, *Clinical Atlas of 3D Printing Bone Reconstruction*,
https://doi.org/10.1007/978-981-16-2043-0_25

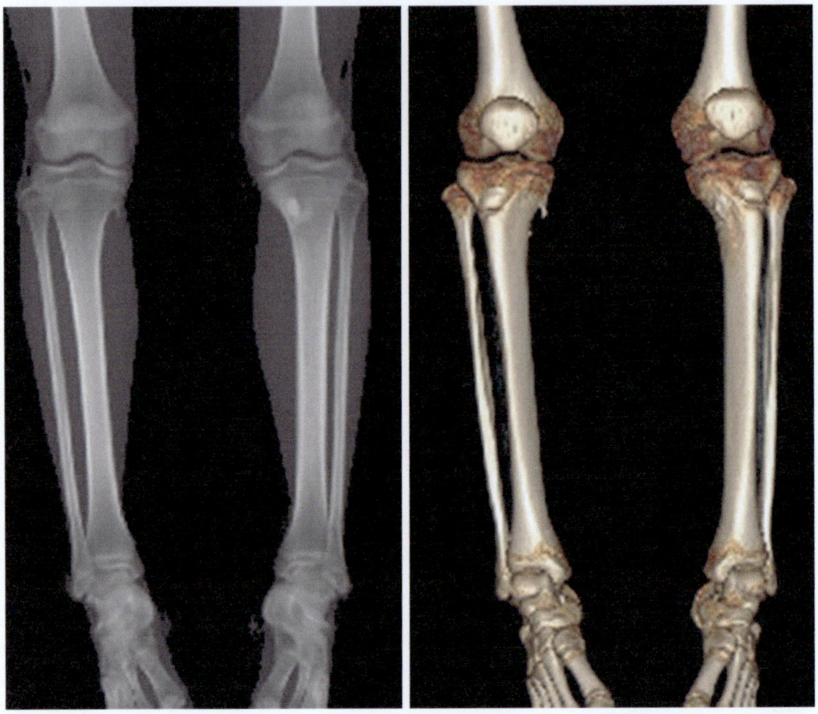

Fig. 25.2 Preoperative CT images

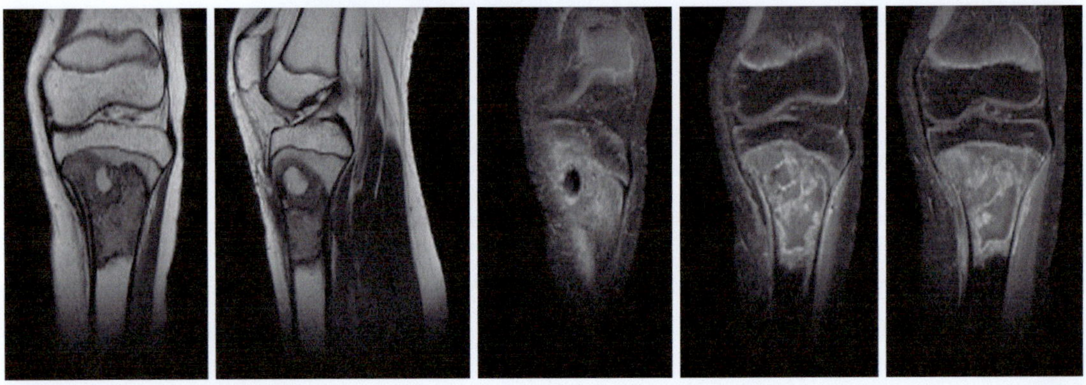

Fig. 25.3 Preoperative MRI images

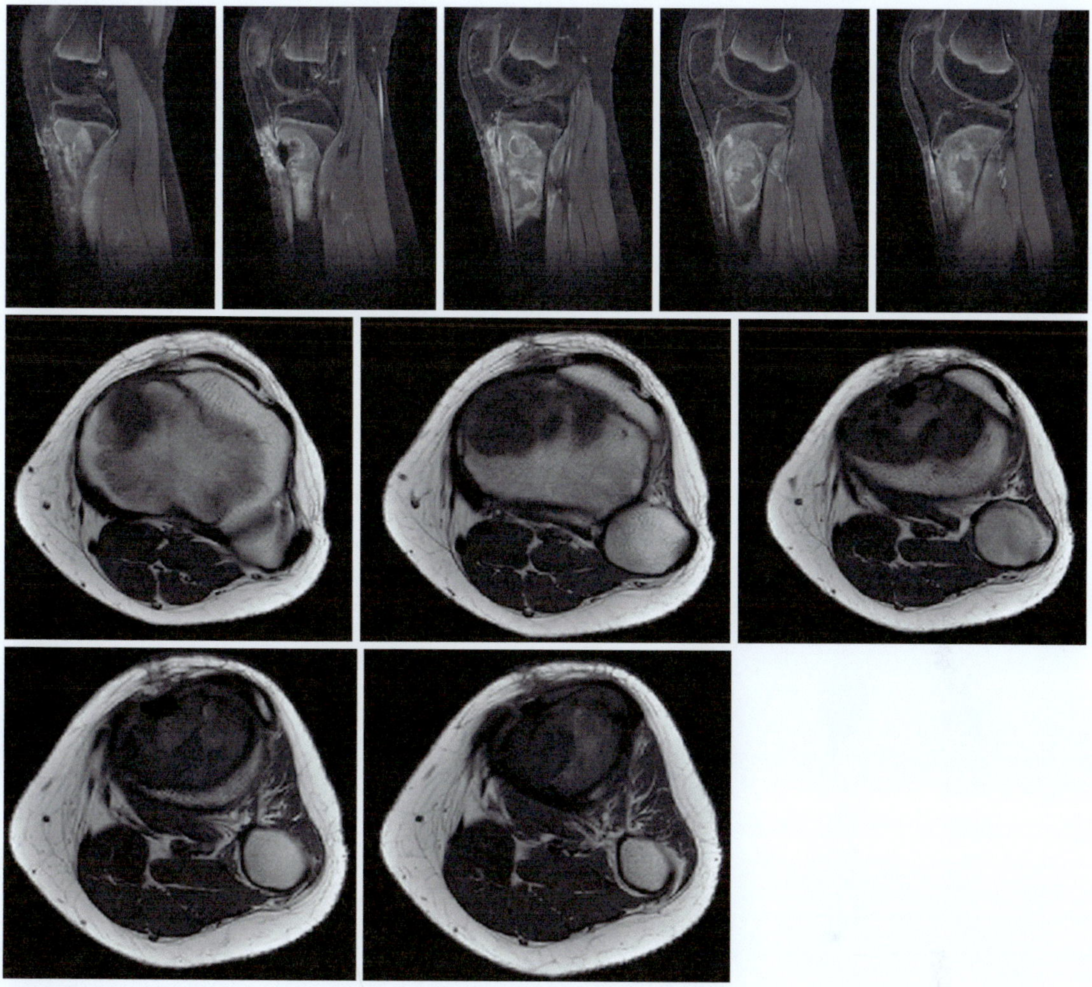

Fig. 25.3 (continued)

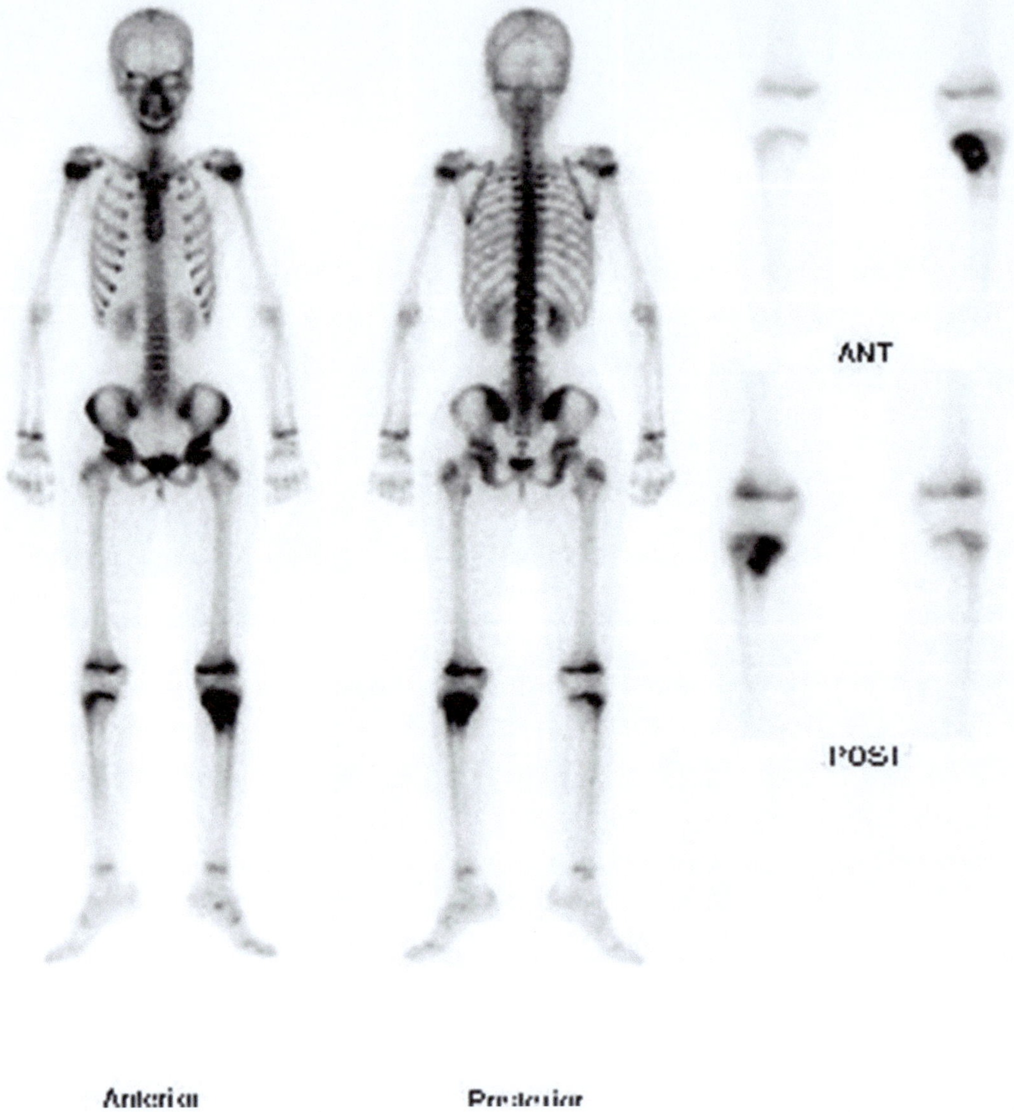

Fig. 25.4 Preoperative bone scan images

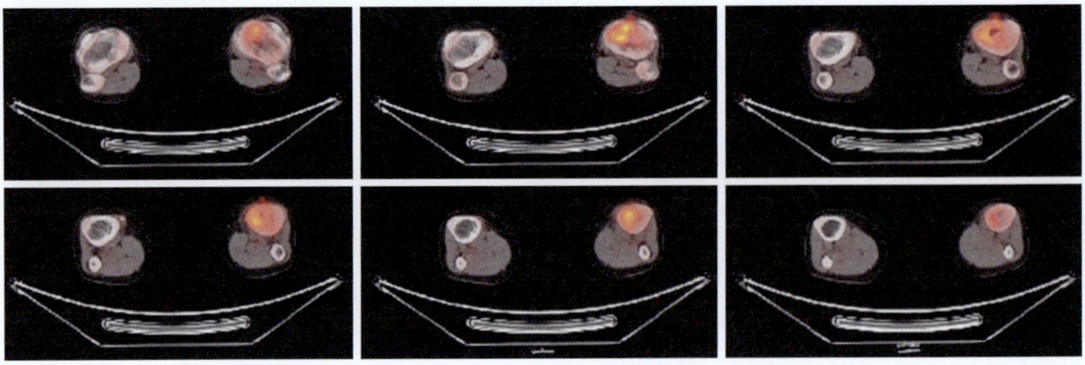

Fig. 25.5 Preoperative PET-CT images

25.3 Planning of Surgery

Knee joint save epiphyseal resection
3D-printed proximal tibia implant

25.4 Design and Fabrication

25.4.1 Bone Cutting Guide

- Proximal tibia epiphyseal cutting
- The patellar tendon area of tibial tuberosity cutting
- Since the growth plate is not parallel, saw cutting the three sides of medial, lateral, patellar tendon attachment tuberosity
- The V-shape bone cutting of the distal tibia

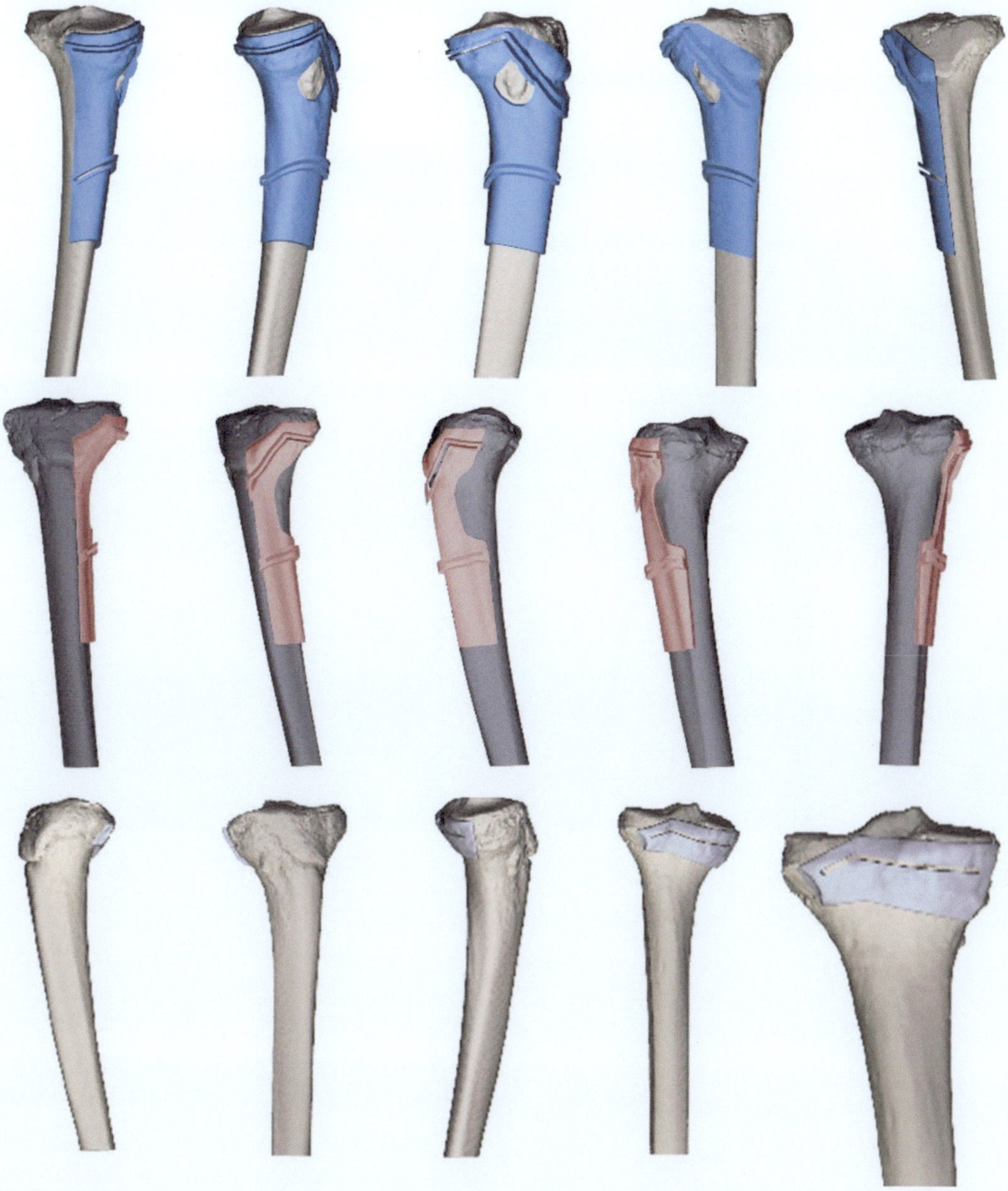

Fig. 25.6 Bone cutting guides: medial, lateral, and posterior application

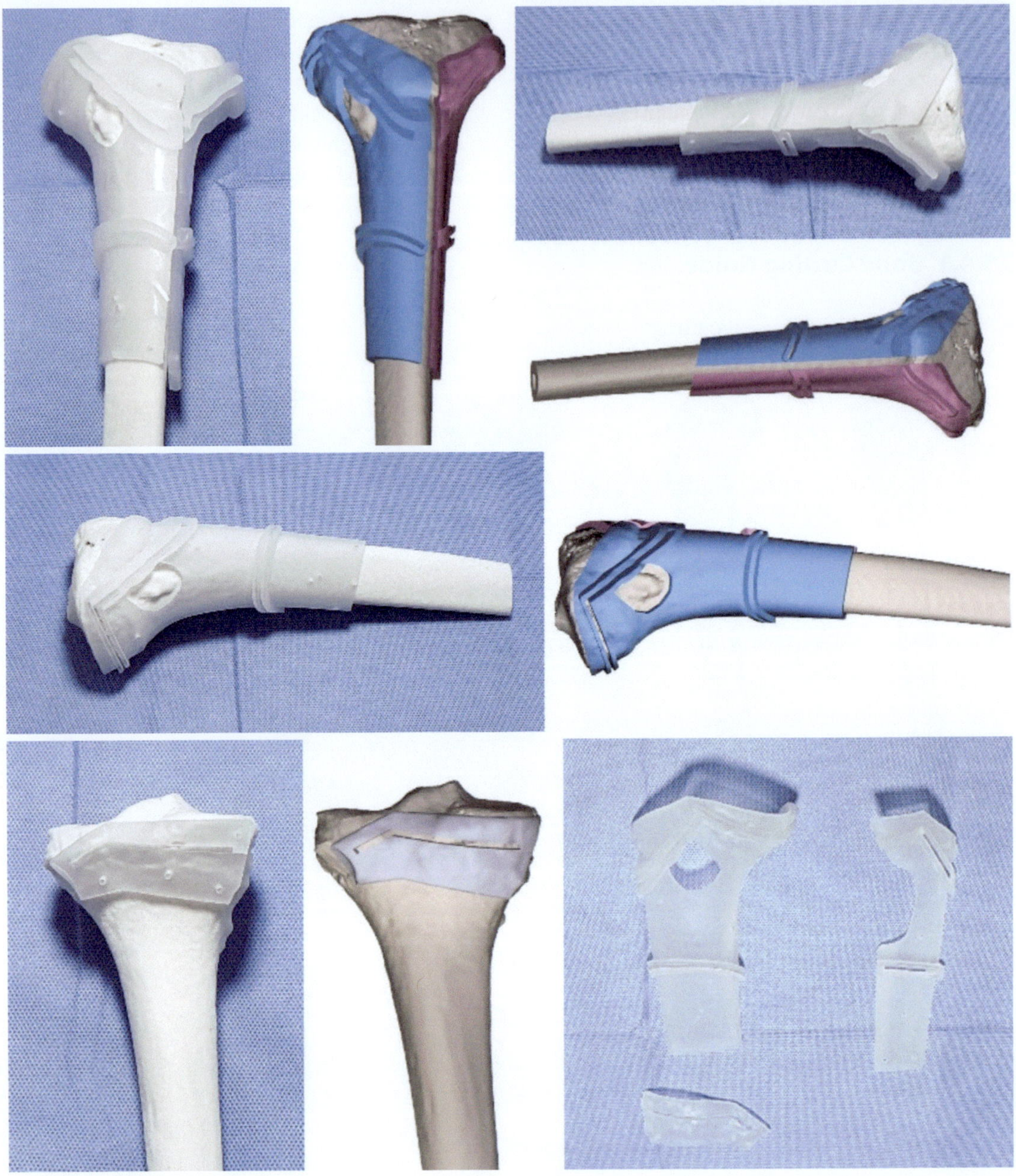

Fig. 25.6 (continued)

25.4.2 Implant

- Mesh style body
- Many suture holes for tendon and joint capsule
- Many screw holes for tibial tuberosity and epiphysis fixation
- Mesh style of inner surface of plate
- The V-shaped mesh implant connect to the distal tibia.

- Implant measurement
- Implant weight (g): 285
- Size (mm): 199

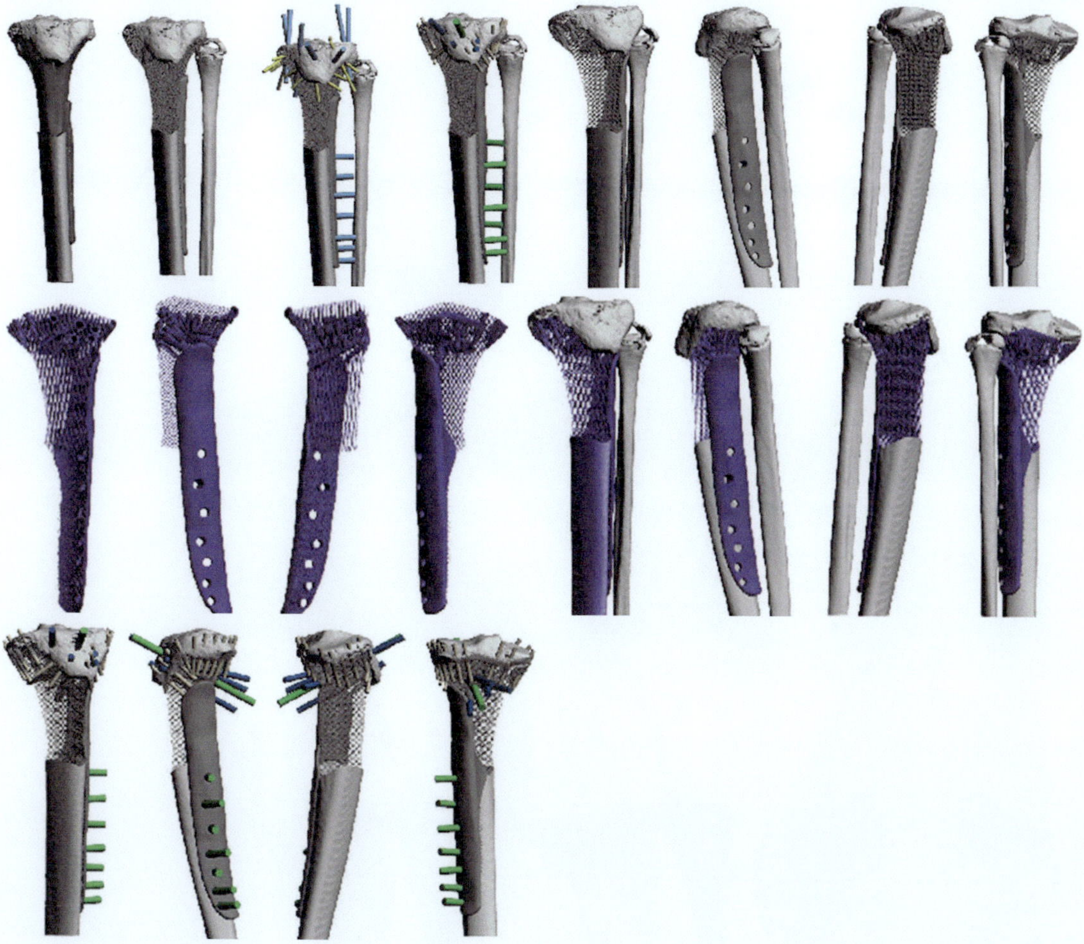

Fig. 25.7 Implant design

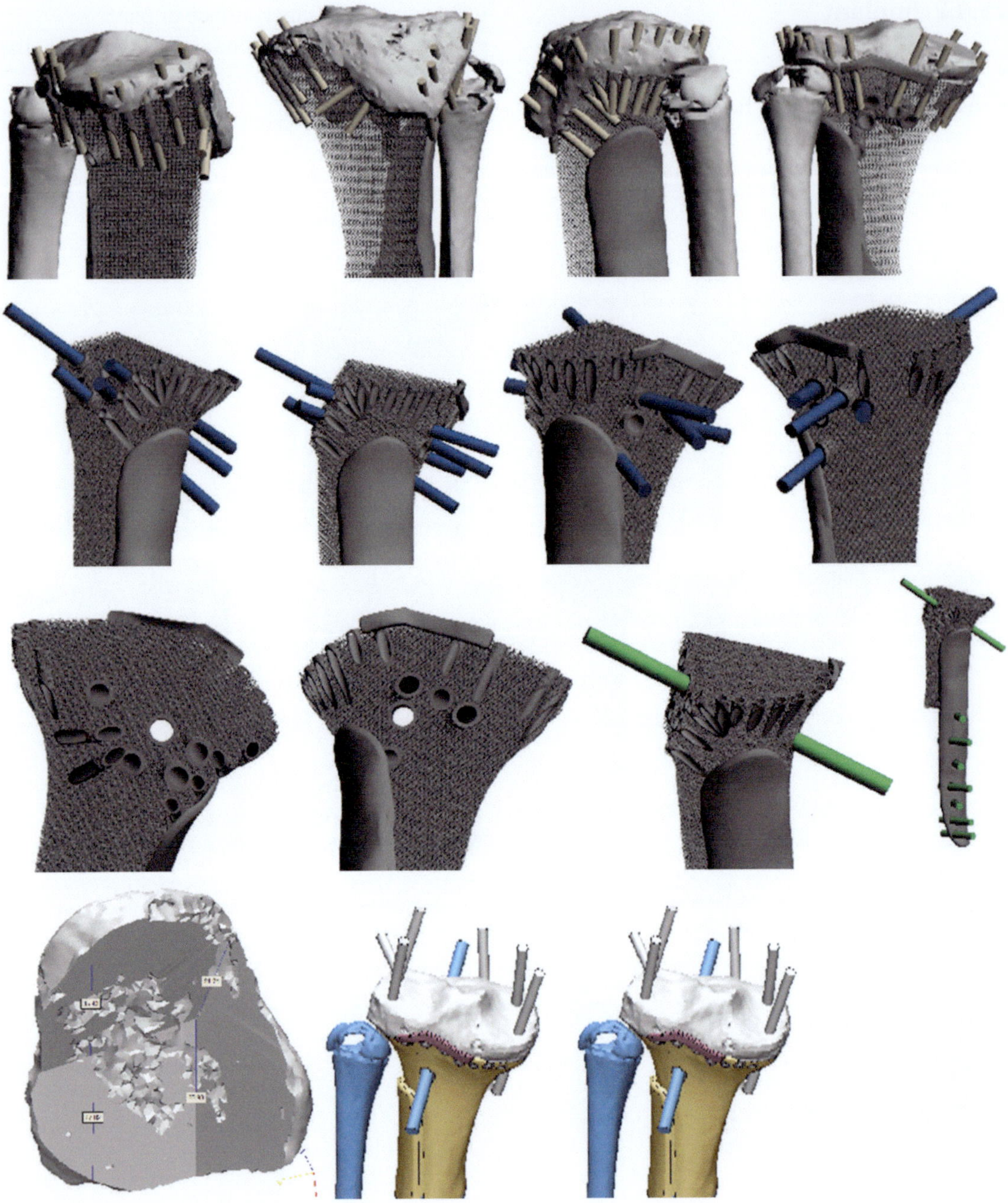

Fig. 25.7 (continued)

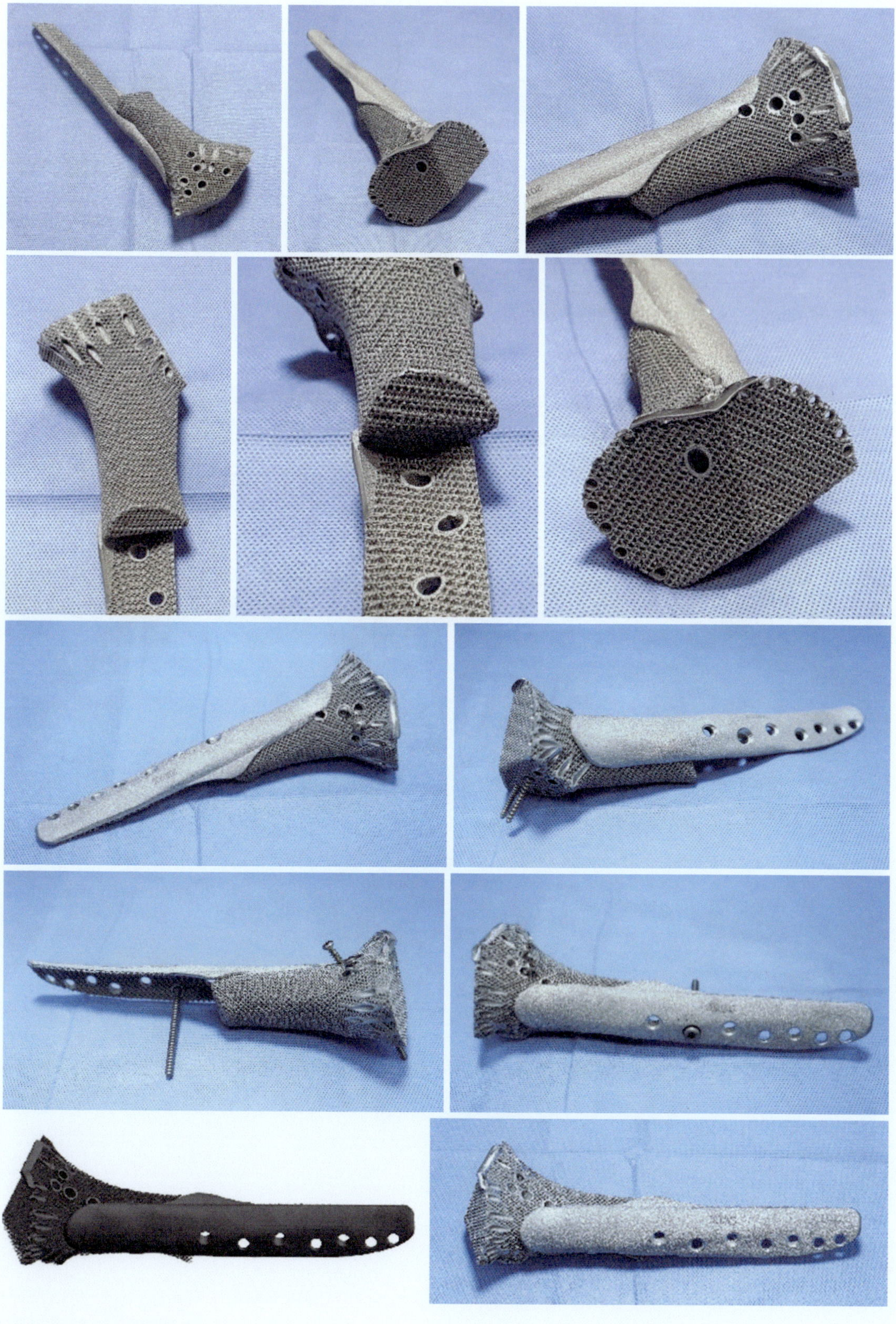

Fig. 25.8 Printed implant

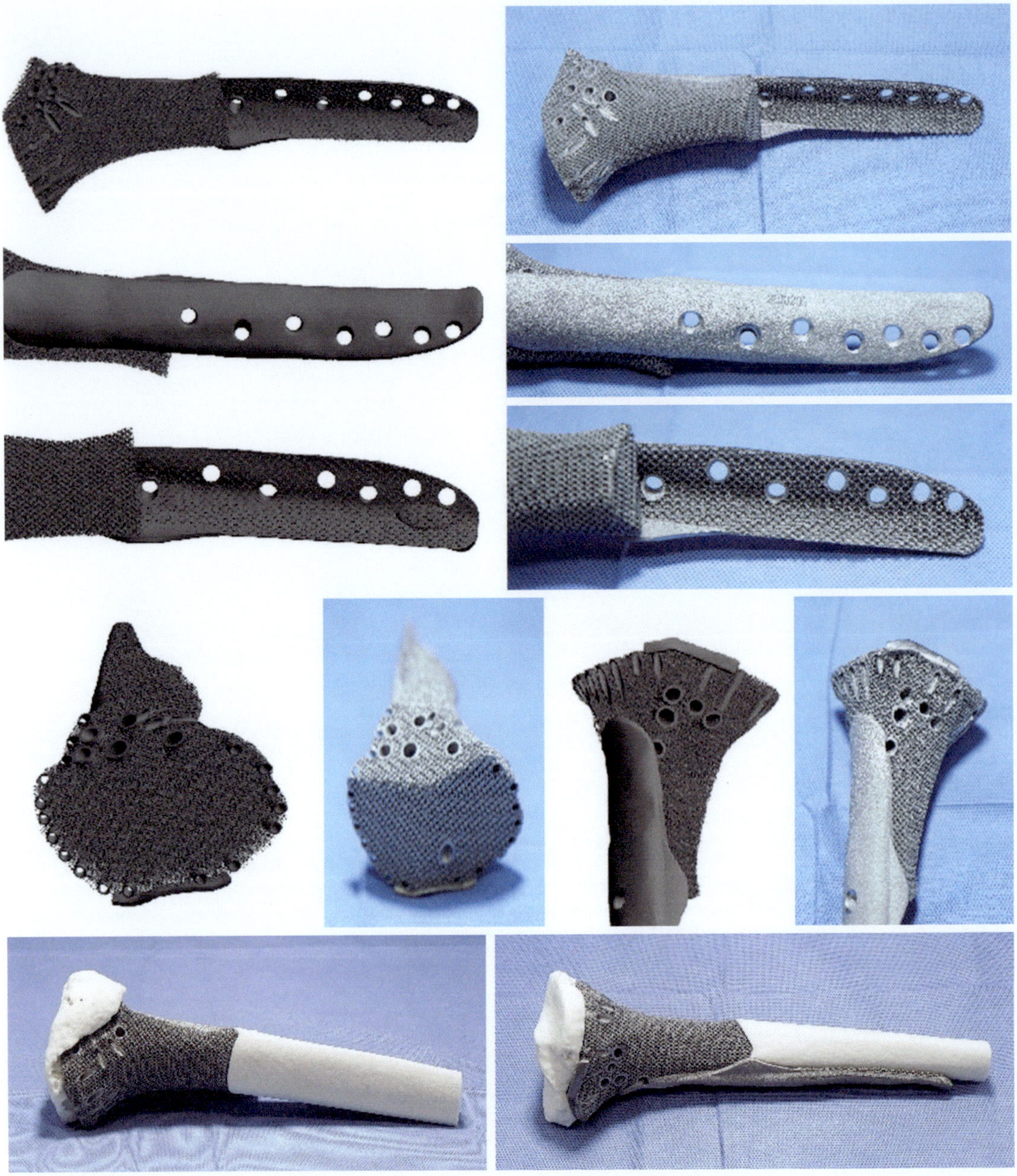

Fig. 25.8 (continued)

25.5 Operation

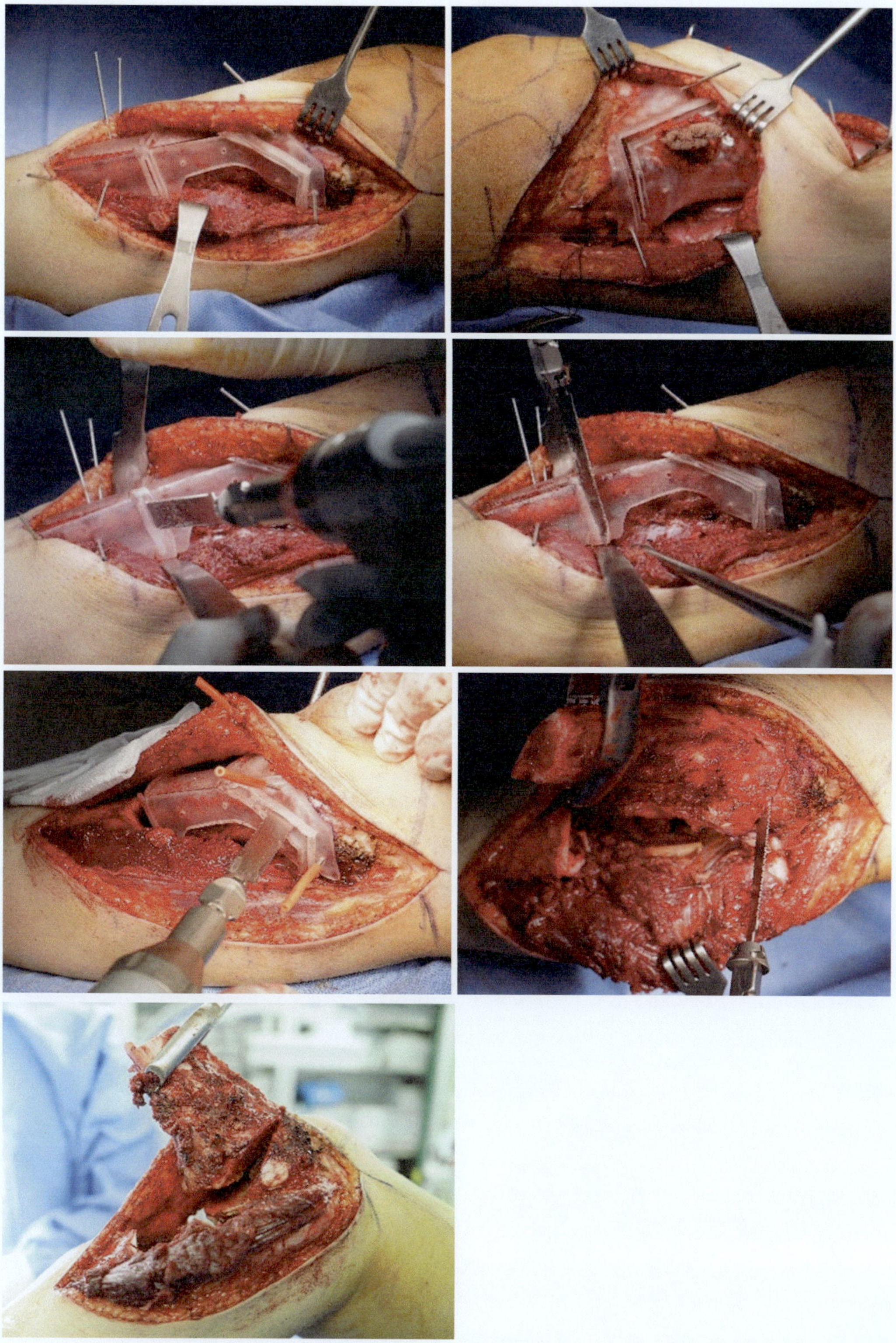

Fig. 25.9 Intraoperative photographs: medial, lateral, and anterior bone cutting of epiphysis proximally, V-shaped bone cutting diaphysis distally

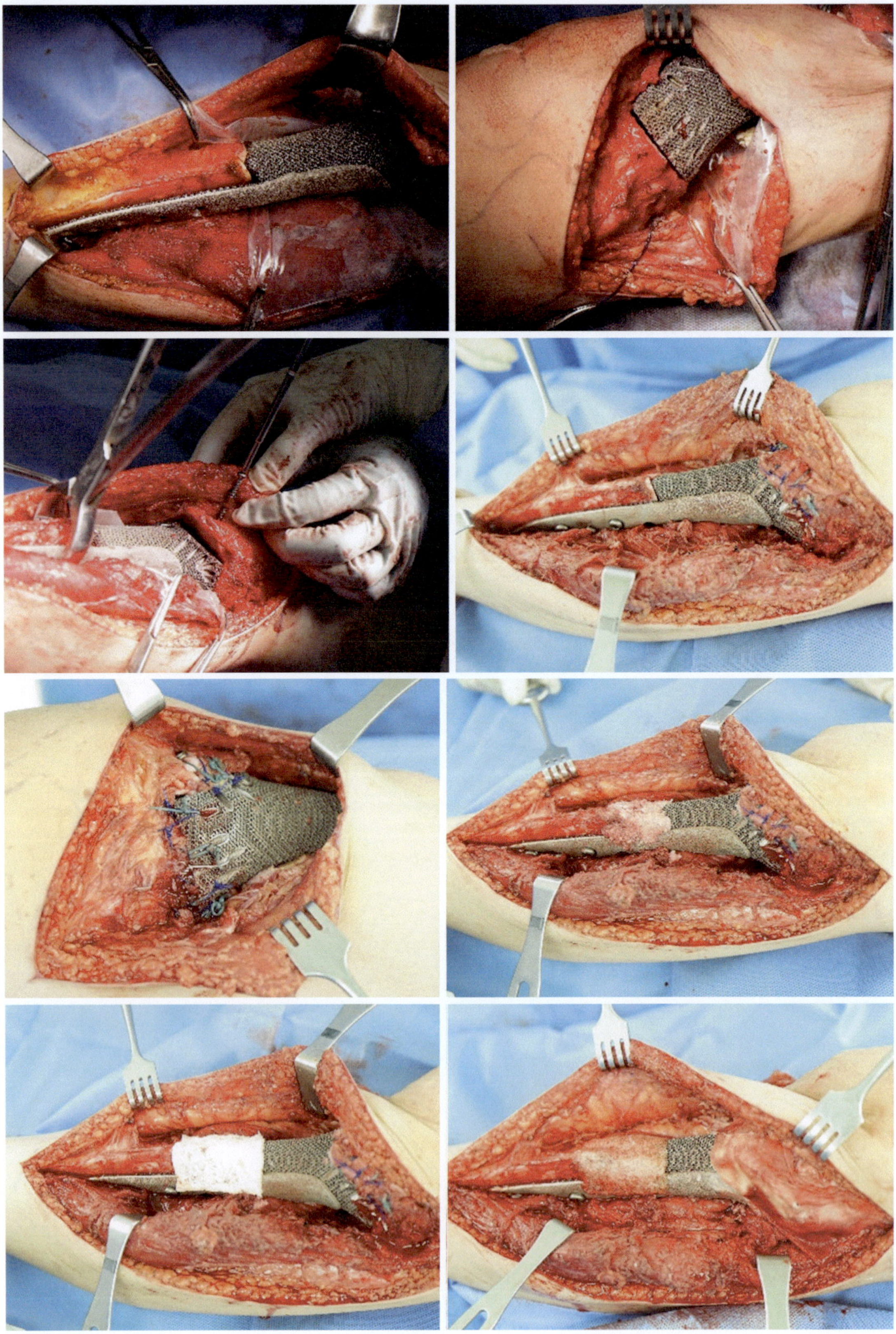

Fig. 25.10 Intraoperative photographs

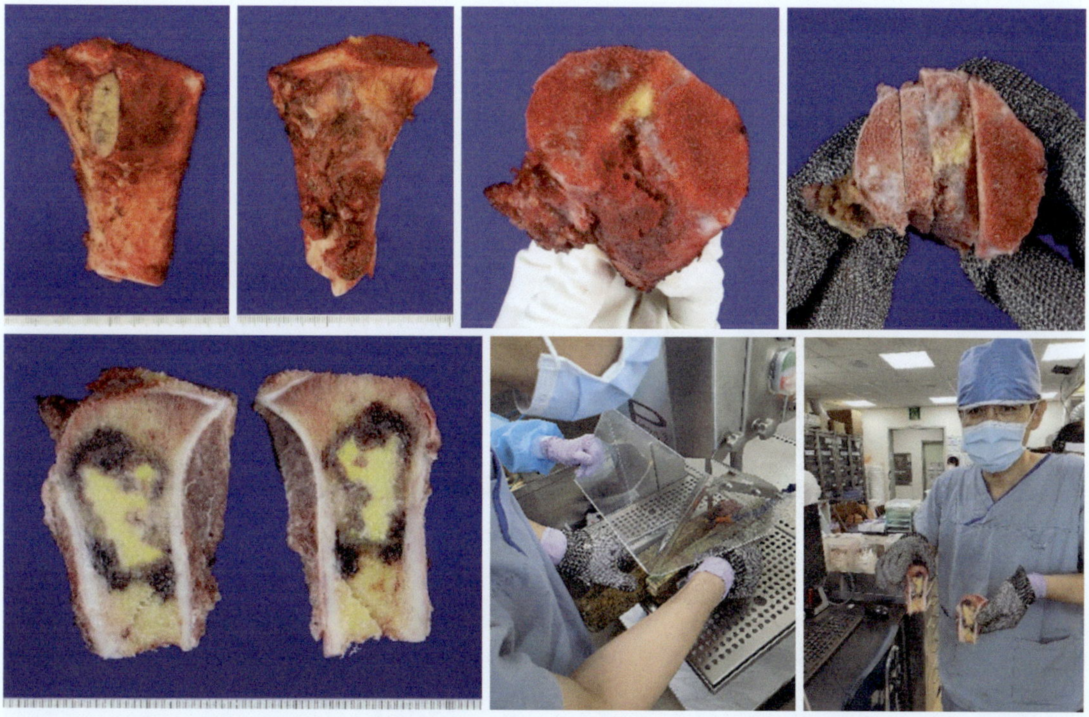

Fig. 25.11 Resected bone tumor: surgeon cuts the resected tumor directly in the pathology room after surgery

25.6 Postoperative Images

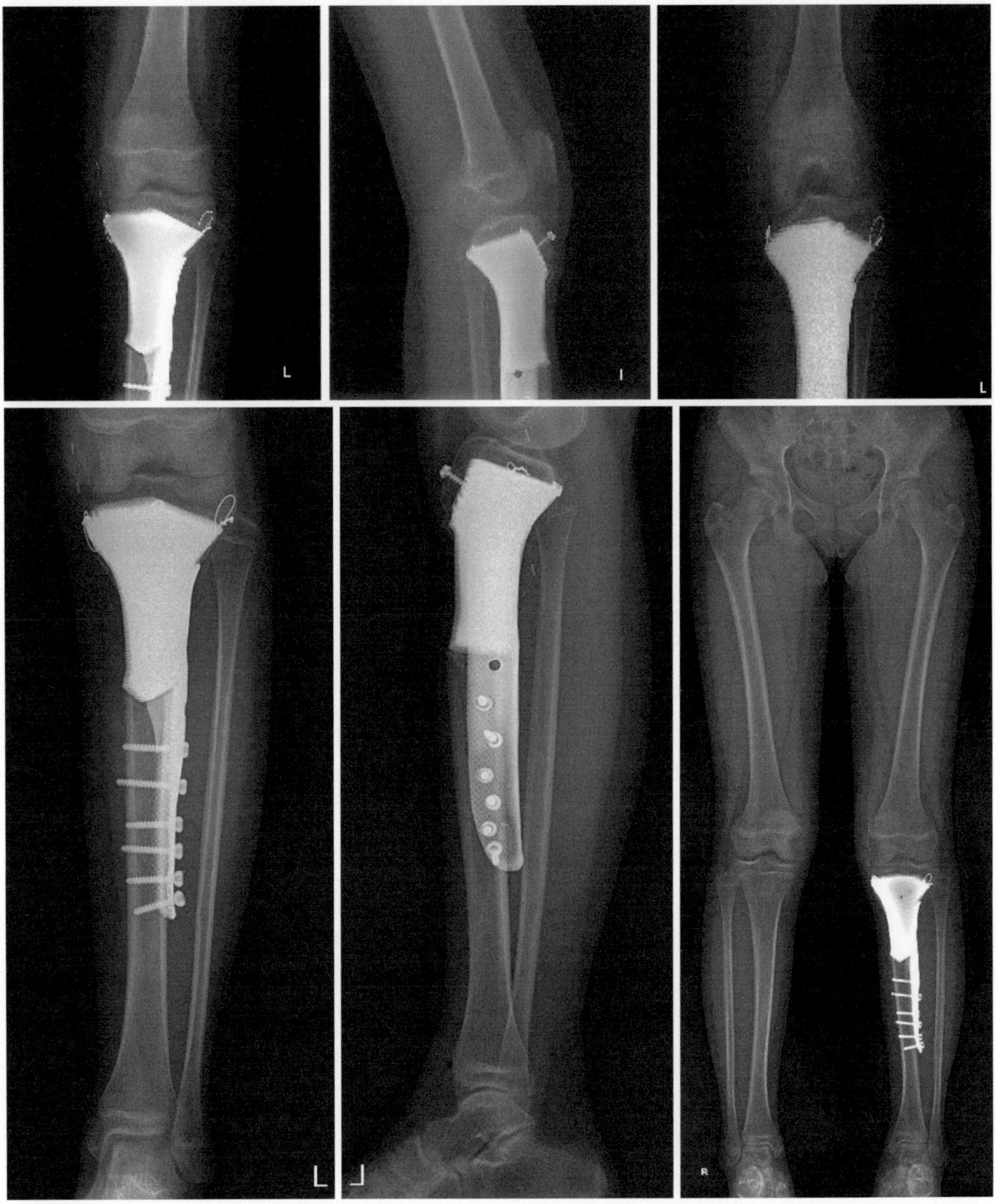

Fig. 25.12 Postoperative X-ray images

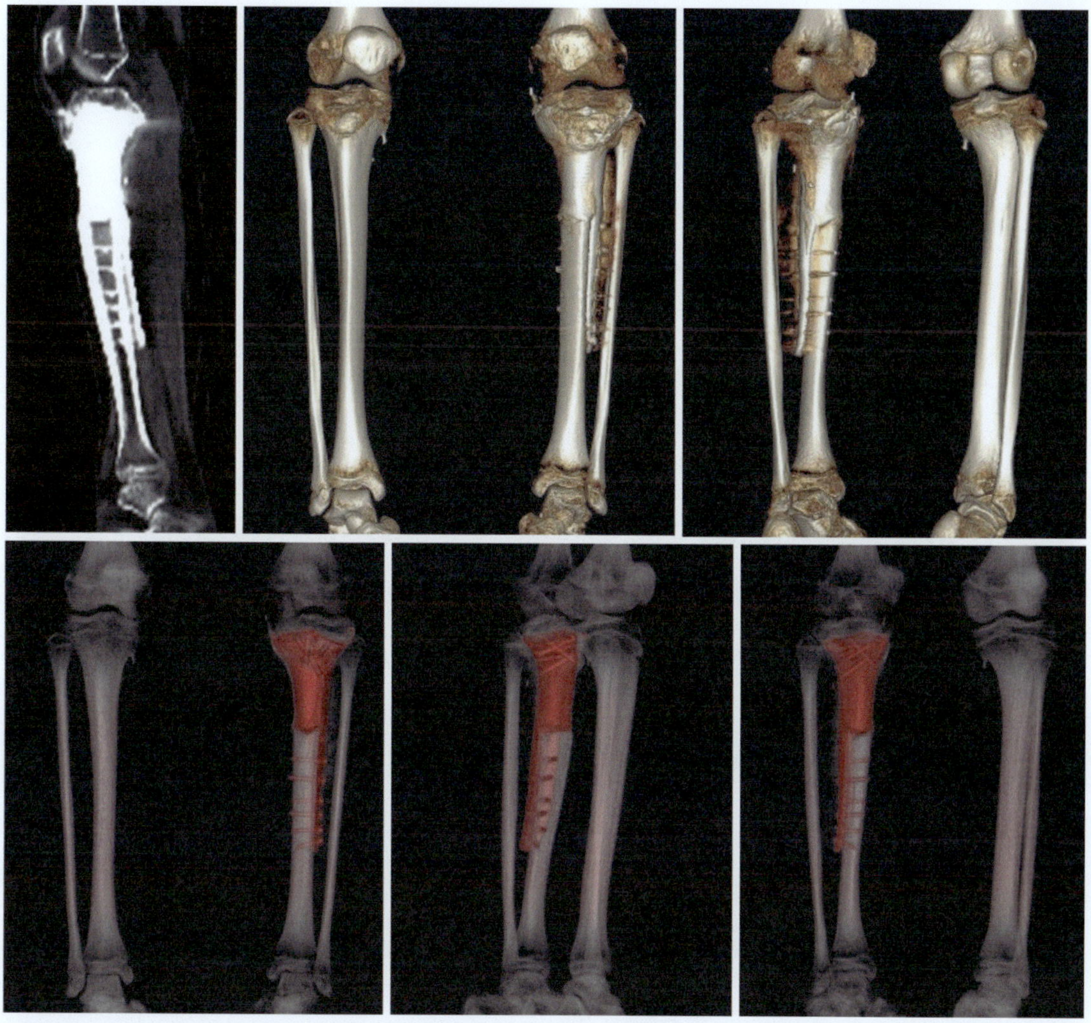

Fig. 25.13 Postoperative CT images

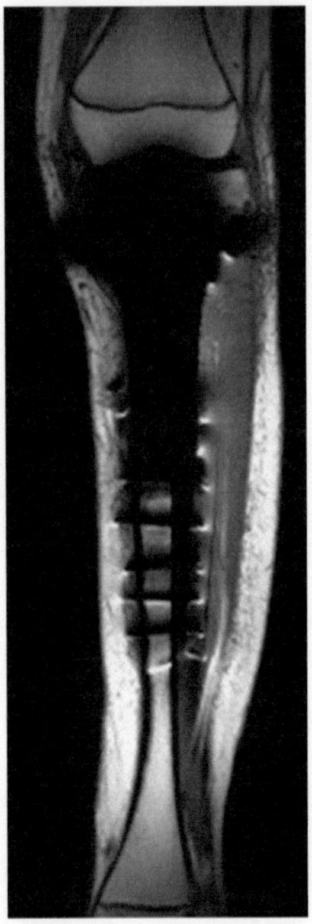

Fig. 25.14 Postoperative MRI image

Fig. 25.15 Post-operative bone scan images

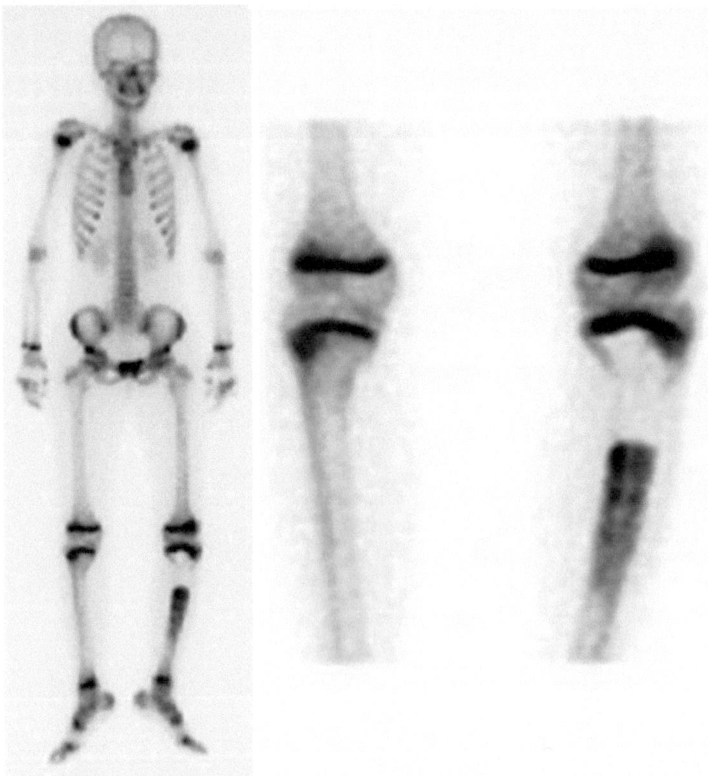

26 Patient Case 26: Tibia Assembled with Knee Artificial Joint Surface

26.1 Patient Case 26

Age/sex	14/female
Location/site	Tibia proximal/left
Diagnosis	Osteosarcoma
Preoperative symptom	Antalgic gait
Preoperative pain score	Resting 2/Activity 5
BMI (height/weight)	17 (154.7/40.7)
Past history	Diagnosed by incisional biopsy
Present illness	Two times preoperative chemotherapy Want to save femur side knee joint

H.-G. Kang, *Clinical Atlas of 3D Printing Bone Reconstruction*,
https://doi.org/10.1007/978-981-16-2043-0_26

26.2 Preoperative Images

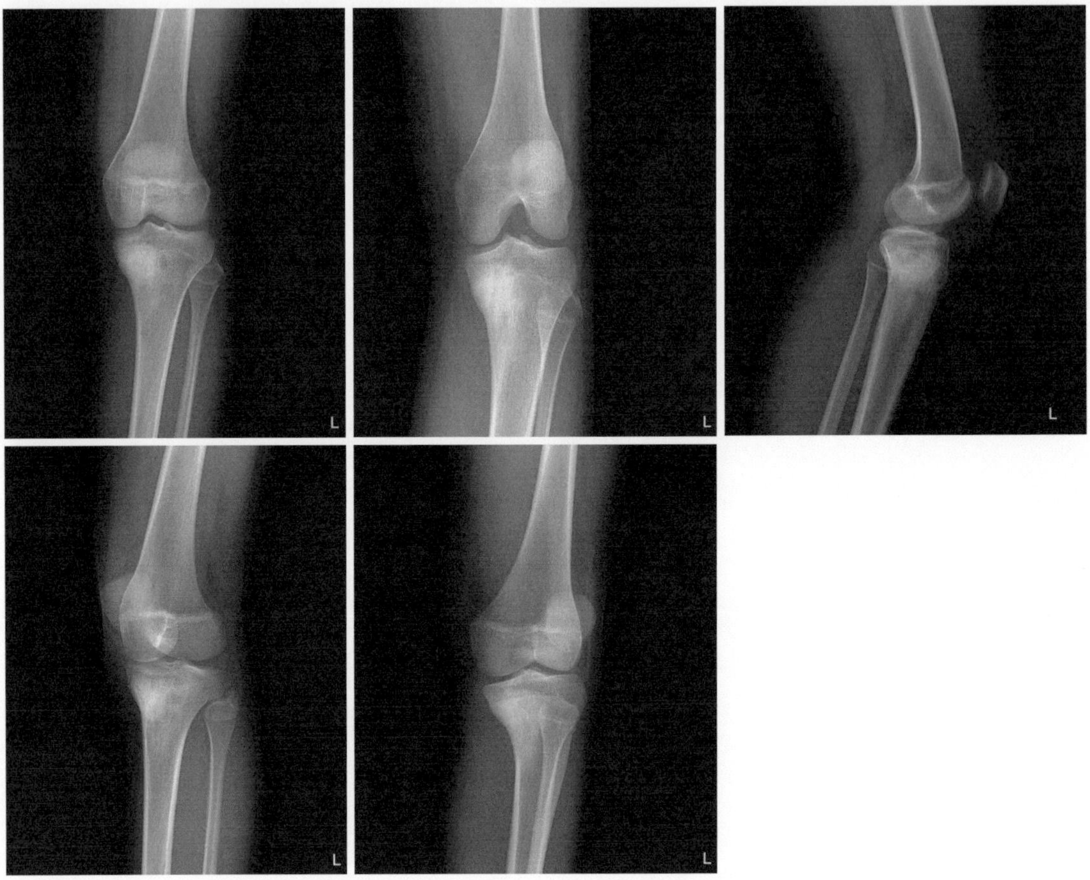

Fig. 26.1 Preoperative X-ray images

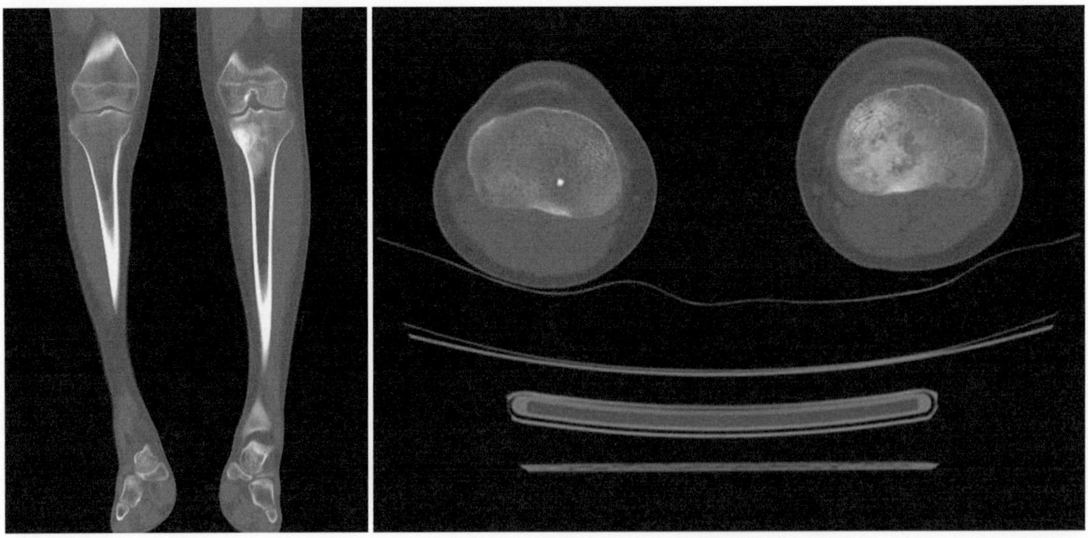

Fig. 26.2 Preoperative CT images

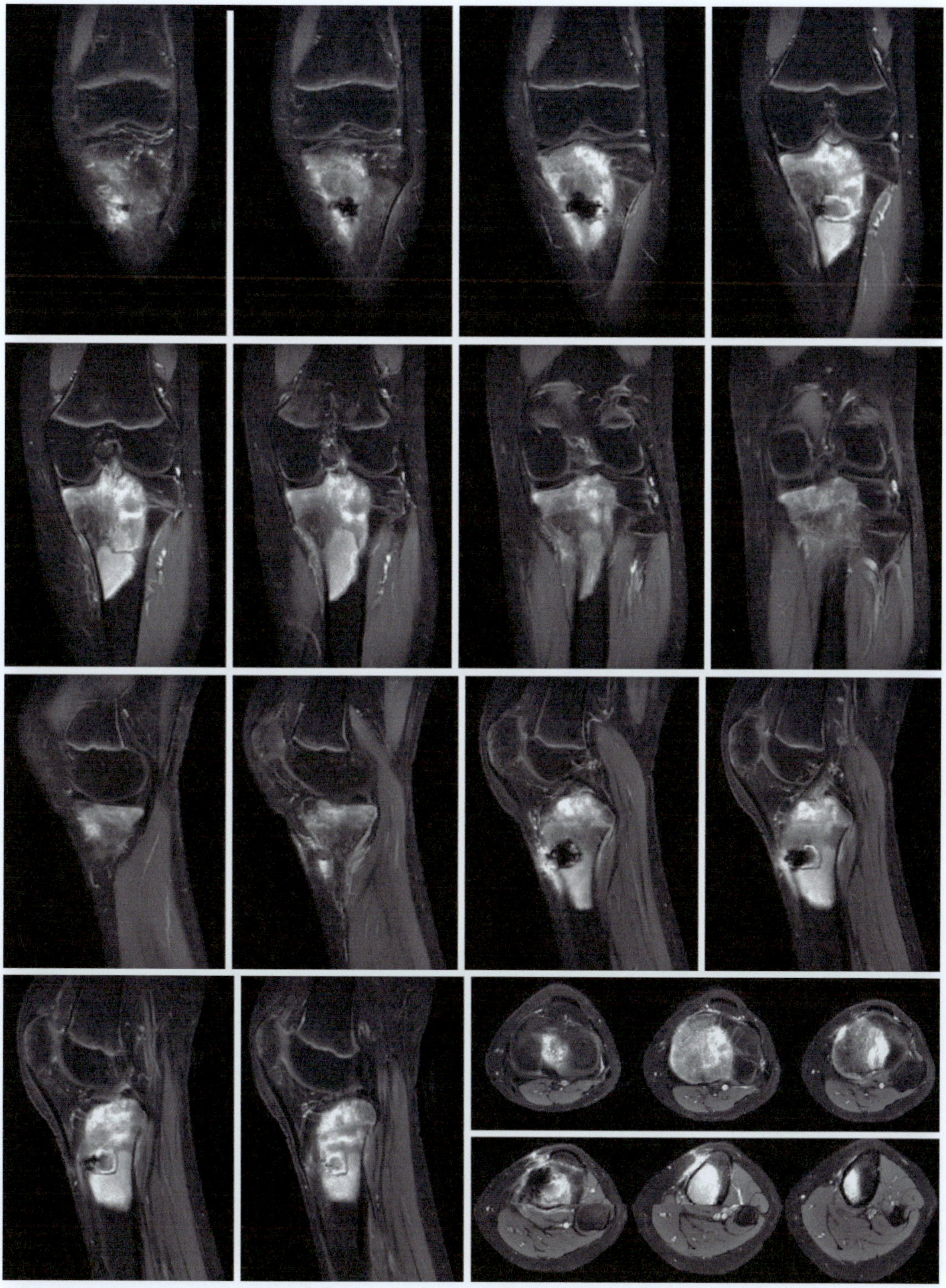

Fig. 26.3 Preoperative MRI images

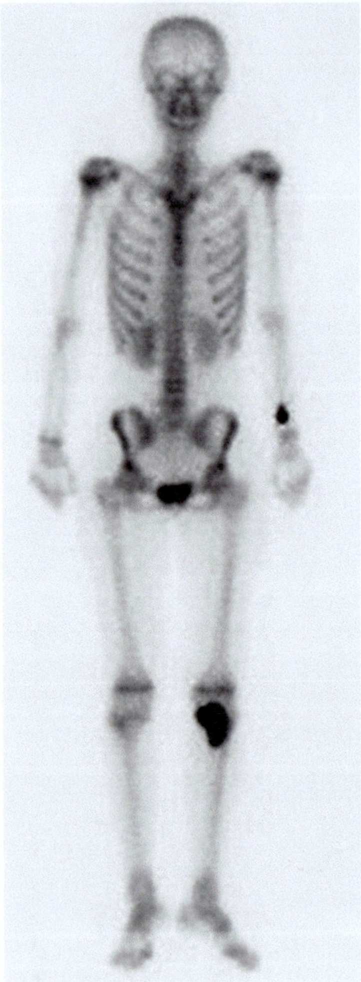

Fig. 26.4 Preoperative bone scan image

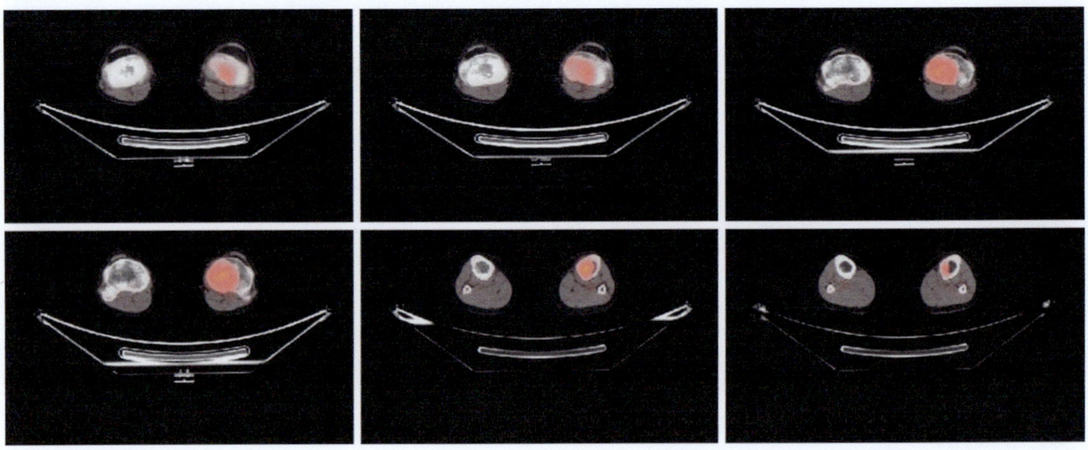

Fig. 26.5 Preoperative PET-CT images

26.3 Planning of Surgery

Wide resection including tibial joint

Hemiarthroplasty tibial side of knee

3D-printed proximal tibia implant + Total knee arthroplasty system

The ATTUNE® DePuy Synthes

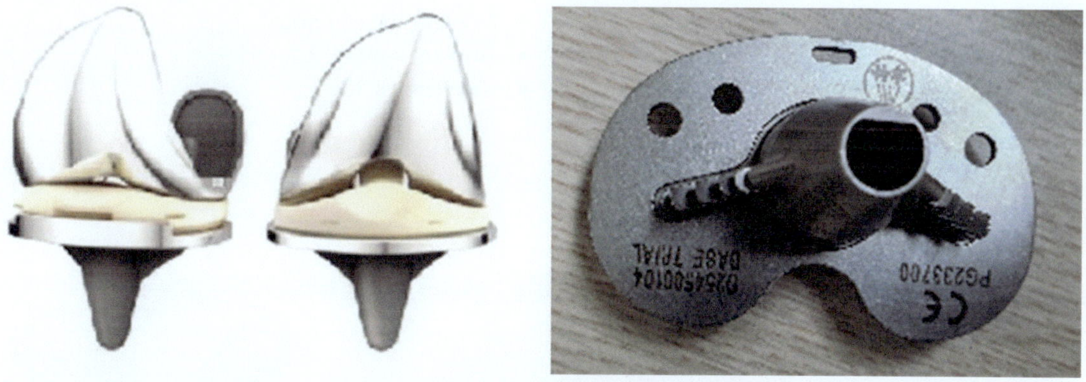

Fig. 26.6 The selected total knee system and its tibial trial for 3D printing design

26.4 Design and Fabrication

26.4.1 Bone Cutting

- Saw cut of tibial tuberosity of the patella tendon attachment part
- Distal tibial bone cutting is transverse
- Transverse bone cutting is easier than V-shape cutting
- 3D-printed instrument for conical medullary reaming

26.4.2 Implant

ATTUNE artificial joint of DePuy was selected for tibia joint hemiarthroplasty.
Proximal surface is designed to be combined with tibial metal plate of ATTUNE.

- Implant measurement
- Implant weight (g): 153
- Size (mm): 196

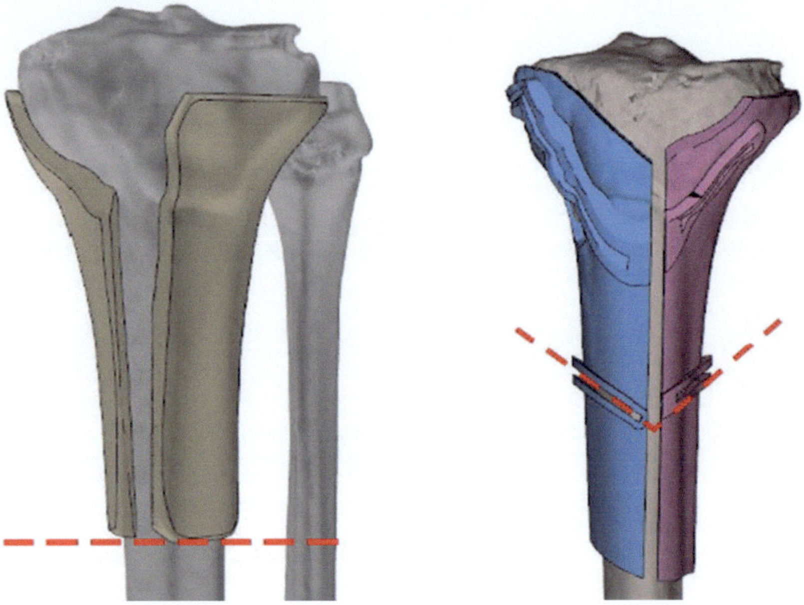

Fig. 26.7 Transverse bone cutting is easier than V-shaped bone cutting

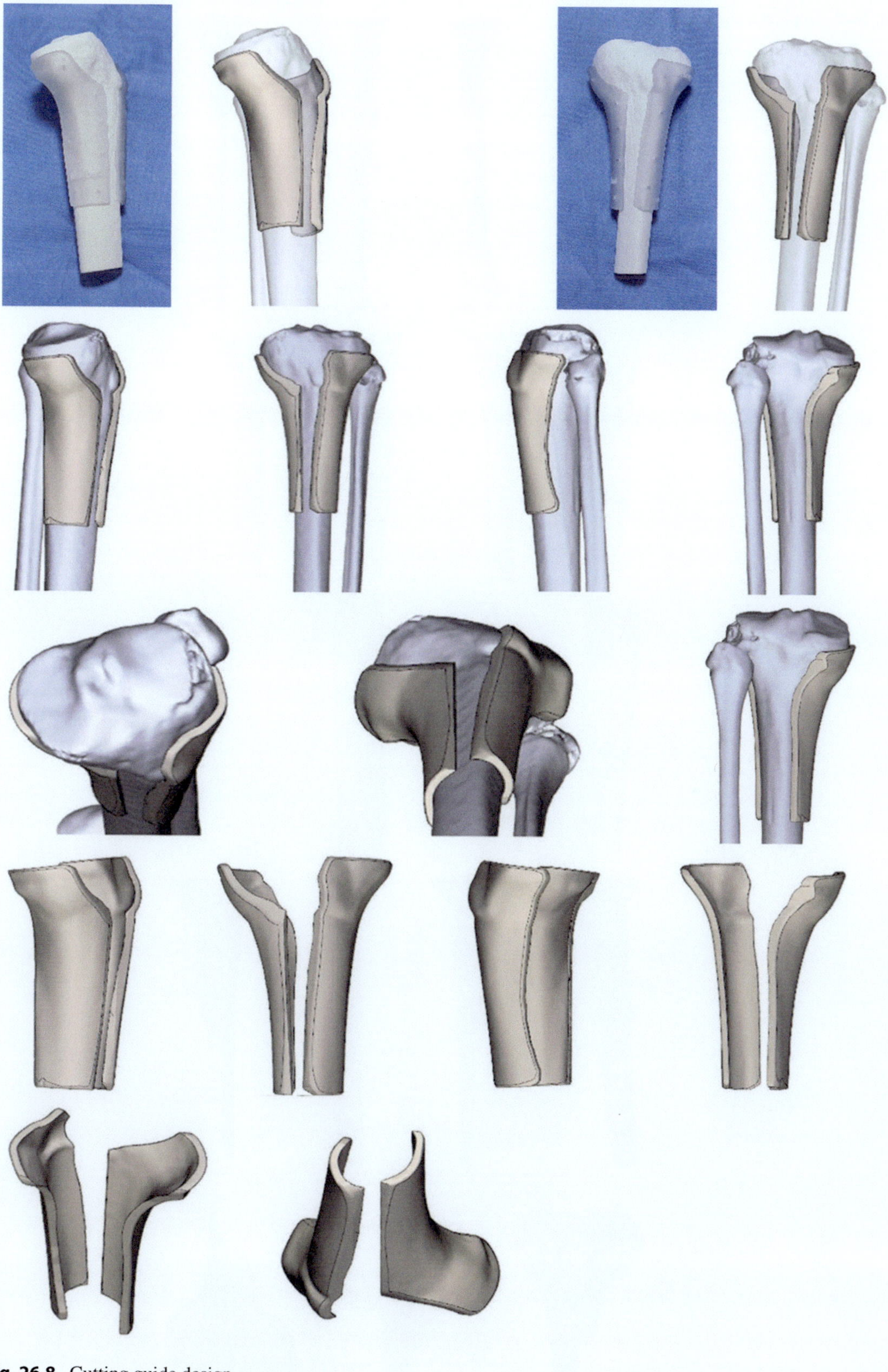

Fig. 26.8 Cutting guide design

Fig. 26.9 Implant design

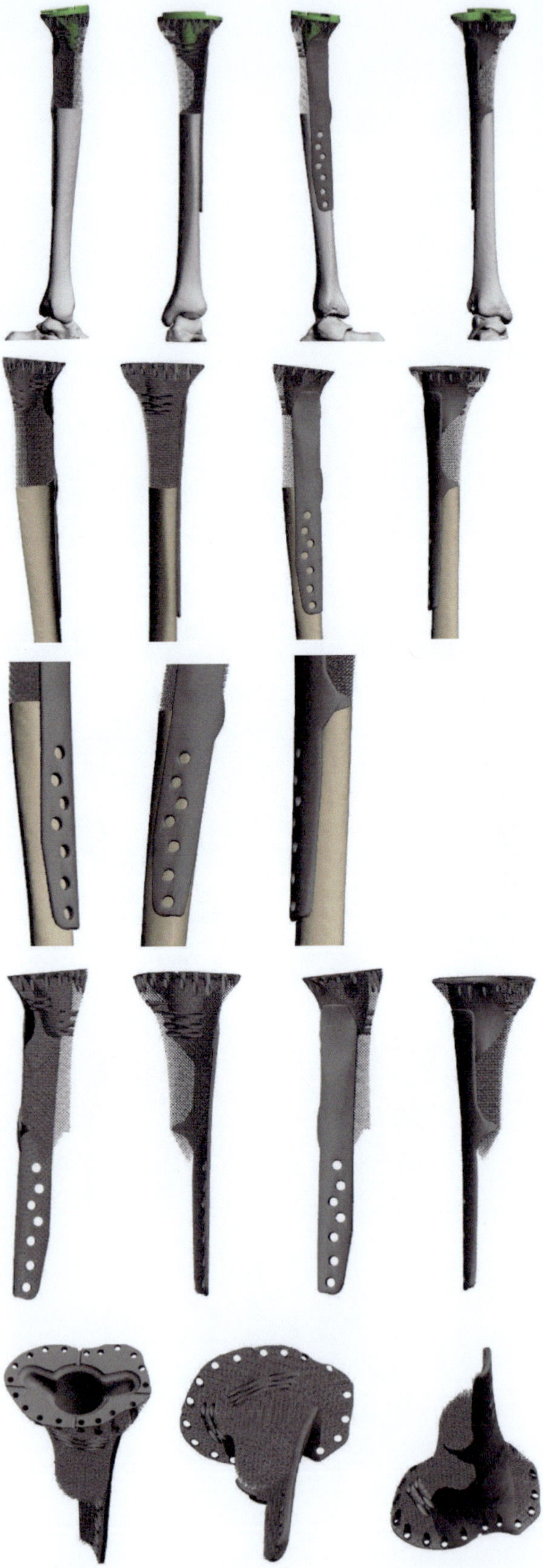

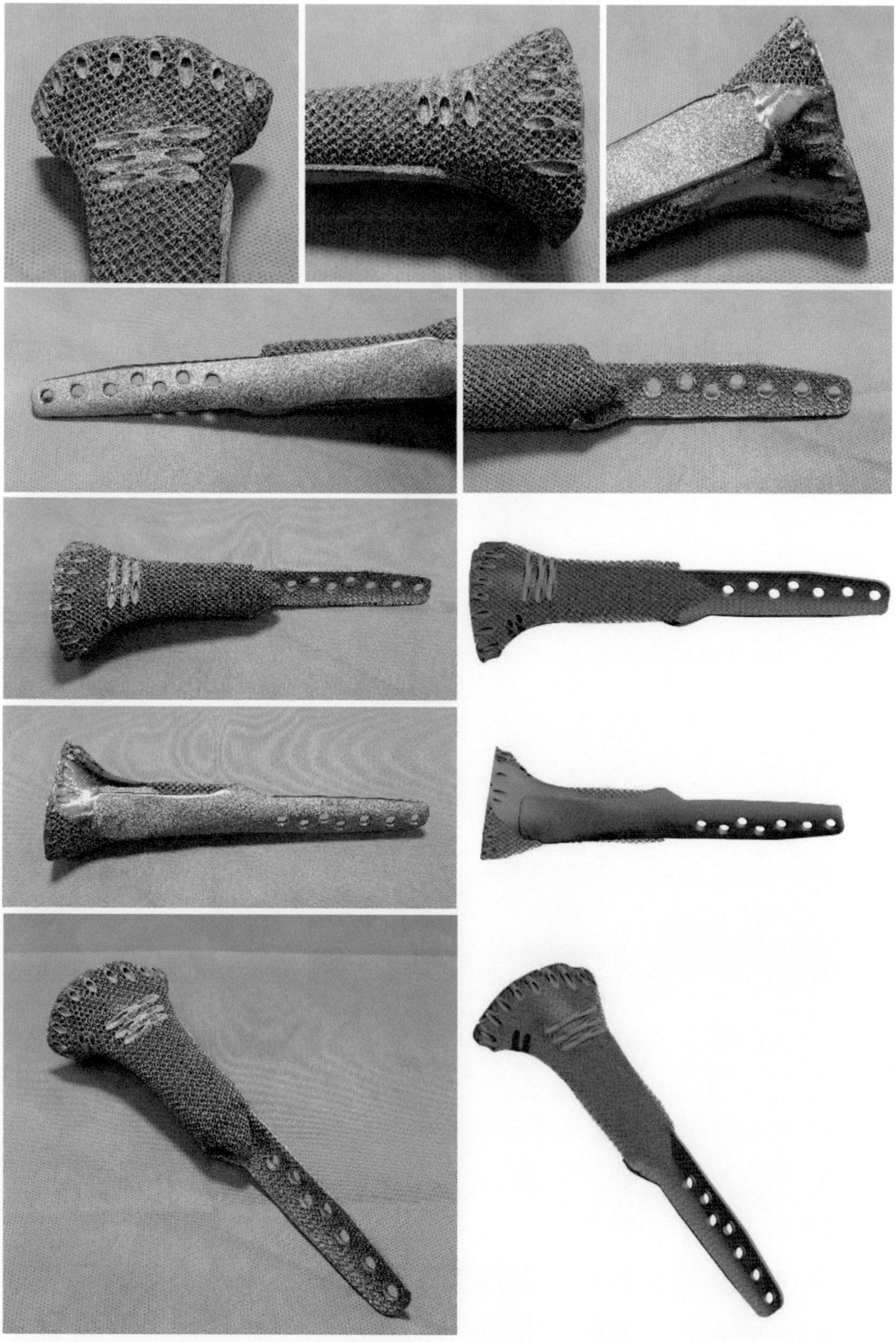

Fig. 26.10 Printed implant

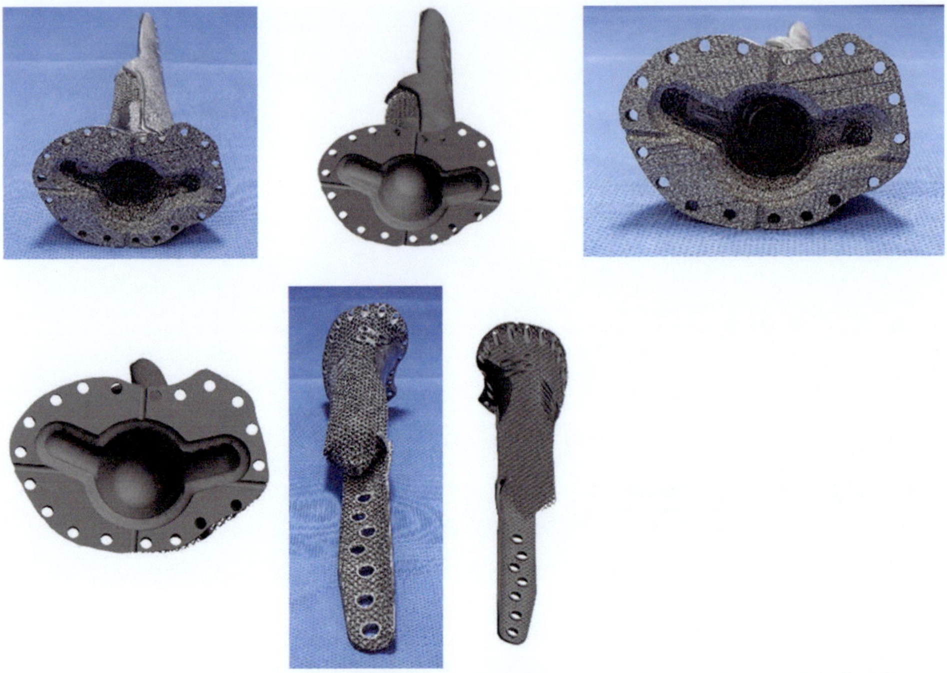

Fig. 26.10 (continued)

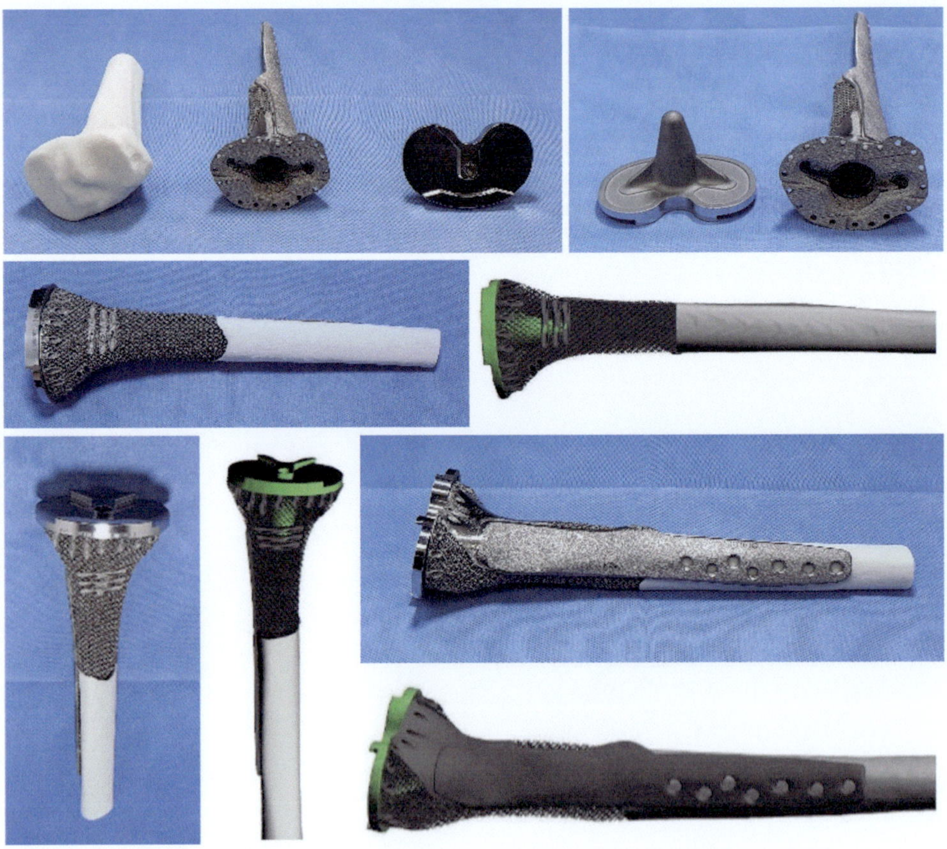

Fig. 26.11 3D-printed implant and tibia plate of arthroplasty combination and modeling

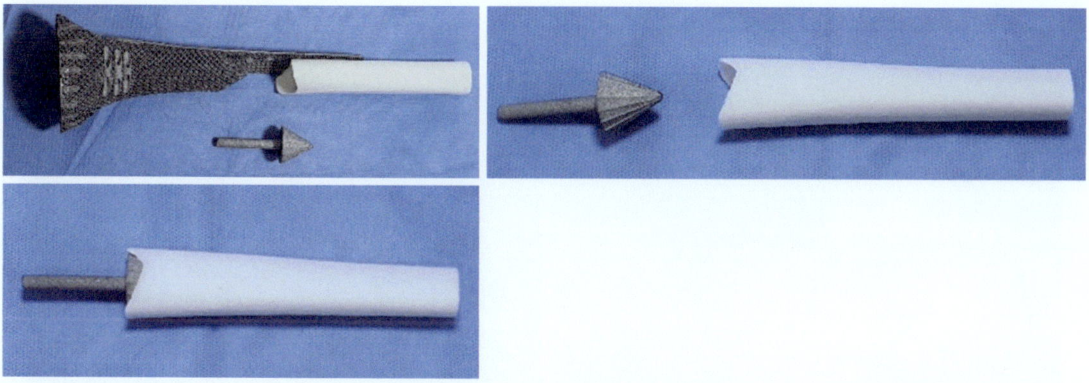

Fig. 26.12 3D-printed conical reamer instrument for deep seating implant at the junction of bone

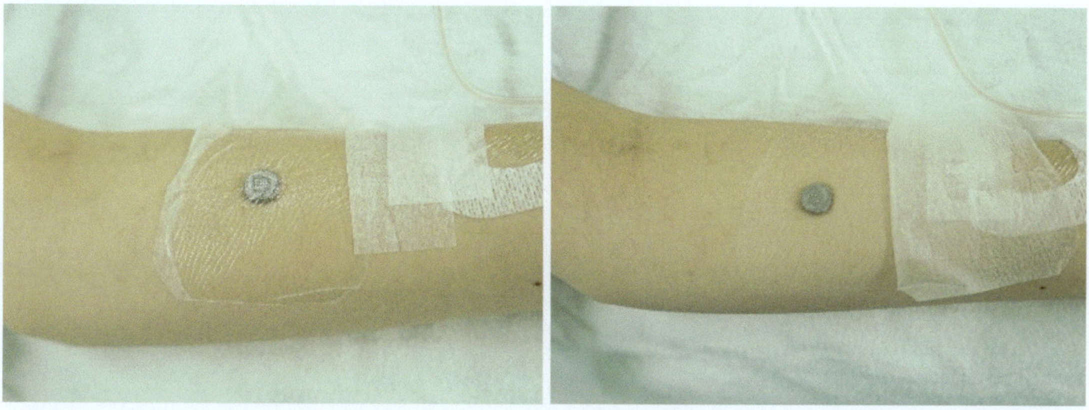

Fig. 26.13 Titanium alloy metal is applied to the patient's forearm the day before surgery to determine the metal allergic reaction

26.5 Operation

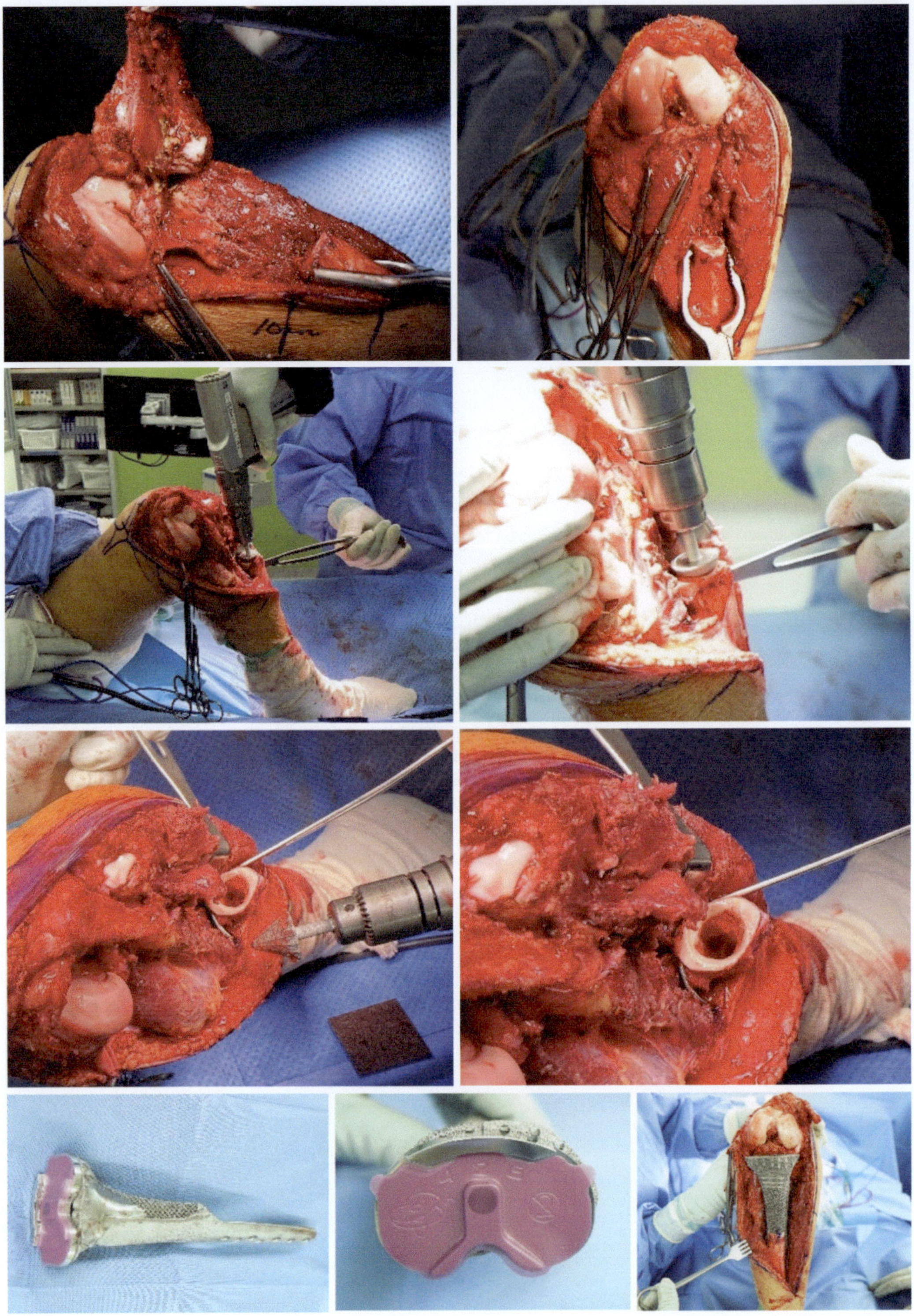

Fig. 26.14 Intraoperative photographs

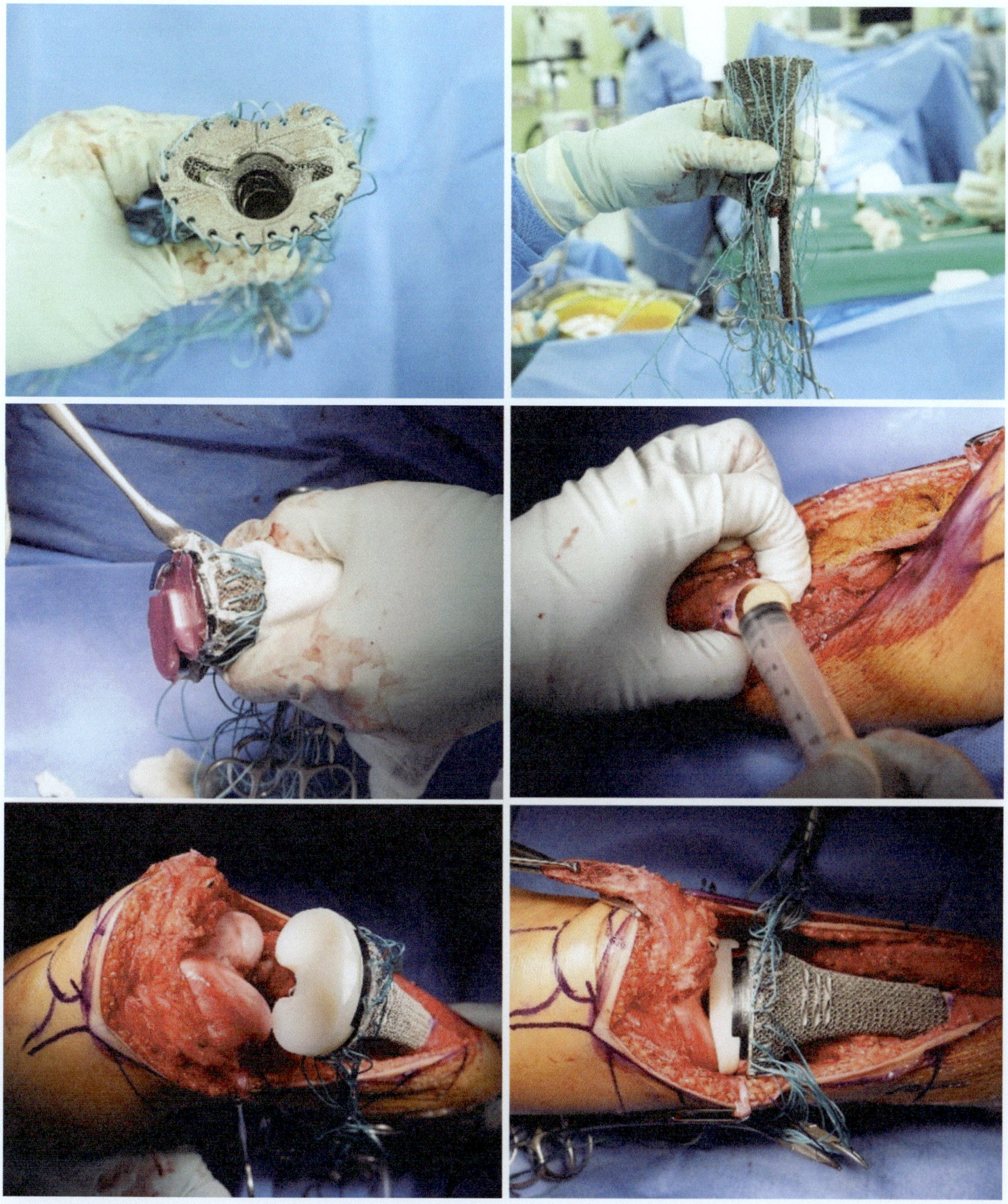

Fig. 26.14 (continued)

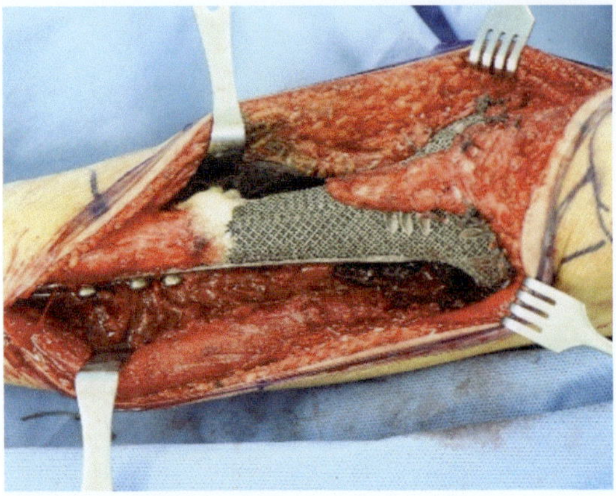

Fig. 26.14 (continued)

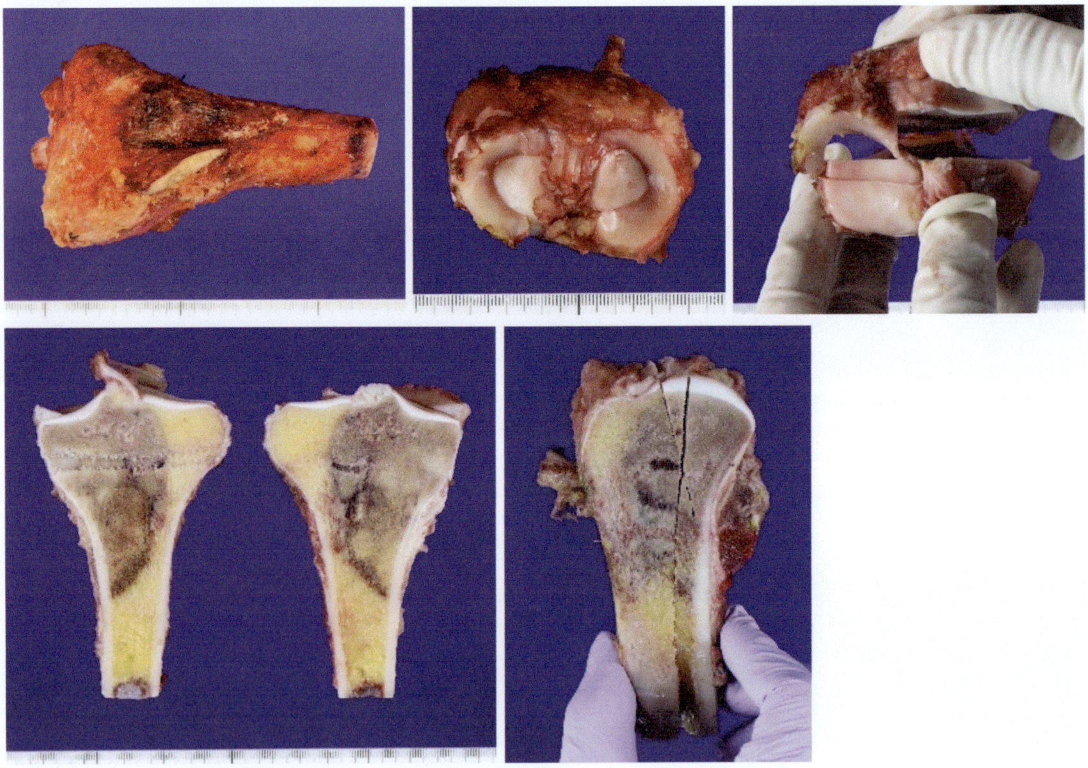

Fig. 26.15 Resected bone tumor

26.6 Postoperative Images

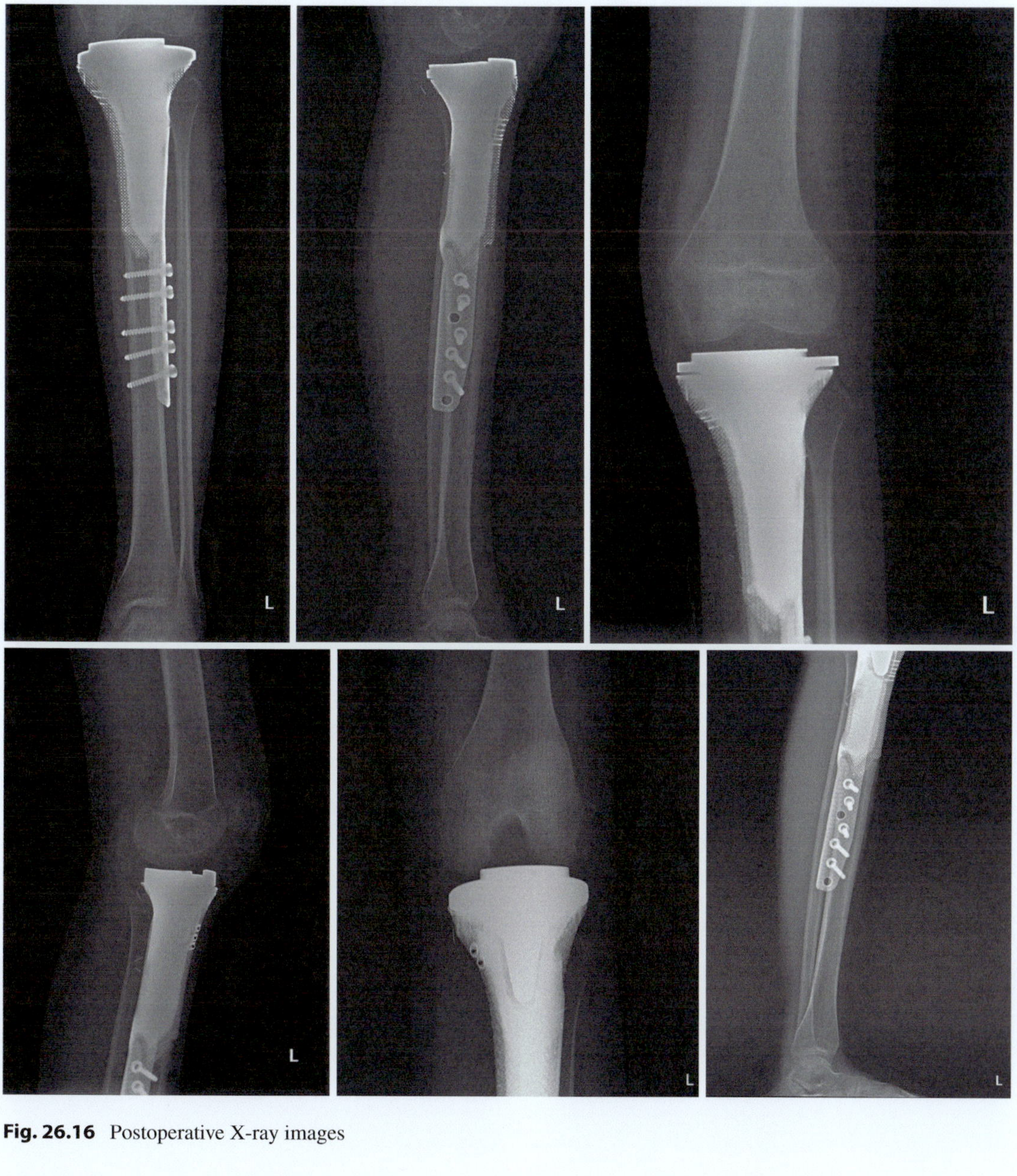

Fig. 26.16 Postoperative X-ray images

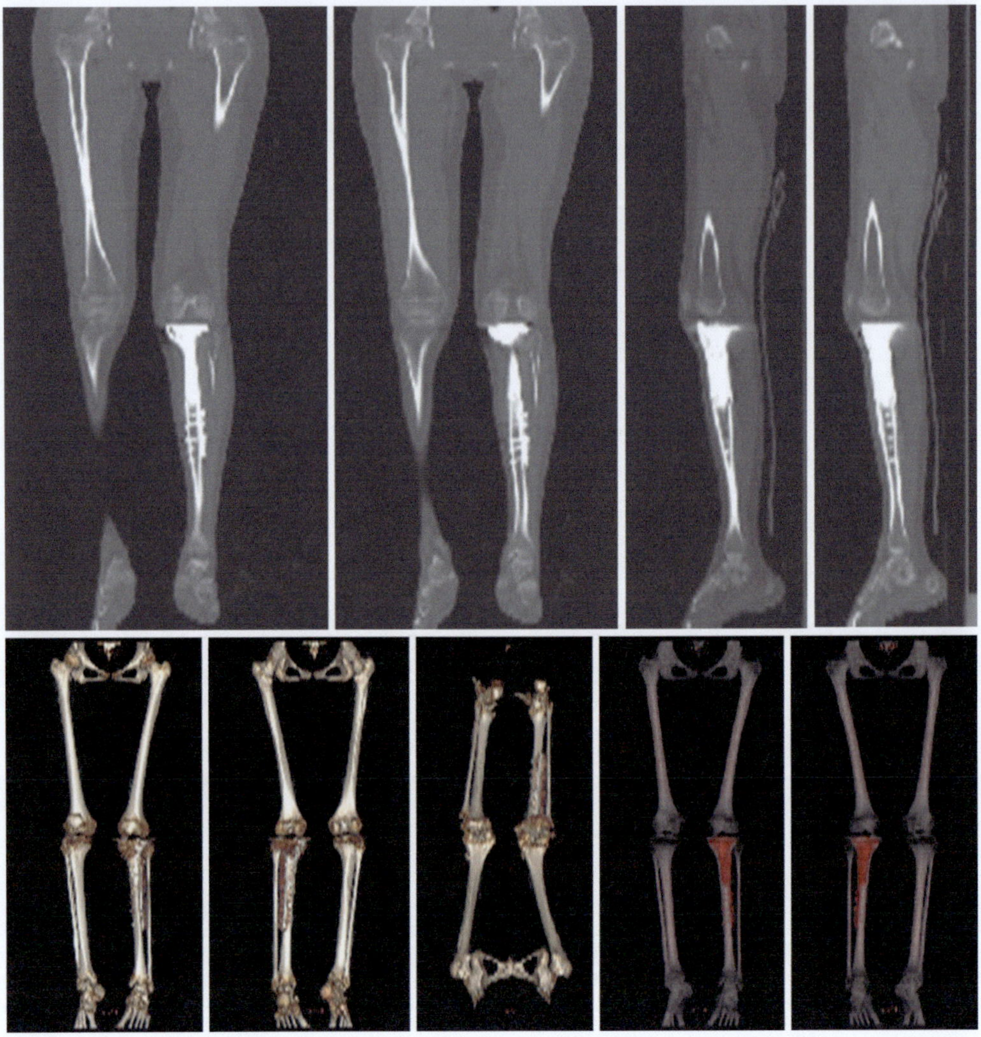

Fig. 26.17 Postoperative CT images

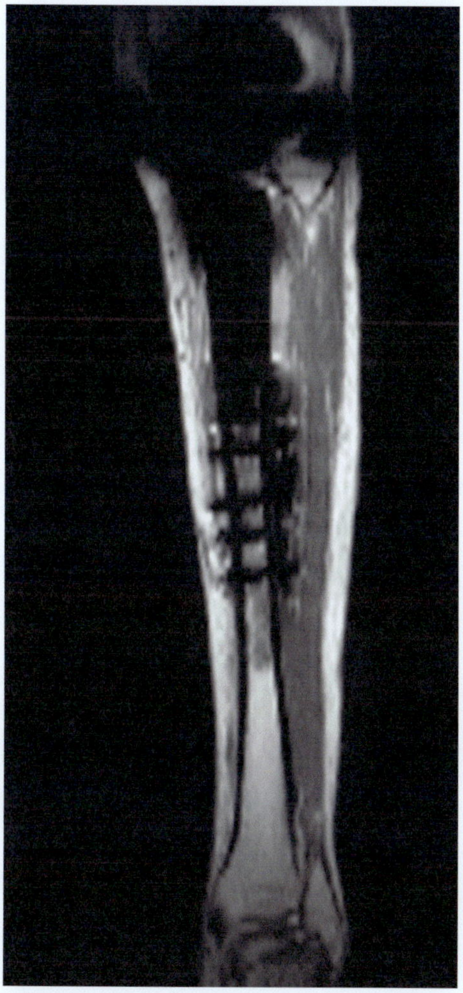

Fig. 26.18 Postoperative MRI image

Part IV

Calcaneus

Patient Case 27: Calcaneus Considering Possible Factors

27

27.1 Patient Case 27

Age/sex	24/male
Location/site	Calcaneus/left
Diagnosis	Desmoid tumor of bone
Preoperative symptom	Difficult walking with heel strike
Preoperative pain score	Resting 2/Working 7
BMI (height/weight)	21.18 (175.2/65)
Past history	Physical therapy at a local clinic at 15 months ago
Present illness	No trauma history Visited after radiologic examination due to worsening foot pain while on military duty in the Air Force Diagnosed by incisional biopsy

27.2 Preoperative Images

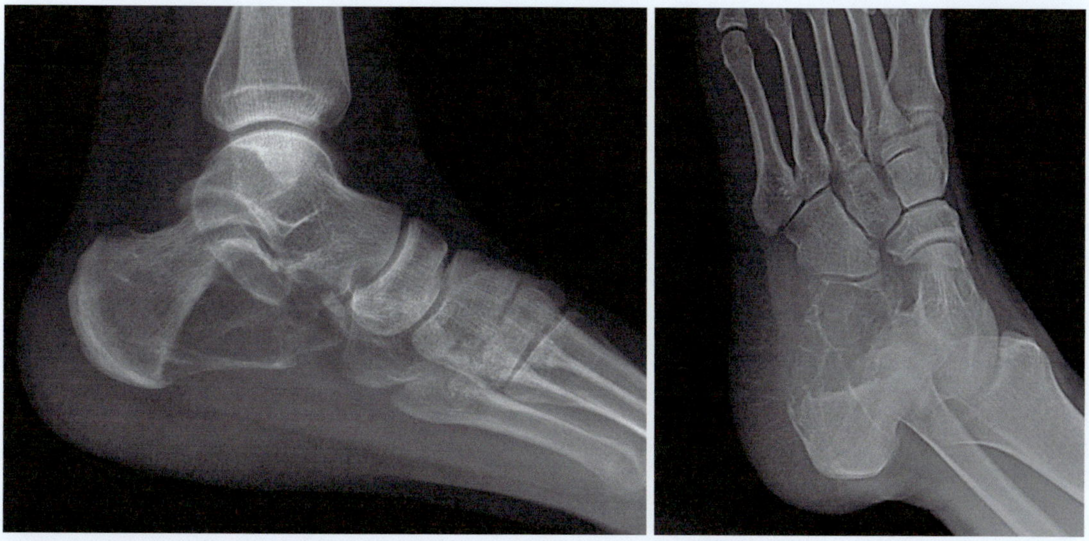

Fig. 27.1 Preoperative X-ray images

H.-G. Kang, *Clinical Atlas of 3D Printing Bone Reconstruction*,
https://doi.org/10.1007/978-981-16-2043-0_27

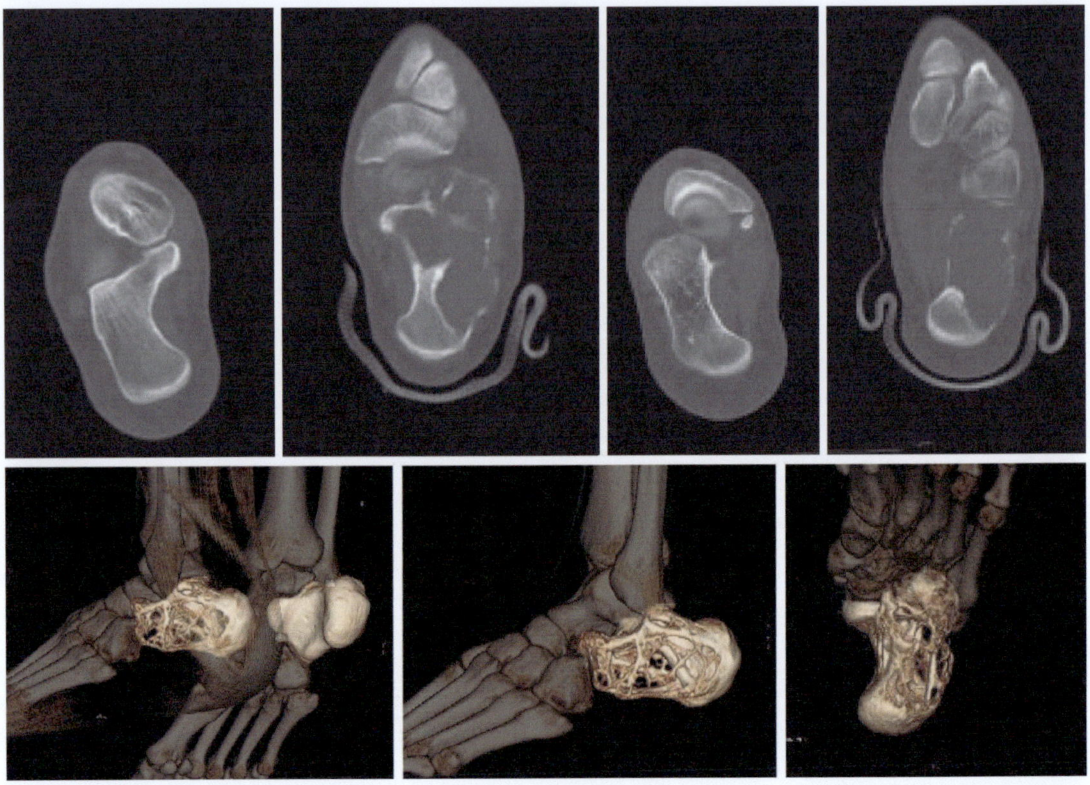

Fig. 27.2 Preoperative CT images

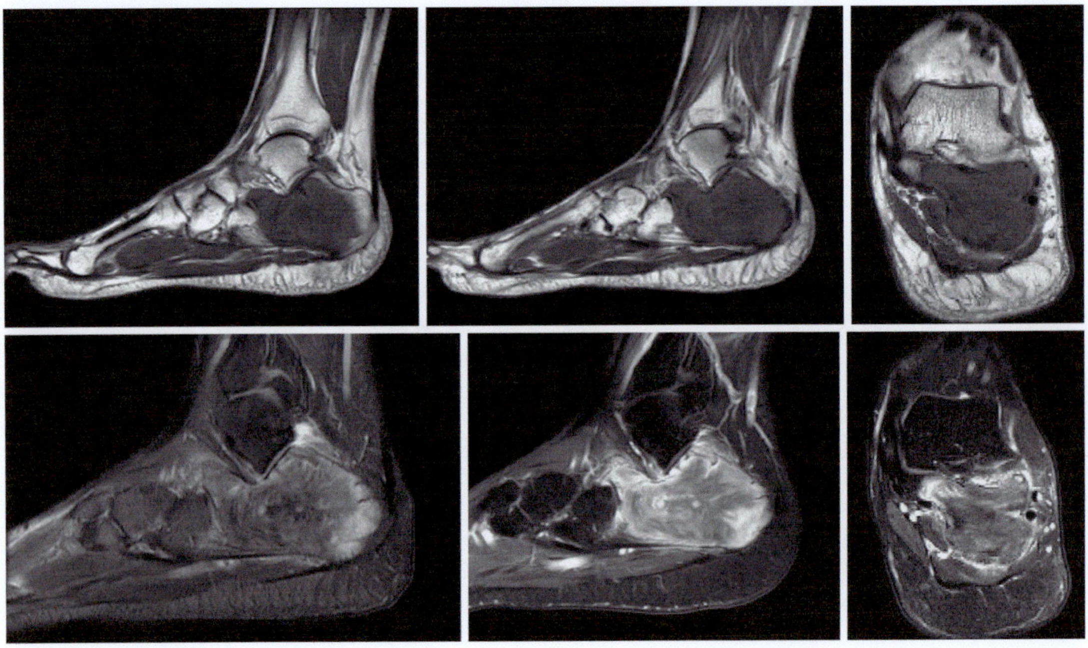

Fig. 27.3 Preoperative MRI images

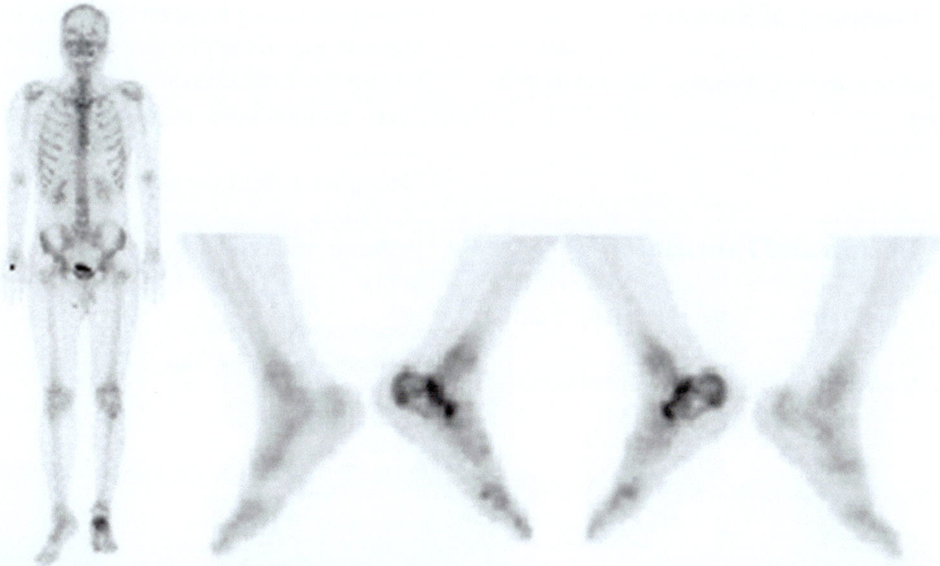

Fig. 27.4 Preoperative bone scan images

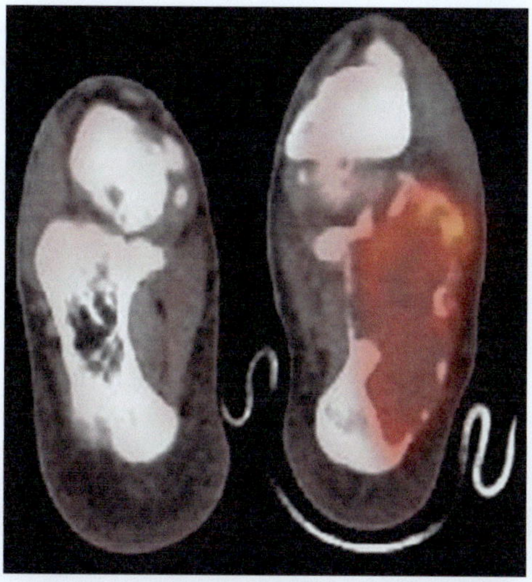

Fig. 27.5 Preoperative PET-CT image

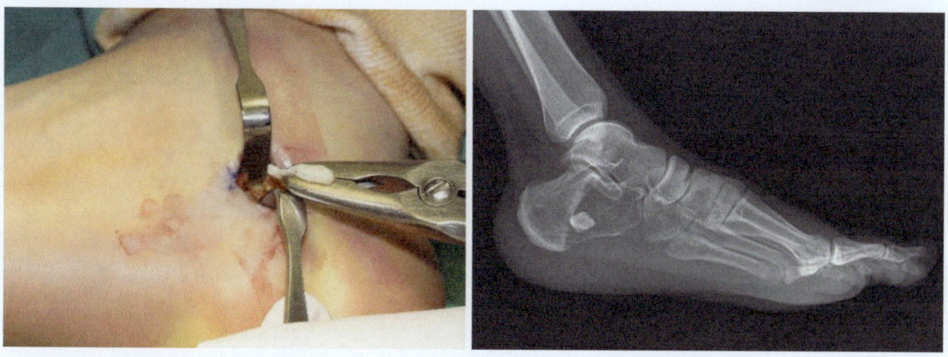

Fig. 27.6 PMMA cementing for sealing of bone biopsy track

27.3 Planning of Surgery

Total excision except Achilles' tendon attachment area

3D-printed calcaneus implant

27.4 Design and Fabrication

- Using the normal side calcaneus (mirror images)
- Save the Achilles' tendon attachment bone
- Slightly reducing the anteroposterior length
- Mesh shape enough to pass the suture needle for soft tissue attachment
- Screw fixation holes in preparation for subtalar arthritis
- Flatten the sole of the calcaneus to reduce the arch angle.
- Reduced front-to-back length to avoid heel injury

- Implant measurement
- Implant weight (g): 104
- Size (mm): 63

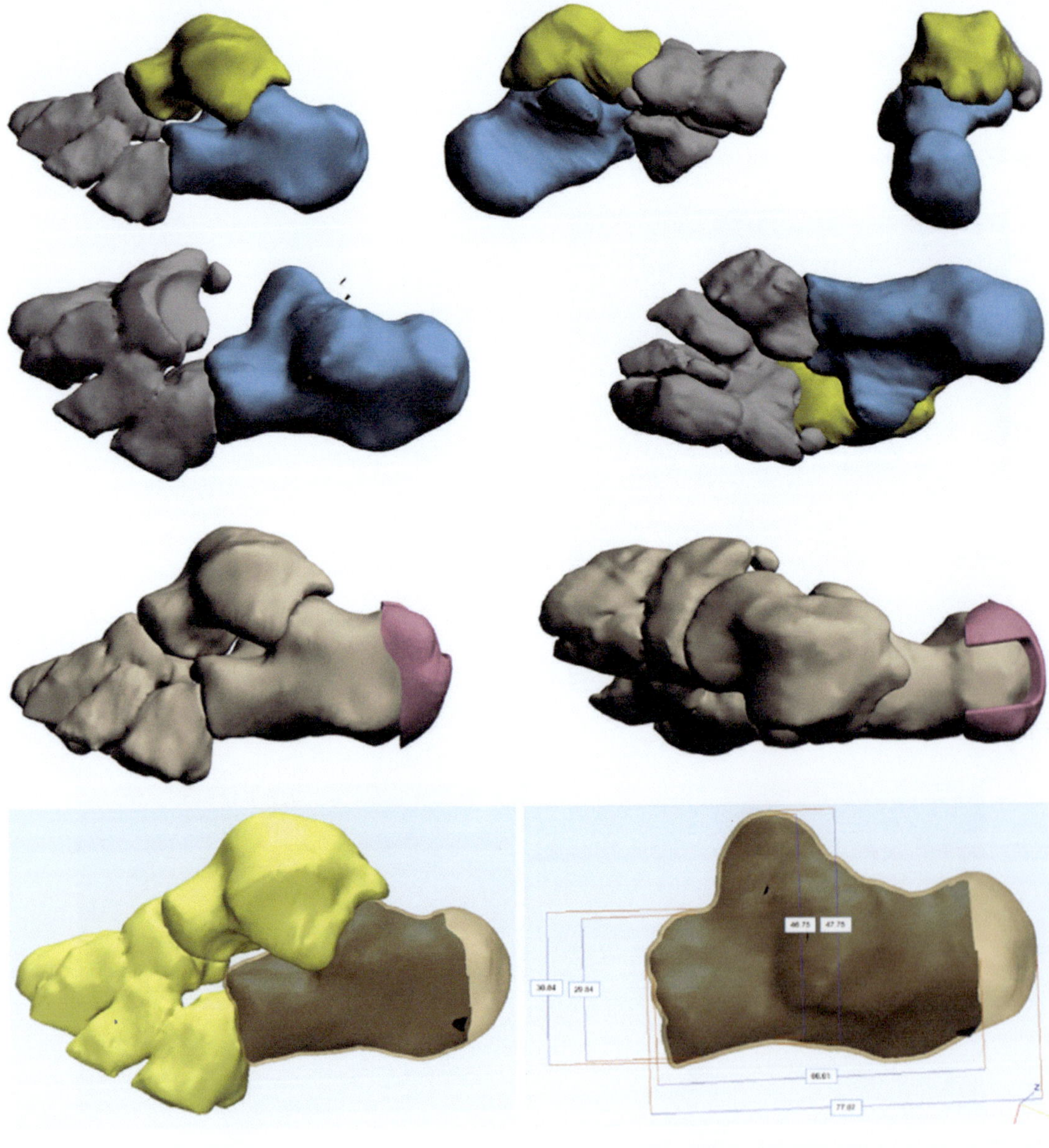

Fig. 27.7 Cutting guide design

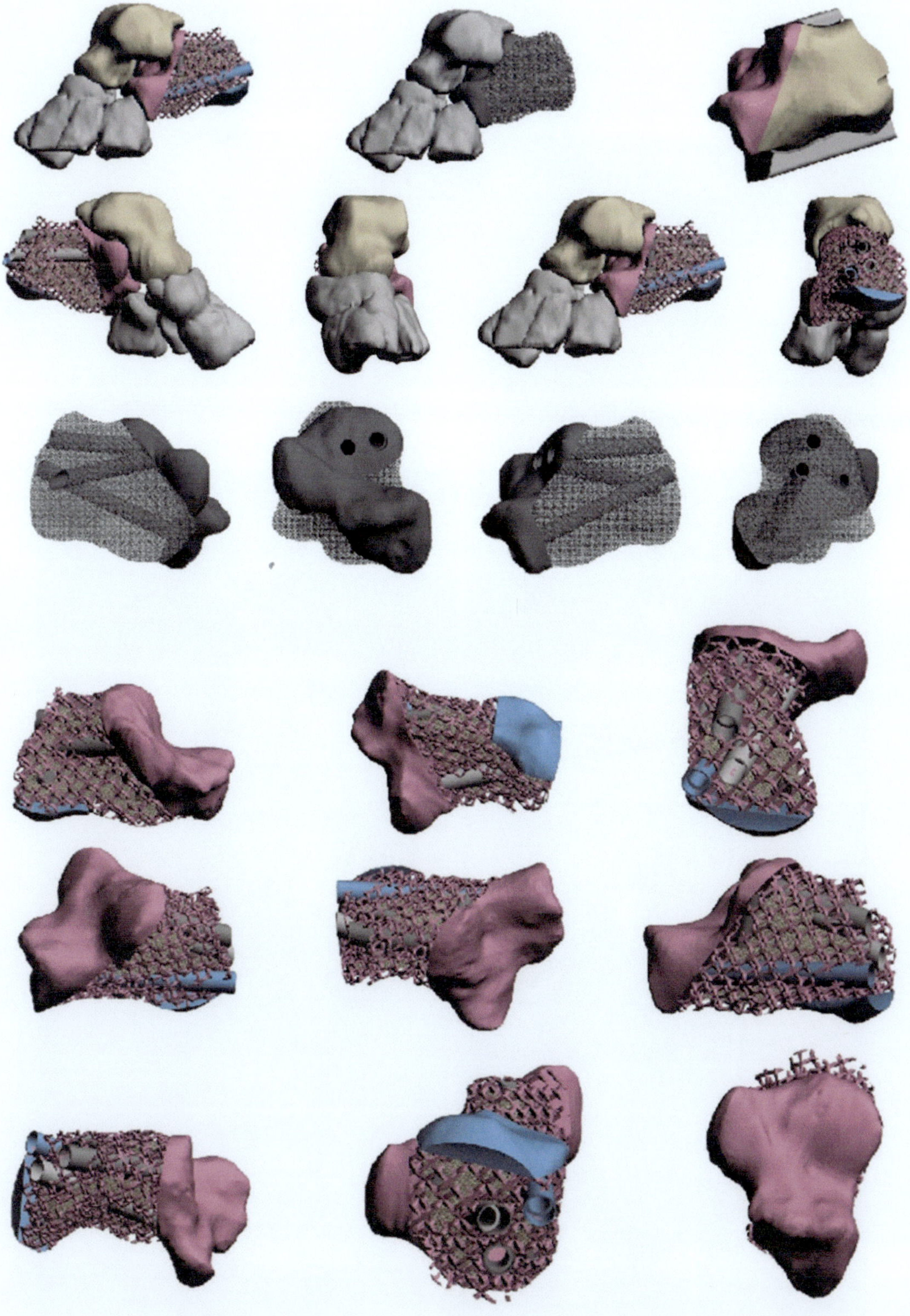

Fig. 27.8 Implant design

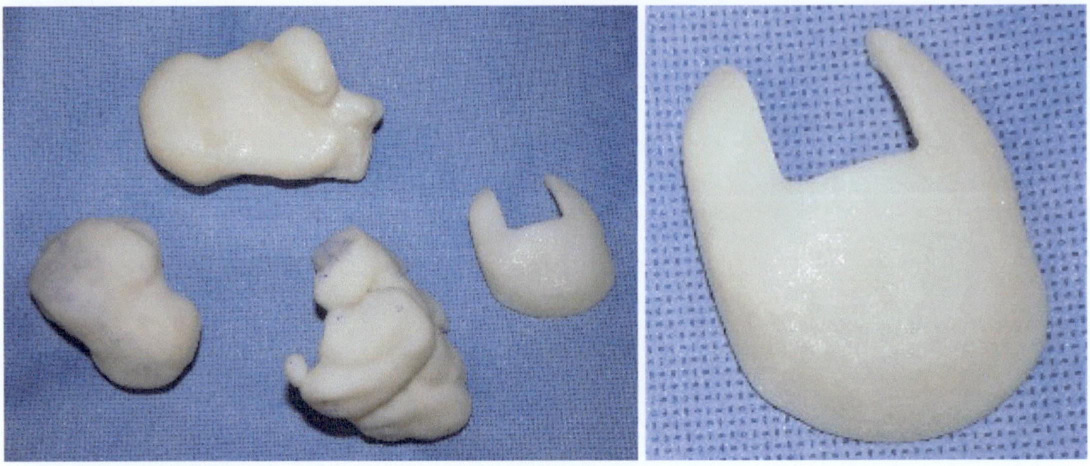

Fig. 27.9 Printed cutting guide and models

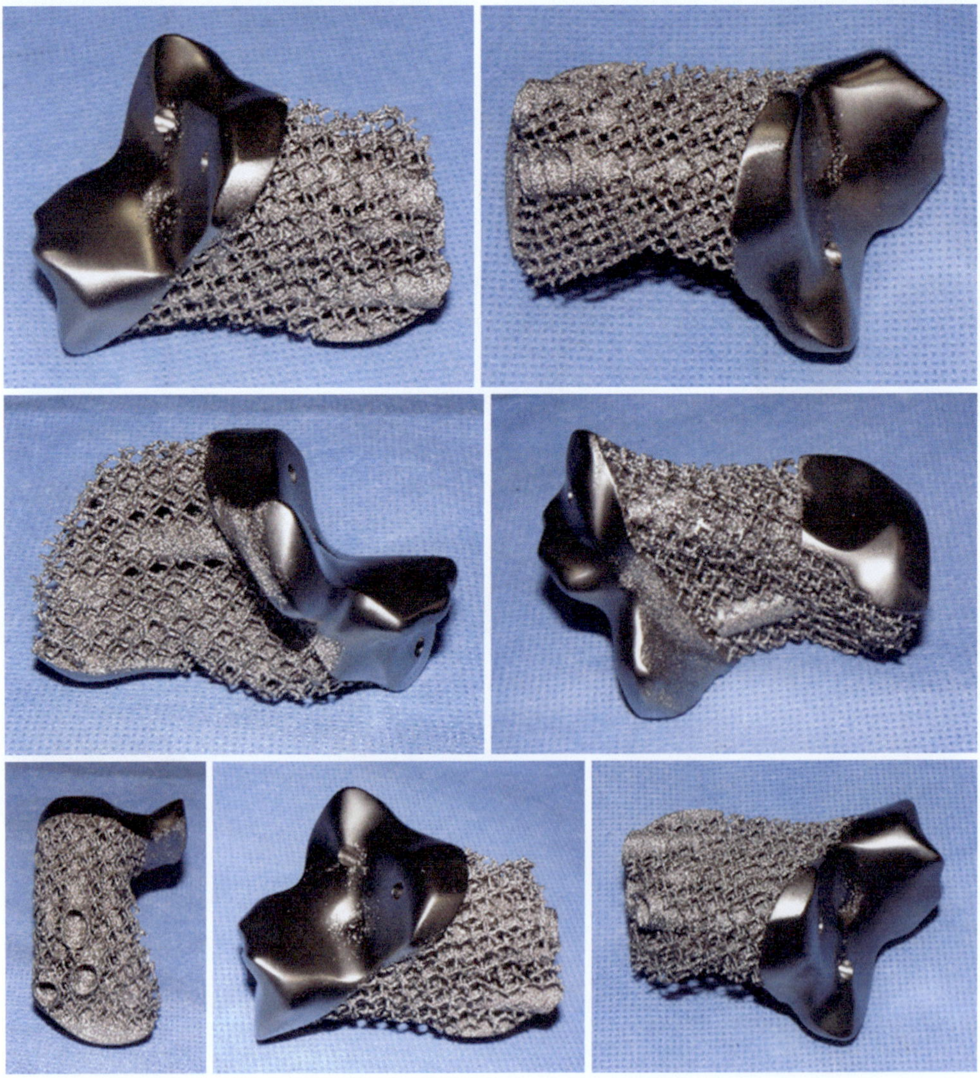

Fig. 27.10 Printed implant

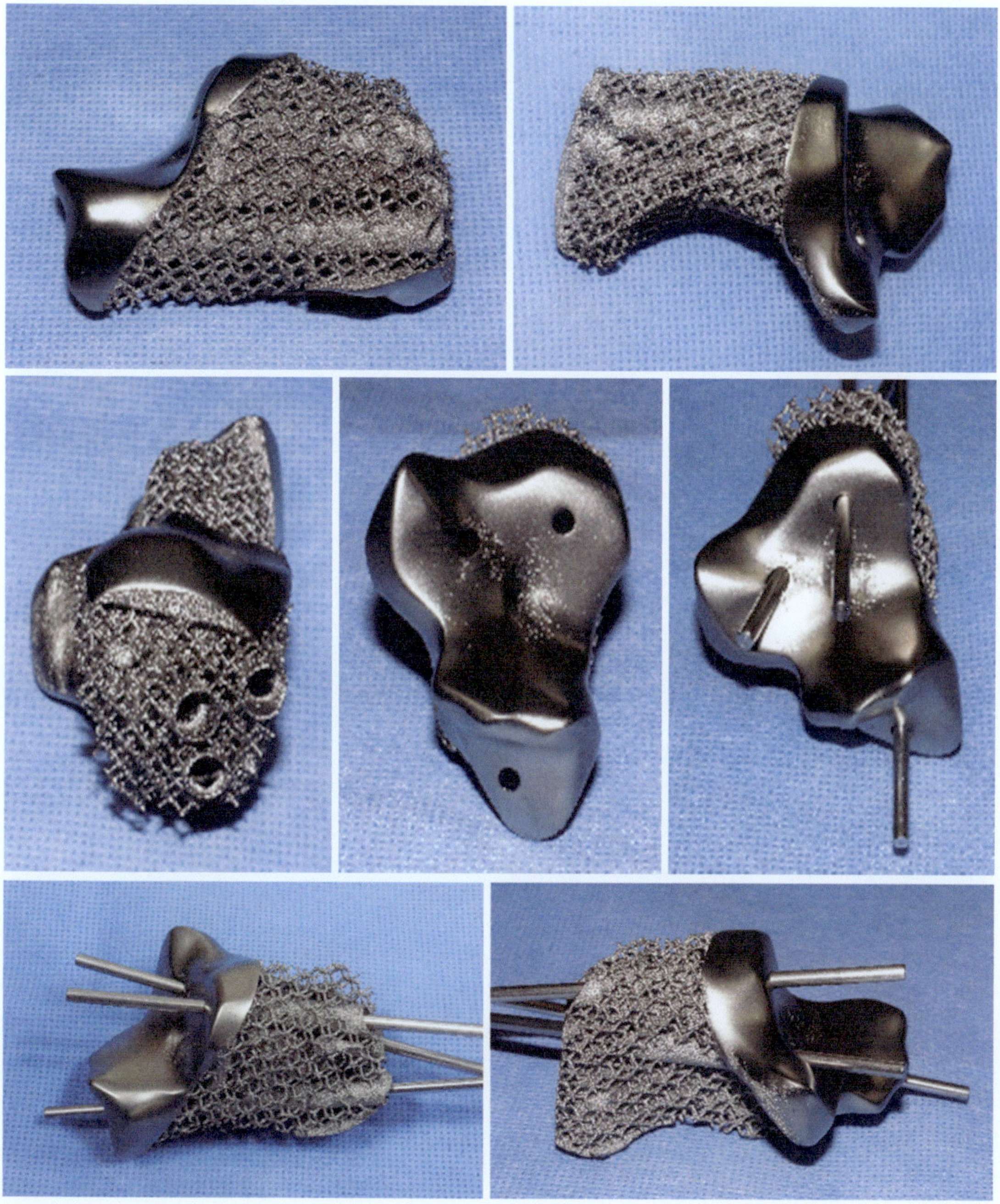

Fig. 27.10 (continued)

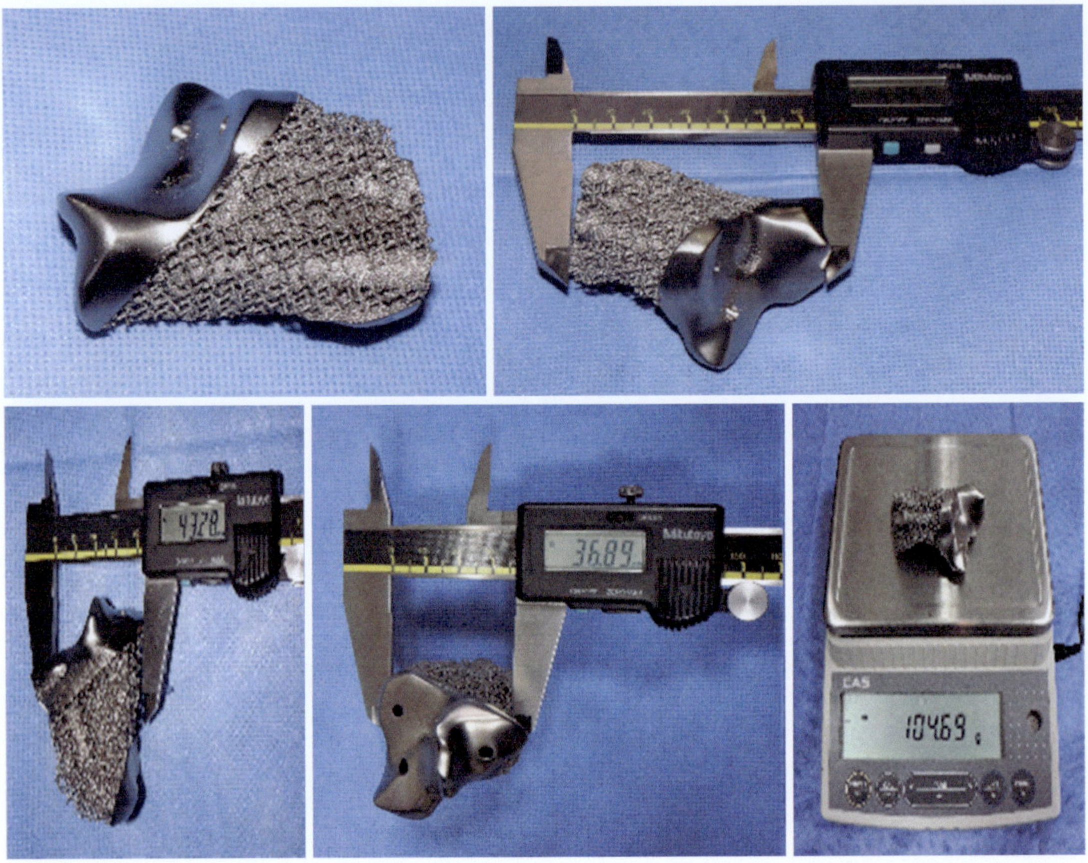

Fig. 27.10 (continued)

27.5 Operation

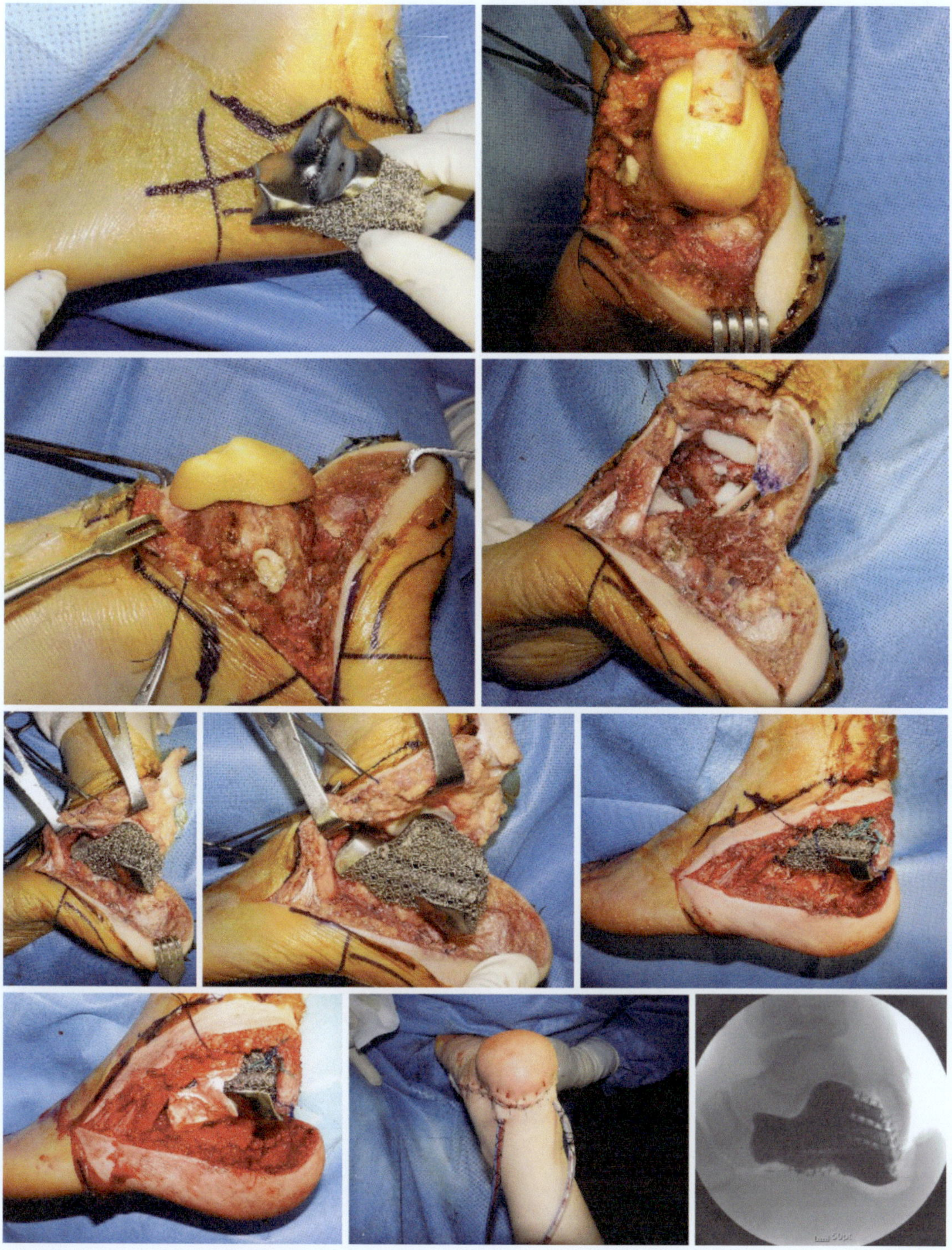

Fig. 27.11 Intraoperative photographs

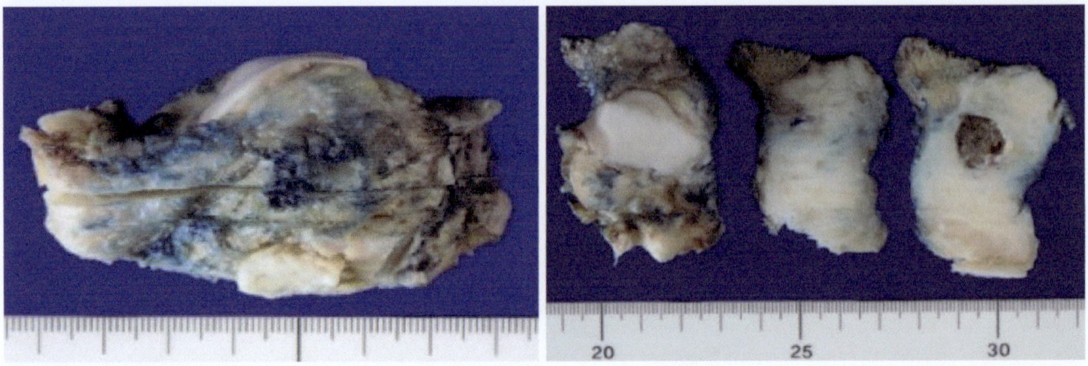

Fig. 27.12 Resected tumor

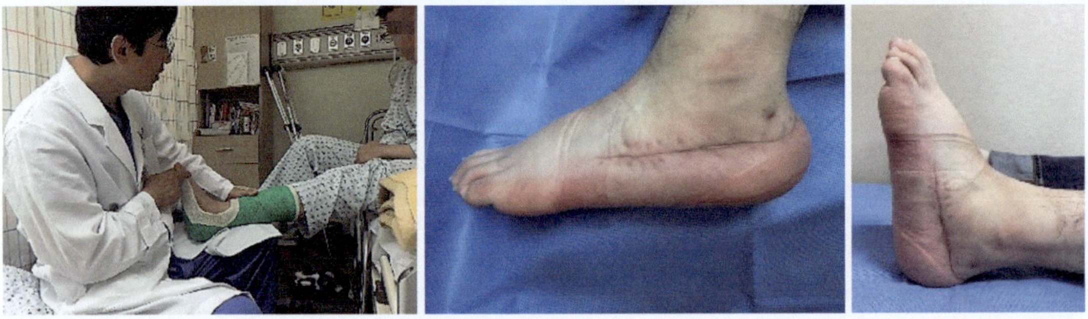

Fig. 27.13 Postoperative care photographs

27.6 Postoperative Images

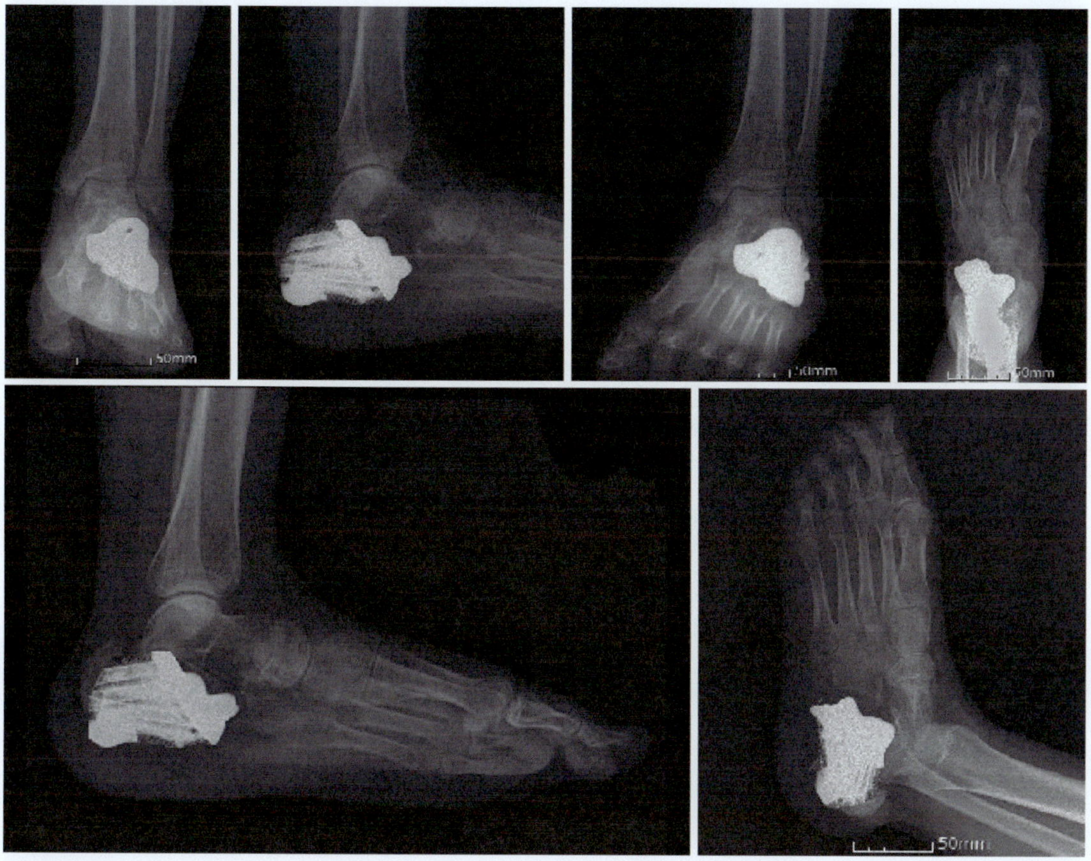

Fig. 27.14 Postoperative X-ray images

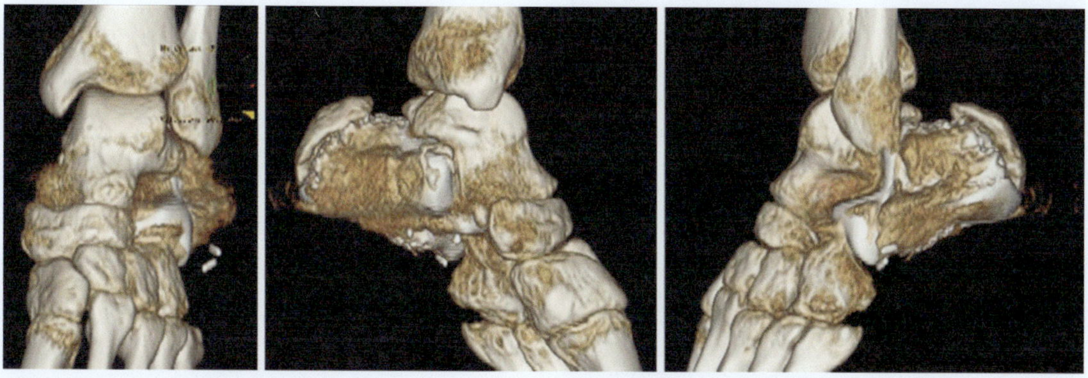

Fig. 27.15 Postoperative CT images

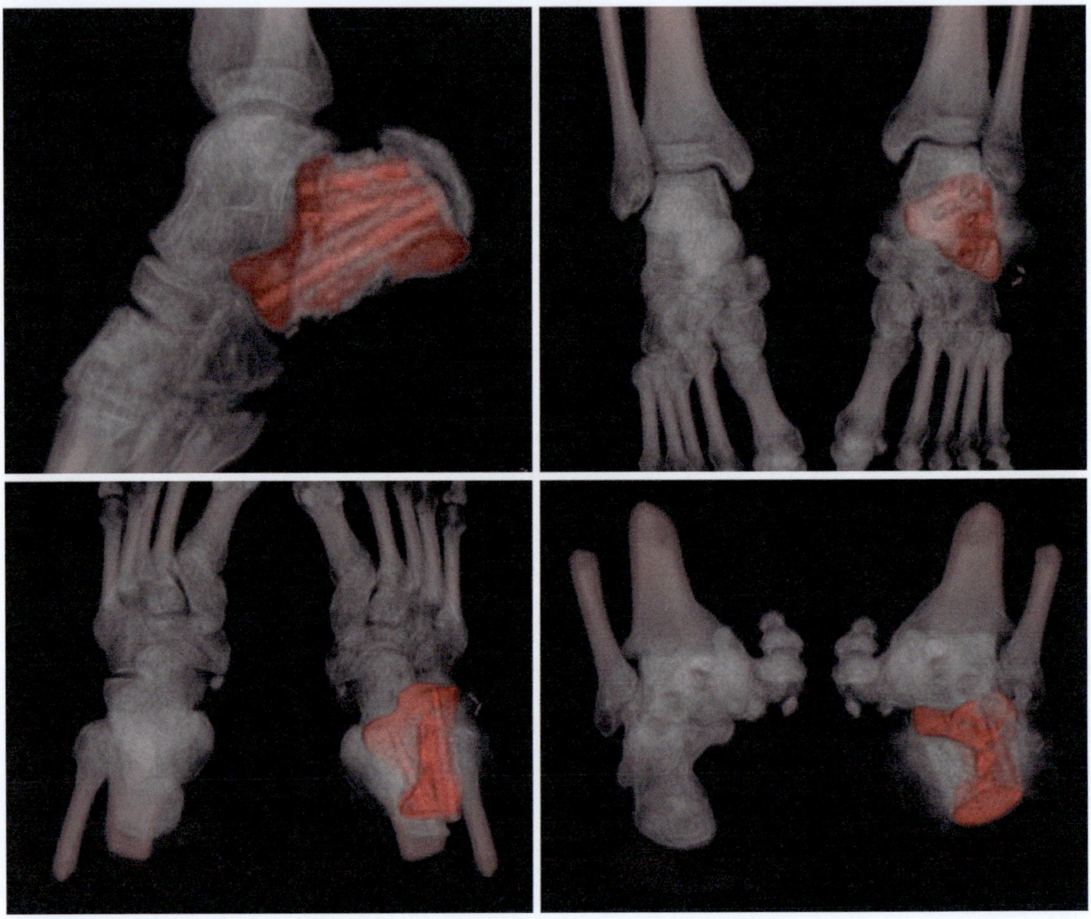

Fig. 27.15 (continued)

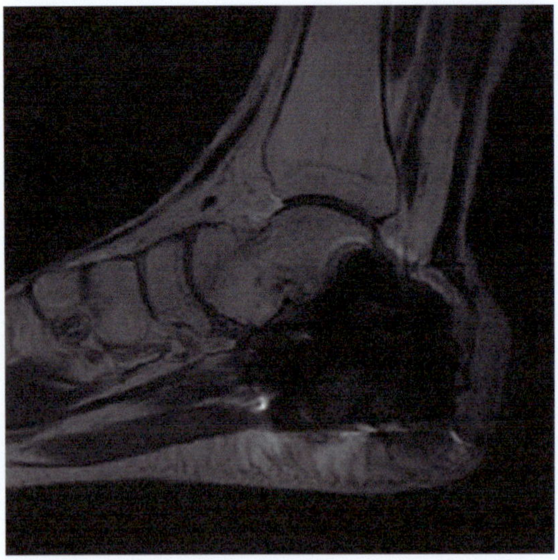

Fig. 27.16 Postoperative MRI image: walking well even though it has been more than 5 years after surgery

Part V

Scapula

Patient Case 28: Scapula Combined with Reverse Shoulder Arthroplasty

28

28.1 Patient Case 28

Age/sex	61/female
Location/site	Scapular/right
Diagnosis	Chondrosarcoma, grade 2
Preoperative symptom	Palpable mass
Preoperative pain score	Resting 0/Working 6
BMI (height/weight)	18.18 (154.7/43.5)
Past history	Considered a frozen shoulder Treated with oriental medicine for 6 months
Present illness	Planning surgery with radiological diagnosis

H.-G. Kang, *Clinical Atlas of 3D Printing Bone Reconstruction*,
https://doi.org/10.1007/978-981-16-2043-0_28

28.2 Preoperative Images

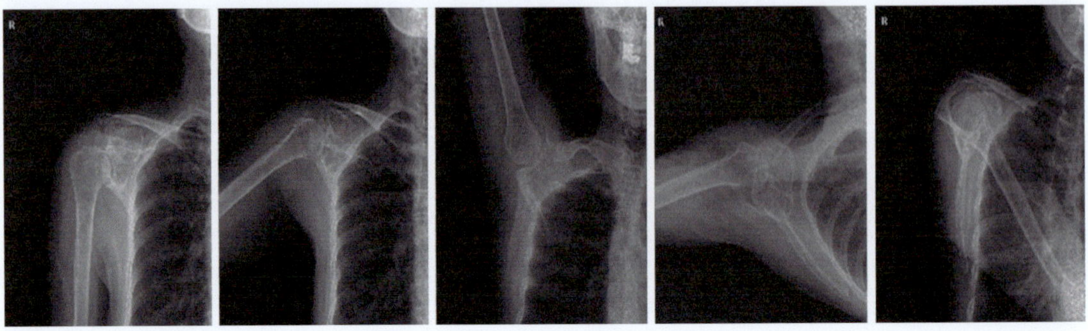

Fig. 28.1 Preoperative X-ray images

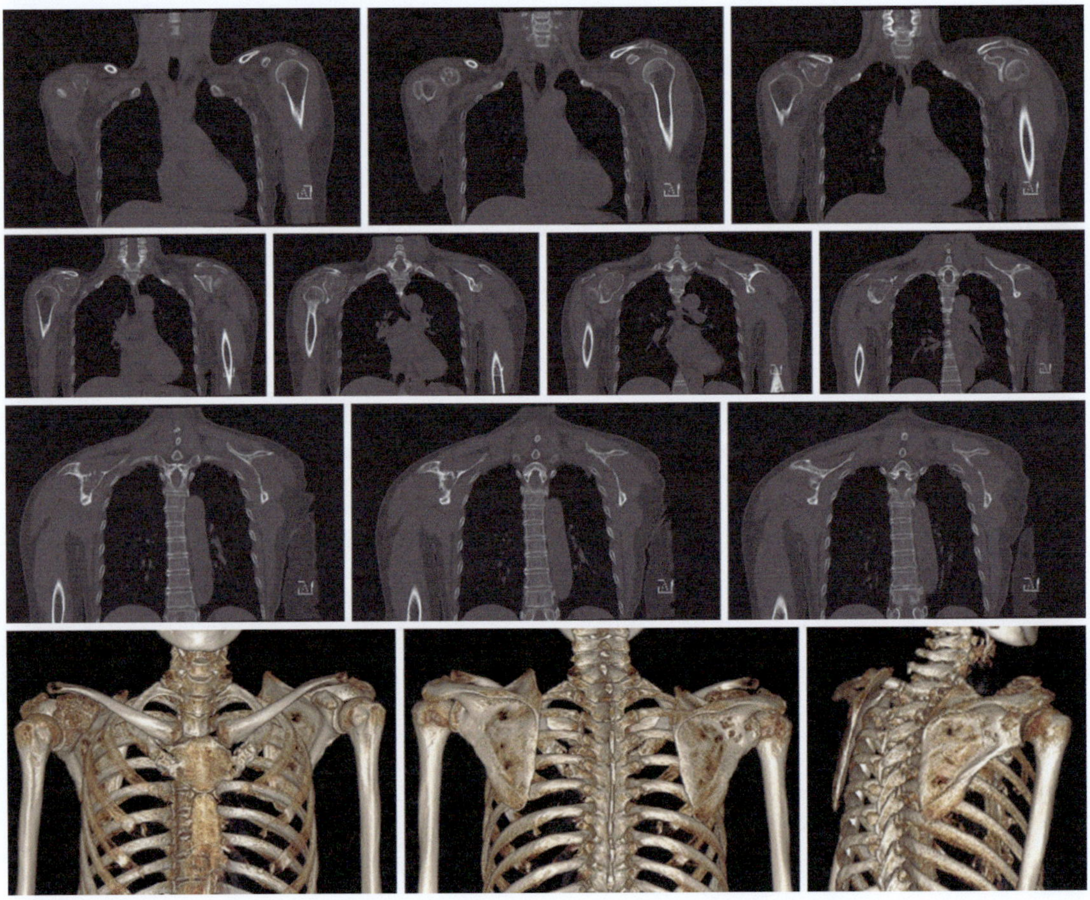

Fig. 28.2 Preoperative CT images

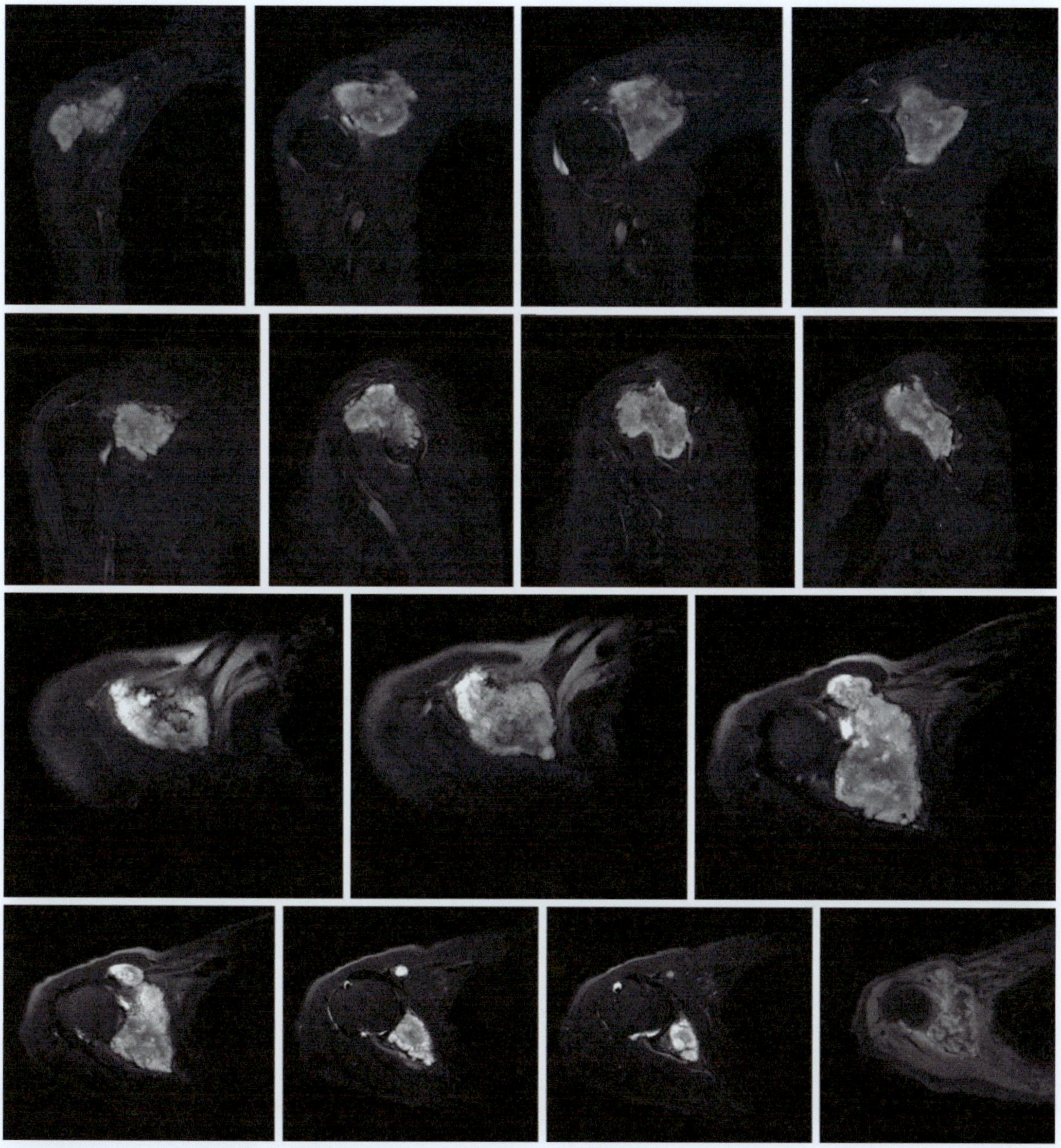

Fig. 28.3 Preoperative MRI images

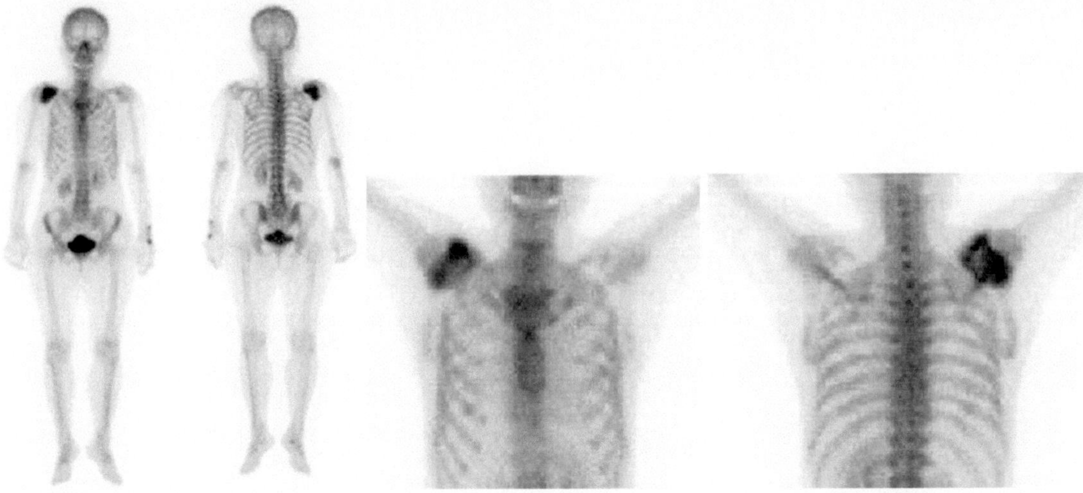

Fig. 28.4 Preoperative bone scan images

28.3 Planning of Surgery

3D printed scapular implant + reverse shoulder arthroplasty

28.4 Design and Fabrication

28.4.1 Resection

- Preserve medial border of scapular with levator and rhomboid muscle attachments
- Preserve acromial end with deltoid muscle partially

28.4.2 Guide

28.4.3 3D-Printed Implant

Glenoid:

- Reverse arthroplasty
- The SMR® Shoulder System of Lima Corporate
- Metal plate of SMR® glenoid component attached 3D-printed scapular with PMMA bone cement

Acromion:

- Size reduction of acromion and scapular spine not to skin irritation
- Acromial end cortical bone preserve to easily connect 3D-printed acromion
- Multiple suture holes
- Thin and smooth polishing of subacromial surface
- Meshed upper surface and clavicular border for easy soft tissue adhesion
- Blunt angle of acromial end

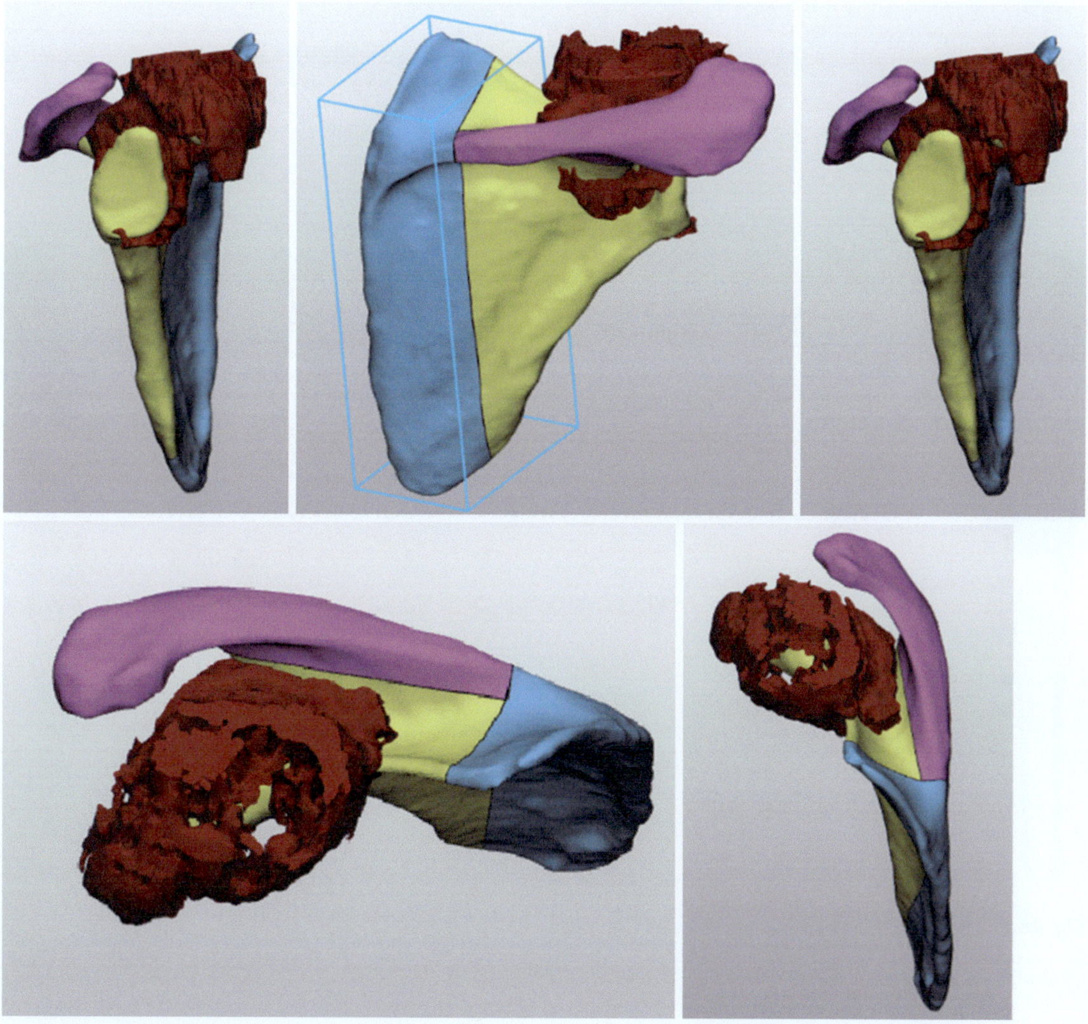

Fig. 28.5 Modeling

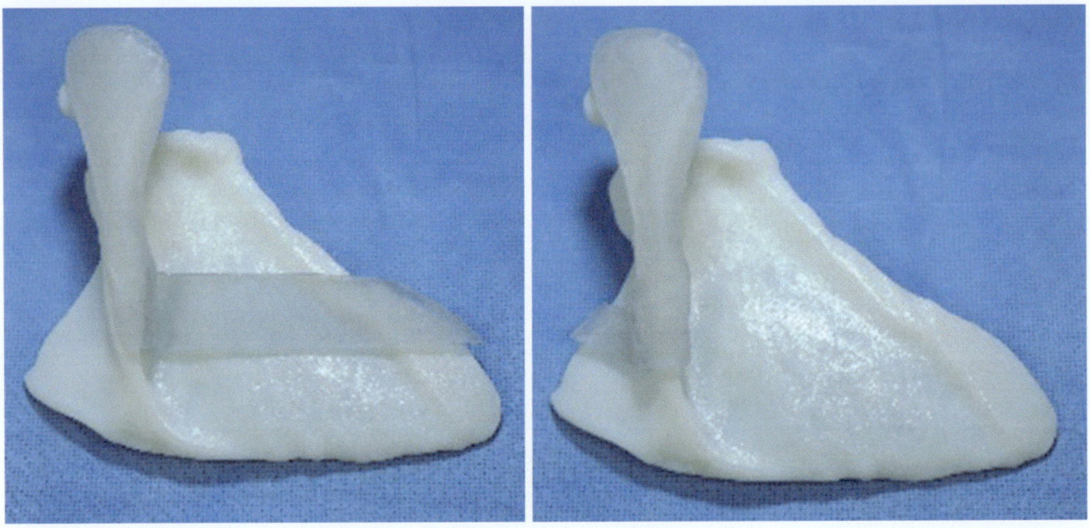

Fig. 28.6 Bone cutting guide: the reference points are scapular back and acromion

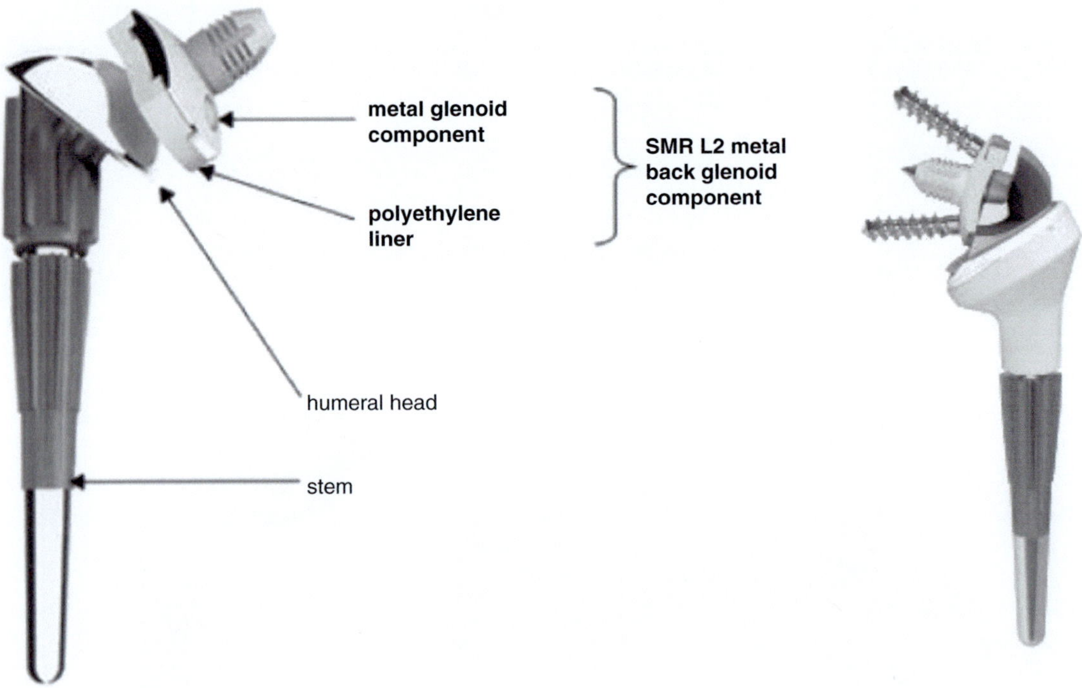

Fig. 28.7 The SMR® Shoulder System of Lima Corporate

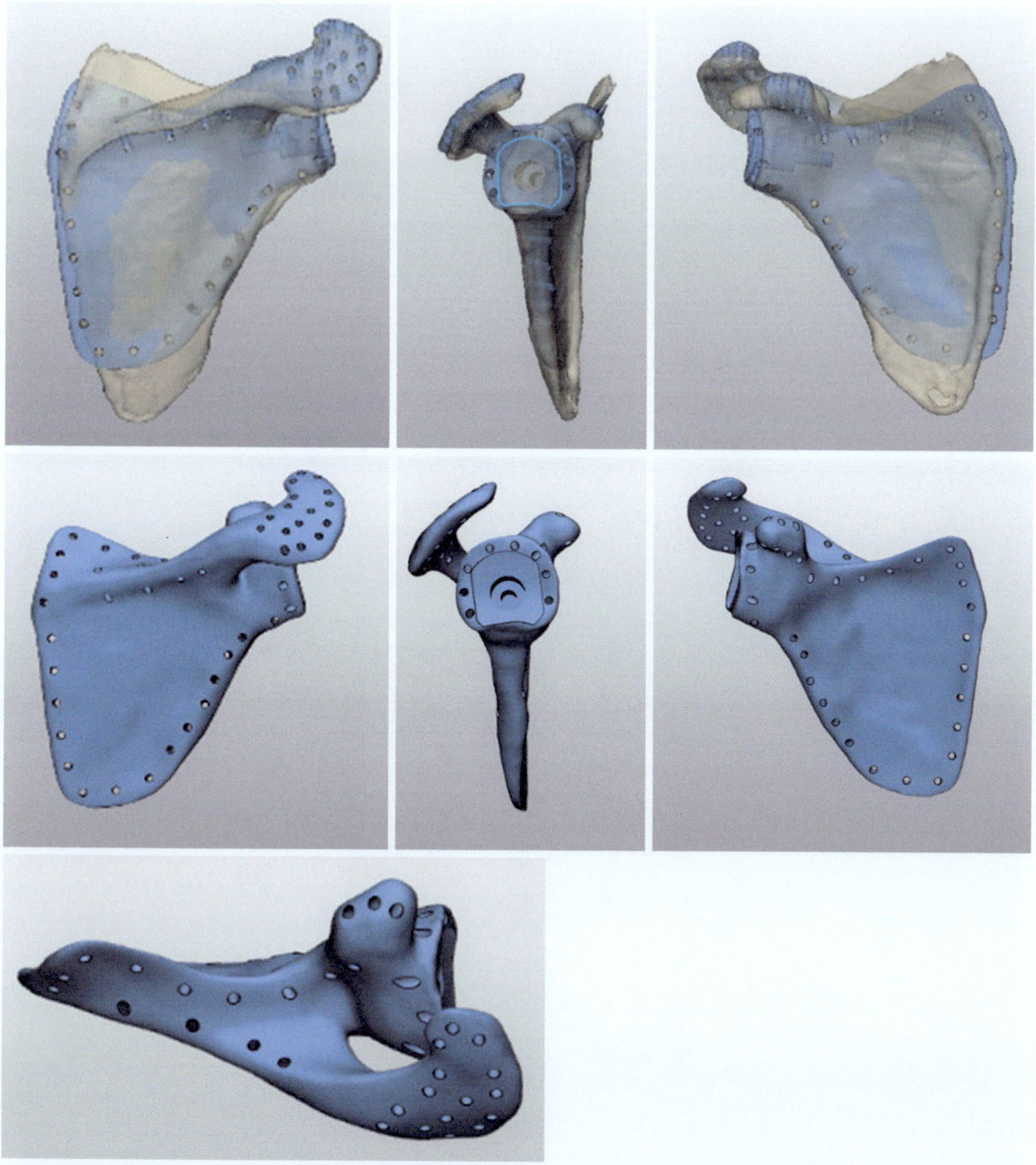

Fig. 28.8 The modeling of 3D-printed implant

Coracoid process:

- Size reduction
- Multiple suture holes
- Meshed surface for soft tissue adhesion

Scapular spine:

- Size reduction
- Wider scapular notch space
- Multiple suture holes

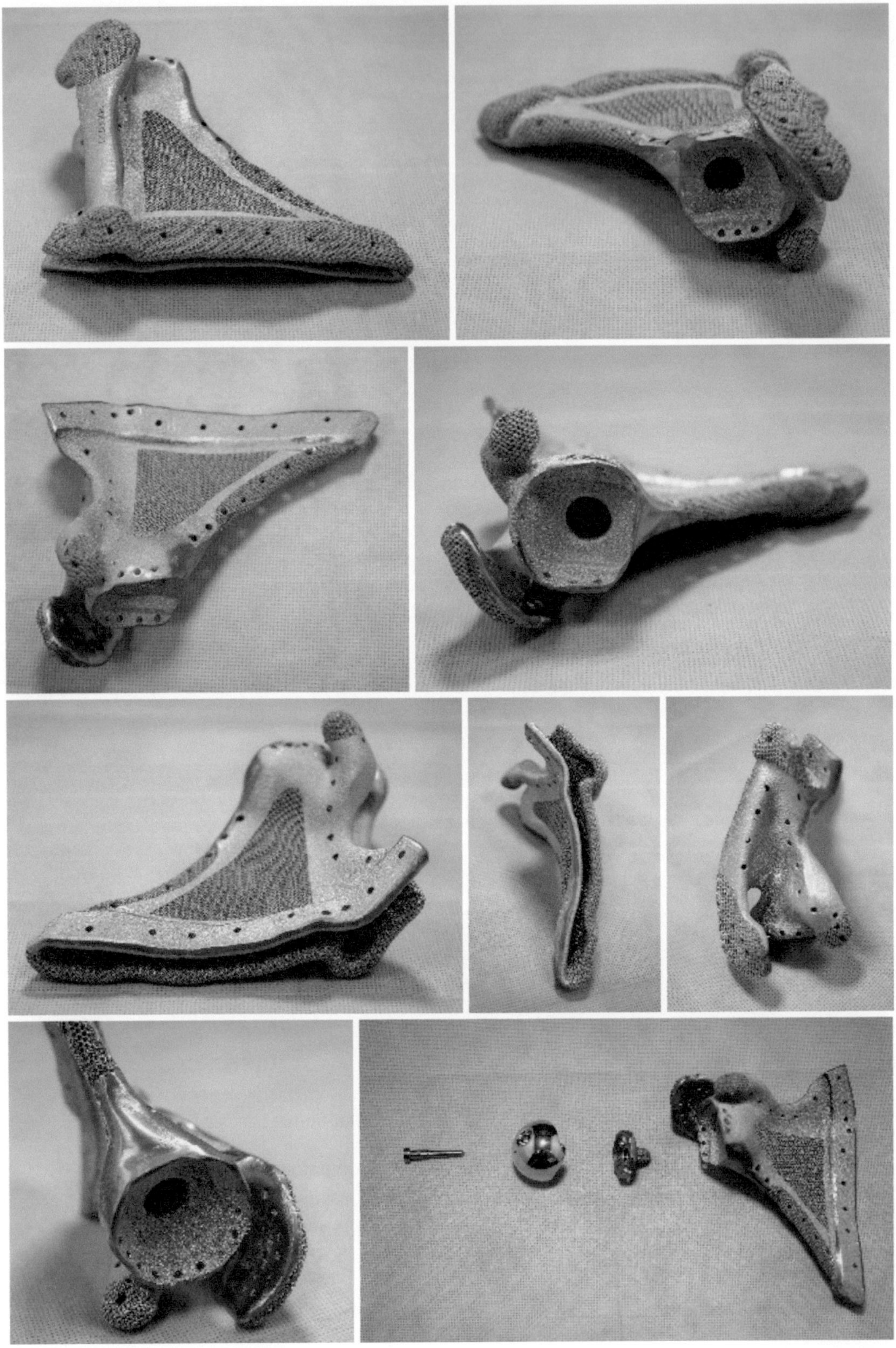

Fig. 28.9 The 3D-printed implant

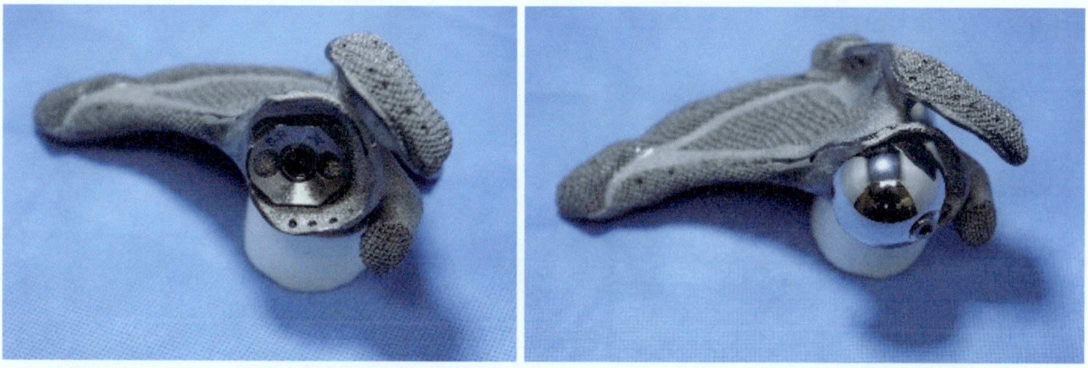

Fig. 28.9 (continued)

Anterior and posterior surface: thin separator border with partial meshed surface

Medial border:

- Groove for insert of medial cut border
- Multiple suture holes

- Implant measurement
- Implant weight (g): 326
- Size (mm): 132

28.5 Operation

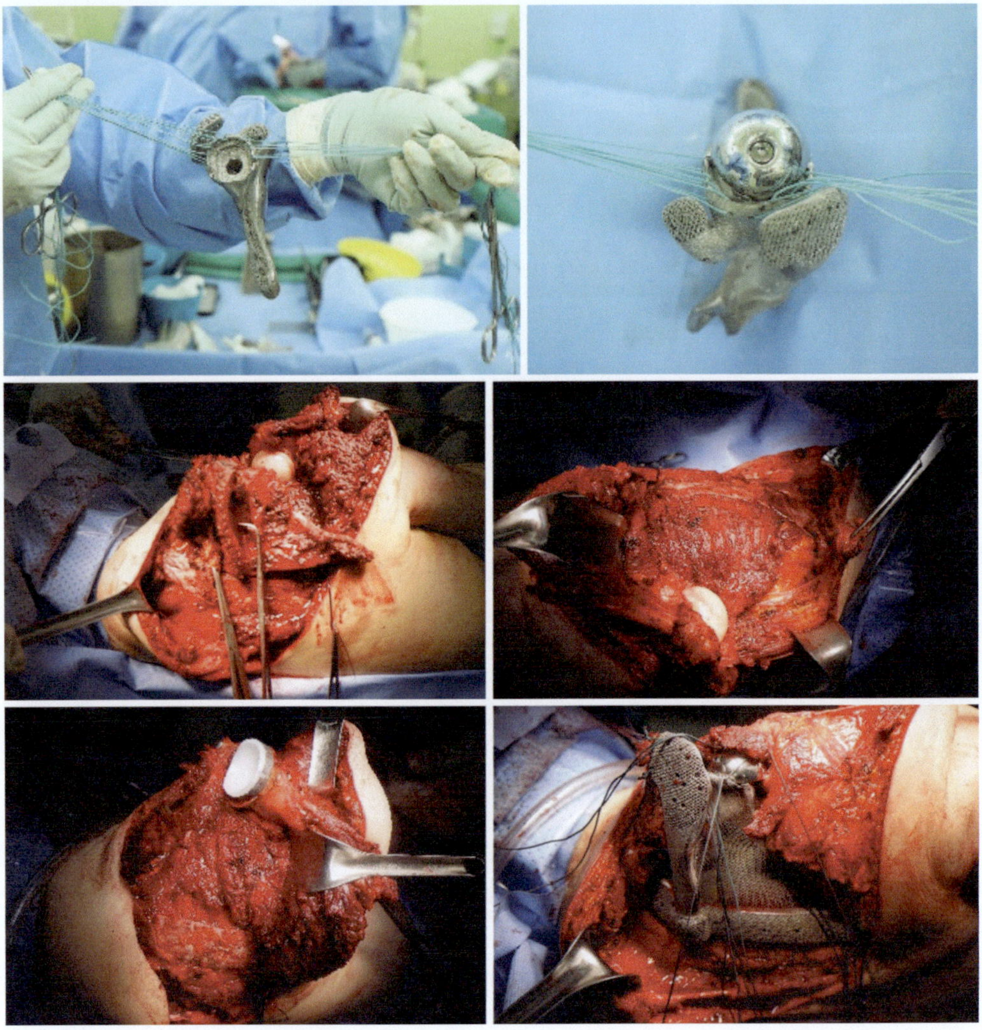

Fig. 28.10 Intraoperative photographs

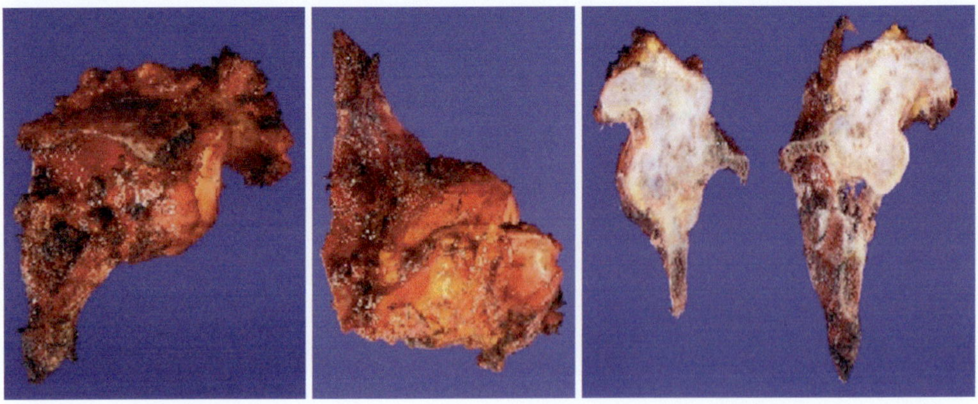

Fig. 28.11 The resected tumor

28.6 Postoperative Images

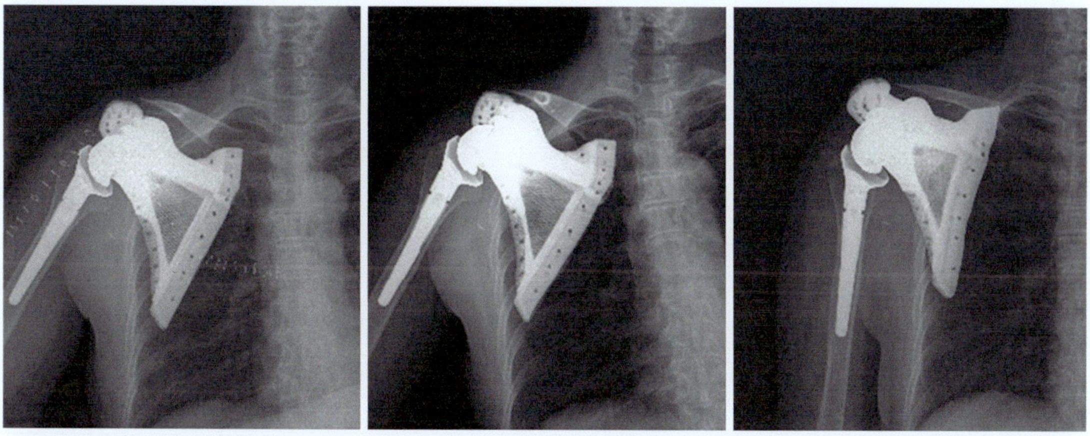

Fig. 28.12 Postoperative X-ray images

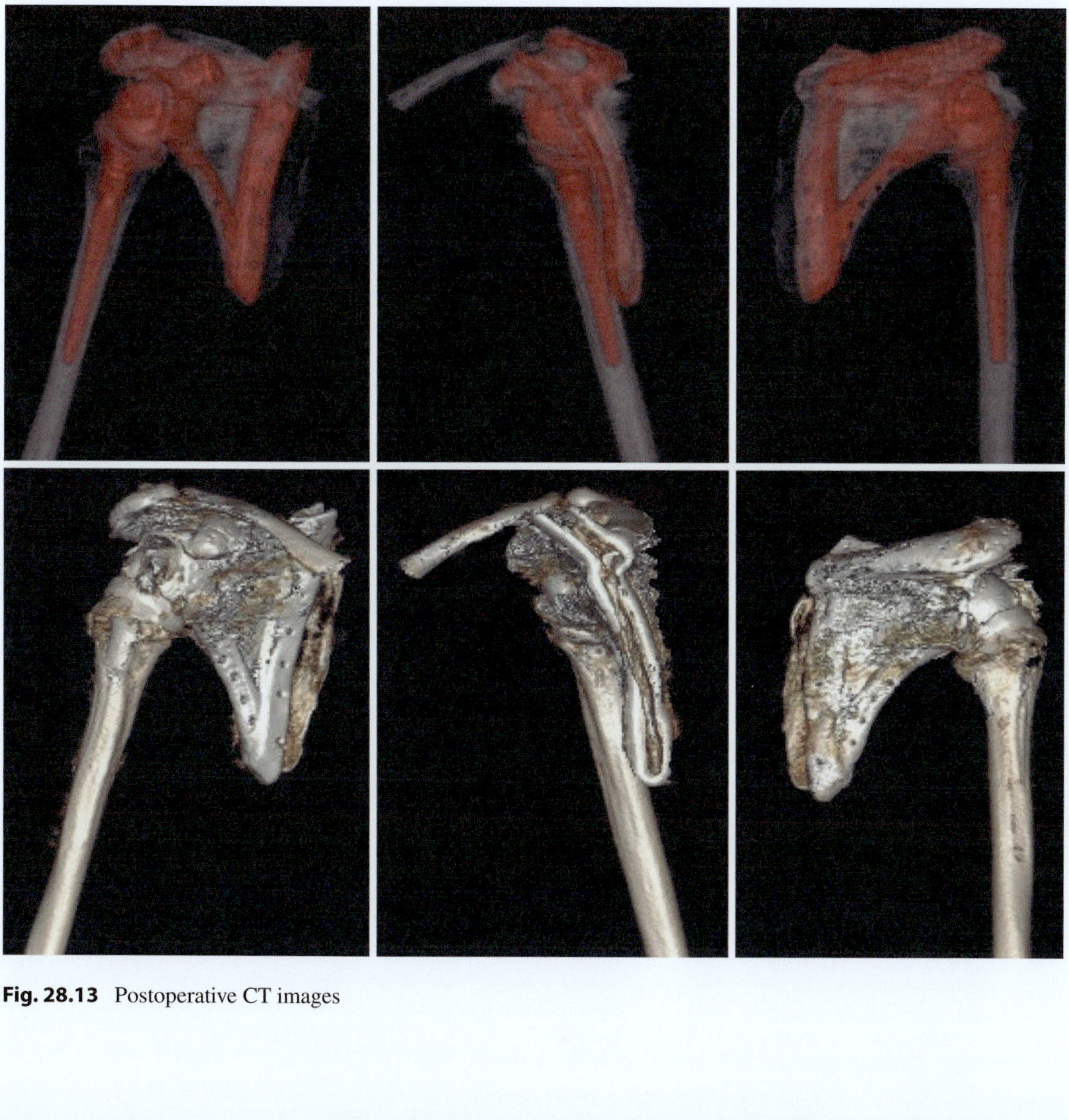

Fig. 28.13 Postoperative CT images

Patient Case 29: Scapula Combined with Glenoid of Conventional Shoulder System

29

29.1 Patient Case 29

Age/Sex	14/male
Location/site	Scapular/right
Diagnosis	Ewing sarcoma
Preoperative symptom	Swelling of right scapular back
Preoperative pain score	Resting 2/Activity 4
Past history	Preoperative chemotherapy 3 times
Present illness	Chemotherapy was less effective

H.-G. Kang, *Clinical Atlas of 3D Printing Bone Reconstruction*,
https://doi.org/10.1007/978-981-16-2043-0_29

29.2 Preoperative Images

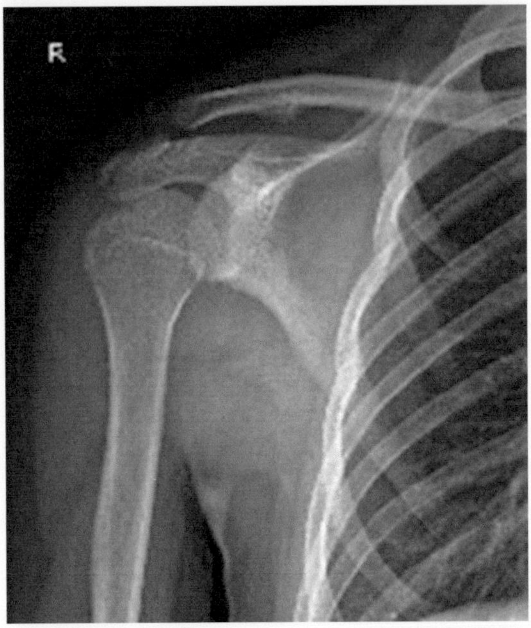

Fig. 29.1 Preoperative X-ray image

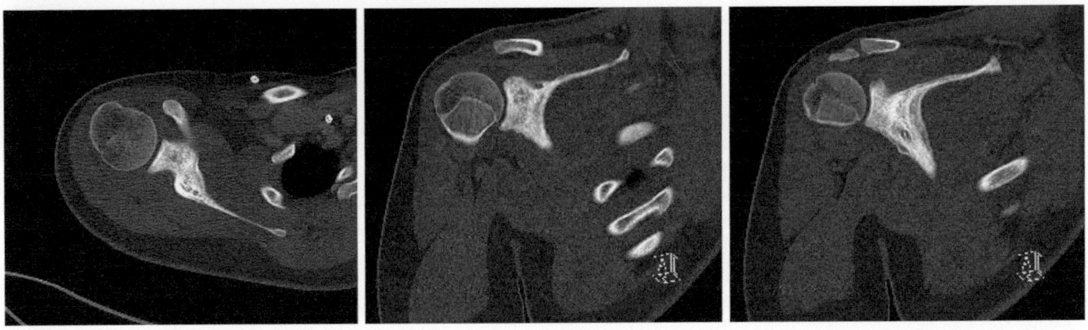

Fig. 29.2 Preoperative CT images

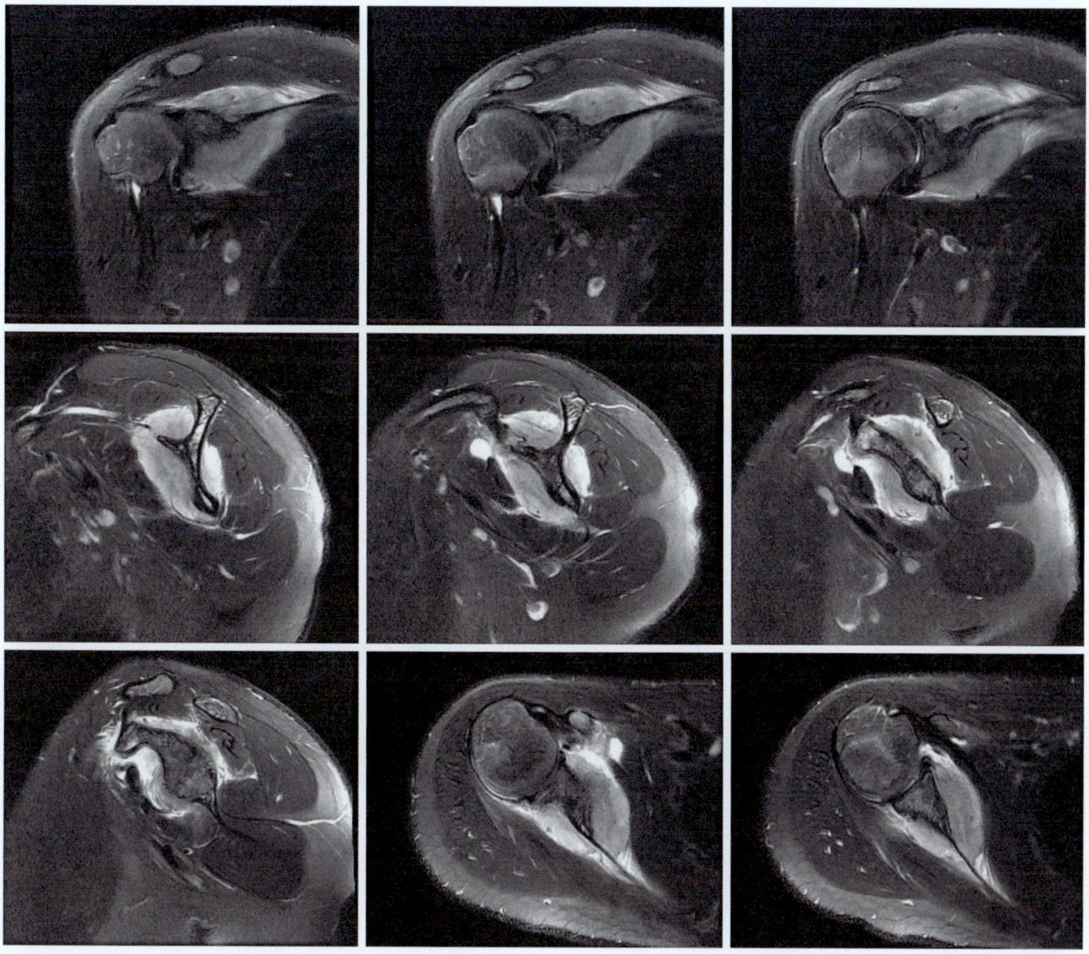

Fig. 29.3 Preoperative MRI images

29.3 Planning of Surgery

3D-printed scapular implant + conventional shoulder glenoid

Preserve humeral head

The SMR® Shoulder System of Lima Corporate

- can easily change conventional and reverse shoulder arthroplasty

29.4 Design and Fabrication

- Implant measurement
- Implant weight (g): 245
- Size (mm): 155

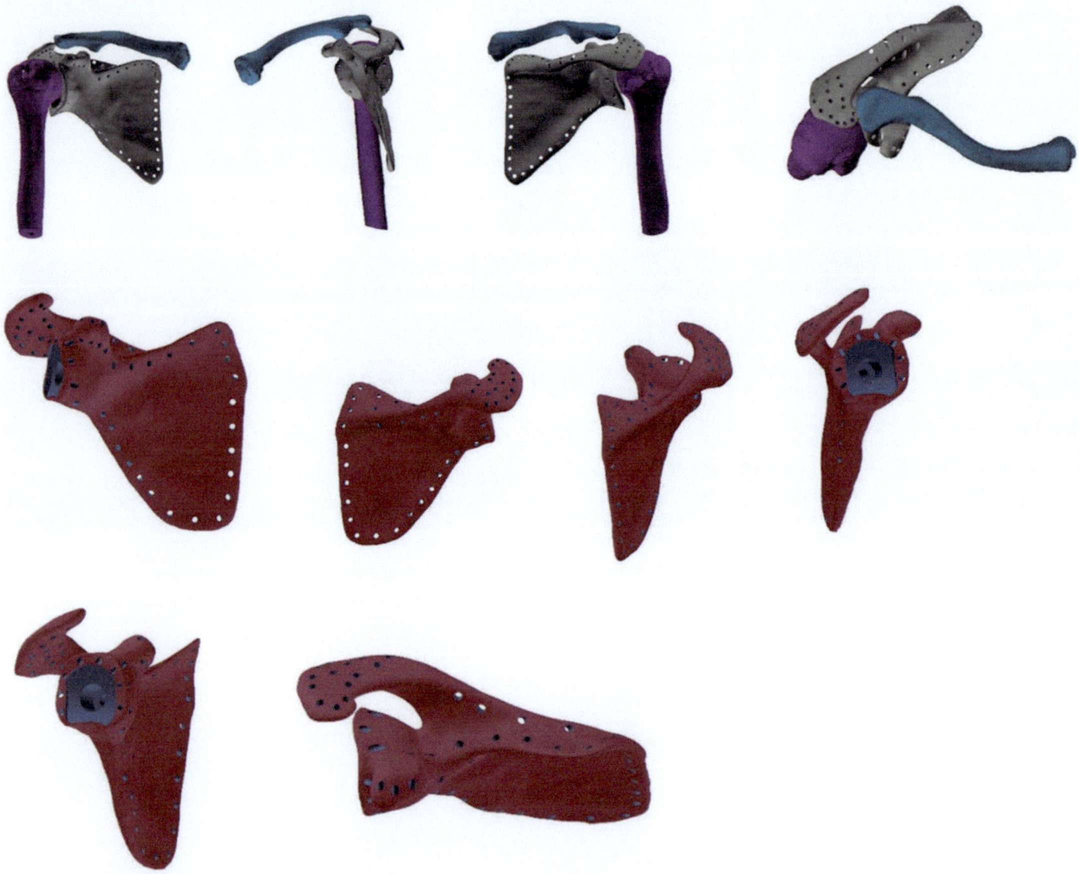

Fig. 29.4 Implant design

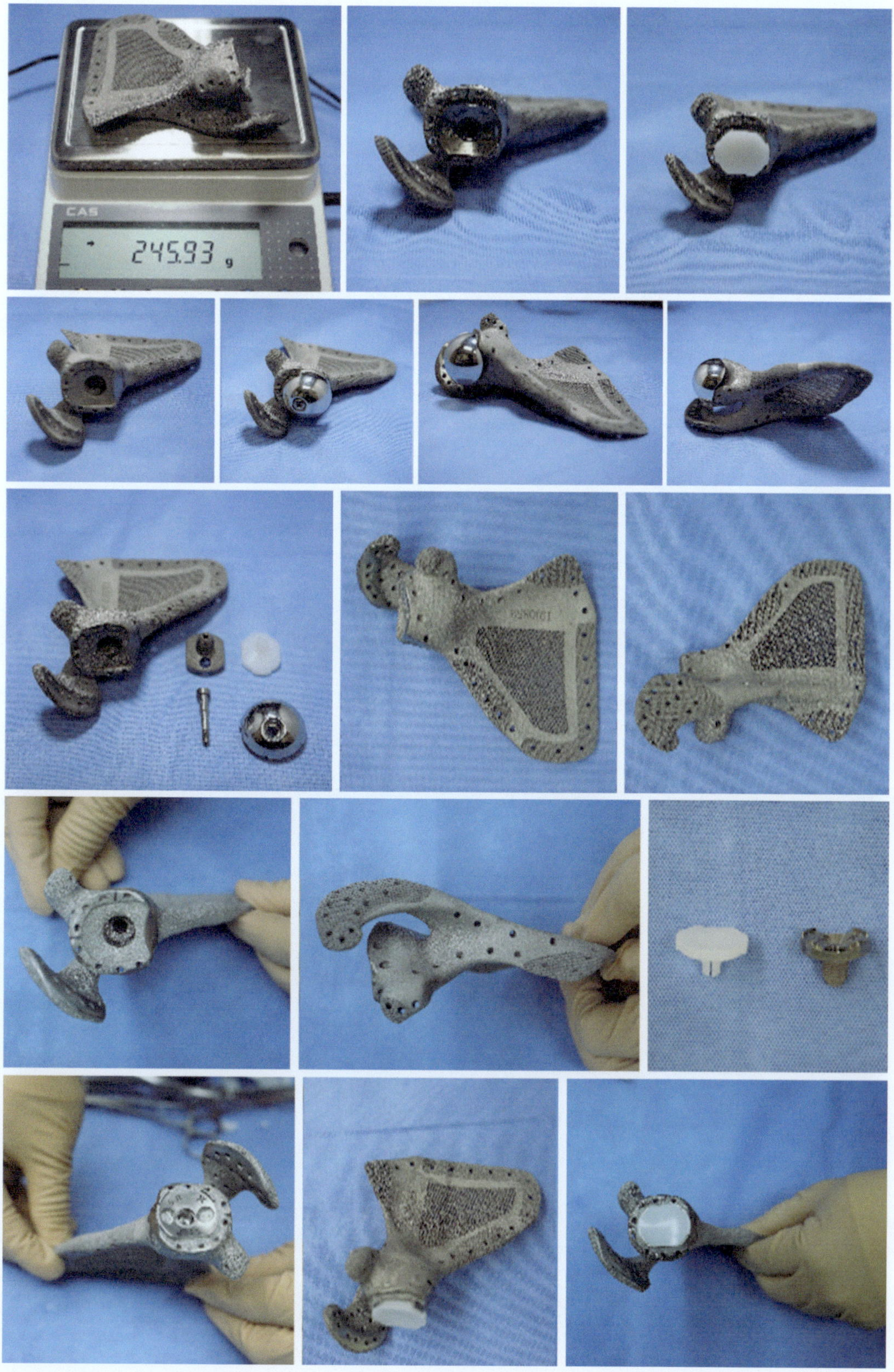

Fig. 29.5 Printed implant: The 3D-printed scapular implant and assembly with glenoid system to conventional total shoulder

29.5 Operation

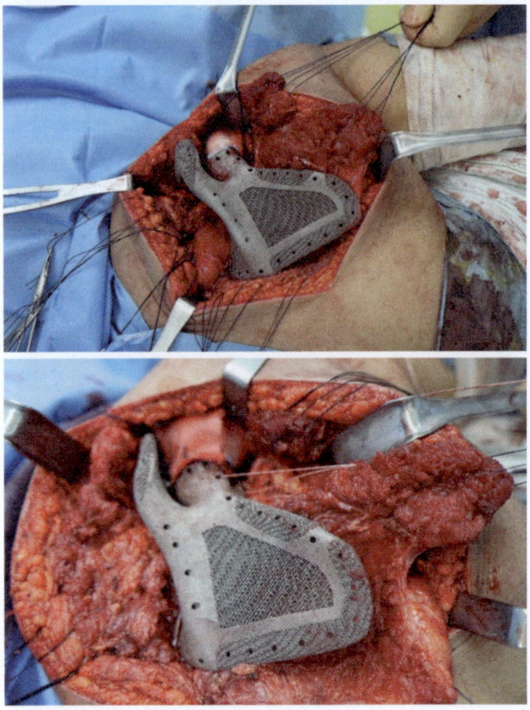

Fig. 29.6 Intraoperative photographs

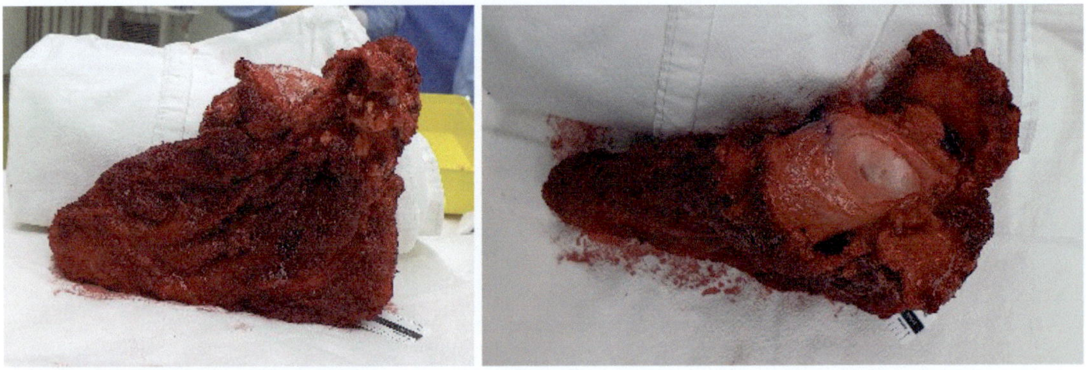

Fig. 29.7 Resected tumor

29.6 Postoperative Images

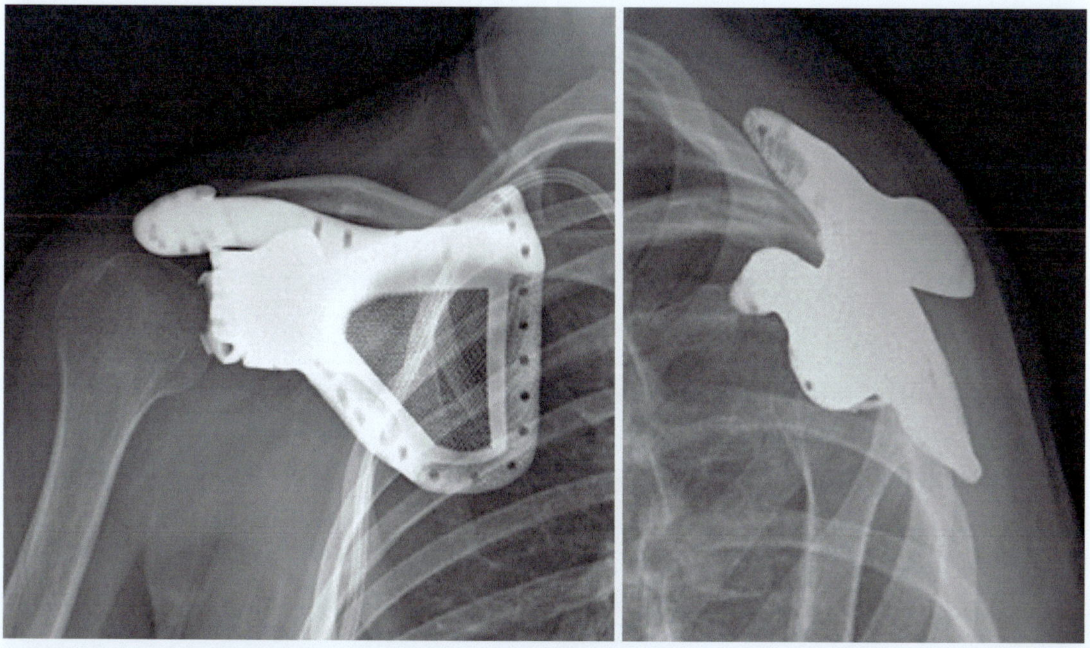

Fig. 29.8 Postoperative X-ray images

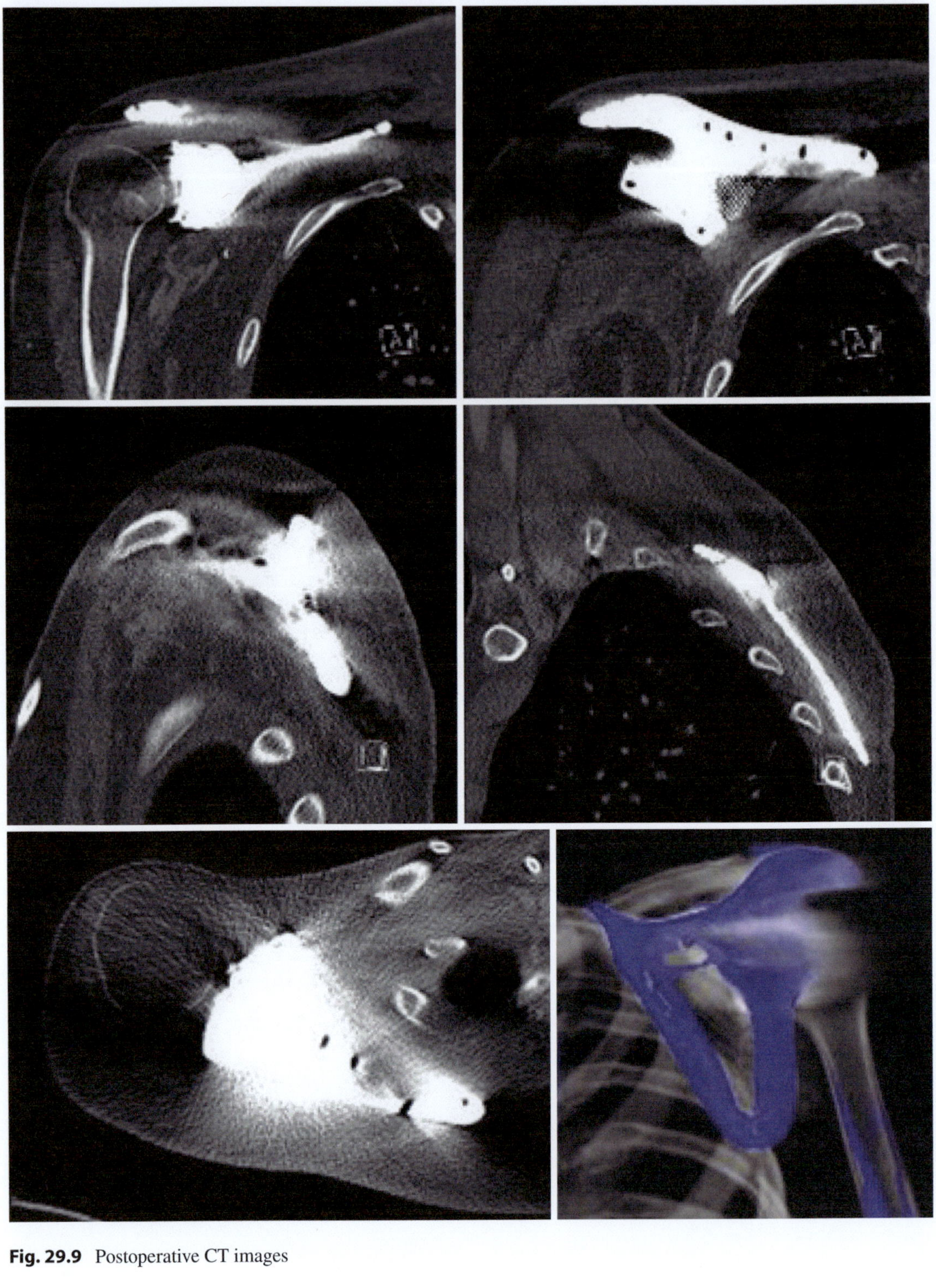

Fig. 29.9 Postoperative CT images

Part VI

Humerus

Patient Case 30: Distal Humerus for Assembly with Tumor Prosthesis

30

30.1 Patient Case 30

Age/sex	20/male
Location/site	Humerus/right
Diagnosis	Osteosarcoma Pathologic fracture
Preoperative symptom	Fractured without external force
Preoperative pain score	Resting 6/Activity 9
BMI (height/weight)	26.99(169/77.1)
Past history	Preoperative chemotherapy 2 times
Present illness	Motor weakness of radial nerve Wants limb salvage surgery and customized reconstruction

H.-G. Kang, *Clinical Atlas of 3D Printing Bone Reconstruction*,
https://doi.org/10.1007/978-981-16-2043-0_30

30.2 Preoperative Images

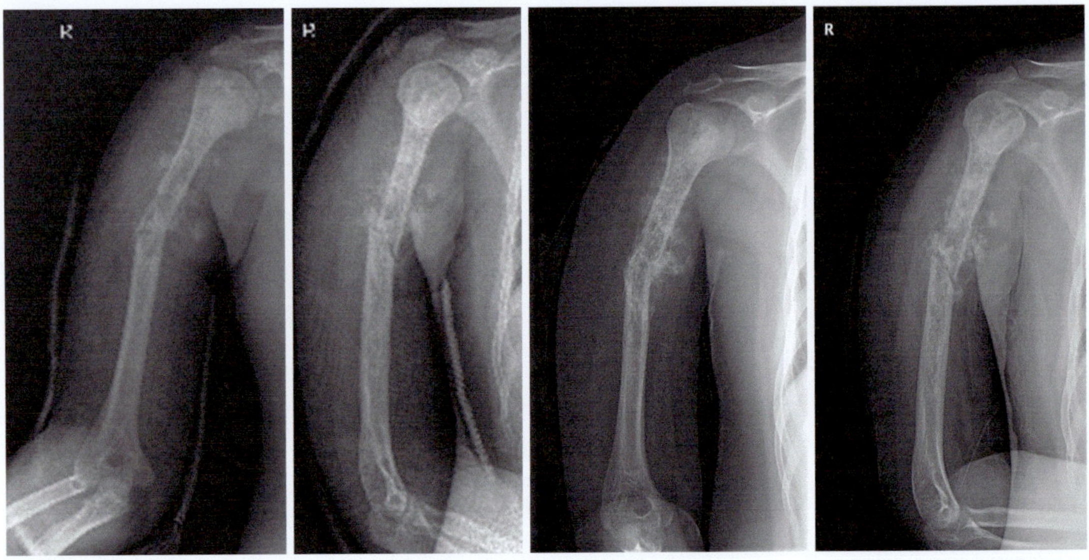

Fig. 30.1 Preoperative X-ray images

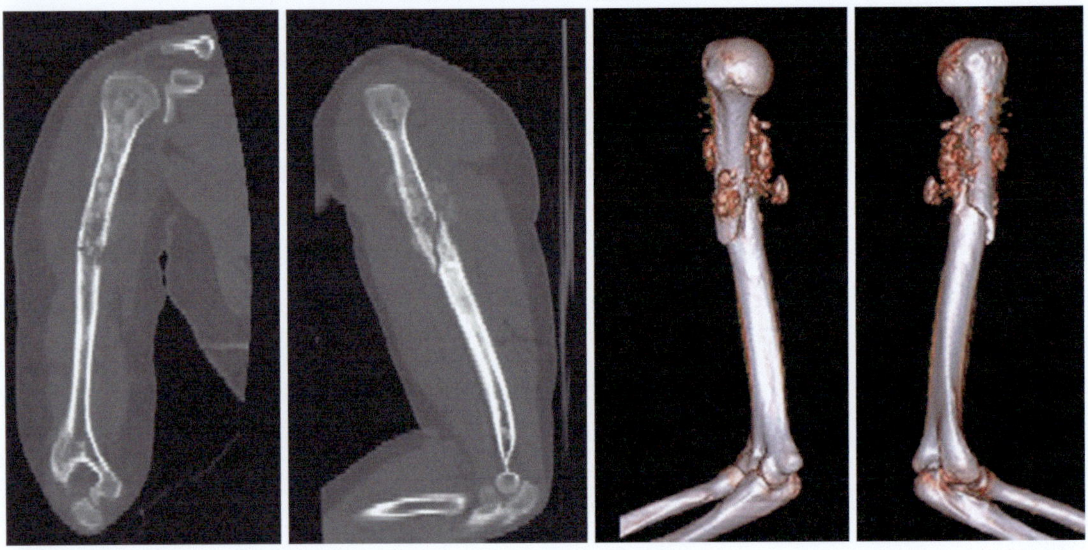

Fig. 30.2 Preoperative CT images

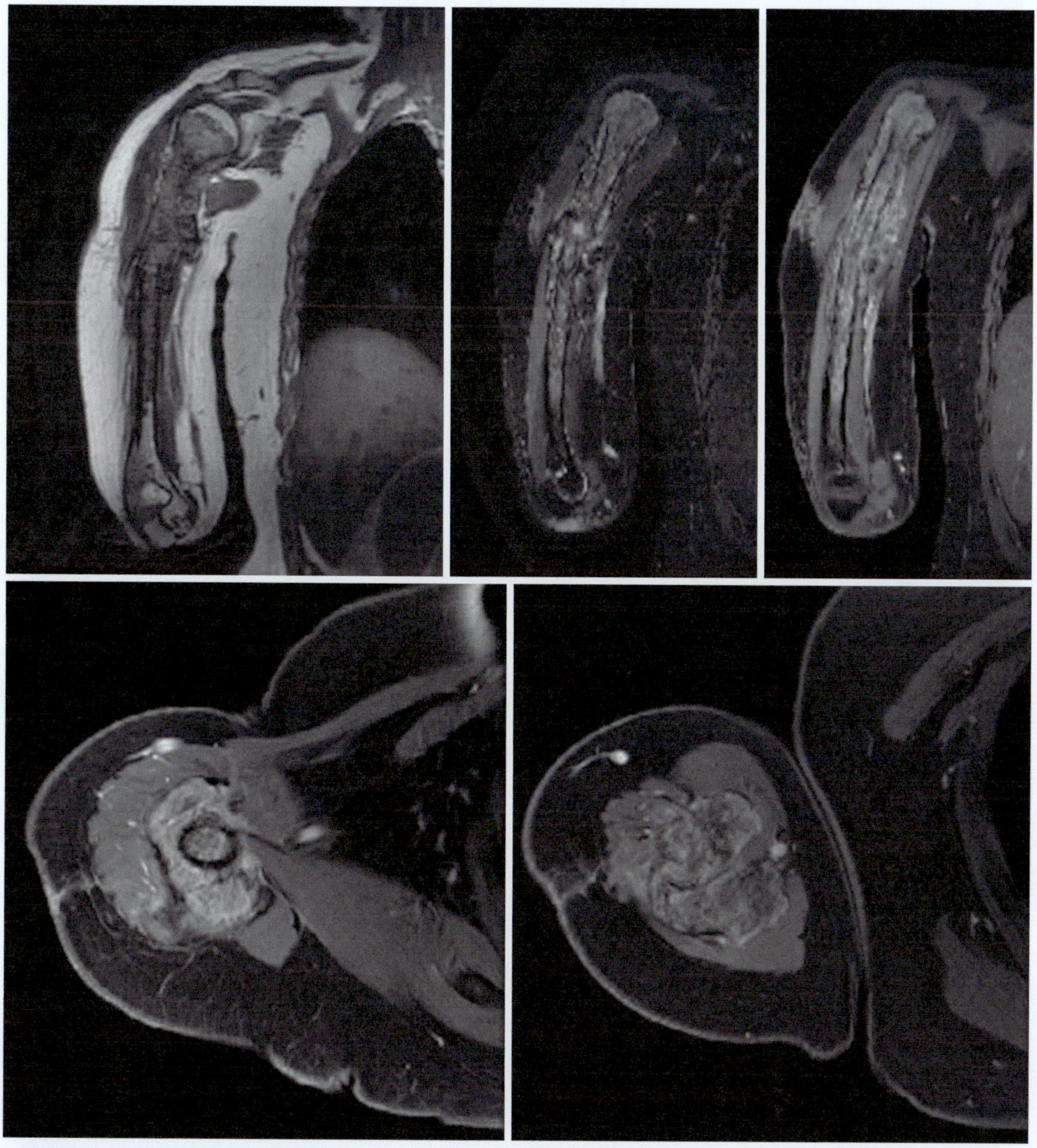

Fig. 30.3 Preoperative MRI images

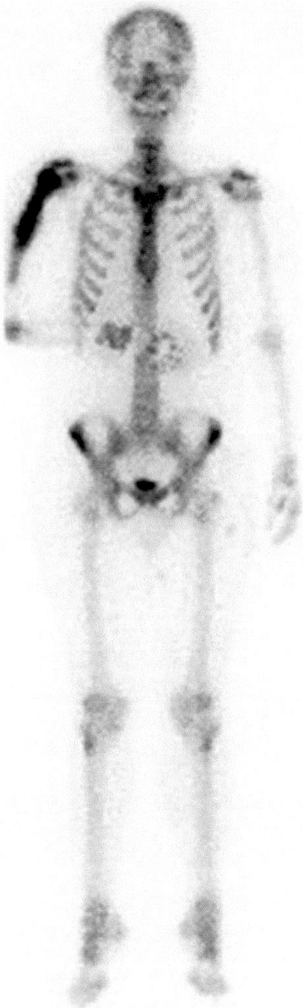

Fig. 30.4 Preoperative bone scan image

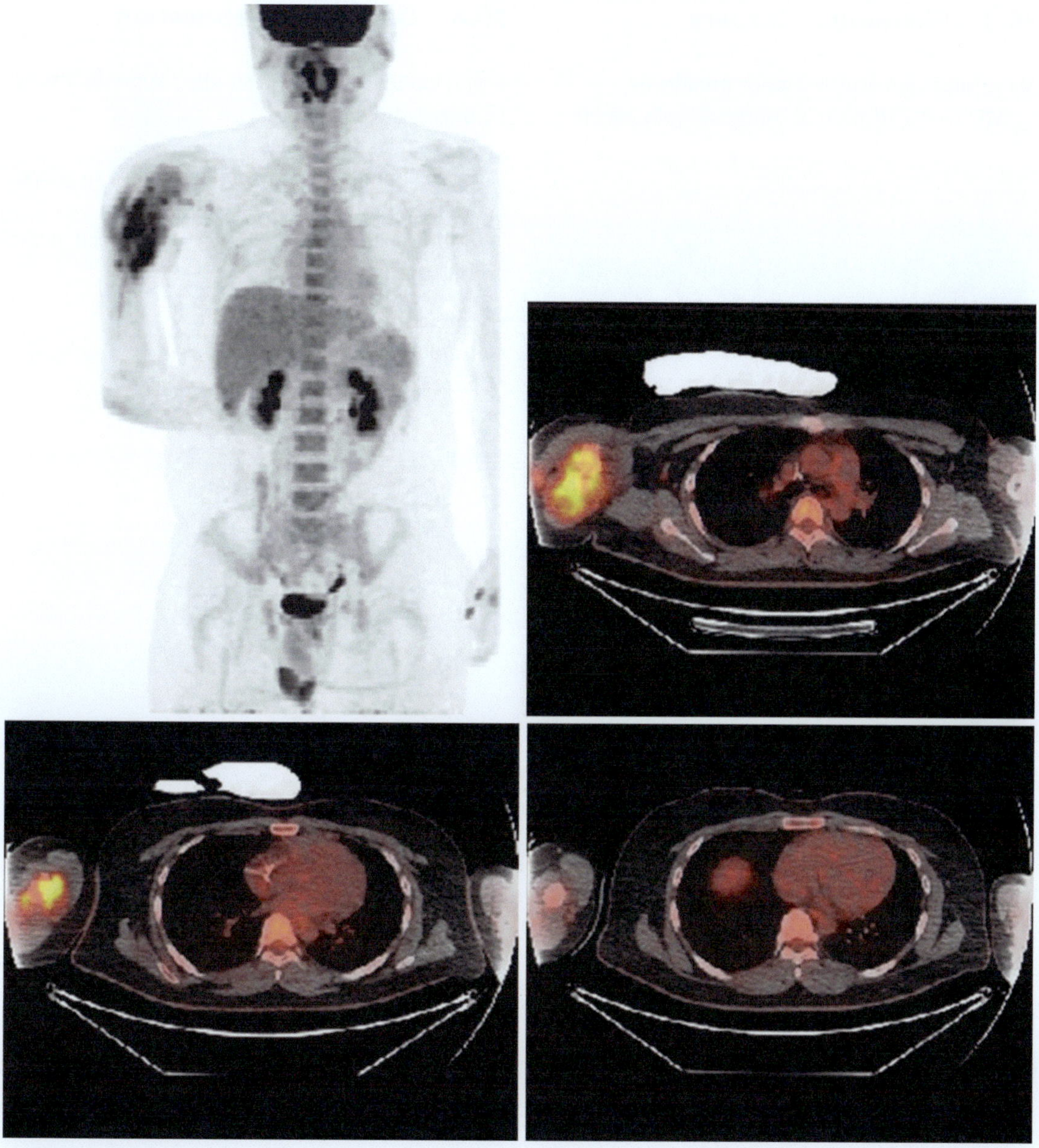

Fig. 30.5 Preoperative PET-CT images

30.3 Planning of Surgery

3D printed humerus + Tumor prosthesis
MUTARS® Proximal humeral replacement

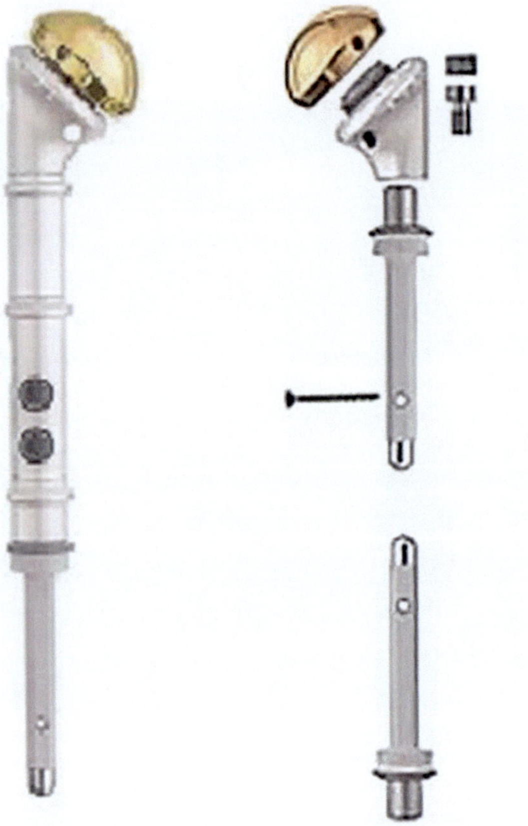

Fig. 30.6 Modular proximal humeral system of MUTARS®

30.4 Design and Fabrication

1-mm cement mantle space than stem thickness: 12 mm, solid canal

Wrap the stem base

Distal humeral condyle plate in a wing shape

Mesh body

Solid surface and polishing for radial nerve driving area

- Implant measurement
- Implant weight (g): 215
- Size (mm): 200

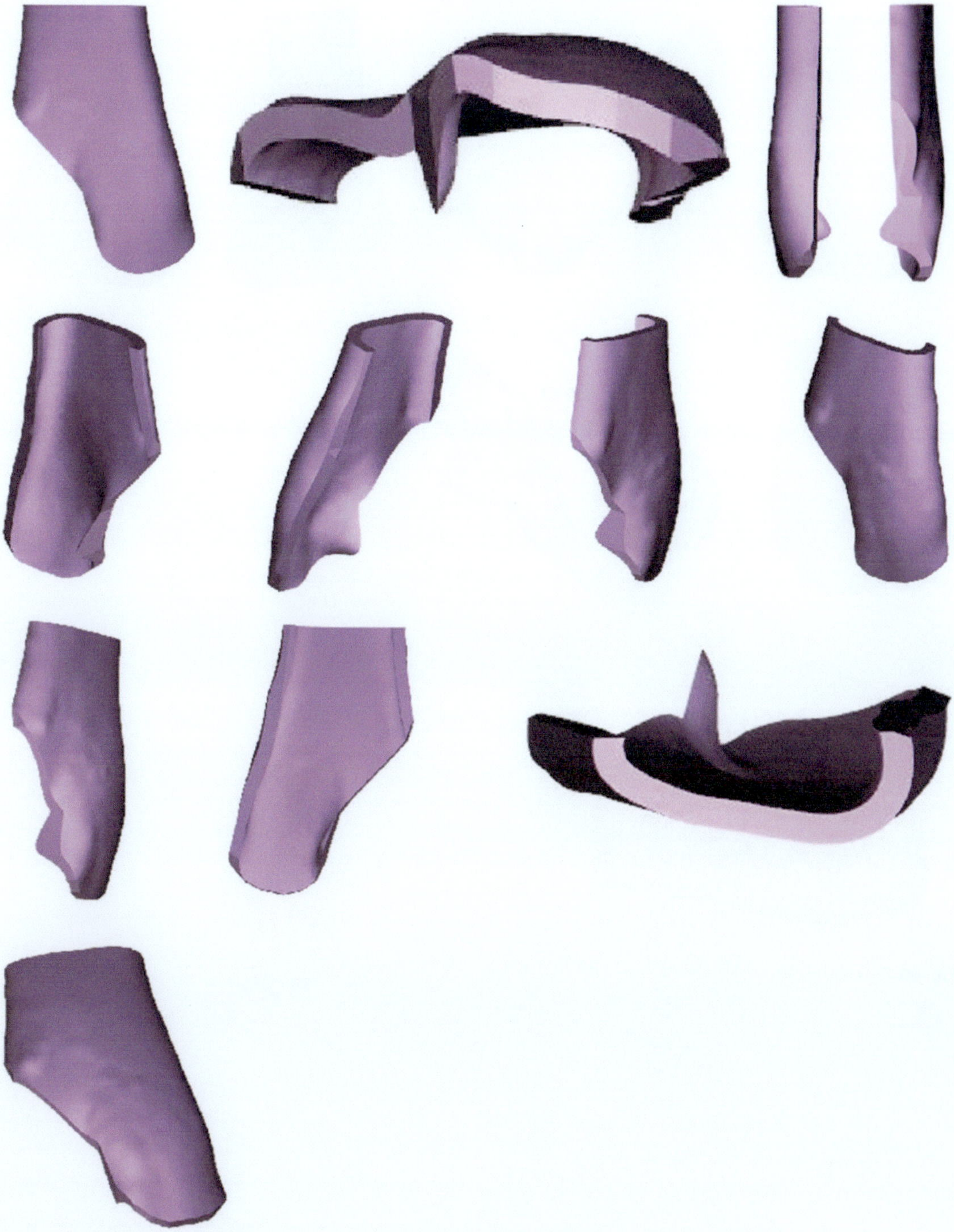

Fig. 30.7 Cutting guide design

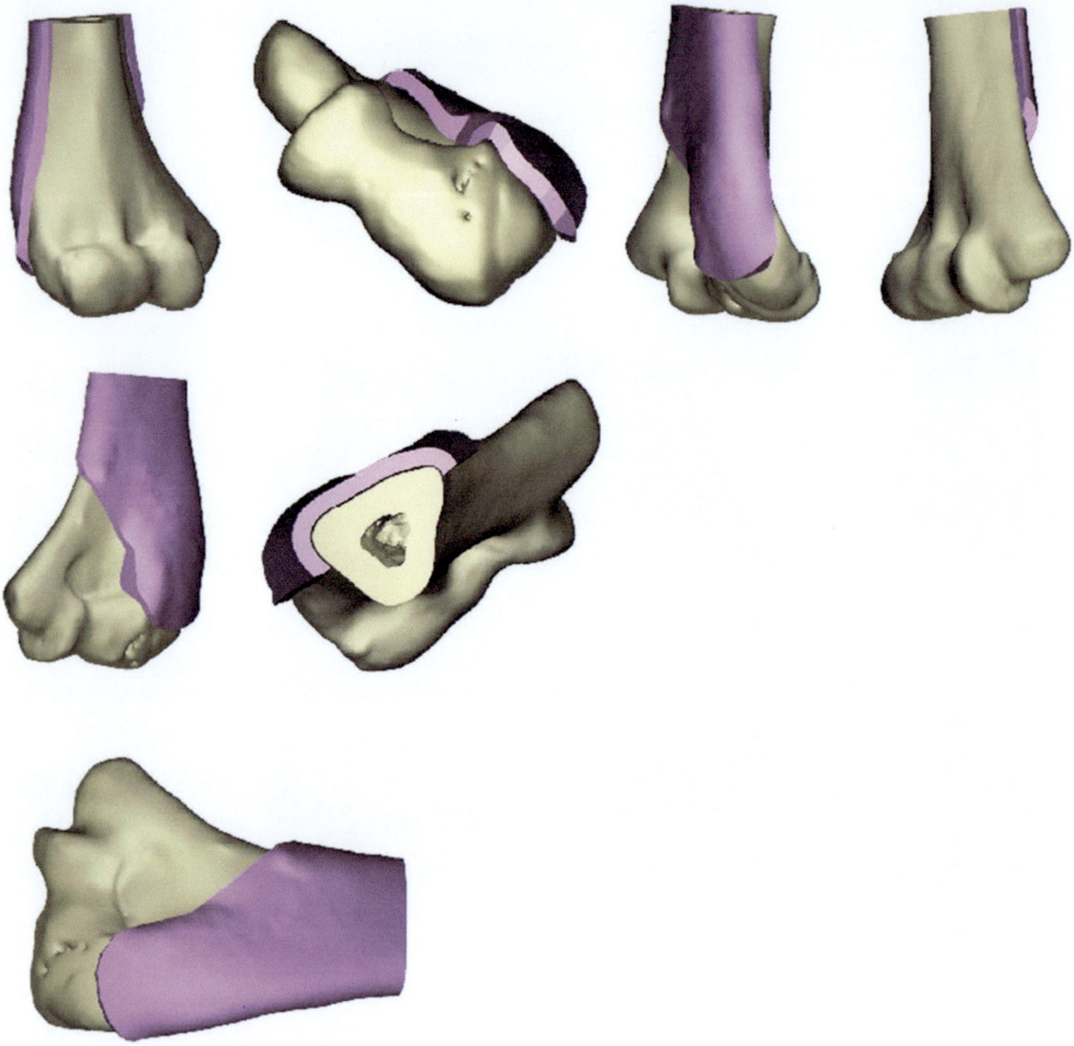

Fig. 30.7 (continued)

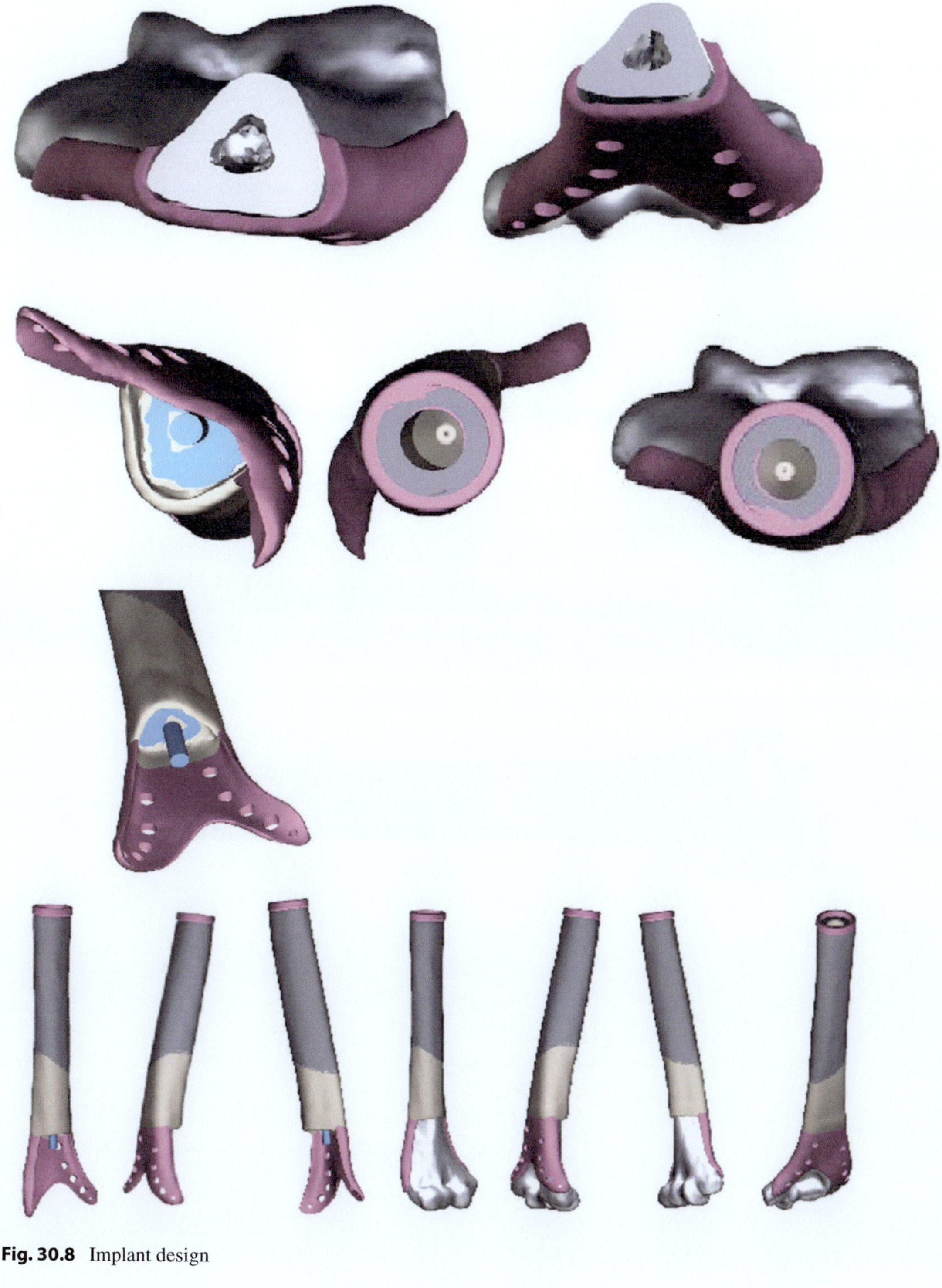

Fig. 30.8 Implant design

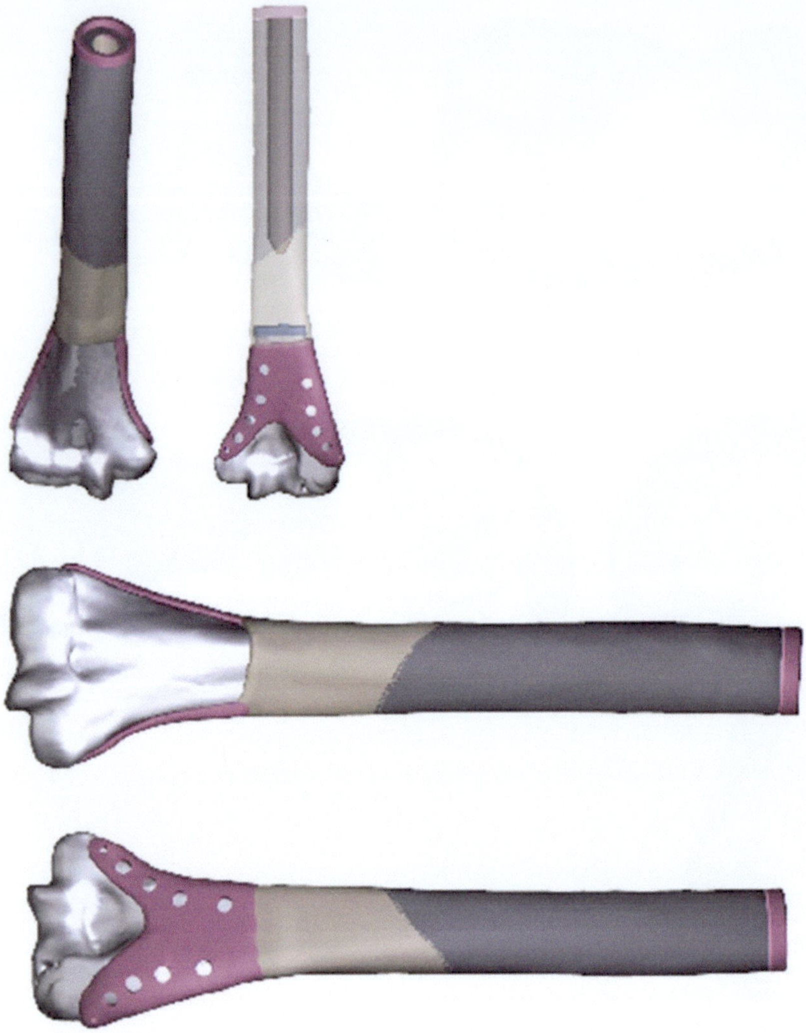

Fig. 30.8 (continued)

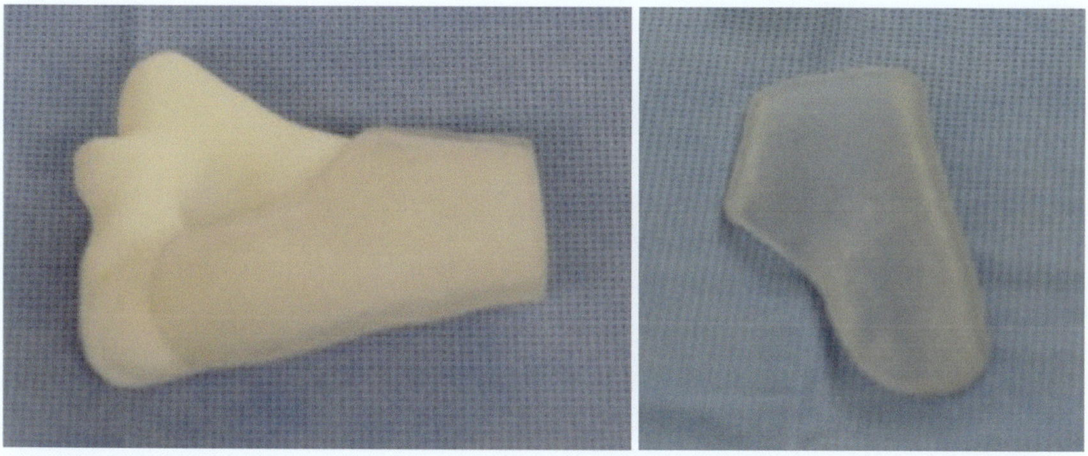

Fig. 30.9 Printed cutting guide

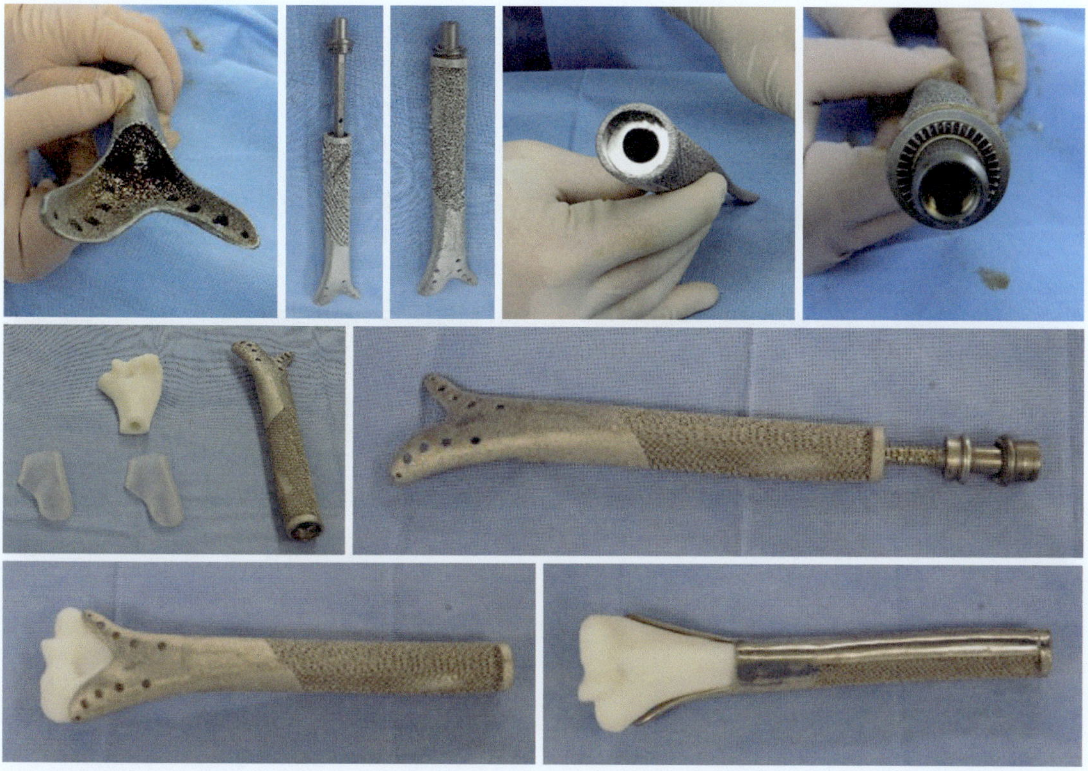

Fig. 30.10 Printed implant

30.5 Operation

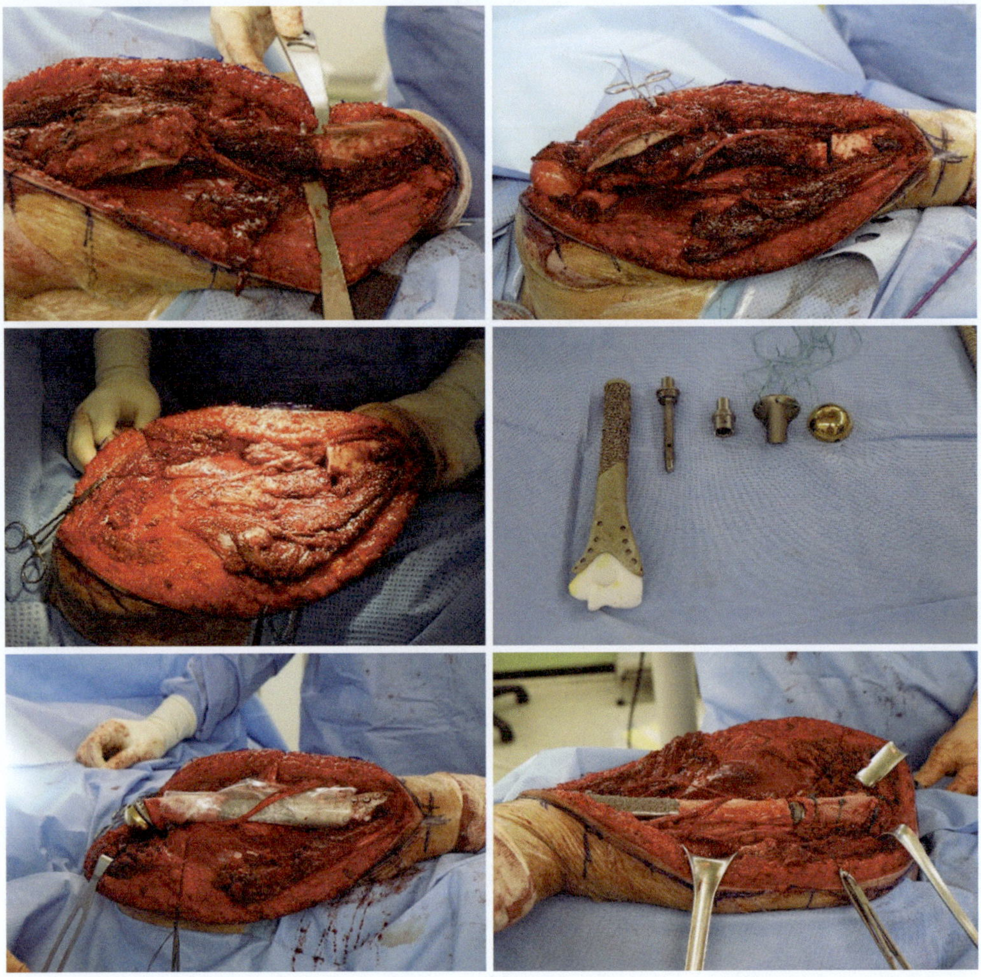

Fig. 30.11 Intraoperative photographs

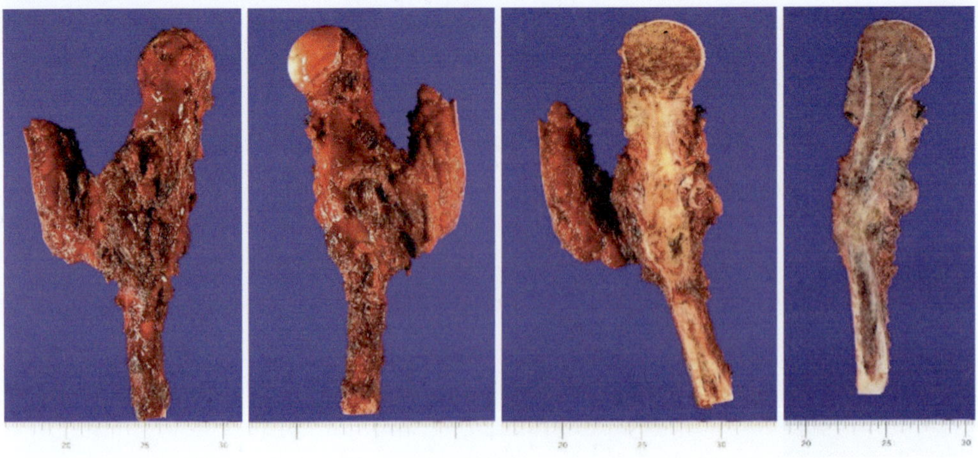

Fig. 30.12 Resected tumor

30.6 Postoperative Images

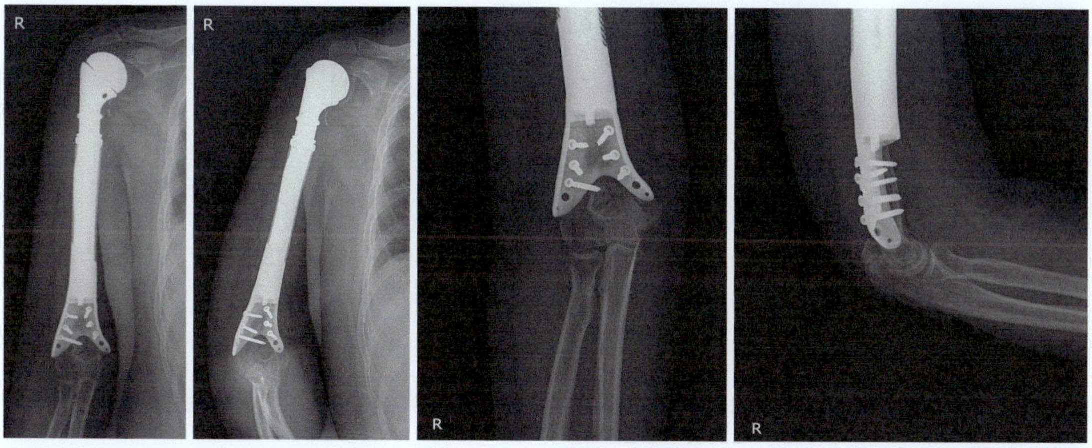

Fig. 30.13 Postoperative X-ray images

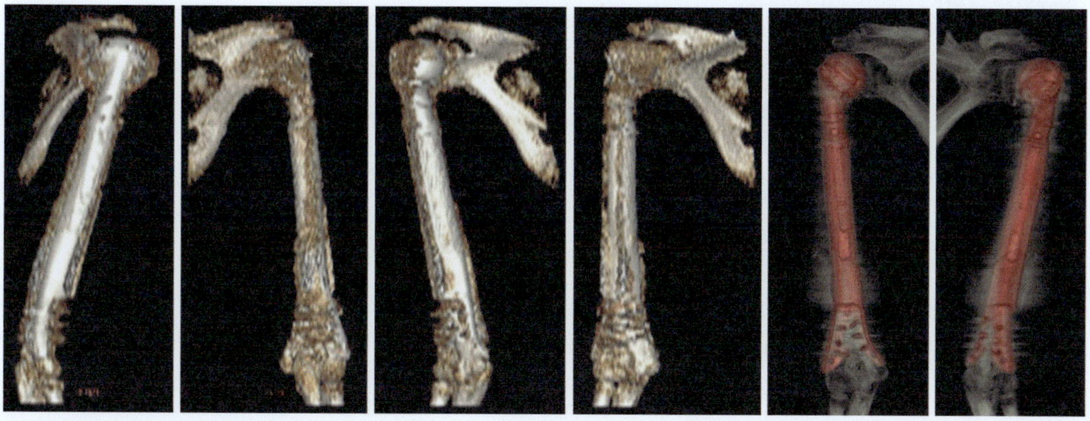

Fig. 30.14 Postoperative CT images

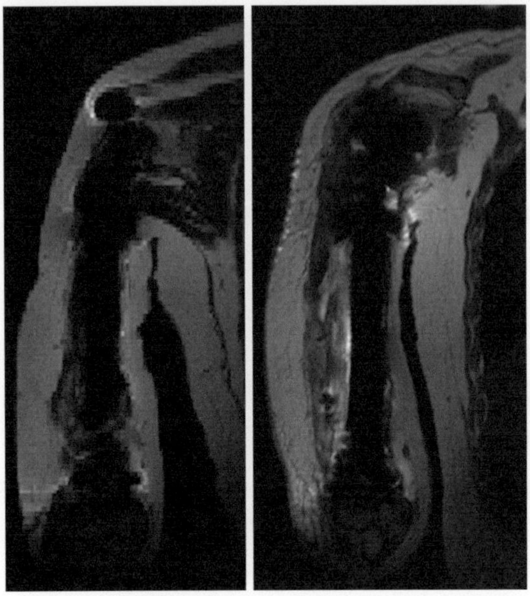

Fig. 30.15 Postoperative MRI images

Patient Case 31: Partial Elbow Joint

31

31.1 Patient Case 31

Age/sex	55/male
Location/site	Humerus, distal/left
Diagnosis	Allograft failure
Preoperative symptom	Elbow joint instability
Preoperative pain score	Resting 0/Activity 4
BMI (height/weight)	22.64 (167.4/63.45)
Past history	Giant cell tumor of bone diagnosed at 4 years ago
Present illness	Medial osteoarticular allograft reconstruction of distal humerus The osteoarticular allograft bone is gradually destroyed

H.-G. Kang, *Clinical Atlas of 3D Printing Bone Reconstruction*,
https://doi.org/10.1007/978-981-16-2043-0_31

31.2 Preoperative Images

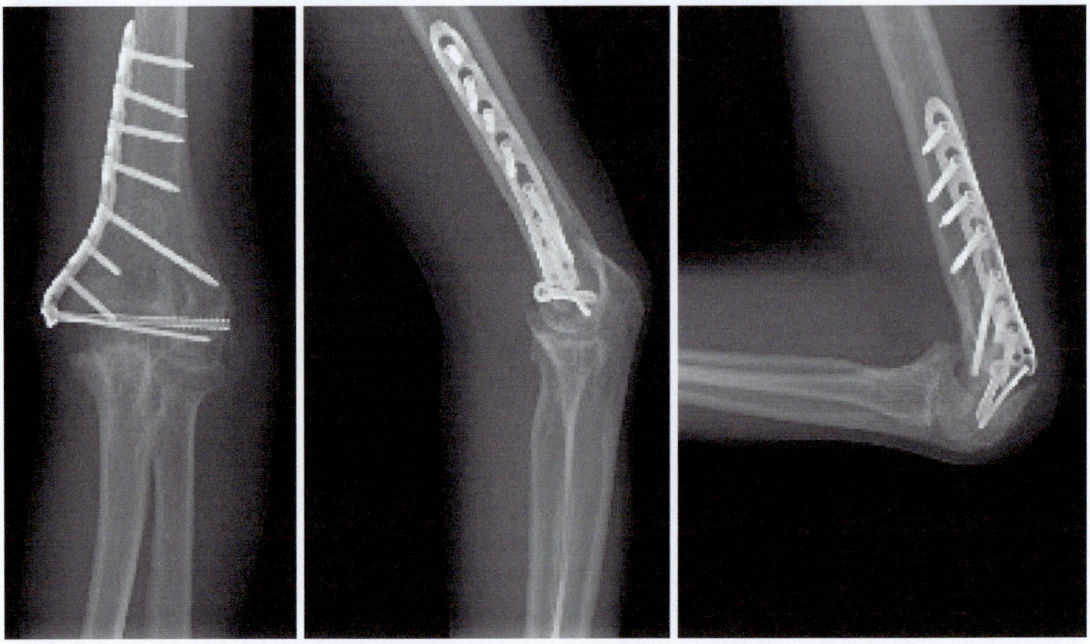

Fig. 31.1 Preoperative X-ray images: medial joint collapse of osteoarticular allograft

Fig. 31.2 Preoperative CT images

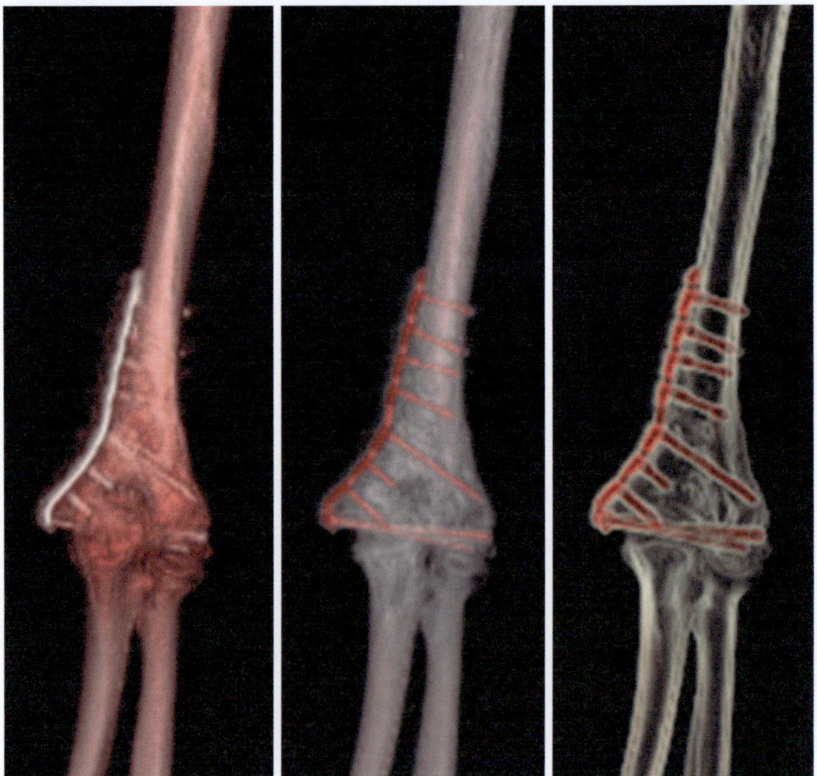

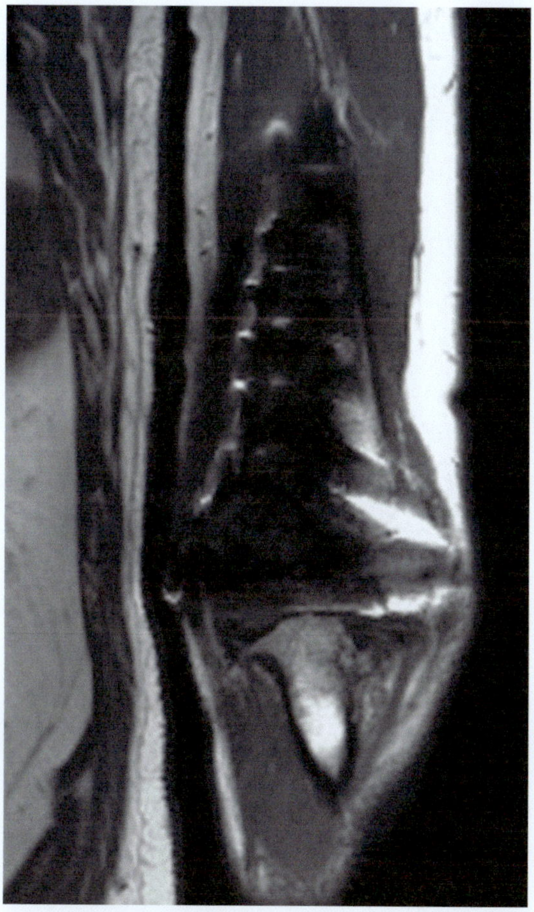

Fig. 31.3 Preoperative MRI image

31.3 Planning of Surgery

3D-printed medial condylar implant of distal humerus

Using the mirror images of contralateral elbow

31.4 Design and Fabrication

- Implant measurement
- Implant weight (g): 90
- Size (mm): 126

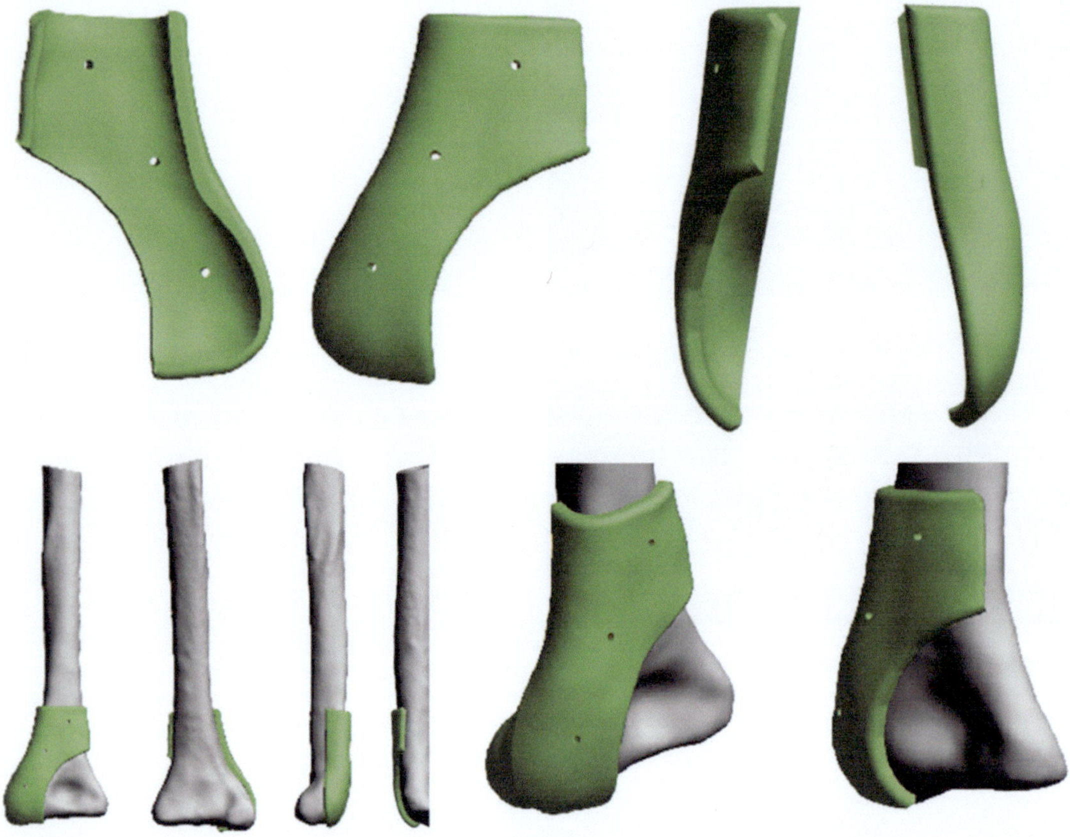

Fig. 31.4 Cutting guide design

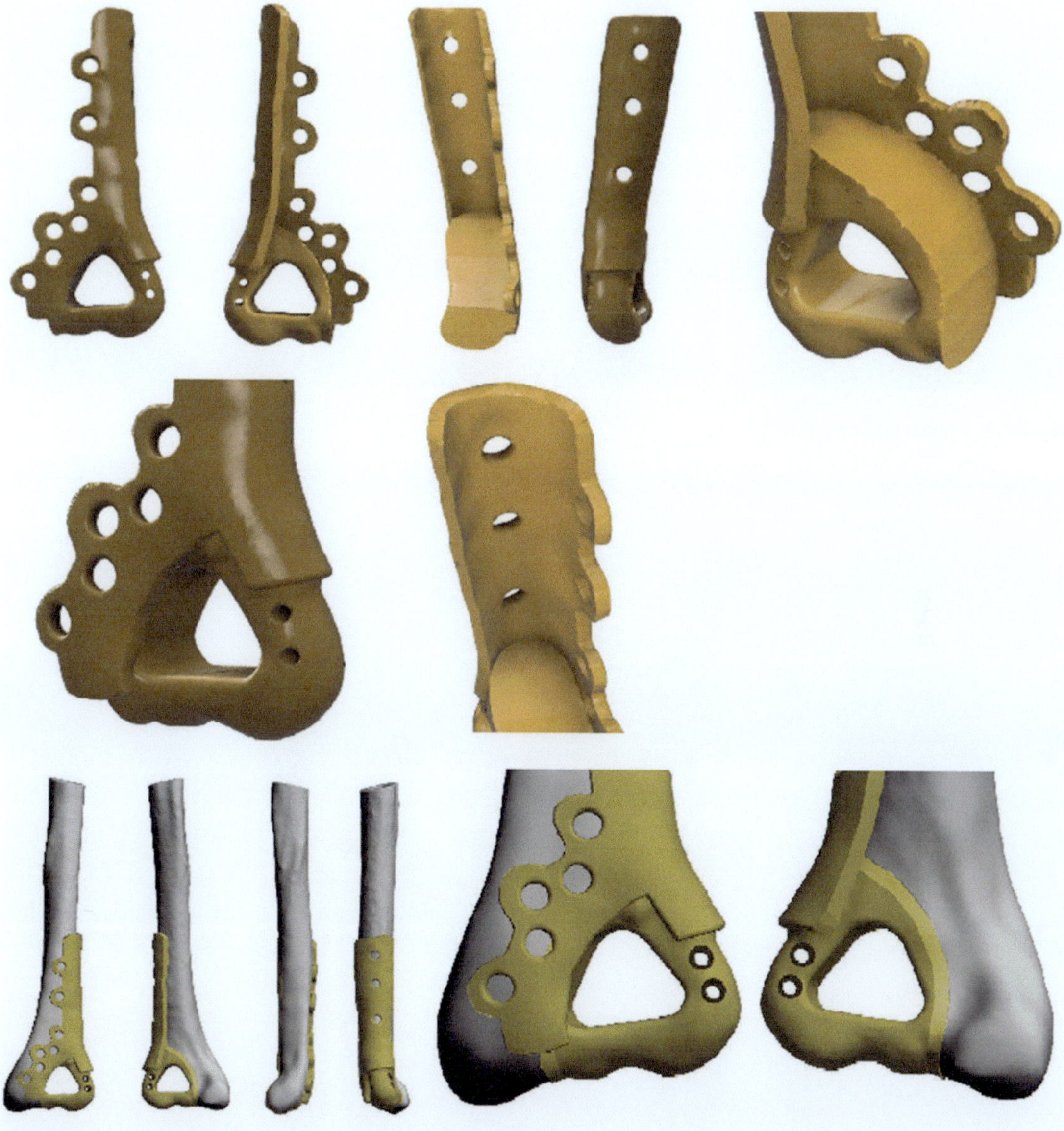

Fig. 31.5 Implant design

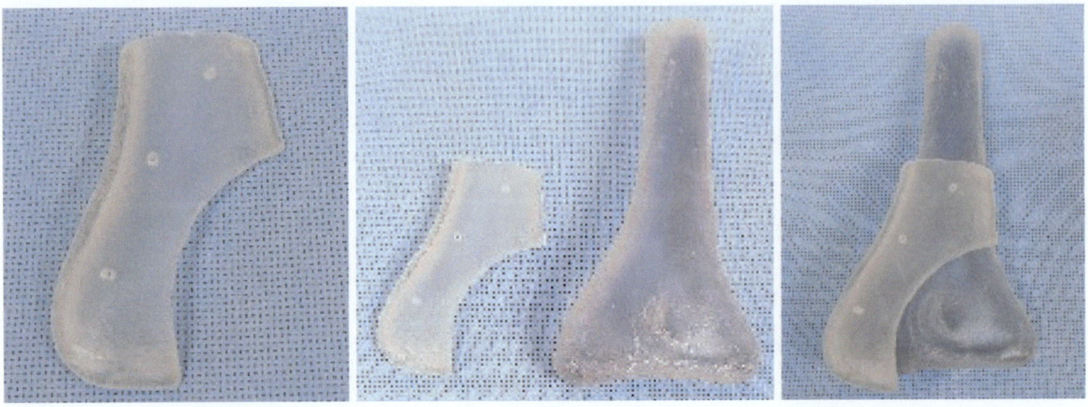

Fig. 31.6 Printed cutting guide

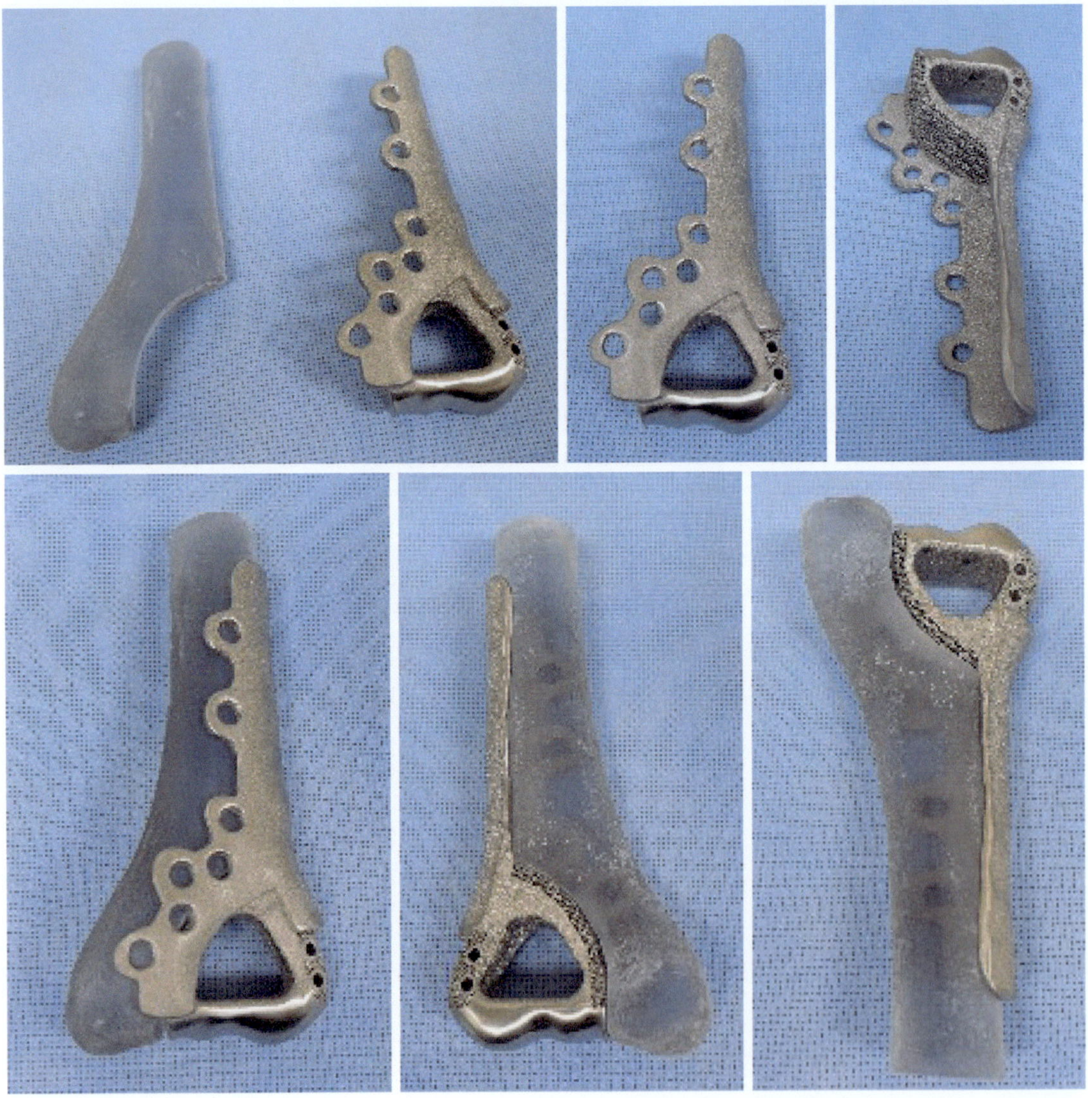

Fig. 31.7 Printed implant

31.5 Operation

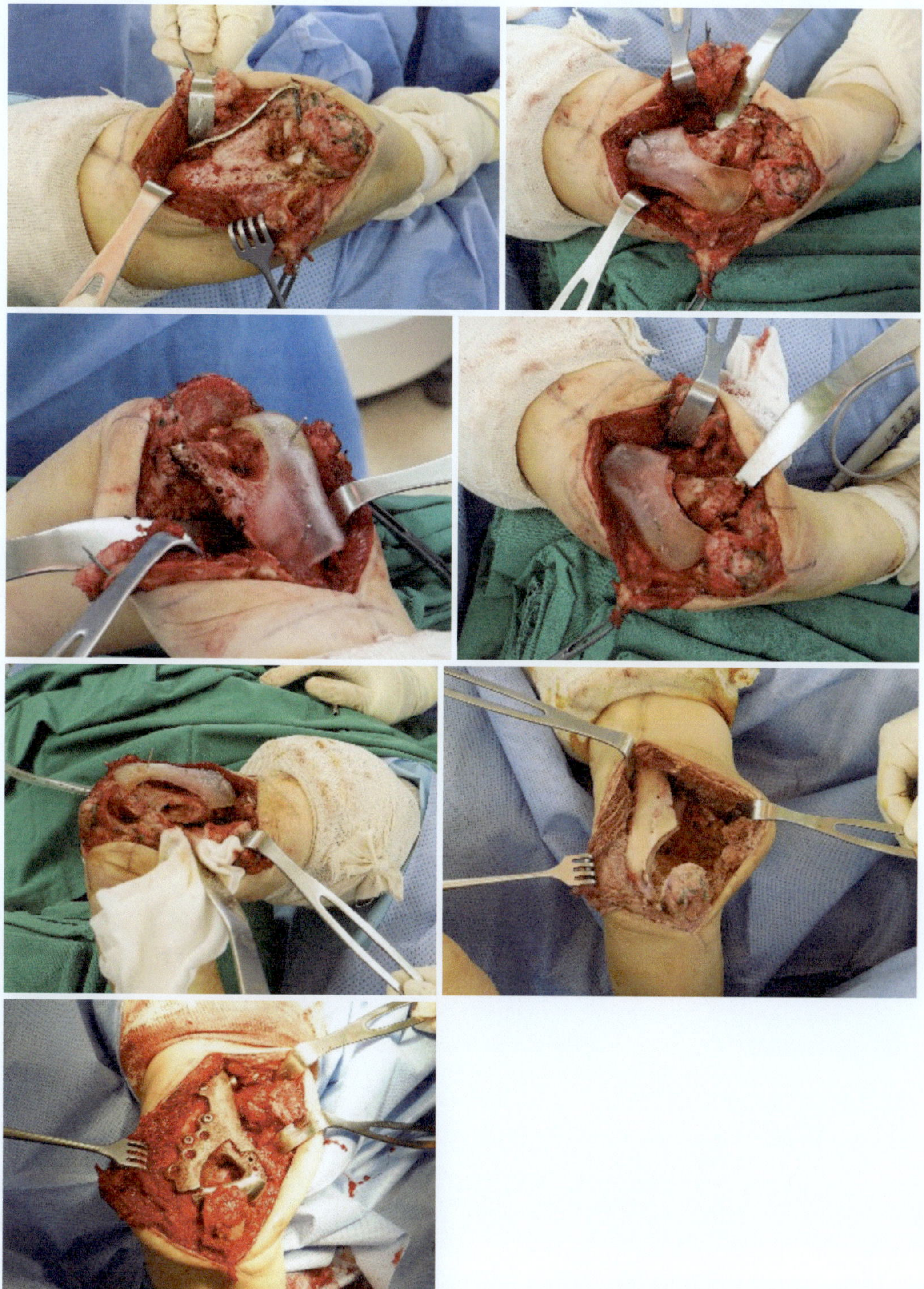

Fig. 31.8 Intraoperative photographs

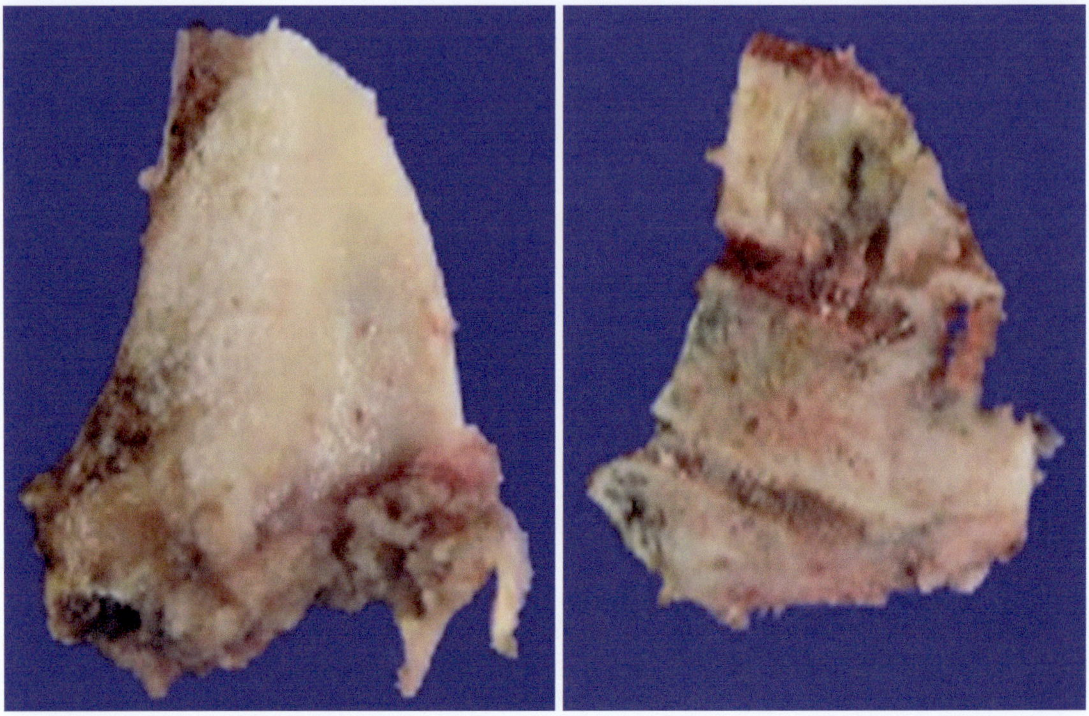

Fig. 31.9 Resected osteoarticular allograft

31.6 Postoperative Images

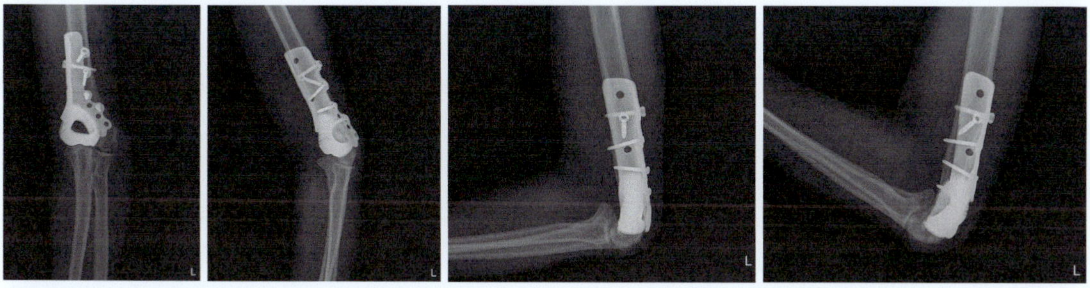

Fig. 31.10 Postoperative X-ray images

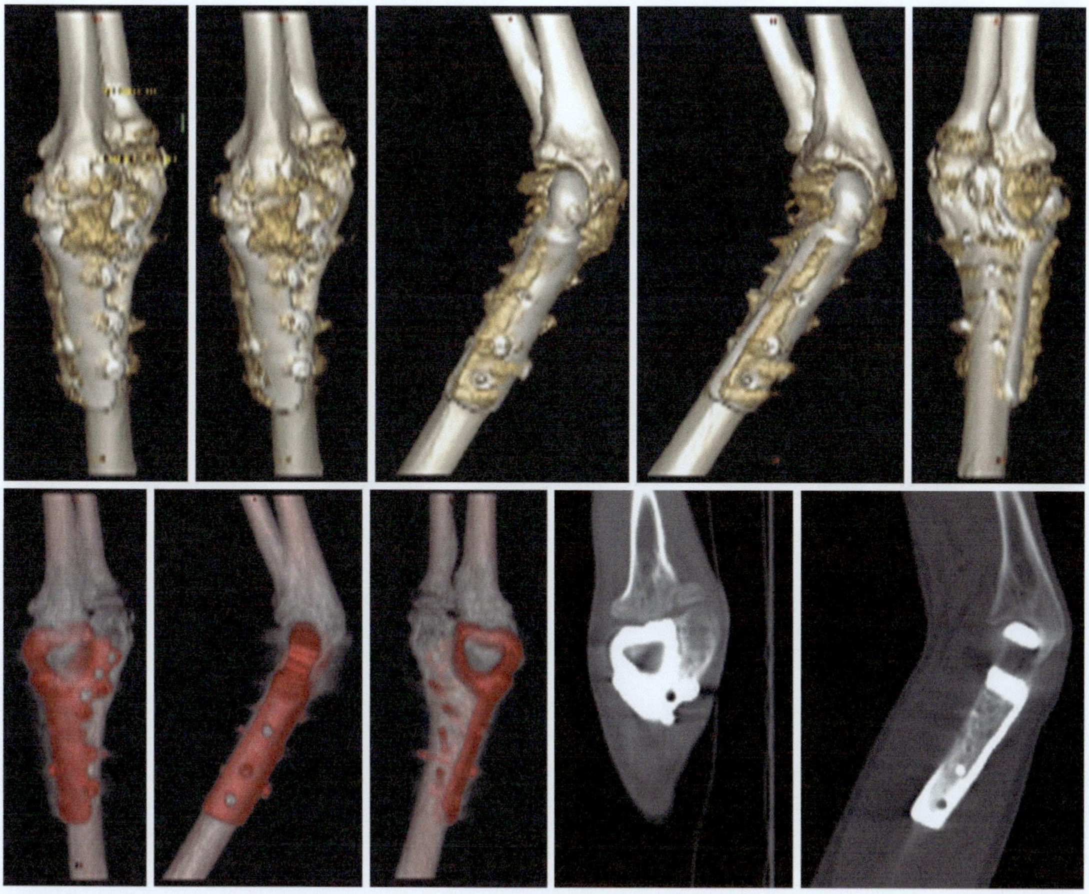

Fig. 31.11 Postoperative CT images

Part VII

Radius and Ulna

Patient Case 32: Radius & Ulna and Implant-Bone Connector

32

32.1 Patient Case 32

Age/sex	40/male
Location/site	Radius and ulnar forearm/right
Diagnosis	Aggressive fibromatosis Bone involvement
Preoperative motion	No specific restriction
Preoperative pain score	Resting 2/activity 5
BMI (height/weight)	23.73 (174.9/72.6)
Past history	Radial head dislocation since childhood
Present illness	Colles fracture on right wrist at 5 years ago Operated with pinning and external fixator The patient wants to preserve the right-hand function

32.2 Preoperative Images

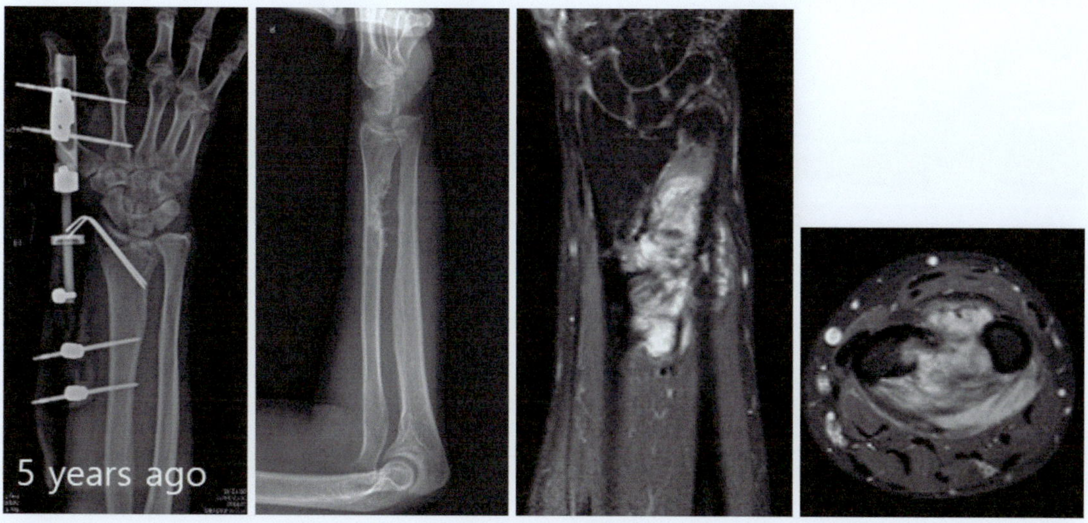

Fig. 32.1 Preoperative X-ray and MRI images bone-destructive tumor develops at the pin site

H.-G. Kang, *Clinical Atlas of 3D Printing Bone Reconstruction*,
https://doi.org/10.1007/978-981-16-2043-0_32

32.3 Planning of Surgery

Patient refuses forearm one bone reconstruction and wants to reconstruct both radius and ulna

Preserve wrist joint

3D-printed radius and ulna

32.4 Design and Fabrication

- Implant measurement
- Implant weight (g): radius 117, ulna 79
- Size (mm): radius 138, ulna 136

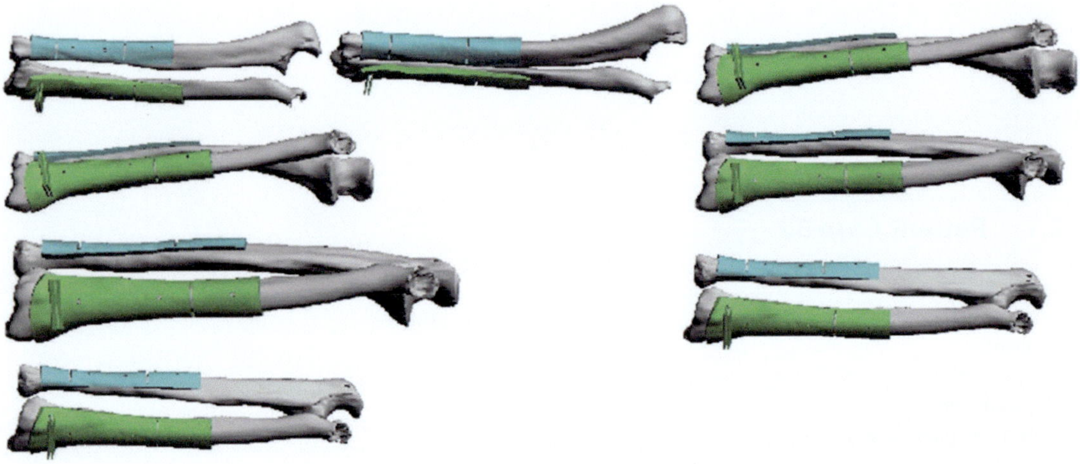

Fig. 32.2 Cutting guide design

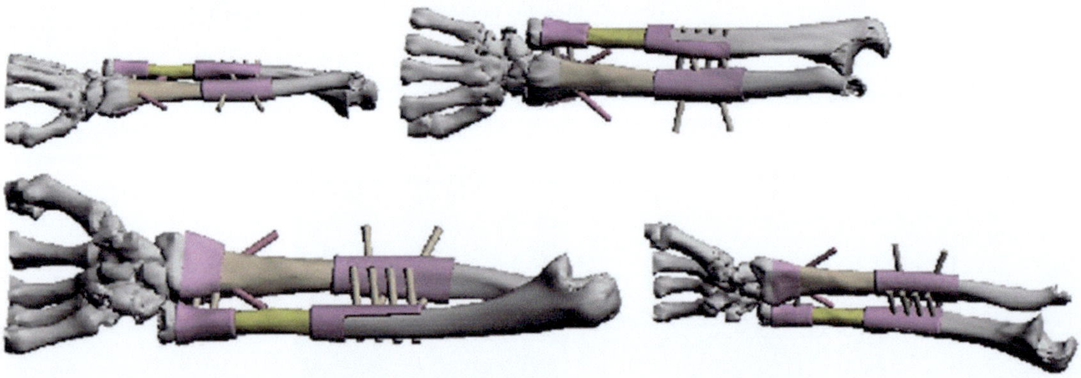

Fig. 32.3 Implant design. All bone contact surfaces were fabricated in a mesh structure

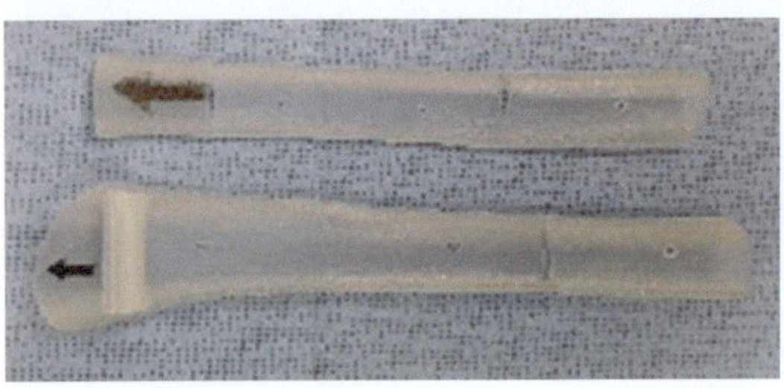

Fig. 32.4 Printed cutting guide

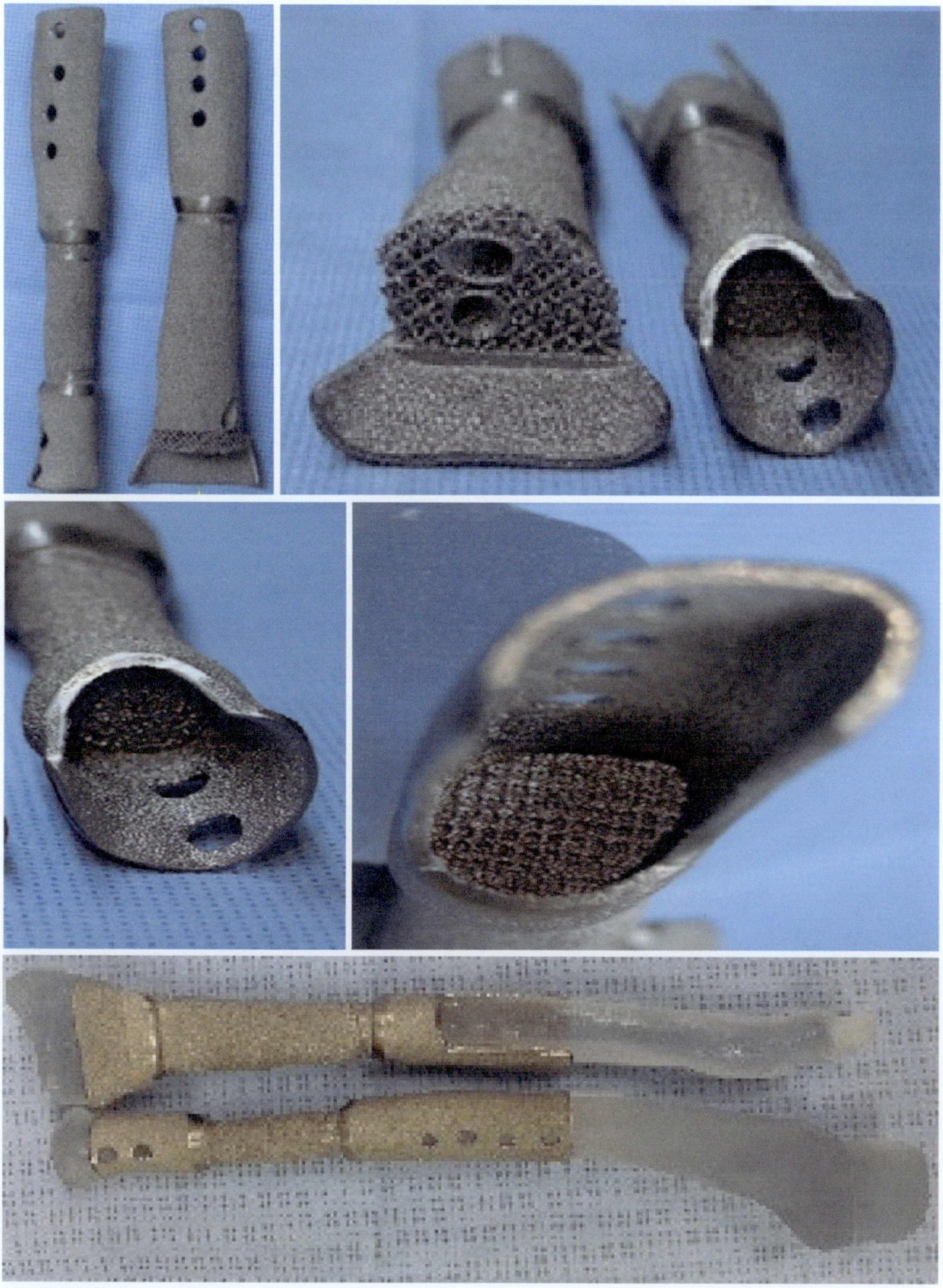

Fig. 32.5 Printed implant

32.5 Operation

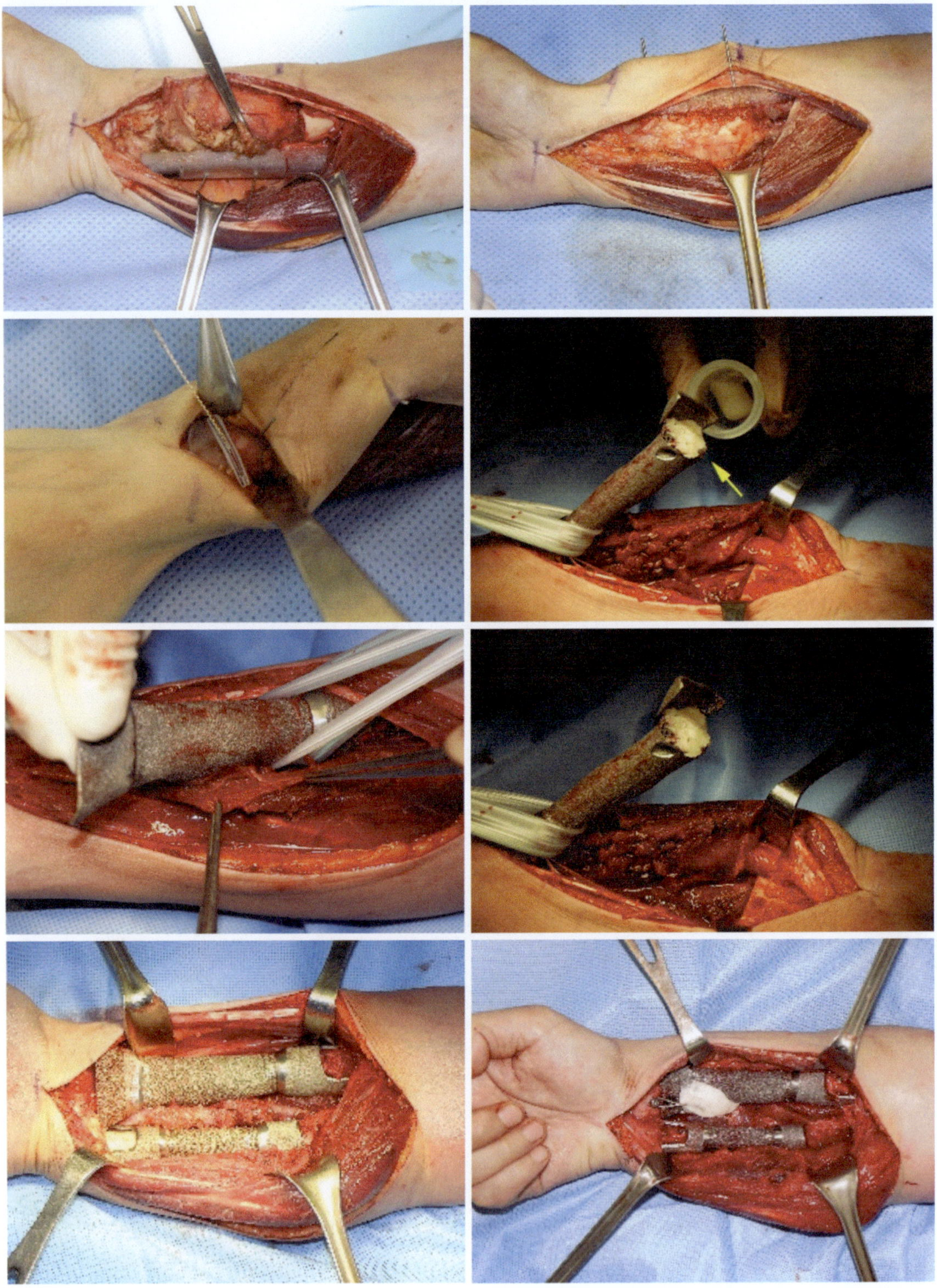

Fig. 32.6 Intraoperative photographs

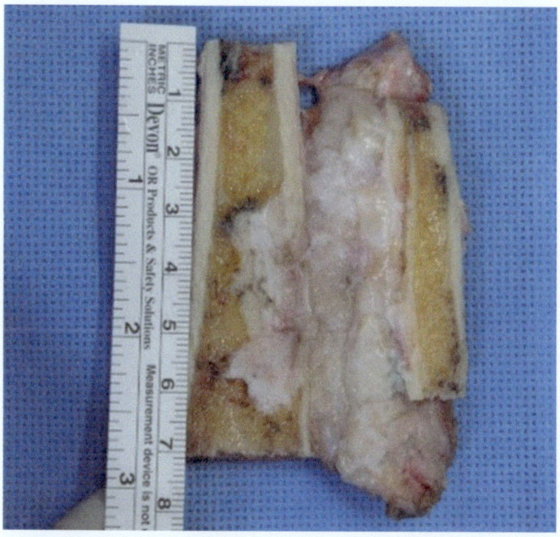

Fig. 32.7 Resected tumor

The demineralized bone matrix (DBM) was attached to the mesh structure part on contact with the bone.

32.6 Postoperative Images

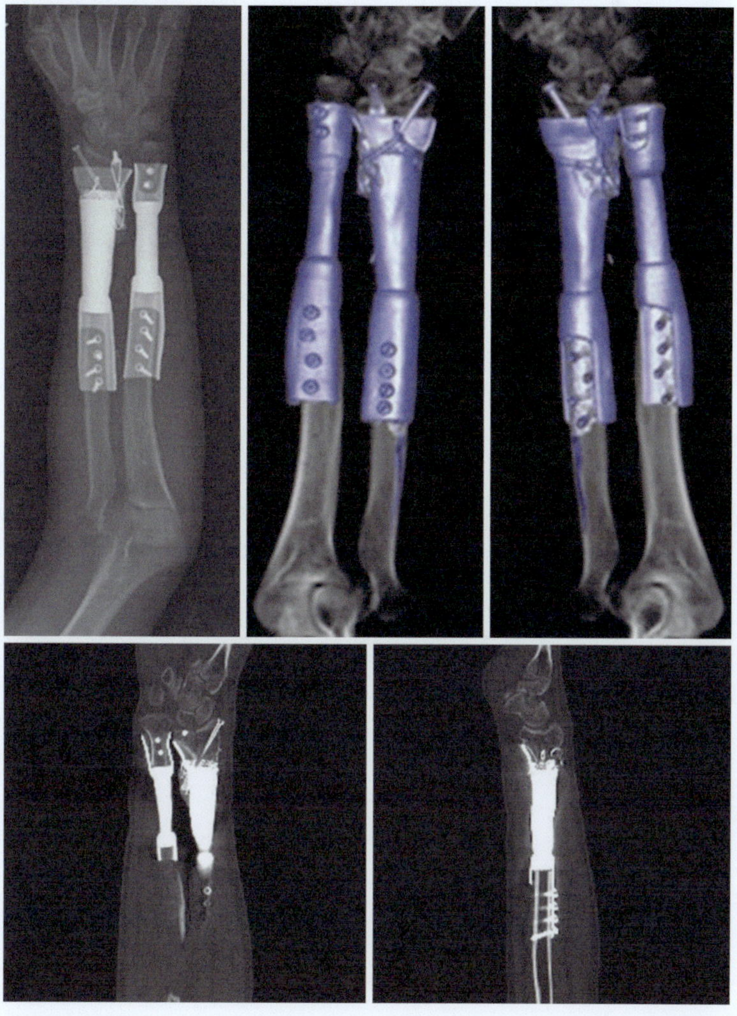

Fig. 32.8 Postoperative X-ray and CT images

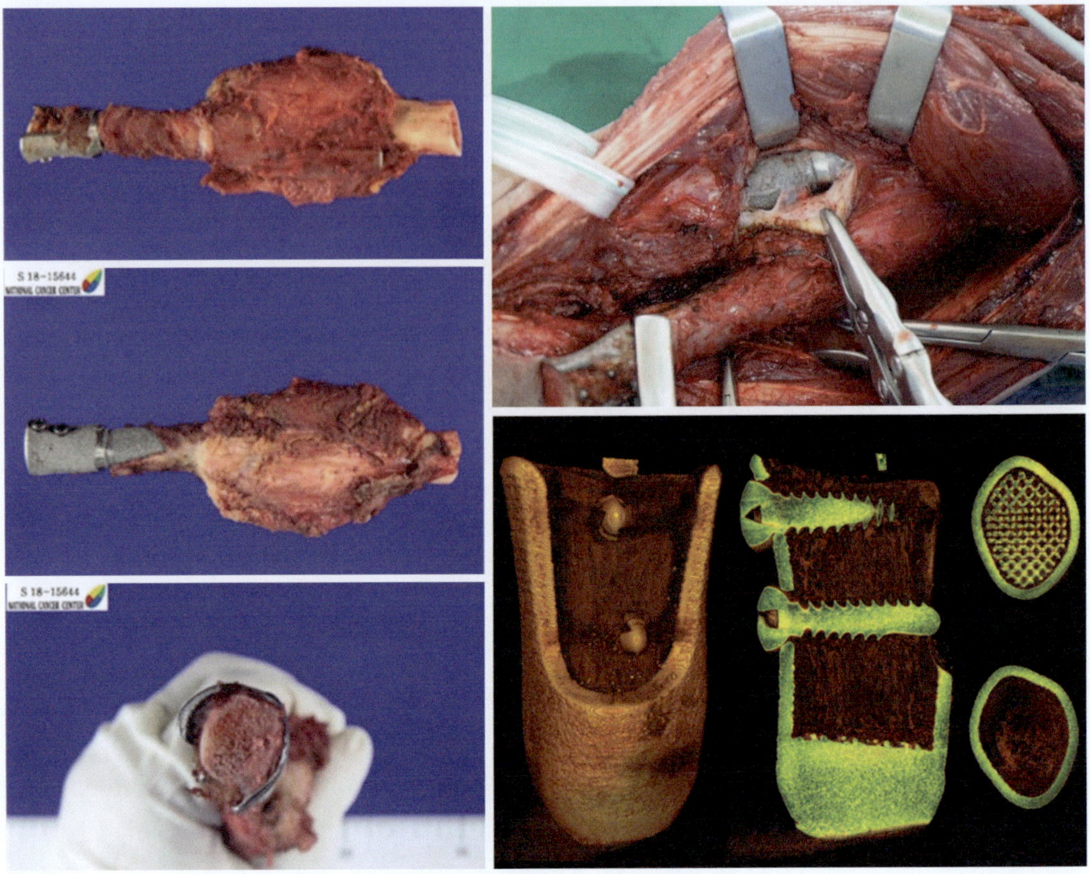

Fig. 32.9 Local recurrent and removal of ulnar implant at one year after

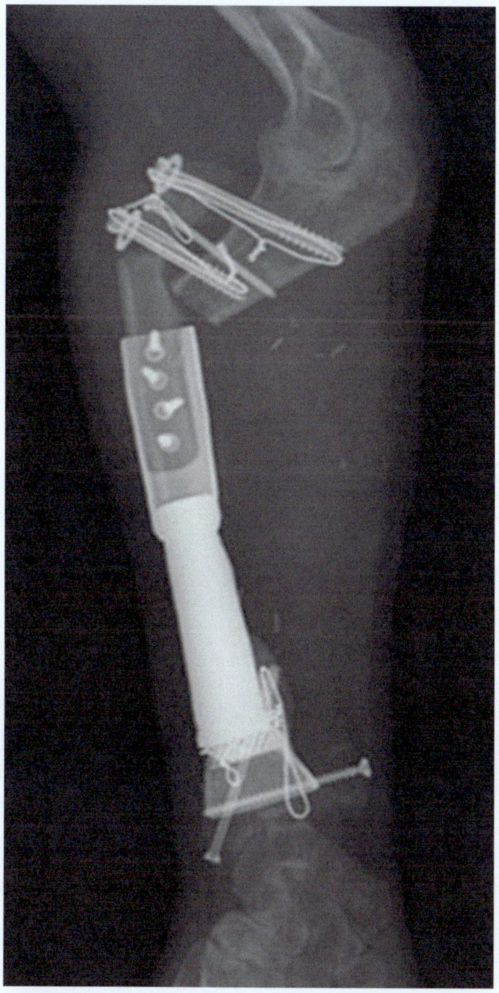

Fig. 32.10 Failure of radius-ulnar fixation at postoperative 4 months

32.7 Planning of 3rd Surgery

3D-printed connecting implant for reconstruction between the previous radial implant distally and the ulnar bone proximally

- Implant measurement
- Implant weight (g): 170
- Size (mm): 146

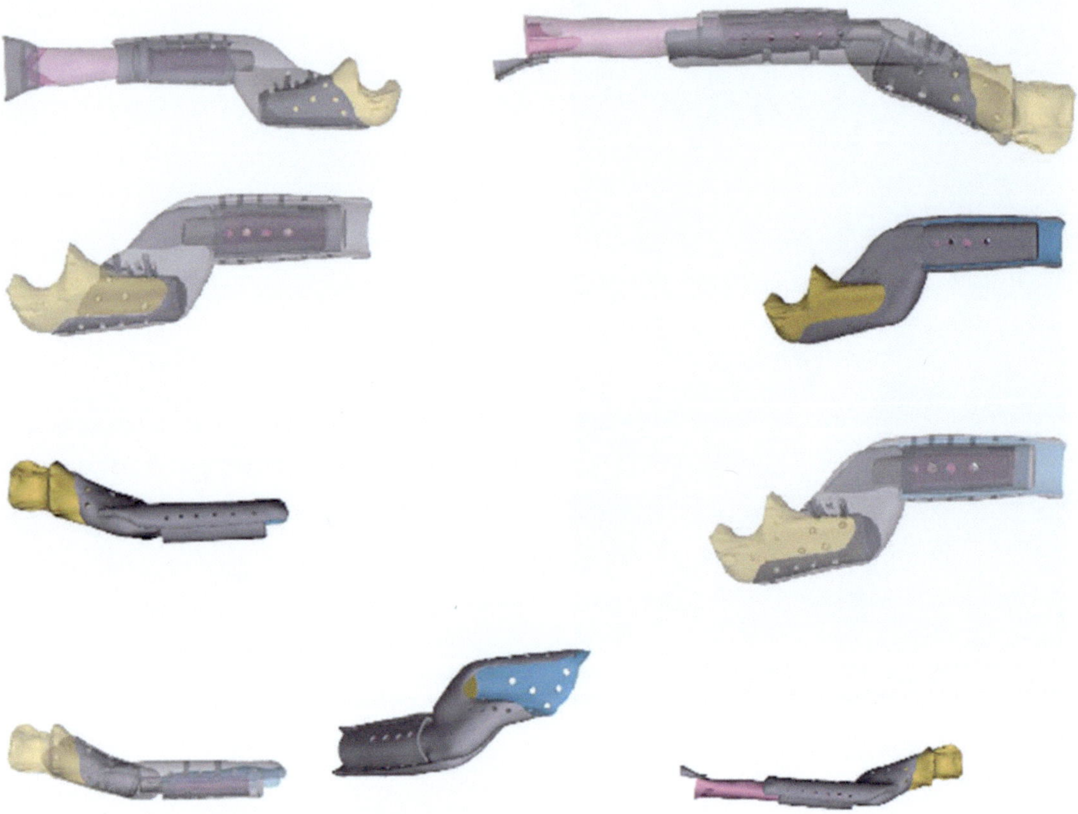

Fig. 32.11 Implant design of 3D-printed connecting implant

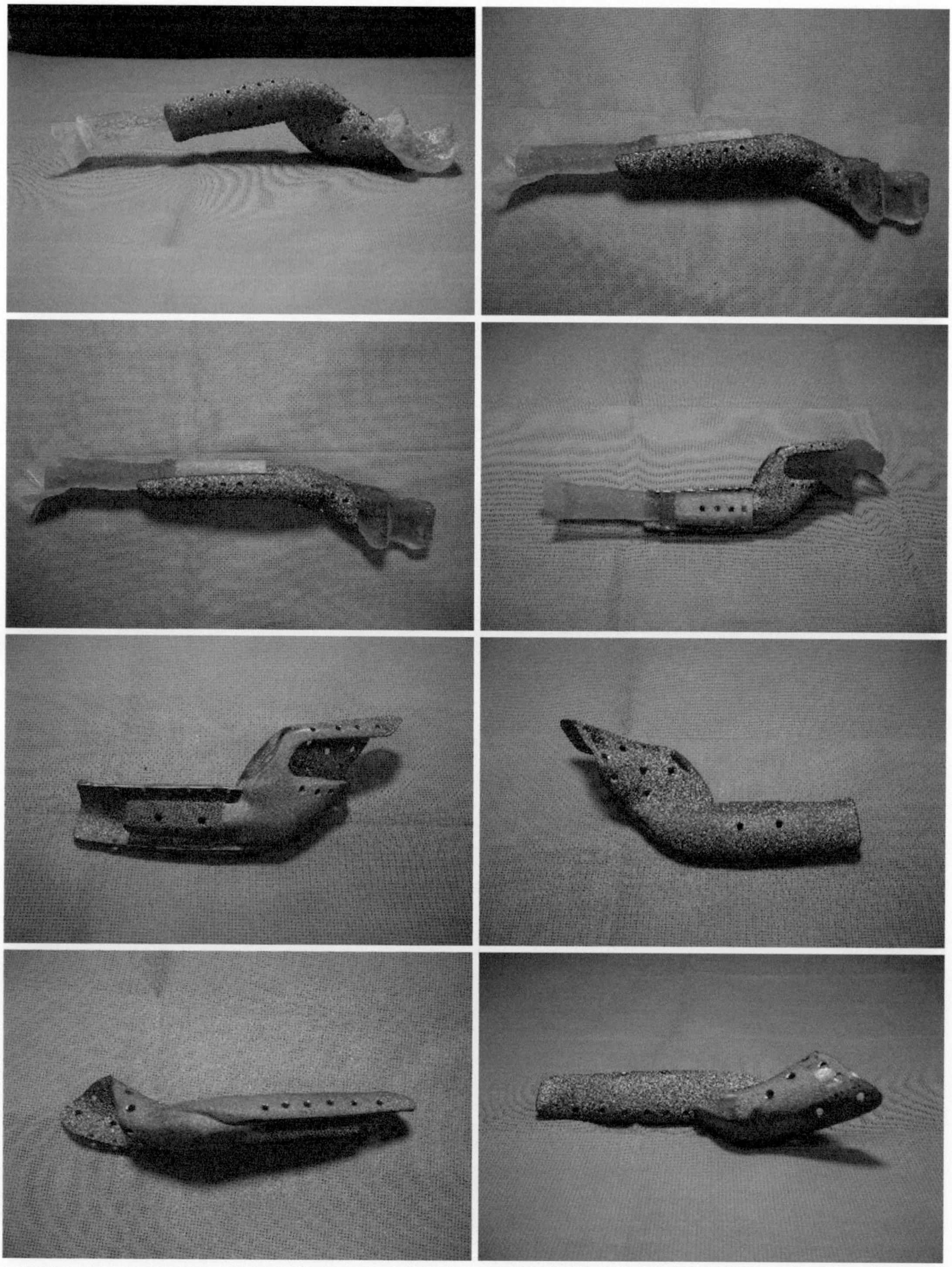

Fig. 32.12 Printed connecting implant

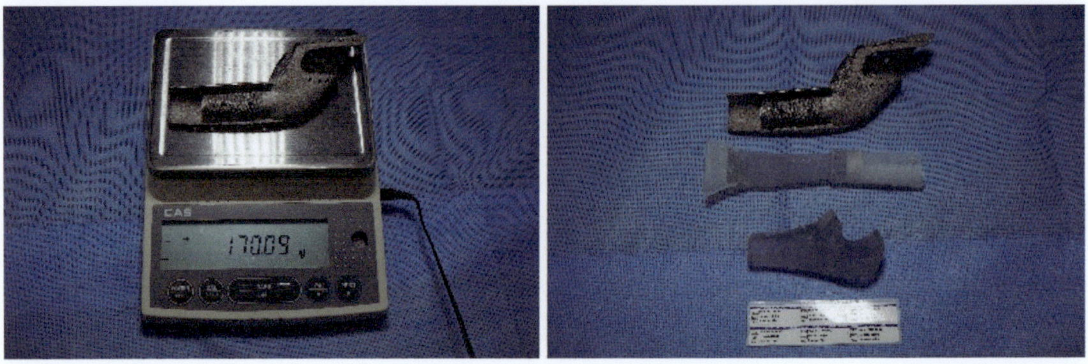

Fig. 32.12 (continued)

32.8 Operation

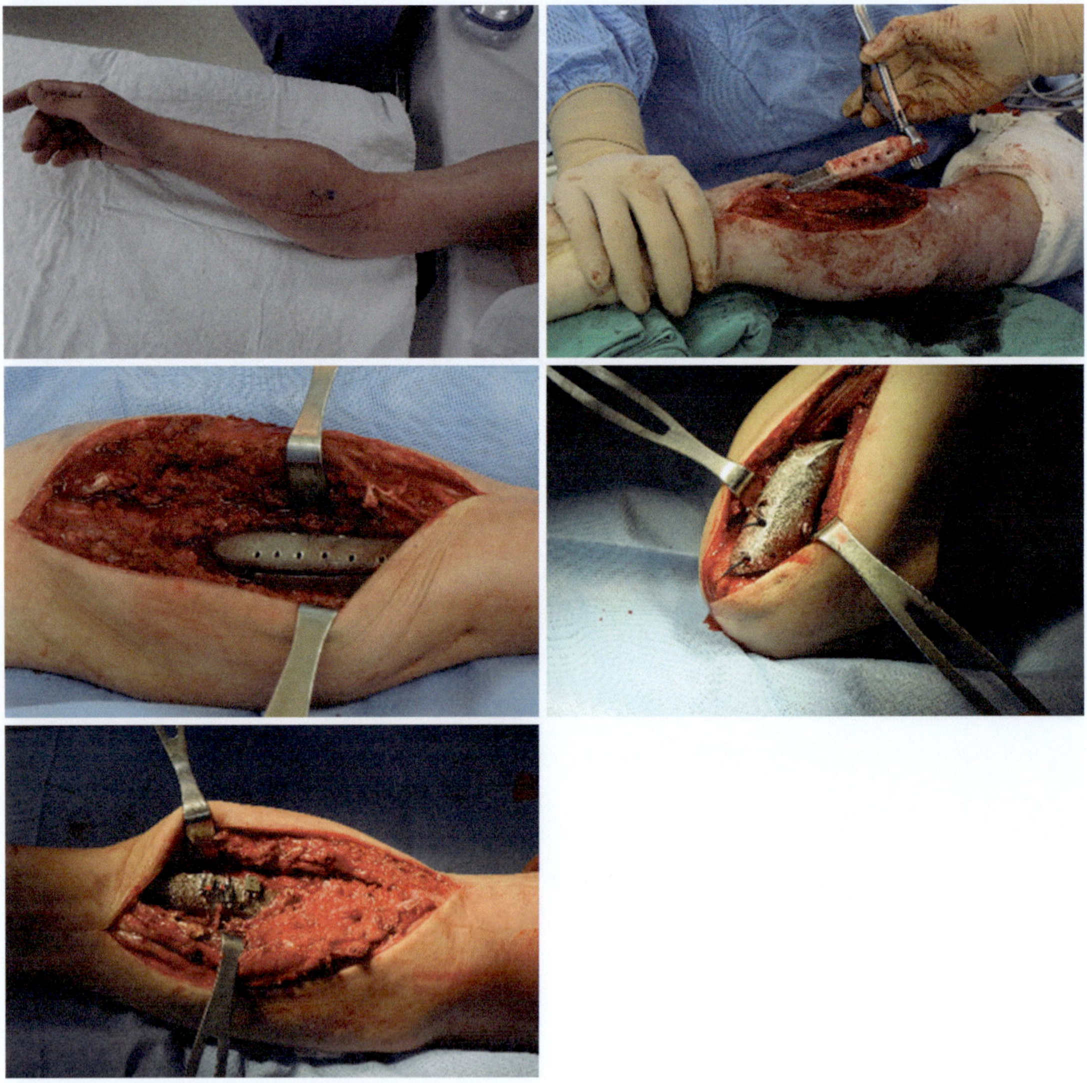

Fig. 32.13 Intraoperative photographs

32.9 Postoperative Images

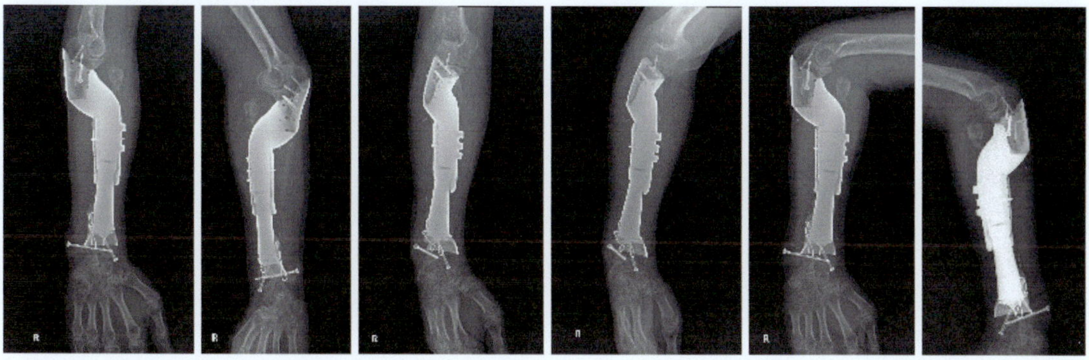

Fig. 32.14 Postoperative X-ray images

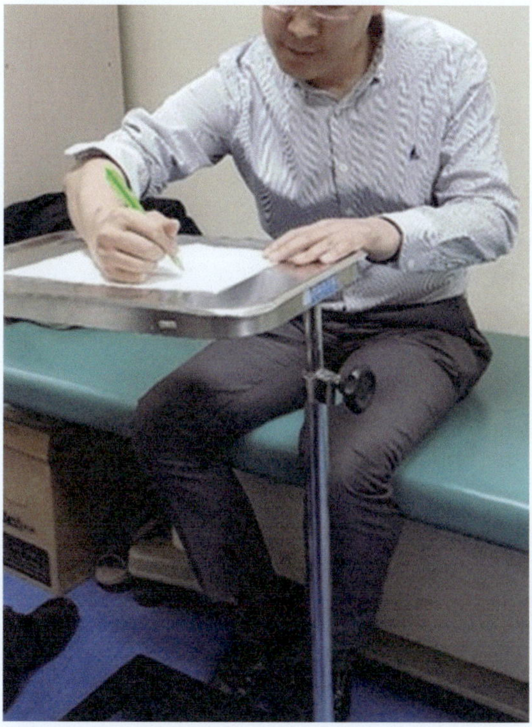

Fig. 32.15 Preserved writing function

Part VIII

High Grade Bone Sarcoma

33 Patient Case 33: Disseminated Metastases after 3D Printing Pelvic Reconstruction

33.1 Patient Case 33

Age/sex	27/male
Location/site	Pelvis/left
Diagnosis	Ewing sarcoma
Preoperative symptom	Limping gate
Preoperative pain score	Resting 3/Activity 6
BMI (height/weight)	21.5 (172/63.6)
Past history	Preoperative chemotherapy 2 times
Present illness	Less effective preoperative chemotherapy

H.-G. Kang, *Clinical Atlas of 3D Printing Bone Reconstruction*,
https://doi.org/10.1007/978-981-16-2043-0_33

33.2 Preoperative Images

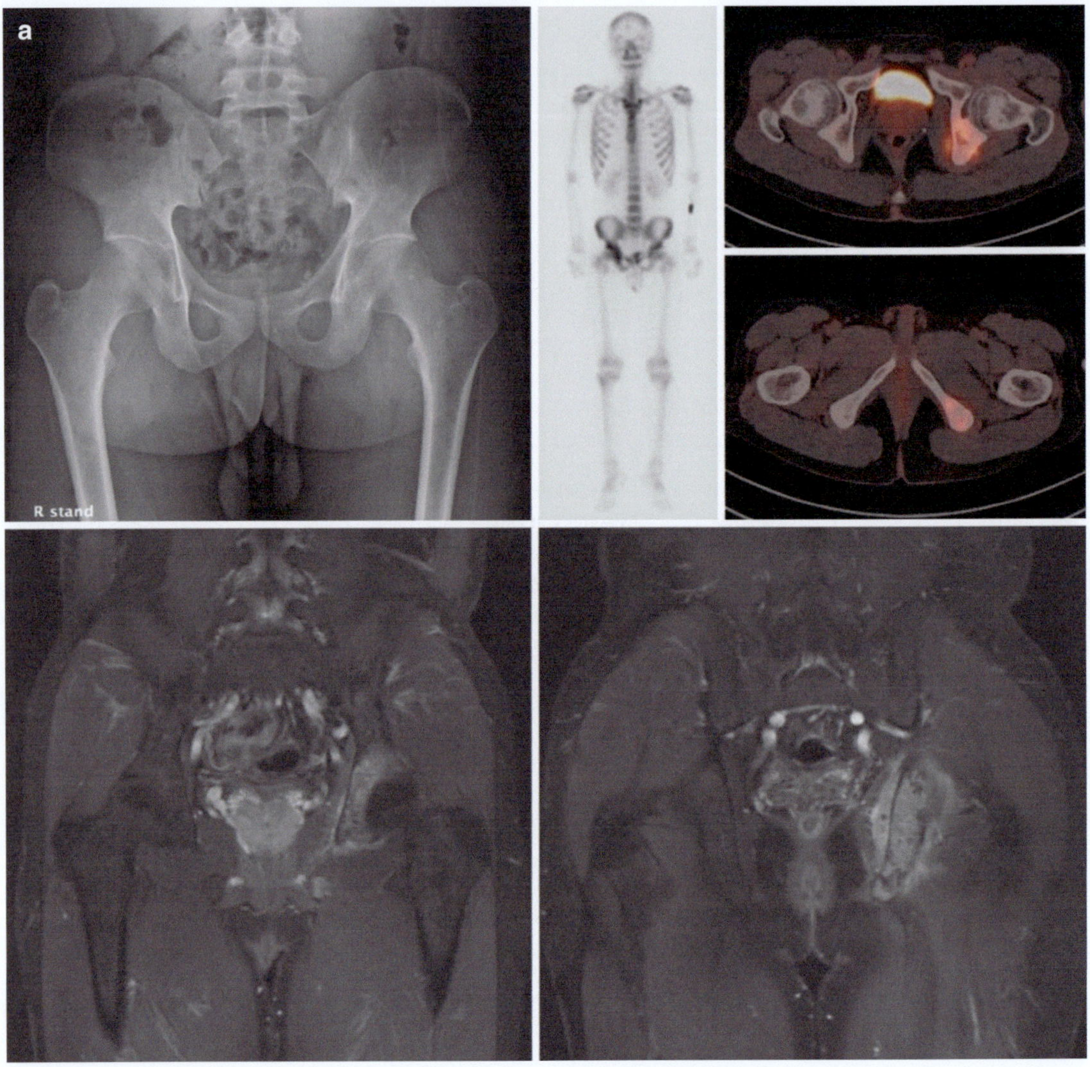

Fig. 33.1 (**a**) Initial images (pre-chemotherapy). (**b**) X-ray images after preoperative chemotherapy

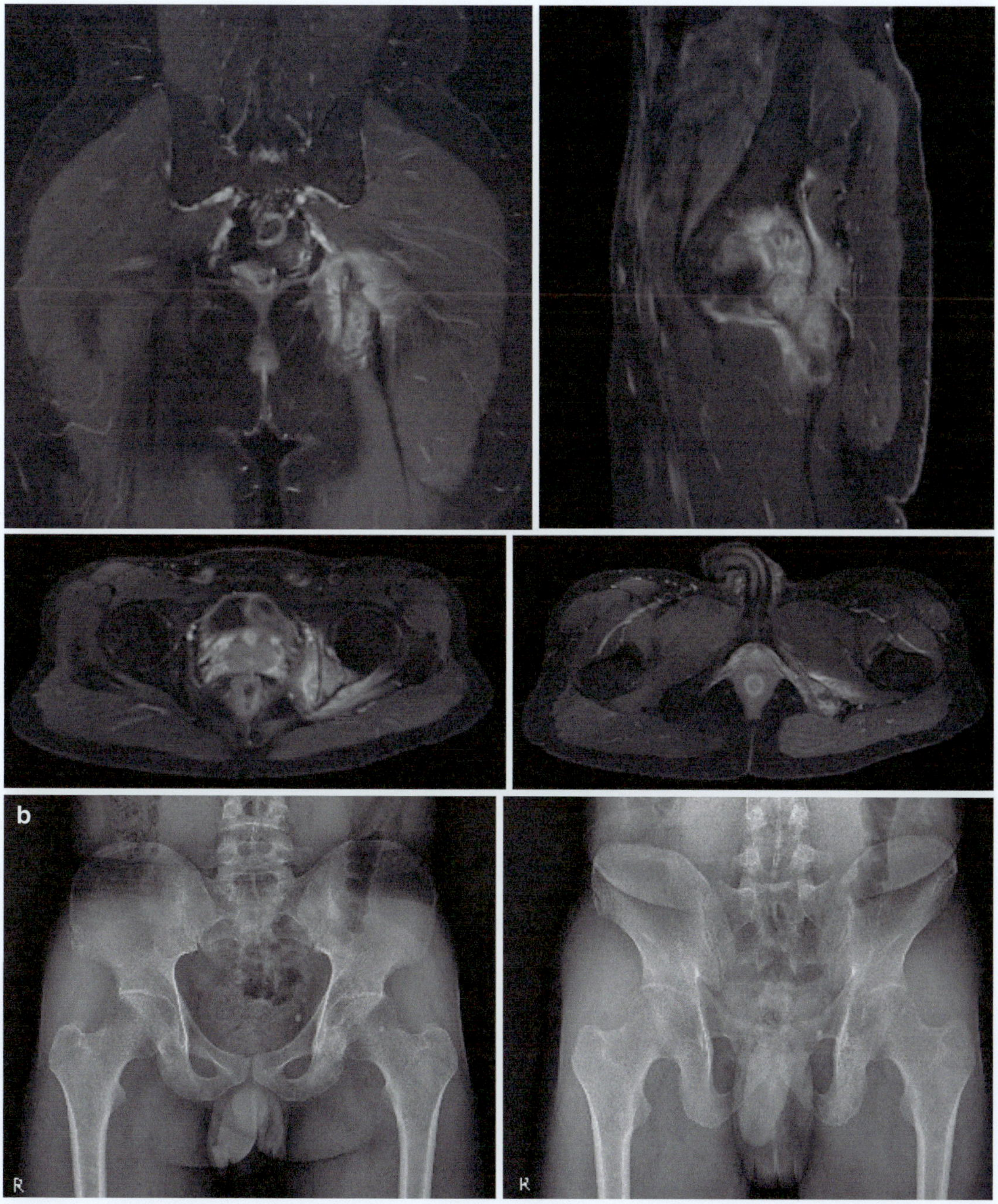

Fig. 33.1 (continued)

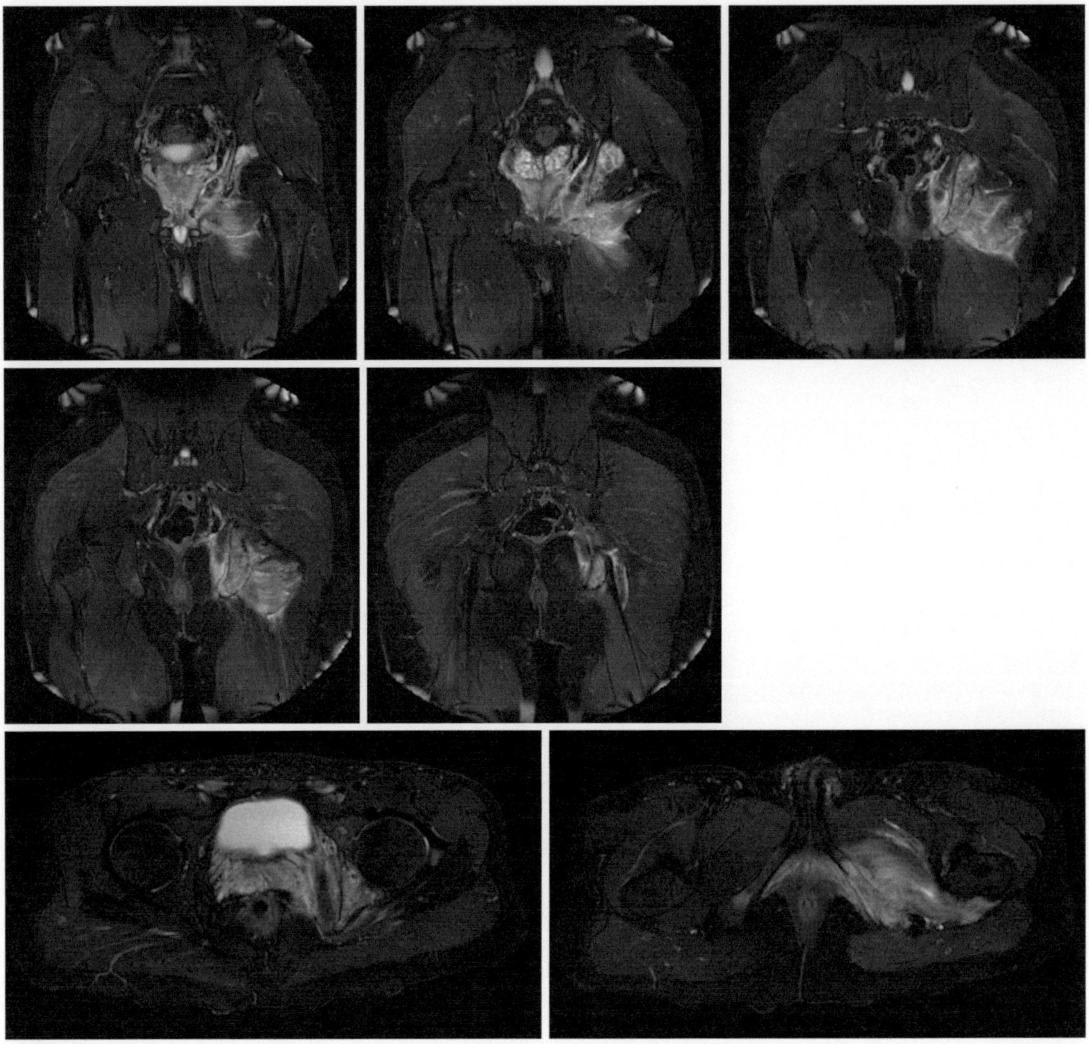

Fig. 33.2 MRI images after preoperative chemotherapy: observation of suspicious lesion on right ischial tuberosity in images taken one day before surgery

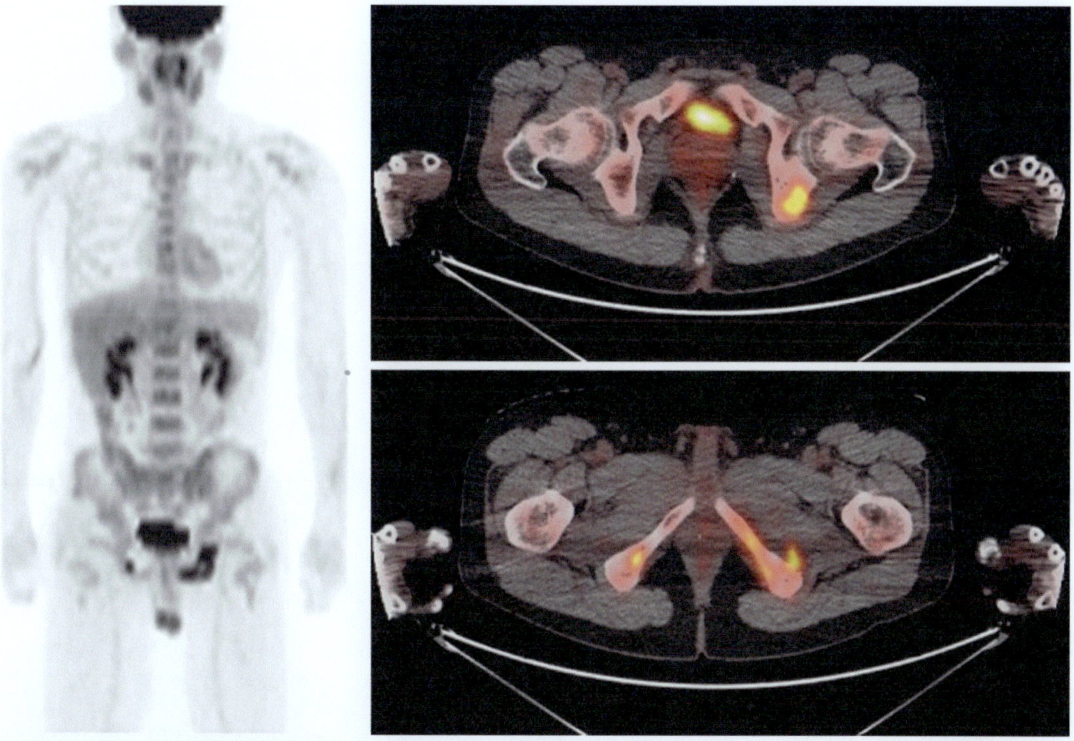

Fig. 33.3 PET-CT taken the day before surgery after chemotherapy: new suspicious right ischial lesion

33.3 Design and Fabrication

- Implant measurement
- Implant weight (g): 462
- Size (mm): 190

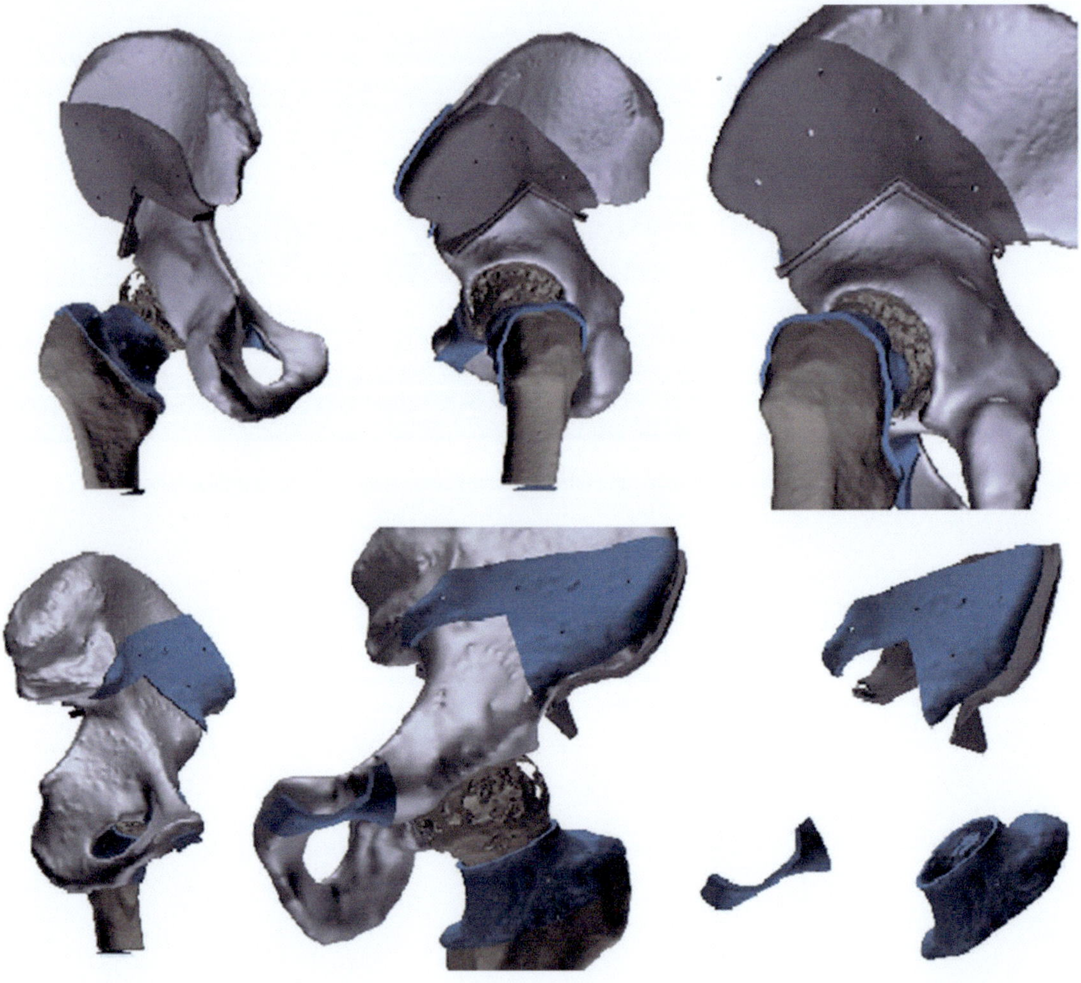

Fig. 33.4 Cutting guide design

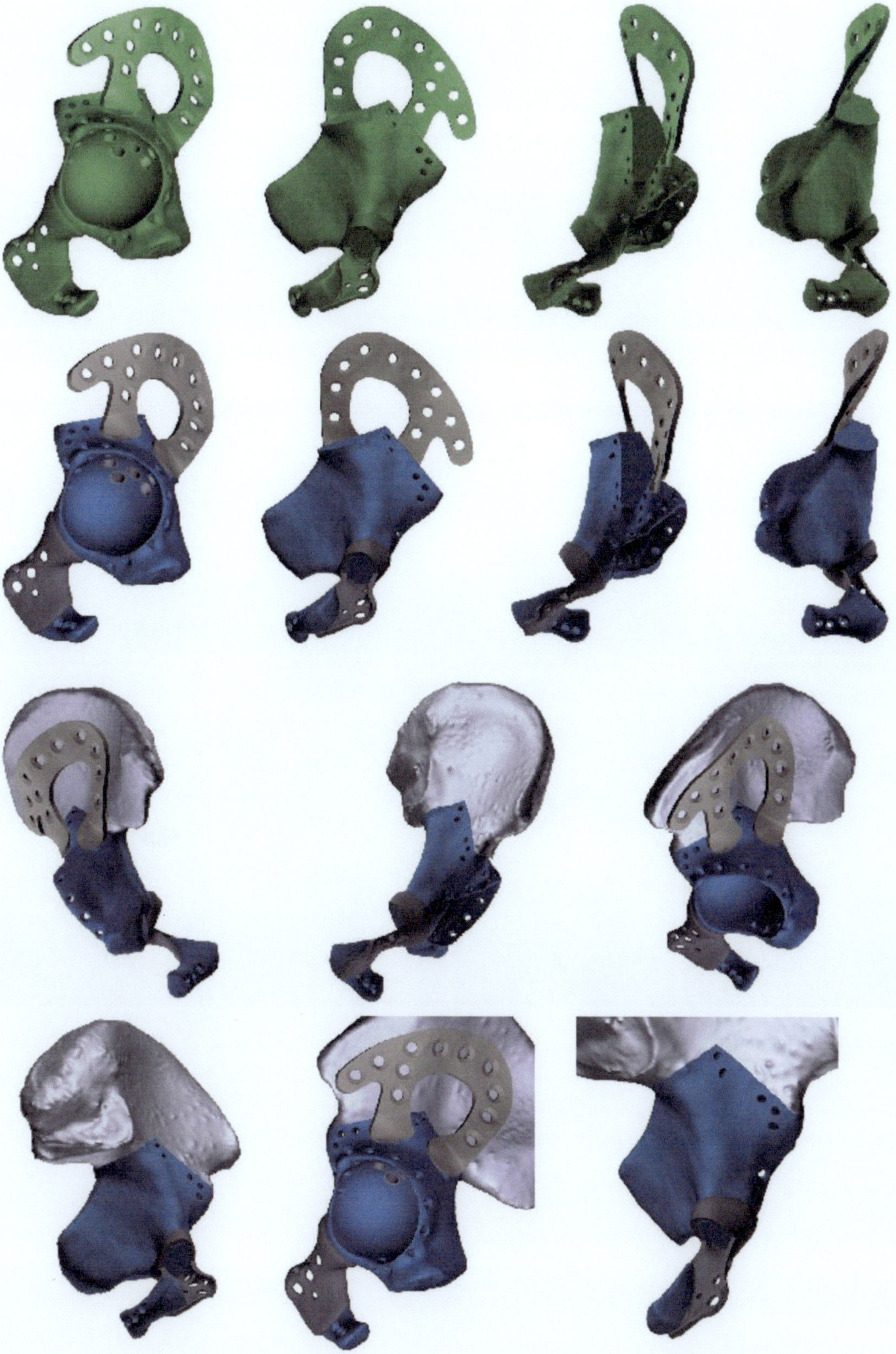

Fig. 33.5 Implant design

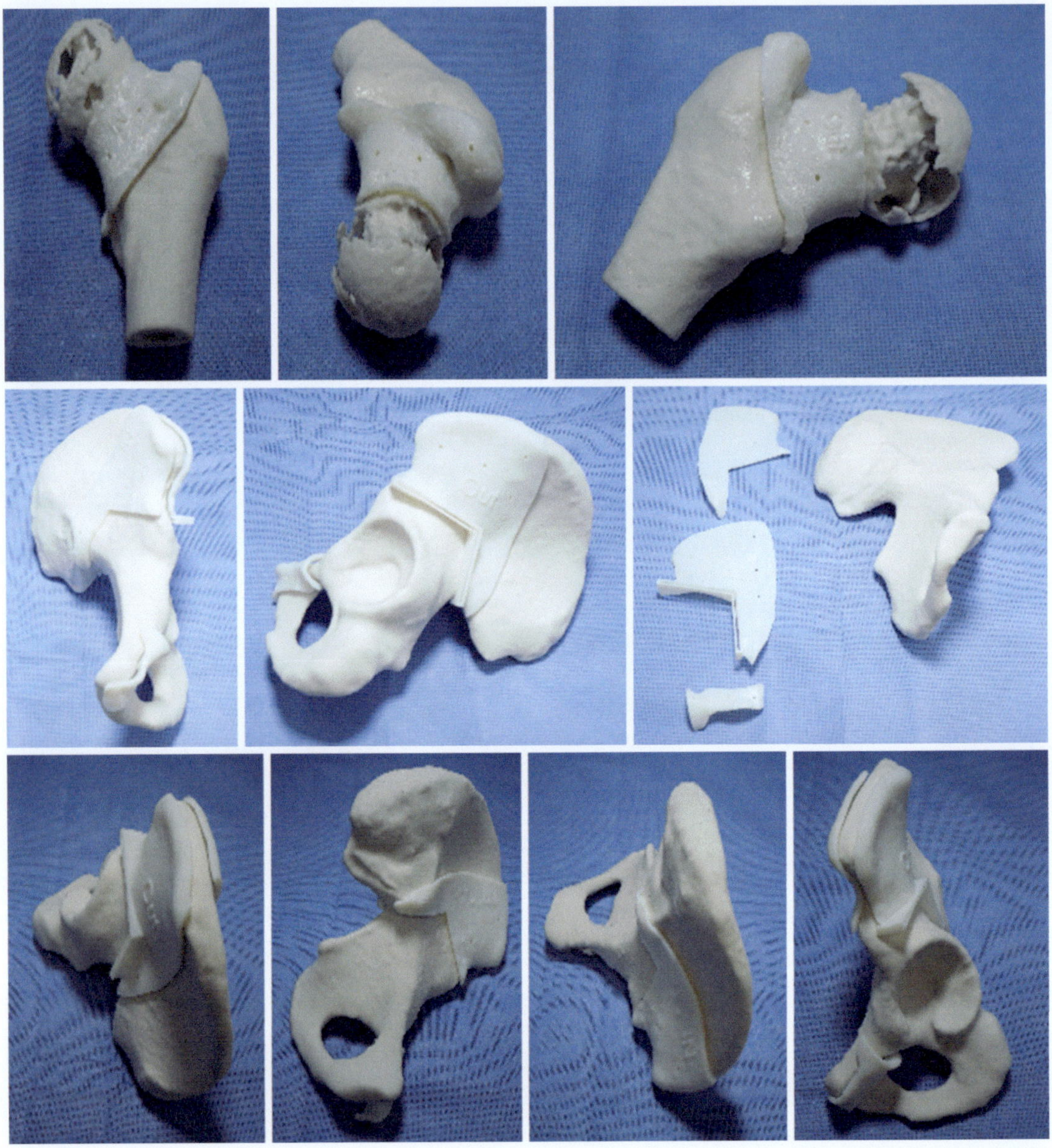

Fig. 33.6 Printed cutting guide

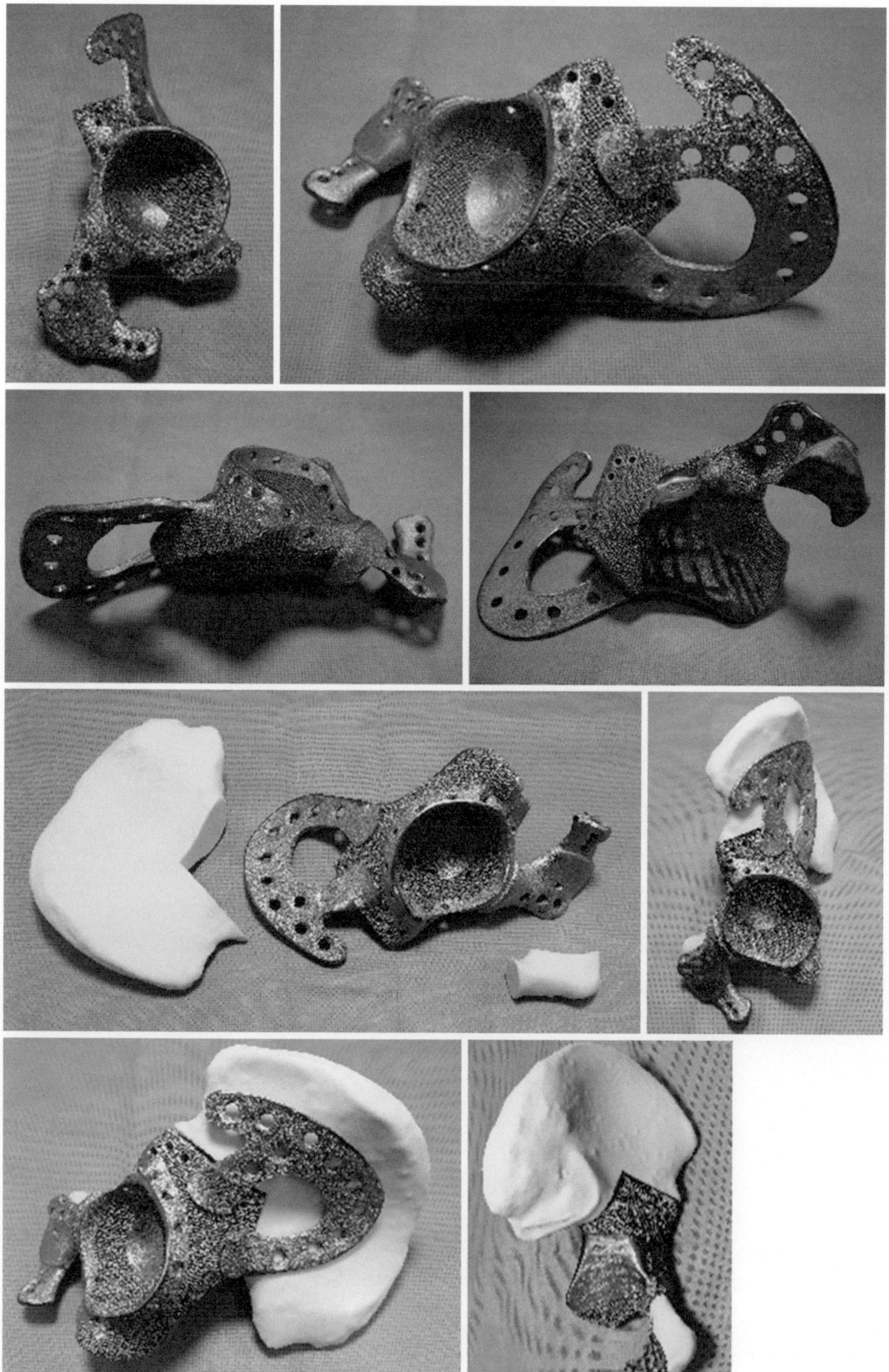

Fig. 33.7 Printed implant

33.4 Operation

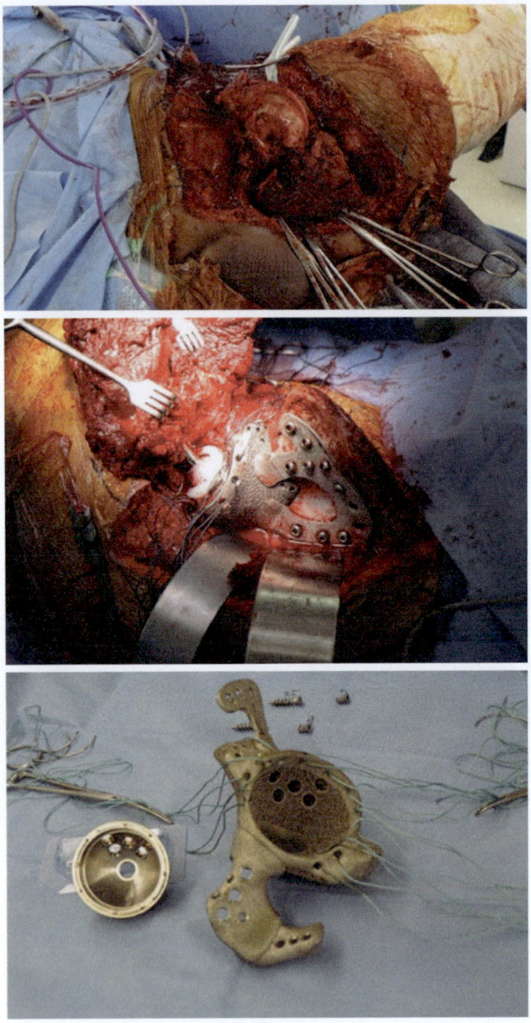

Fig. 33.8 Intraoperative photographs

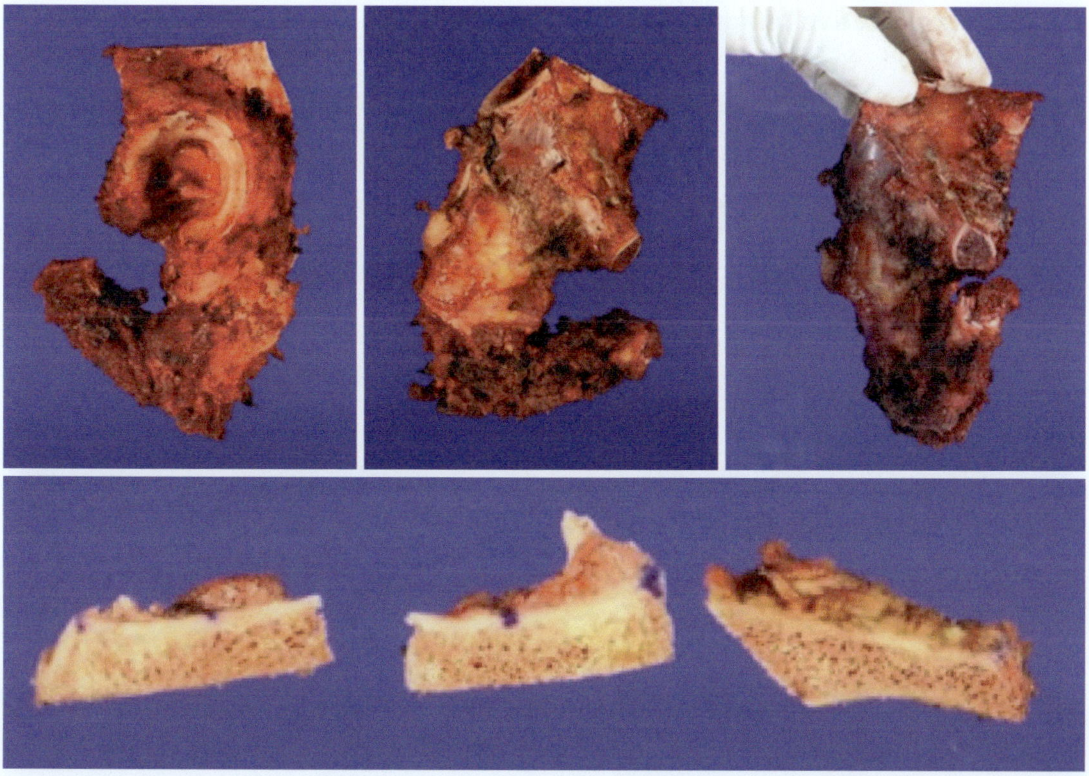

Fig. 33.9 Resected left pelvic tumor and right ischium. The right ischium is also confirmed as an Ewing sarcoma

33.5 Postoperative Images

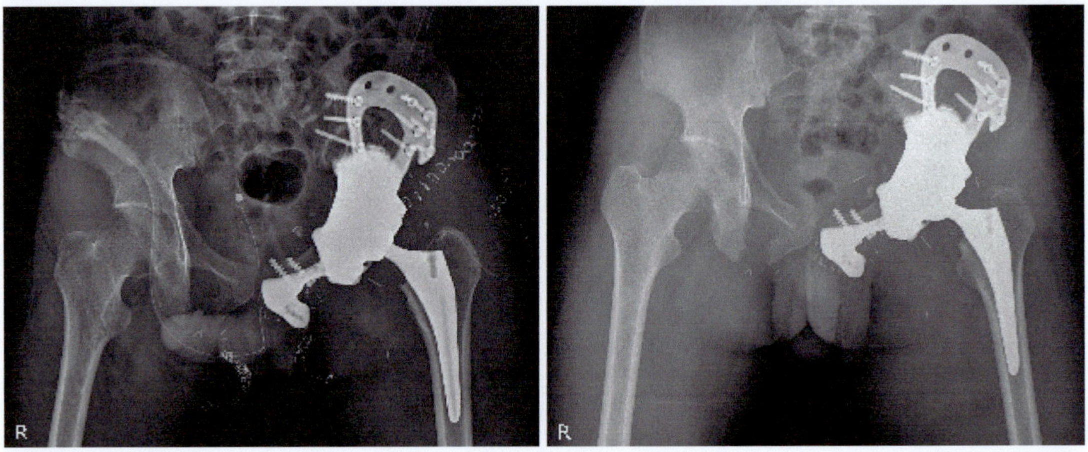

Fig. 33.10 Postoperative X-ray images: right ischial lesion was also excised

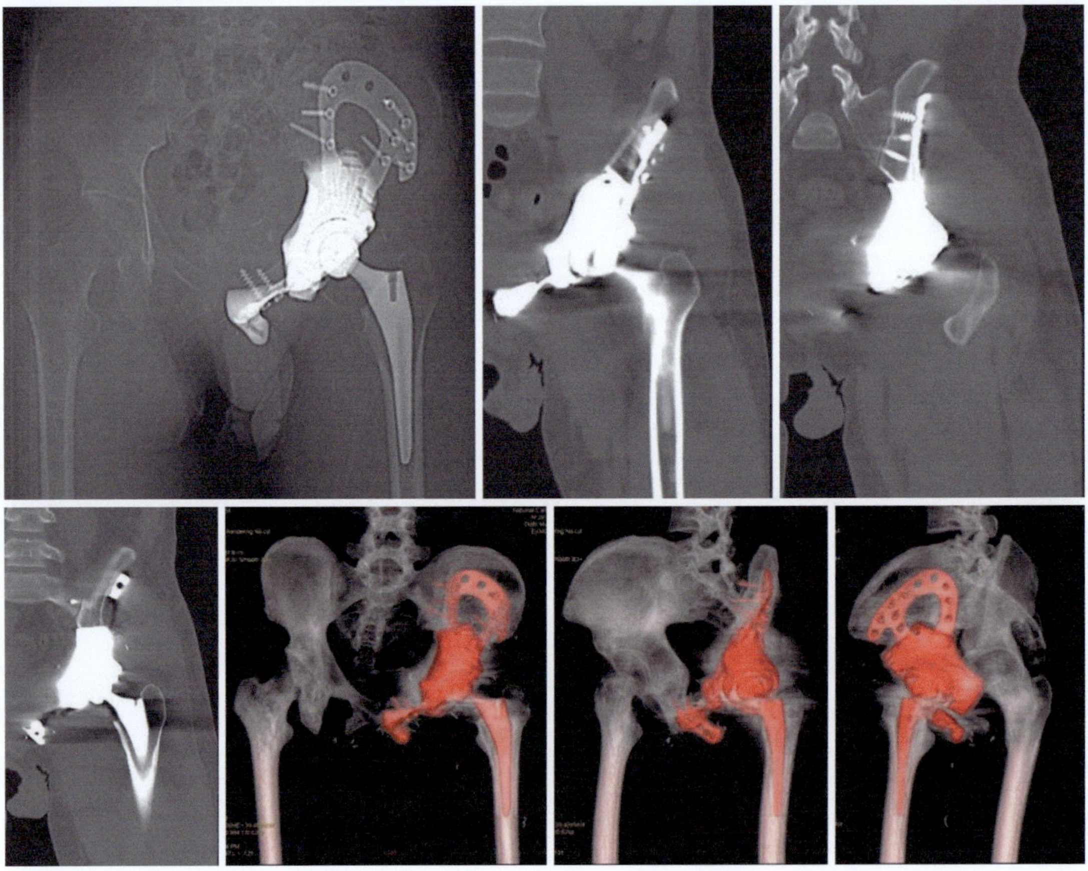

Fig. 33.11 Postoperative CT images

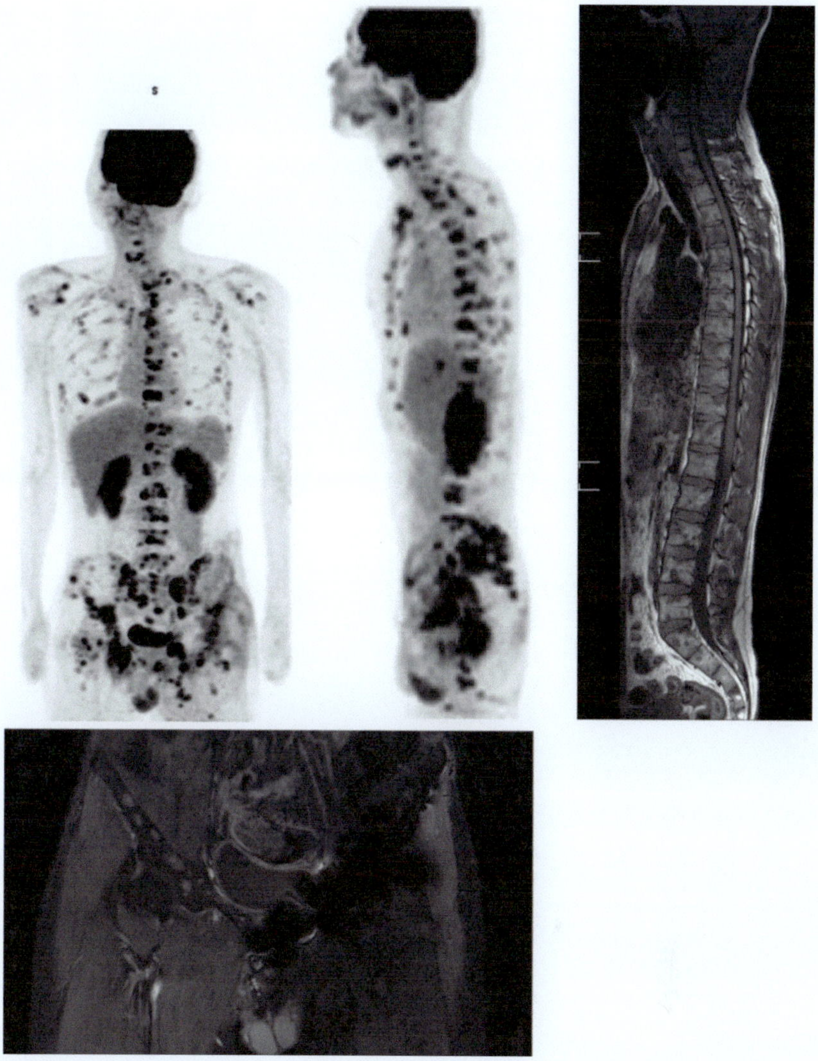

Fig. 33.12 Disseminated metastases at two months follow-up after surgery

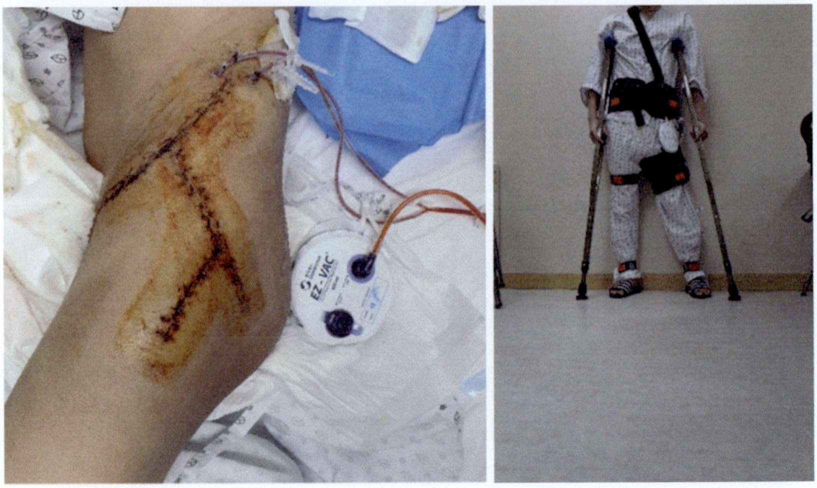

Fig. 33.13 The patient tried to walk with bone reconstruction, but unfortunately, he could not overcome the oncological problem

Part IX

Perioperative Times

34 Preparations and Postoperative Cares of 3D Printing Bone Reconstruction

34.1 Process of 3D Printing Implant

34.1.1 IRB Consent Sign

34.1.1.1 Preoperative Radiology

CT: less than 1-mm thin section as possible
MRI: less than 3 mm thin section as possible
PET-CT check: tumor margin check, recurrence surveillance after surgery
Bone scan: recurrence surveillance after surgery

34.1.2 Dicom Files Send to Engineering Team

CT, MRI, and/or PET-CT: axial images

34.1.3 Engineering Team of Company

3D rendering

Design as Surgeon's plan of implant and cutting guide

Communication can use the Cell Phone—3D PDF Reader (App, https://play.google.com)

3D printing bone model, cutting guide, and implant

- **EBM (Electron Beam Melting) machine**: ARCAM A1
- **Ti6Al4V** ELI (Extra Low Interstitials)

Implant printing time: 12–48 h

- Depending on the size and direction of output

Post printed processing

- Cooling (700 °C ➔ 40 °C, 4 h)
- Blow out the titanium powder (Powder recovery system)
- Supporter removal
- Inspection
- Polishing
- Product marking with laser
- Cleaning and Packaging

H.-G. Kang, *Clinical Atlas of 3D Printing Bone Reconstruction*,
https://doi.org/10.1007/978-981-16-2043-0_34

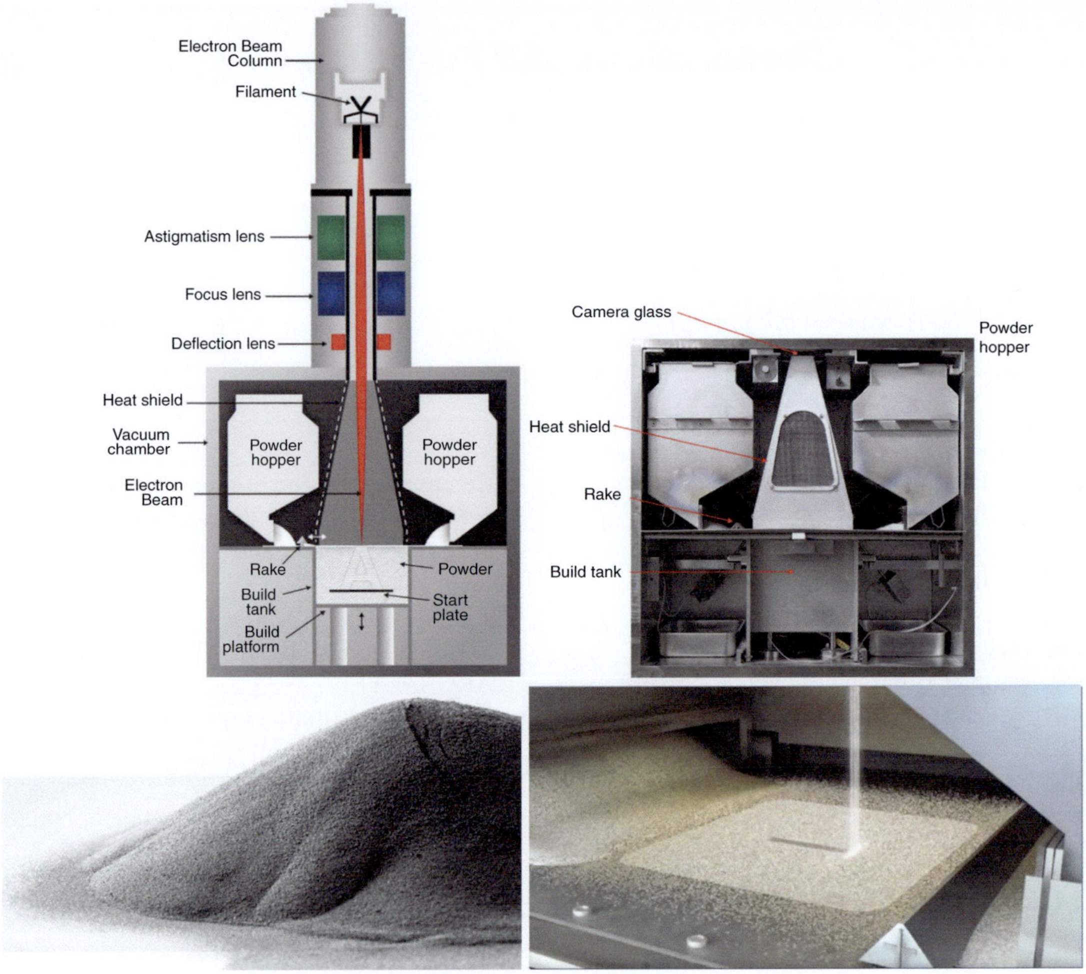

Fig. 34.1 EBM (electron beam melting) machine and Titanium alloy powder

34.1.4 Delivery to the Hospital

Measurement of weight and size of printed implant

Surgical simulation with printed implant and guide

- Sterilization: Implant—Autoclave
- Guide, Bone model—Ion gas or Plasma gas

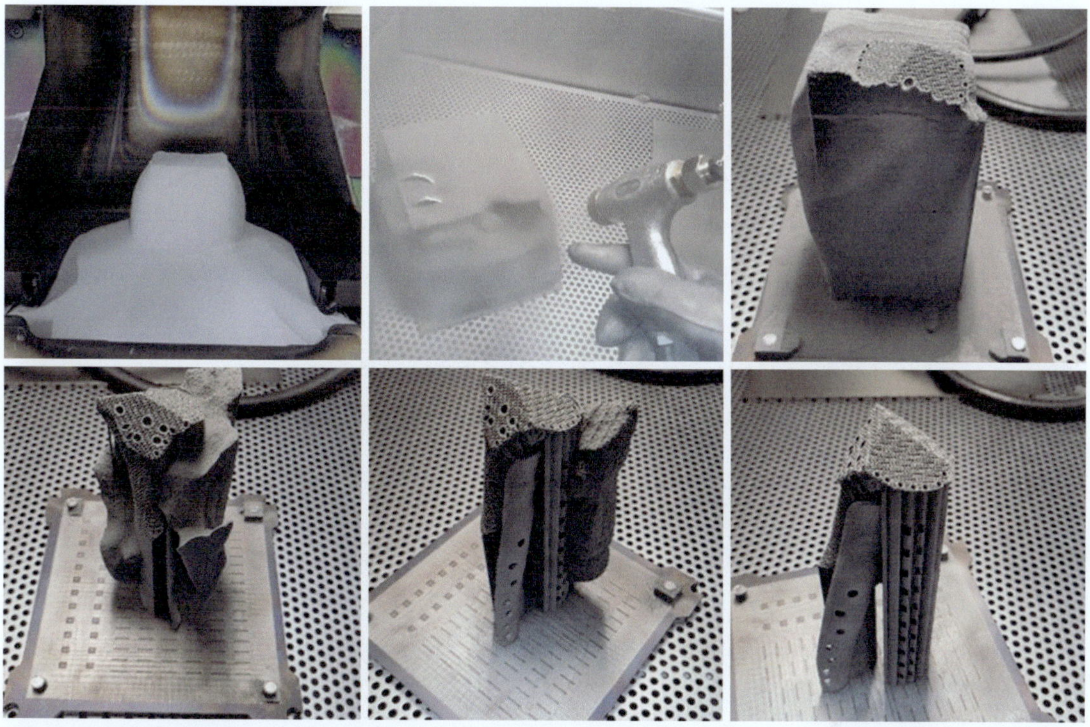

Fig. 34.2 Post-printed processing

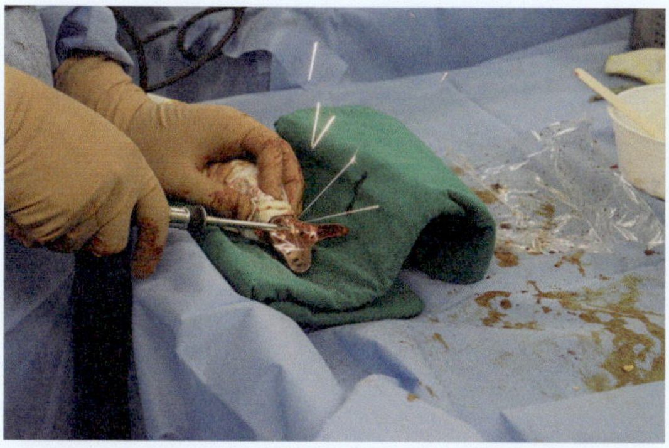

Fig. 34.3 Intraoperative trimming unsuitable areas using high-speed metal or stone burr

34.2 Postoperative Cares

Wound bag or Hemovac drainage: Maintain for 7–21 days

Antibiotic use period: Usually 1–3 weeks until close to normal CRP

Exercise: Started earlier than other bone reconstruction methods

- Consideration of postoperative chemotherapy

Follow-up surveillance for recurrence

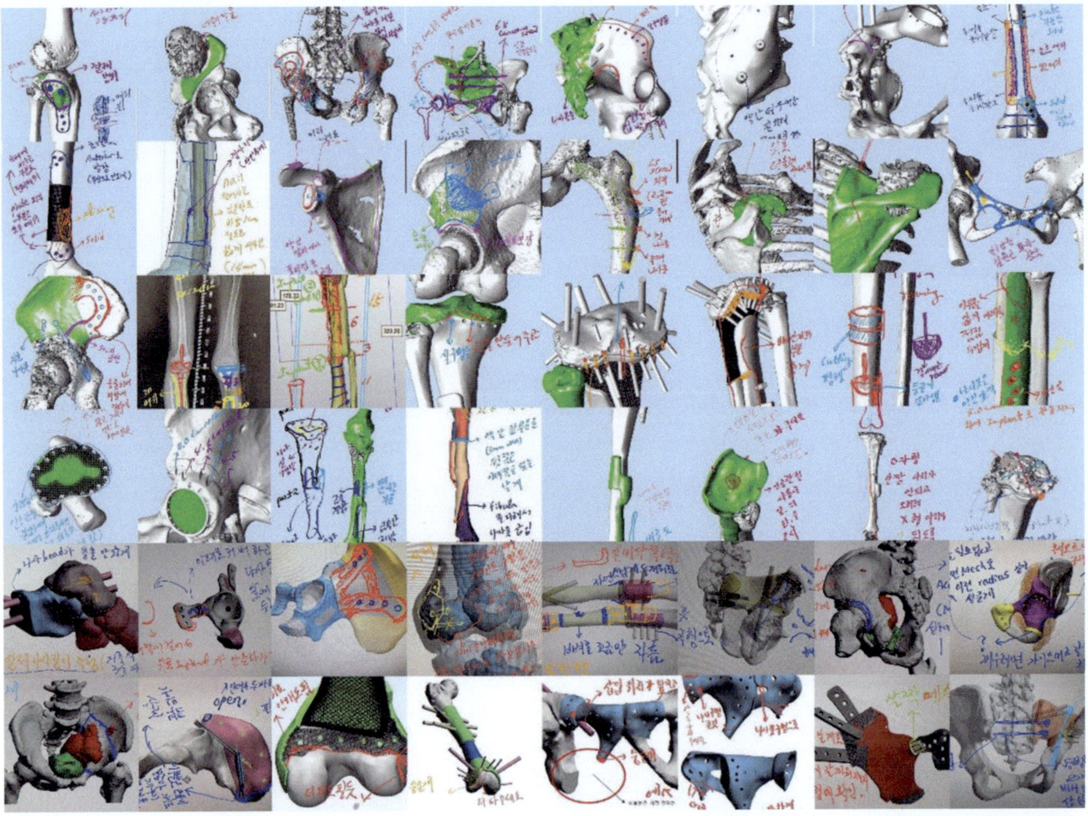

Fig. 34.4 Art of 3D printing design

MIX
Papier aus verantwortungsvollen Quellen
Paper from responsible sources
FSC® C105338

If you have any concerns about our products,
you can contact us on
ProductSafety@springernature.com

In case Publisher is established outside the EU,
the EU authorized representative is:
Springer Nature Customer Service Center GmbH
Europaplatz 3, 69115 Heidelberg, Germany

Printed by Libri Plureos GmbH
in Hamburg, Germany